Barrett's Esophagus

Barrett's Esophagus

Edited by

H.W. TILANUS

Professor of Surgery,
Erasmus University Medical Centre,
Rotterdam, The Netherlands

and

S.E.A. ATTWOOD, F.R.C.S.

Consultant Surgeon,
Hope Hospital, Salford, The United Kingdom

KLUWER ACADEMIC PUBLISHERS

DORDRECHT / BOSTON / LONDON

Library of Congress Cataloging-in-Publication Data

Barrett's esophagus / edited by H.W. Tilanus and A.E. Attwood.
    p. ; cm.
  Includes index.
  ISBN 1-40200-102-9 (HB : alk. paper)
   1. Esophagus--Diseases. 2. Esophagus--Cancer. I. Tilanus, H. W. (Hugo W.) II.
Attwood, A. E.
   [DNLM: 1. Barrett Esophagus. 2. Esophageal Diseases. 3. Esophagus--physiology. WI
250 B27413 2001]
  RC815.7 .B355 2001
  616.3'2--dc21
                                                                        2001050222

  ISBN 1-4020-0102-9

Published by Kluwer Academic Publishers,
P.O. Box 17, 3300 AA Dordrecht, The Netherlands.

Sold and distributed in North, Central and South America
by Kluwer Academic Publishers,
101 Philip Drive, Norwell, MA 02061, U.S.A.

In all other countries, sold and distributed
by Kluwer Academic Publishers,
P.O. Box 322, 3300 AH Dordrecht, The Netherlands.

Printed on acid-free paper

Printed in the Netherlands.

*This work is dedicated
to Madeleine
and to Ann*

CONTENTS

SECTION 4: BARRETT'S ESOPHAGUS – TREATMENT

SECTION 5: ADENOCARCINOMA IN BARRETT'S

SECTION 6: TREATMENT OF ADENOCARCINOMA

SECTION 7: QUALITY OF LIFE

BARRETT'S ESOPHAGUS

Foreword

Tom R. DeMeester

In the latter half of the twentieth century, gastro-esophageal disease emerged as the most common upper gastrointestinal disease of the western world. The disease is a major contributor to the rise in the war of endoscopy and acid suppression therapy. Despite the almost universal availability of both, we find ourselves in the midst of an epidemic of Barrett's esophagus, and an alarming rise in the incidence of adenocarcinoma of the esophagus. This happened within the lifetime of most readers of this book and for no apparent reason that a general consensus will accept. Consequently, physicians today are faced with a linkage between the most common benign foregut disease in the western world and the most lethal carcinoma known to man. Obviously, an in-depth book on Barrett's esophagus is both timely and needed.

I remember Stephen Attwood in his early days as a research fellow in our department. He published some of the first work confirming that bile was a common component of the gastric juice refluxed into the esophagus of patients with Barrett's. This led to studies that proved bile reflux responsible for both an increase yield of tumors and a change in their histology from squamous cell carcinoma to adenocarcinoma in an animal model both he and Sidney Mirvish developed. He has continued to stalk the disease and now has collaborated with Hugo Tilanus, a clinical investigator of reputation on both sides of the Atlantic, to organize and edit a book on Barrett's esophagus. The table of contents is a list of the most renowned investigators in the field making reading of this book a must for all those who have a serious interest in the disease.

PREFACE

Two years ago we developed the idea of the edition of a book regarding Barrett's esophagus including the extensive field of the early pathophysiologic features leading to this condition and the late sequelae eventually resulting in malignant degeneration. As adenocarcinoma of the distal esophagus and the gastro-esophageal junction has the fastest growing incidence of all tumors today and it's development is closely related to Barrett's esophagus we thought that the timing for such a book was optimal.

These facts stimulated us to invite over 30 authors with an extensive knowledge in their field of interest, combined with a great international reputation in the diagnosis and treatment of esophageal disease. The result was overwhelming as all authors produced without any exception "state of the art" chapters, which were placed in one of the 7 sections of "Barrett's Esophagus". All aspects like anatomy, physiology and pathophysiology as well as biology, epidemiology and molecular pathology are covered in the first 3 sections. The last 4 sections are entirely devoted to diagnosis and treatment. The number of diagnostic and therapeutic options for Barrett's esophagus is expanding rapidly and this book discusses the place of all of the current technologies. The issues covered include the whole range of pathologies including preceding conditions such as reflux esophagitis, right through multi modality therapy for adenocarcinoma in Barrett's esophagus.

We are very grateful to all contributors who kept their word resulting in this extensive, well-written, profusely illustrated and comprehensively referenced work.

We are greatly indebted to Carla Capel-Scheel, Head of the Editorial Office. Without her enthusiasm from the first idea, during the whole preparation until the last sentence, this project would never have resulted in "Barrett's Esophagus".

Hugo W. Tilanus.   Stephen A.E.Attwood.
Rotterdam, The Netherlands, 2001   Manchester, U.K., 2001

CONTRIBUTORS

M.S. Allen
Dept. of General Thoracic Surgery
Mayo Clinic and Foundation
Rochester MN, USA

S.E.A. Attwood
Consultant surgeon
Hope Hospital
Manchester, United Kingdom

H. Barr
Professor of Surgery
Gloucestershire Royal Hospital
Gloucester, United Kingdom

A. Berstad
Dept. of Medicine
University of Bergen
Bergen, Norway

R. Bumm
Consultant Surgeon
Technischen Universität
München, Germany

P. Burdiles
Dept. of Surgery
Clinical Hospital University
Santiago, Chile

J.P. Byrne
Consultant Surgeon
Hope Hospital
Manchester, United Kingdom

A. Cats
Dept. of Gastroenterology
Academic Hospital Vrije Universiteit
Amsterdam, the Netherlands

A. Cameron
Professor of Medicine
Div. of Gastroenterology, Mayo Clinic
Rochester MN, USA

G.W.B. Clark
Senior Lecturer in Surgery
St. James's Univ. Hospital
Leeds, United Kingdom

L. Coia
Dept. of Radiotherapy
Community Medical Center
Toms River, New Jersey, USA

J.M. Collard
Consultant Surgeon
University Hospital Saint-Luc
Brussels, Belgium

A. Csendes
Professor of Surgery
Clinical Hospital University
Santiago, Chile

H. van Dekken
Associate Professor of Pathology
Erasmus Medical Center Rotterdam
Rotterdam, the Netherlands

A.S. DeNittis
Dept. of Radiation Oncology
Hosp. of the Univ. of Pennsylvania
Philadelphia, USA

C. Deschamps
Associate Professor of Surgery
Mayo Clinic and Foundation
Rochester MN, USA

W.N.M. Dinjens
Dept. of Pathology
Erasmus Medical Center Rotterdam
Rotterdam, the Netherlands

G. Falk
Staff Gastroenterologist
Cleveland Clinic Foundation
Cleveland, Ohio, USA

P.M.A. Fisichella
Fellow in Gastrointestinal Surgery
Univ. of California
San Francisco, USA

J.G. Hatlebakk
Assistant Professor Dept. of Medicine
University of Bergen
Bergen, Norway

J.R. Headrick
Dept. of General Thoracic Surgery
Mayo Clinic and Foundation
Rochester MN, USA

A.H. Hölscher
Professor of Surgery
University of Cologne
Cologne, Germany

J.B.F. Hulscher
Dept. of Surgery
Academic Medical Center
Amsterdam, the Netherlands

G.G. Jamieson
Professor of Surgery
University of Adelaide
Adelaide, Australia

J.A.Z. Jankowski
Reader in Medicine
University of Birmingham
Birmingham, United Kingdom

M.B. de Jong
Dept. of Surgery
Erasmus Medical Center Rotterdam
Rotterdam, the Netherlands

B.T. Johnston
Consultant Gastroenterologist
Royal Victoria Hospital
Belfast, United Kingdom

O. Korn
Dept. of Surgery
Clinical Hospital University
Santiago, Chile

E.J. Kuipers
Professor of Gastroenterology
Erasmus Medical Center Rotterdam
Rotterdam, the Netherlands

J.J.B. van Lanschot
Professor of Surgery
Academic Medical Center
Amsterdam, the Netherlands

T. Lerut
Professor of Surgery
University Hospital Gasthuisberg
Leuven, Belgium

D. Liebermann – Meffert
Professor of Surgery
Technische Universität
München, Germany

R.V.N. Lord
Consultant surgeon
Univ. of Southern California
Los Angeles, USA

A.H.G. Love †
Consultant Gastroenterologist
Royal Victoria Hospital
Belfast, United Kingdom

L. Lundell
Professor of Surgery
Sahlgrenska University Hospital
Göteborg, Sweden

D. Maguire
Senior Registrar in General Surgery
Univ. College Hospital
Cork, Ireland

R.E.K. Marshall
Consultant Surgeon
Gu's Hospital
London, United Kingdom

A.J. McLarty
Dept. of General Thoracic Surgery
Mayo Clinic and Foundation
Rochester MN, USA

D.M. Miller
Dept. of General Thoracic Surgery
Mayo Clinic and Foundation
Rochester MN, USA

S.P. Mönig
Dept. of Surgery
University of Cologne
Cologne, Germany

C.D. Morris
Dept. of Surgery
Hope Hospital
Manchester, United Kingdom

F.C. Nichols
Dept. of General Thoracic Surgery
Mayo Clinic and Foundation
Rochester MN, USA

G.C. O'Sullivan
Professor of Surgery
University College Cork
Cork, Ireland

W.J. Owen
Consultant Surgeon
Guy's Hospital
London, United Kingdom

P.C. Pairolero
Dept. of General Thoracic Surgery
Mayo Clinic and Foundation
Rochester MN, USA

M.G. Patti
Assistant Professor of Surgery
University of California
San Fransisco, USA

S.R. Preston
Specialist Registrar
Dept. of Surgery
St. James's Univ. Hospital
Leeds, United Kingdom

V. Rempe-Sorm
Dept. of Surgery
Erasmus Medical Center Rotterdam
Rotterdam, the Netherlands

R.E. Sampliner
Professor of Pathology
University of Arizona
Tucson, USA

W. Schröder
Dept. of Surgery
University of Cologne
Cologne, Germany

F. Shanahan
Professor and Chairman
Dept. of Medicine
Univ. Collega Hospital
Cork, Ireland

N.A. Shepherd
Professor of Histopathology
Gloucester Royal Hospital
Gloucester, United Kingdom

P.D. Siersema
Staff Gastroenterologist
Erasmus Medical Center Rotterdam
Rotterdam, the Netherlands

J.R. Siewert
Professor of Surgery
Technischen Universität
München, Germany

A.J.P.M. Smout
Professor of Gastrointestinal Motility
University Medical Center
Utrecht, the Netherlands

H.W. Tilanus
Professor of Surgery
Erasmus Medical Center Rotterdam
Rotterdam, the Netherlands

V.F. Trastek
Dept. of General Thoracic Surgery
Mayo Clinic and Foundation
Rochester MN, USA

D.I. Watson
Consultant Surgeon
University of Adelaide
Adelaide, Australia

B.P.L. Wijnhoven
Dept. of Surgery
Erasmus Medical Center Rotterdam
Rotterdam, the Netherlands

A.C. Woodman
Lecturer, Inst. of Biosciences and
Technology, Cranfield University
Bedfordshire, United Kingdom

NORMAN BARRETT AND THE ESOPHAGUS.

Reginald V. N. Lord

This chapter includes sections from a manuscript entitled "Norman Barrett, Doyen of Esophageal Surgery" published by the author in Annals of Surgery, Vol. 229, No. 3, March 1999.

1. INTRODUCTION

The pioneer thoracic surgeon Norman Barrett is chiefly remembered for his description of the esophagus lined by columnar epithelium, a condition subsequently referred to as Barrett's esophagus. Barrett made important contributions in several areas of thoracic surgery, and among his many personal gifts can be listed an incisive intellect, an elegant use of language, and an often brilliant wit, balanced by a deprecatory cynicism, features which add to his attractiveness as a biographical subject.

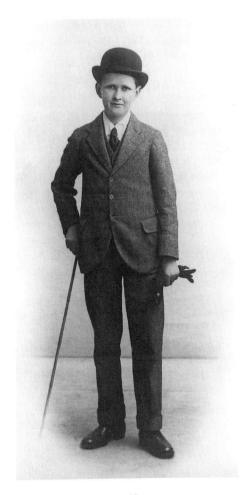

Figure 1. Norman Barrett, age 13

2. EARLY LIFE

Barrett's ancestors were Quaker maltsters and yeastmakers who lived near Adderbury in the Banbury region of Oxfordshire, England. In the 1880s, two brothers, George William Barrett, a maltster, and James Barrett, a doctor, sailed for Australia with their families. Although Norman was the grandson of George Barrett the maltster, it seems likely that he was influenced in his choice of career by Dr. James Barrett and his family. Four of James Barrett's children became doctors, including Sir James Barrett, who was influential in many areas of Australia's development. Sir James was one of the founders of the Royal Australasian College of Surgeons, a Chancellor of Melbourne University, and President of the British Medical Association when it met in Australia in 1935. He also founded the Victoria Bush Nursing Association, which at the time of his death was a famous group with sixty-seven hospitals[1]. Amongst numerous other interests and achievements, Sir James Barrett was also an early environmentalist who was responsible for the founding of a National Park and a wildlife sanctuary and who was among those who saved the koala bear from extinction[1-5]. Norman Barrett was very aware of Sir James' achievements, and in one article included him in a list of "brilliant men"[6].

George William Barrett, the grandfather of Norman Barrett, settled in Adelaide, South Australia, with his wife Emma and their thirteen children. Alfred, Norman Barrett's father, was the ninth child. George William and his sons established Barrett Brothers malt producers, which was successful enough to enable Norman's father Alfred Barrett to retire while still young to manage his investments. Alfred Barrett married Catherine "Katie" Hill Connor, an Irishwoman from Geelong in Australia. Alfred and Katie had two children, Norman Rupert (born May 16, 1903 in North Adelaide) and Alison Barrett, born three years later. At about ten years of age Norman Barrett left Australia, travelling with his father and an Australian nurse, Gwen Chaplin. Norman's mother and sister followed later.

1

rather than as an Australian talking about home"[6].

Barrett was educated at Eton and Trinity College Cambridge. At Eton (1917-1922) he excelled academically, was a member of the Eton Society (Pop), and played in the cricket XI. He hit a great six in the annual Eton versus Harrow cricket match at Lord's, a shot that was recalled even by several of his obituarists[7,8]. At Eton, he was perversely given the nickname "Pasty" because of his somewhat florid complexion, and despite losing the color in his cheeks as an adult, he was widely known as "Pasty" for the rest of his life.

At Trinity College Cambridge (1922-1925), despite a very full social calendar, he obtained a first in the Natural Science Tripos (Physics, Chemistry, Geology, Physiology, Zoology, Botany). No details of Barrett's medical studies are available, except that he successfully took the Part I exams in 1922, the Part II in 1924, and after three years on the wards as a student at St Thomas's Hospital, London, the Part III in 1928. At both Eton and Cambridge Barrett was known as a practical joker. At Trinity College, he prepared a friend's room for a smart party by placing a very large fish in a chair. The fish was obscured from view and was wearing a hat; it was not until the guests approached to engage the fish in conversation that they realized the cause of its quietude and offensive odor.

3. SURGICAL TRAINING

Barrett remained at St Thomas's Hospital for his resident years, progressing to the position of resident assistant surgeon (RAS) for two years. The RAS job was much sought after, despite its restrictions: Barrett was advised by C.R. Nitch, one of the consultant surgeons "Barrett you are only RAS for two years-there can be no reason to go out in that time"[9]. Nitch had earlier reported Barrett to the hospital governors for leaving the ward to take a short walk in hospital grounds.[9] The RAS was on call every day, and a later RAS recalls averaging three hours sleep for the two year RAS period (R.H.R. Belsey, personal communication, May 1998). Within three years of graduation Barrett was elected to Fellowship of the Royal College of Surgeons (1930) and had been awarded the postgraduate degree M.Chir.(1931). He joined the surgical staff of St Thomas's as Consulting Surgeon in 1935, and remained there throughout his career.

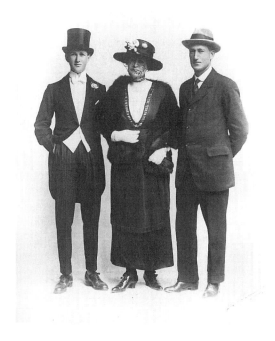

Figure 2. Norman with parents Katie and Alfred Barrett, 1917

The family lived first in Switzerland, moving to England with the outbreak of World War 1. The domestic arrangements were somewhat unusual; Norman stayed mostly with his father and Miss Chaplin, whilst his mother and sister were housed nearby. His parents formally separated when Norman was in his late teens, and Norman's father eventually married Miss Chaplin. His mother and sister went back to Australia, returning to England only when Katie, Norman's mother, was diagnosed with incurable cancer in the late 1930s. Norman Barrett returned to Australia only once, when he was invited to lecture in Sydney in 1963. In London in 1966 he spoke about medicine in Australia for a "Symposium on *The History of Medicine in the Commonwealth*" but examined his subject "through the eyes of a critic in a distant country,

4. DOMESTIC LIFE

The 28 year old Barrett married Annabel Elizabeth "Betty" Warington Smyth, one year his senior, on April 21, 1931. They had met six years previously when Barrett was invited by Betty's brother, an old school friend, to help sail their yacht from Cornwall to the Baltic Sea. The Warington Smyths were a prominent Cornwall family and Betty's father had been Minister of Mines in South Africa. Betty had studied English at London University and art at the Slade School. She became a writer and published five well received novels under her maiden name.

Barrett was obliged to keep his marriage secret from the senior men at St Thomas's because junior surgical staff was not permitted to marry. Barrett consequently spent his early married life living in quarters at the hospital, seeing his wife only on weekends.

The Barretts had two children, Julia and Althea. Although a fond father, Barrett's professional obligations meant that parenting was often limited to just one hour on Sunday afternoons, when he would take tea with the nannies in the children's playroom.

After Norman was appointed to the staff at St Thomas's, the Barretts leased an attractive Georgian terrace at 2 Dorset Street in the Marylebone area of central London. They lived here for about 20 years, surviving a bomb blast during World War II that completely destroyed the terrace next door. One of Betty's novels "London Village" (1960) was set in this area. In 1954 they moved into the magnificent red brick house "Old Palace Place", Richmond Green. Barrett purchased this modernized Tudor house (built c.1500) from Lord Kenneth Clark, Director of the National Gallery. The house had ten large bedrooms and a hall where the Barretts entertained regularly. Junior medical staff invited by Barrett to an evening at home were sometimes surprised to find themselves in the company of famous members of society. Many of the guests were Betty's literary friends from the "Pen" (Poets, Essayists, Novelists) club, but prominent musicians, politicians, businessmen and artists frequently visited as well.

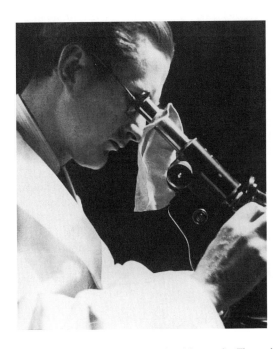

Figure 3. Norman Barrett, surgical resident at St. Thomas' Hospital, aged about 24

Many who worked at St Thomas' have commented on Barrett's "strong, delightful personality"[9] and his "disregard for sham and humbug and his search for truth",[9] features which were apparent from his earliest days at the hospital. Sir Thomas Holmes Sellors wrote that "Pasty Barrett brought to St Thomas's from Cambridge the reputation of a wit and humorist whose outward respect for needless authority was not deeply rooted. He was the complete debunker of anything in medicine that savored of pomposity, and would criticize the pointless and unnecessary in a disarmingly amusing and accurate manner"[8].

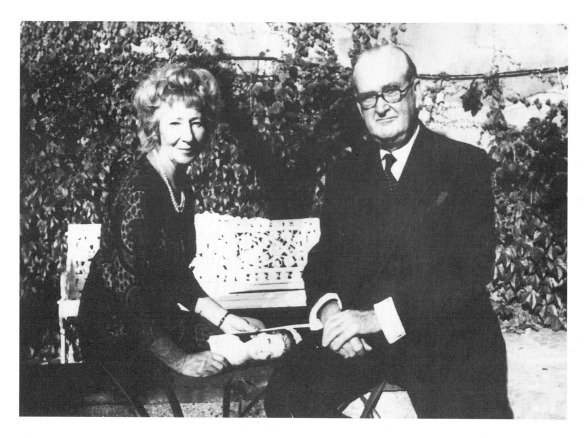

Figure 4. Norman and Elizabeth Barrett, 1969

5. U.S. CONNECTIONS

In 1935-1936 Barrett traveled to the United States, supported by a Rockefeller Travelling Fellowship. A period of US training was somewhat unusual for a British doctor at the time, although five years previously another thoracic surgeon Russell (later Lord) Brock had also received a Rockefeller Fellowship to train with Evarts Graham. Barrett's experience inspired others to visit the United States, and he encouraged and assisted his own trainees to study there[9]. Hector Goadby, who was Resident Assistant Physician to Barrett's Resident Assistant Surgeon, recalled that "Of all the men I worked with in St Thomas's, Pasty Barrett was the most stimulating, and also the most original in big ways, as witness his being the first to go to the USA to work for a year, his setting up the Thoracic Surgical Unit, and his work on the examination of the sputum for malignant cells."[9] Barrett had intended to study upper

gastrointestinal surgery in the U.S., but was dissuaded by Donald C. Balfour at the Mayo Clinic, who urged him to apply himself to a newer field, one more "open" with opportunities[10]. Impressed by the work of Churchill in Boston and Harrington and Moersch at the Mayo Clinic, Barrett settled on thoracic surgery. He spent most of his time at these two centers, but he also visited Graham in St. Louis and Alexander in Michigan[10].

Barrett greatly appreciated his time in the United States. In a 1959 lecture "Wealth, Power and Philanthropy. John Davison Rockefeller",[11] Barrett commented that a research fellowship "gives a chance for young scientists to step outside their own hedged-in community, and to appreciate the international society of science and scholarship. It broadens horizons. It results in friendships that remain useful throughout a man's professional life; and later on, when he himself is responsible for the direction of younger men, it helps him to direct them upon useful roads of endeavour"[11]. In another article he applauded the American system by writing "The importance of research, as a part of the education of every doctor who aspires to higher things, was accepted and implemented a long time ago in the United States. In England the emphasis is still on patient care, and research is reserved for a minority"[6]. He noted, however, that "Modern methods [of US-style training], excellent though they are, often produce men who are not primarily interested in treating patients"[6].

Barrett returned to the United States every few years, both for the reciprocal dissemination of knowledge and to meet with his good friends. Amongst these were, in particular, O.T. "Jim" Clagett, Max Chamberlain, Dwight Harken, Ralph D. Alley, F. Henry Ellis, Jr., and Robert L. Replogle. There is a story that Barrett and Philip Allison were invited to the US to speak on surgical management of carcinoma of the esophagus, with Barrett to speak first for 30 minutes on the upper third of the esophagus, and Allison filling the allotted one hour with management of lower two-thirds cancers. Barrett took the podium, stating "there is no surgical treatment for cancer of the upper third; it is all radiotherapy" and sat down, leaving Allison considerably more speaking time than he had anticipated.

6. PROFESSIONAL LIFE

Returning to the UK, Barrett pioneered the then "unrecognized and somewhat suspect" (Cockett)[9] field of thoracic surgery at St Thomas's and at the Brompton Hospital, London. Other British contributors included Tudor Edwards, Clement Price Thomas, J.E.H. Roberts, George Grey Turner, Ivor Lewis, George Mason, Russell Brock, and Ronald H.R. Belsey. The greatest demand at this time was for surgery for pulmonary tuberculosis, and Barrett was one of several surgeons who traveled, usually on weekends, to regional hospitals and sanatoria to provide surgical care for this disease. "Norman's "parish" was Cornwall (which incidentally was handy for yachting) and Wales....It was from his experiences in South Wales that he became the acknowledged authority on hydatid disease of the lungs"[7]. He was appointed as well to the King Edward VII Sanatorium, Midhurst, when it was a leading center for the treatment of pulmonary TB. Although he specialized in surgery of the

chest, Barrett followed the tradition at St Thomas' Hospital by continuing as a general surgeon and, despite his increasing reputation he did not have a specialist Thoracic Unit at St Thomas's until 1948, when he became a senior surgeon and thus entitled to certain beds. The story of how Barrett established the thoracic ward at St Thomas' illustrates his effective if unorthodox approach: one morning he simply walked onto a ward and announced, without consulting any committees, that it was now a thoracic unit[9].

Barrett took great care managing his patients, as evidenced by reports of some of the desperate but often successful operations he would undertake to wrest cure where none seemed possible[8]. Clagett wrote of his good friend Barrett that, although he was "a brilliant technical surgeon and endoscopist, as good as I have ever seen, his surgical judgement, breadth of knowledge and compassion for patients were even more remarkable"[10]. Clagett's complimentary assessment of Barrett's technical ability is interesting, as others who worked with Barrett have noted that if there was any area in which Barrett was not particularly gifted, it was as a technician, his natural ambidexterity notwithstanding.

7. OFFICIAL WORK

Barrett was retained as a consultant advisor in the Emergency Medical Service during the Second World War and was made consulting thoracic surgeon to the Royal Navy in 1944. He was later also consulting thoracic surgeon for the Ministry of Pensions (Social Security).

Barrett was an original member of the Thoracic Society, and was selected by that Society as the first Surgical Editor of its journal *Thorax*, remaining Editor from 1945-1971, a total of more than 25 years[12]. His Medical Co-Editor recalled how valuable Barrett's energies and good humor were, especially in the early days of *Thorax*, when submitted manuscripts were few. Barrett, he wrote, "would go to immense trouble to help a foreign author to get his paper into acceptable literary style if it contained material scientifically worth publishing"[8]. As an editor, Barrett particularly disliked the practice of publishing similar material in more than one journal[13].
In 1962, as the honored guest of the Annual Meeting of the American Association for

Thoracic Surgery, he discussed surgical writing and the editor's role. In this address he suggested that "too many papers that are unworthy of publication are being written, and important information is often swamped...young men driven to publish or perish find their inspiration in laboratories and write many of these immature works"[13]. He went on to suggest "that surgeons in their headlong surge toward science have lost something" and he recommended, quoting the philosopher Whitehead, some familiarity with the humanities to attain "Mastery of knowledge, which is wisdom...The ancients saw clearly - more clearly than we do - the necessity for dominating knowledge by wisdom"[13]. In this address Barrett also offered suggestions on how to write. Barrett's own prose was superb, if a trifle florid by current standards. Belsey considers that "Everything that Barrett wrote was a literary masterpiece" (R.H.R. Belsey, personal communication, May 1998). Barrett himself acknowledged the influence of his novelist wife Betty in the development of his writing style[14].

Barrett was the President of both the Thoracic Surgeons of Great Britain and Ireland (1962) and the Thoracic Society (1963). He was a member of the Court of Examiners of the Royal College of Surgeons, eventually as Chairman, and was examiner at different times to the universities of Oxford, Cambridge, London, Birmingham, and Khartoum. Sir Thomas Holmes Sellors noted that he had "never listened to a better examiner-his questions were simple and without ambiguity and he invariably got a smile out of the most timorous candidate"[7]. He was careful never to examine on aspects of thoracic diseases, confining his questions to general surgery subjects.

In appreciation of his fostering of relations between thoracic surgery on both sides of the Atlantic, Barrett was elected an honorary member of the American Association for Thoracic Surgery, receiving that Association's presidential chain of office, and he was awarded the Gold Medal of the American College of Chest Physicians.

Barrett served on the councils of the Imperial Cancer Research Fund and the General Medical Council, and on the Council of the Royal College of Surgeons from his election in 1963 until 1974, the last two years as Vice-President of the College. He was appointed CBE (Commander of the British Empire) in 1969 in recognition of his

official work. Health concerns prompted him not to allow his name to go forward for President of the College (with its inevitable knighthood), distinctions he would otherwise undoubtedly have received.

8. TEACHING

Barrett was regarded as an excellent teacher and some have commented that his greatest abilities were as a teacher. His lectures were reportedly always full and his open ward rounds "of vast proportions, crammed with students, who appreciated the wit and enthusiasm with which he imparted his very personal view..."[9] Dr. William Thomson wrote of him that "A pretty gift for cynicism, linked with a pleasing degree of disrespect for authority - or at least a joy in debunking it, combined with a gift for exposition, made him one of the best surgical teachers of his time. Heaven help any of his colleagues who tried to be pompous, but the learner in search of knowledge always found him accessible and clarity personified"[15]. Sir Ronald Belsey, who was a resident under Barrett, recalled that Barrett "cultivated a sardonic sense of humor" and that one of his favourite teachings was "Never, under any circumstances, give way to the illusion that you are doing any good" (R.H.R. Belsey, personal communication, May 1998). Other favorite aphorisms were "Know the measure of your luck" (Balthasar Gracian)[13] and "When you make pronouncements, listen for the still small voice that whispers 'Fiddlesticks' " (Jonathan Hutchinson)[16].

Barrett took care to teach and involve the ancillary members of the Thoracic Unit. Many years before this would be standard practice, he promoted the development of a skilled and harmonious team, with nursing, social work, physiotherapy, and clerical staff all accorded attention and importance. Barrett asked for a social work report on all his patients, a most unusual request at the time. He took a particular interest in the career of Cicely (later Dame Cicely) Saunders, who was for three years Barrett's medical social worker, doubling up in the last year as his secretary[17]. Cicely Saunders wanted to do more for the dying, and she would eventually found the modern hospice movement. She writes "In the summer of 1951 I was driving with Mr. Barrett down to one of the hospitals where he worked and I told him I would have to get back into nursing in order to help dying patients. His response is etched in my memory –

he said "Go and read medicine, it's the doctors who desert the dying and there's so much more to be learnt about pain. You will only be frustrated if you don't do it properly and they won't listen to you…As well as encouraging me to take the step of taking medicine at the relatively late age of 33, he helped me get into the Medical School at St. Thomas's and took an interest in what I was doing thereafter…He was a most stimulating person to work for and I owe him a great deal" (C. Saunders, personal communication, May 1998).

9. CONTRIBUTIONS TO THORACIC SURGERY

Barrett had little involvement in the new field of cardiac surgery, but in most other areas of thoracic surgery he was influential. He advised his residents to follow, as he did, John Hunter's methods: observe, record, deduce, and put to the test. As Belsey notes, "his observations were meticulous", (R.H.R. Belsey, personal communication, May 1998) and Cicely Saunders recalls how she was inspired by Barrett's careful records to keep her own detailed and ultimately very important records (C. Saunders, personal communication, May 1998). A list of Barrett's principal publications indicates the wide range of his interests,[6,11,13,16,18-82] and in many of these articles he made important original contributions. His papers customarily began with a detailed historical review. A 1950 article on foreign bodies in the cardiovascular system, for example, included a summary of all recorded cases, with 200 references[56].

Although remembered principally for his achievements in esophageal surgery, Barrett did impressive work in other areas of thoracic surgery. He worked with Leonard S. Dudgeon, the Professor of Pathology at the University of London, on the cytological examination of tumors[40,83,84]. In particular, Barrett helped demonstrate the accuracy of the "wet-film method" of cytological examination of the sputum in the diagnosis of malignancy[40]. Barrett's other major contribution to pulmonary surgery was in the management of patients with pulmonary hydatid disease[18,27,41,51,53,69]. Barrett treated many patients with this disease because of his attachments to Sully Hospital, Cardiff, and Horton War Hospital, Epsom. He advocated enucleation of hydatid cysts without aspiration to avoid spillage and contamination, and this method of removing pulmonary hydatid cysts

was known at one time as "the Barrett technique"[85]. He also wrote authoritative articles on primary tumors of the rib[63] on fibrous diseases of the pleura[81] and mediastinum,[67] and on the use of drainage tubes in the chest and elsewhere[33,37,44]. In 1933, when infants with congenital diaphragmatic hernia were still denied operation by some doctors, Barrett stated that for the more common types of hernia "an attempt to repair the defect must certainly be made as soon as the diagnosis is established."[30] He also correctly advised, based on others' reports, that the repair should usually be made via laparotomy rather than by thoracotomy[30].

10. STUDIES ON THE ESOPHAGUS

The lower esophagus was, however, Barrett's area of particular expertise. For the first issue of *Thorax* in 1946, Barrett and his medical co-editor Scadding were faced with insufficient articles for publication. Barrett, wrote Scadding, "resolved our problems by writing a paper, more or less to order, on spontaneous rupture of the esophagus. Two of his interests, the esophagus and the history of medicine, were combined in this scholarly and informative paper, which remains a pleasure to read"[8]. Barrett included in this paper Morell Mackenzie's amusing abstract of Boerhaave's original case, and after reviewing this and all other recorded cases of spontaneous perforation of the esophagus, Barrett commented that "in the byways of surgery there can be few conditions more dramatic in their presentation and more terrible in their symptoms than spontaneous perforation of the esophagus. No case has yet been treated successfully and diagnosis has only been achieved in a very few before death, and yet there is no fundamental reason why this unsatisfactory position should not be improved in the future"[48]. Having studied all aspects of this condition so thoroughly, Barrett had only to await the presentation of a suitable case, and one year later, on March 7, 1947, he performed the first successful repair of this condition[50]. Olsen and Clagett carried out the second successful operation, only two months later[86]. Barrett also reported the first successful transthoracic resection of a thoracic esophageal diverticulum, although this was during his training years, and he was not the principal surgeon in that case[31].

Along with Maingot,[87] Barrett promoted Heller's operation for achalasia in the UK, with the result that this operation was accepted there earlier than in other countries. In 1949 Barrett and R.H. Franklin published a paper on the late results of esophagogastrostomy and cardioplasty, then standard operations for achalasia[22]. They found that after esophagogastrostomy and cardioplasty there was eventually "almost constant development of 'esophagitis'" due to "regurgitation of gastric contents from the stomach into the lower esophagus…as a result of temporary or permanent incompetence of the cardia"[22]. They stated that "Heller's operation is a sound procedure whereas the two operations at present under consideration are unsound"[22] In 1950[55] and again in 1964,[74] when he published his results for Heller's procedure, Barrett's belief in the superiority of myotomy for the treatment of achalasia was further confirmed. "There are no people more grateful than those whose dysphagia has been cured" he concluded. "Indeed, the results of a successful Heller's operation can be far reaching; it is not unusual for divorce proceedings to be settled out of court, for bags to be packed and the family to go away for a holiday, for father to put on weight and mother to become pregnant"[55].

Despite Barrett's publications, considered by Hurt "the deciding factors"[88] in establishing the superiority of Heller's operation, esophagogastrostomy or dilatation continued to be the preferred treatments for achalasia in the United States and even in Heller's native Germany[88,89]. This was probably because of influential papers written by Ochsner and DeBakey,[90] by Clagett et al.,[91] and by Kay[88,92]. These papers reported good results for esophagogastrostomy or dilatation, but they were based on collected series or had only very short follow-up periods. Only much later, following in particular papers from Okike et al (1979)[93] and from Ellis et al (1980)[94], was the worth of Heller's operation (1913)[95] finally widely accepted in the United States. Barrett was justified in writing, many years after his first publications on this subject, that his own early observations "disputed at the time, are now accepted as correct"[74].

Barrett's writings on gastroesophageal reflux, hiatus hernia, and the complications of these conditions contain many important original findings and some remarkably accurate speculations. It is apparent now, however, that Barrett was confused or incorrect on some points, with the result that these subjects were confusing ones for many doctors for many years

afterwards. Barrett's 1950 article "Chronic peptic ulcer of the esophagus and 'esophagitis' " is usually cited as the first report, by Barrett at least, of the columnar-lined or "Barrett's" esophagus[57]. In this article, Barrett attempted to clarify the "chaos" which already existed regarding the two conditions "esophagitis" and "peptic ulcer of the esophagus". He introduced the term "reflux esophagitis" in this article, stated that it was a common condition, and observed that a benign stricture due to inflammation in the muscularis propria layers may develop in patients with this condition. Eventually, he stated, there may be contraction in both longitudinal and transverse directions, with shortening of the affected segment (short esophagus). He observed the presence of a pouch of stomach (which was "partially enveloped by peritoneum" and thus true stomach) below the stricture, but he thought the stomach was "drawn up by scar tissue into the mediastinum", rather than the result of a hiatus hernia. The two X-rays illustrated by Barrett, however, show the presence of hiatal hernias below the strictures[57].

Why Barrett preferred at this stage to think of the stomach as being drawn up by contraction of the esophagus rather than herniating through the hiatus is unclear[57]. In the same article he recognizes that hiatal hernia is an important cause of gastroesophageal reflux. He also refers to Allison's 1946 publication[96] confirming the association between gastroesophageal reflux, peptic injury to the esophagus, and hiatus hernia, and discusses Allison's study in which, by screening patients with metal clips positioned at the squamocolumnar junction, pouches of stomach above the "cardiac sphincter" were demonstrated. Barrett would also have edited Allison's 1948 publication[97] on this subject in *Thorax*. Barrett himself, obviously aware of earlier European work,[88] had written as early as 1933 that "The acquired type of [hiatus] hernia is much more common than the congenital, and in this the general lines of diagnosis have been studied and agreed upon"[30].

Barrett may have been overly impressed by Keith's[98] and Lawford Knagg's[99] descriptions of congenital hiatus hernias, which they reasoned were due to congenital short esophagus. Barrett had discussed these authors' descriptions of this condition some years earlier, writing that "If the [embryonal] esophagus does not elongate [the stomach] may remain in the chest. The sac is not formed by the protrusion of the organ but by the downward movement of the diaphragm over the stomach which is stationary"[30]. Allison had also described ten cases of "congenitally short esophagus" in 1942,[100] although by 1948 he believed that "short esophagus is usually an acquired condition..."[97] In deciding on the congenital short esophagus etiology, Barrett was probably also influenced by the main case presented to him, that of a 13 year old boy "who had several other congenital deformities",[57] in whom columnar mucosa was found up to the level of the aortic arch, and who died of perforation into a pulmonary vein.

It should therefore not be considered such a remarkable error as it now appears that in the second part of his 1950 article Barrett reviewed all published cases and four new cases of "Chronic peptic ulcer of the esophagus" and concluded that they were chronic gastric ulcers in association with congenital short esophagus[57]. These were the ulcers which Allison termed "Barrett's ulcers"[101]. The gastric type epithelium surrounding these ulcers came to be known, through no effort of Barrett's, as Barrett's esophagus.

Although the question is of historical interest only, it may be wondered whether the cases described by Barrett were in fact cases of columnar-lined Barrett's esophagus. In favor of the possibility that he was describing true cases of Barrett's esophagus is the fact that in order to account for his observations he found it necessary to redefine the esophagus as "that part of the foregut...which is lined by squamous epithelium"[57] and his comment that "in cases of congenital short esophagus...the bare area is larger than usual"[57].

Despite these statements, it seems quite possible that the patients described in this 1950 article, which is widely regarded as the first report of Barrett's esophagus, did not have Barrett's esophagus. Rather, he may have been describing cases of chronic peptic ulcer in an intrathoracic stomach, just as he stated at the time, although the underlying abnormality was almost certainly herniation of the stomach through the esophageal hiatus rather than congenital short esophagus. In support of this possibility, Barrett stated that some cases of congenital short esophagus had a partial covering of peritoneum above the crura (indicating that they were part of the stomach), the mucosa is described as "histologically gastric in type" with no mention of goblet cells, which would be expected with such an extensive area of true Barrett's esophagus, and the case illustrated shows gastric folds around the ulcer[57]. Finally, there is Barrett's later reassessment of these ulcers and the columnar lining which surrounded them, written when he had a much greater understanding of both hiatus hernia and the columnar lined esophagus. In 1960 Barrett wrote the following:

> Ulcers that occur in the pouch of stomach that forms a sliding hiatal hernia are true gastric ulcers (Barrett, 1950) and have nothing to do with reflux. They were originally described by Rokitanski ...[71].

In 1962 he wrote:

> Some years ago I pointed out that when a piece of stomach passes into a sliding hiatal or a paraesophageal hernia, it is not unusual for a typical peptic ulcer to develop in the abnormally placed segment of the stomach. Such an ulcer (Barrett's ulcer) has the character of a typical gastric ulcer..."[16].

Barrett did not claim to be the first to describe the columnar lined esophagus, and he mentions nine previous possible reports, with at least one probable case (reported by Lyall[102]) of extensive columnar lined esophagus[57]. He would later acknowledge that the Lortat-Jacobs in Paris were making similar observations,[103-105] and he also later referenced the 1951 case report by Lewis H. Bosher Jr. and Frederick H. Taylor from St. Louis, Missouri[66,106]. Bosher and Taylor clearly described a case of extensive Barrett's esophagus and they noted and illustrated the presence of goblet cells in the columnar epithelium[106]. Barrett generously acknowledged Allison's work, particularly on hiatus hernia. In one article he wrote "I wish to record my debt to P. R. Allison and his colleagues, who have contributed so much to this subject"[61]. In an article in the British Medical Journal he credits his colleague again, patriotically stating that "It was an Englishman, Philip Allison, who strung the isolated threads [of hiatus hernia] into one story"[71]. Lecturing in the United States, he emphasized the help he had received from his American colleagues, in particular Ellis and Wangensteen[16].

In several subsequent articles on "The lower esophagus lined by columnar epithelium",[66]

"Benign stricture in the lower esophagus"[16] and on hiatus hernia[61,71] Barrett corrected many of his earlier errors regarding these conditions and he made some impressive observations. In a 1954 article he admitted the importance of sliding hiatus hernia and his own error in this regard, stating: "The explanations which came first to mind are not correct. It was thought that the stomach was dragged into the mediastinum by contraction of fibrous tissue in the wall of the esophagus. But the hernia precedes and causes the esophagitis and not the reverse"[61]. He made the original observation in this article that "severity of symptoms does not always tally with the extent of the esophagitis; and, in particular, pain is not proportional to visible inflammation"[61].

Observing that patients with achlorhydria and with duodeno-esophageal anastomosis developed esophageal injury, Barrett concluded that duodenal contents, along with acid and pepsin, were an important component of the injurious refluxate[61]. In 1954 he advised that the ideal treatment for gastroesophageal reflux disease "eliminates reflux from the stomach *and from the duodenum*" (Barrett's italics)[61]. He therefore rejected both partial gastrectomy and vagotomy, advocated by others because they reduce acid secretion, as essentially unsound. In a subsequent article (1960) he referenced the early experimental work of other groups on this subject[71].

Barrett also noted that depression of the fundus allowed incompetence of the cardia (the cardia being, at least until the 1960s, the most distal part of the esophagus or gastroesophageal junction and not a part of the stomach). He therefore agreed with Allison, Lortat-Jacob, and others on the importance of maintaining an acute esophago-gastric angle at a low position within the abdomen. A recent study has demonstrated the correctness of these anatomical theories[107]. In 1960 Barrett recognized that an important component of resistance to gastroesophageal reflux was "having a length of the esophagus that is subjected to positive abdominal pressure below the diaphragm"[71]. This concept has also been supported by more recent studies[108,109].

Barrett eventually indicated his preference for the term "lower esophagus lined by columnar epithelium" over "congenital short esophagus" or "gullet", stating in 1960 that "It would have been better if the term ["congenital short esophagus"]

had never been introduced..."[71] Despite this, he continued to promote a developmental etiology for the columnar lined esophagus, even after Hayward had submitted to Barrett's *Thorax* in 1960 his persuasive argument that the columnar lined esophagus was a metaplastic, potentially reversible process which was secondary to gastroesophageal reflux and which originated in cardiac epithelium normally present in the distal esophagus[110]. Hayward's landmark publication contained no reference to how he reached his conclusions, but in a personal communication Hayward recalled that they were based on examination of the distal esophageal mucosa in more than 200 rigid esophagoscopies and esophageal operations, with histologic examination in many cases (J.I. Hayward, personal communication, May 1998). Hayward and Barrett had worked together at the Brompton Hospital in London, although Hayward worked with JEH Roberts and Russell Brock, while Barrett worked on the other team, with Tudor Edwards and Clement Price Thomas. As a former Brompton colleague, and as Editor of *Thorax*, Barrett offered to amend Hayward's article, which contained, in his opinion, "a lot of nonsense". Hayward refused to make any alterations, and he considers it a credit to Barrett that he published the paper as it stood (J.I. Hayward, personal communication, May 1998).

Had Barrett accepted the acquired theory more readily, he was well positioned to achieve an even more advanced understanding of the columnar lined esophagus, for he recognized as early as 1957 that "if for any reason the squamous lining of the lower esophagus were to be destroyed it could, theoretically, be replaced by columnar cells"[66]. Barrett had even apparently conducted studies in the dog to test this theory,[66,111] but he had omitted to induce the free reflux into the lower esophagus which made Bremner et al.'s later similar experiment successful, and in Barrett's dogs rapid squamous regrowth followed the esophageal injury[111].

The then mysterious Schatzki's rings were also examined by Barrett. He stated in 1962 that these rings were "the end result of inflammation in the mucosa and submucosa. They are caused by reflux esophagitis..."[16]. He also noted, in 1960, that "A lower esophagus lined by columnar epithelium may cause esophagitis and its complications, and it is the usual source of columnar-cell carcinoma that arises in the gullet as opposed to the stomach"[71].

11. OTHER INTERESTS

Barrett was a keen sailor and he built a house named "Lorelei" with a boathouse on the Helford River in South Cornwall, near Falmouth. When not in Cornwall, he often sailed at the Royal Corinthian Yacht Club at Burnam-in-Crouch in Essex. He also enjoyed drawing and painting, especially maritime scenes, and "NRB" can be discerned on many of the illustrations in his medical publications.

Barrett was interested in history, especially medical aspects of British history. In 1958 he delivered a paper entitled "Thoughts about Henry VIII" for the Rowfant Club in Cleveland, Ohio,[73] and in 1970 he addressed the same subject for the 50th Thomas Vicary Lecture for the Worshipful Company of Barbers of London and the Surgeons of the Royal College of England, Vicary having been Serjeant Surgeon for Henry VIII, and for Edward VI, Mary, and Elizabeth also[82]. Contrary to accepted opinion, Barrett contended that Henry VIII had probably not contracted syphilis. He argued that the king's deterioration in temperament, his "sorre legges", and his late-onset obesity could be explained by repeated head injuries sustained in jousting and other martial sports, to chronic osteomyelitis of the lower end of the right femur, and to amyloid disease resulting from the chronic infection in the leg[82].

In "A Paper of No Value", Barrett related in a humorous fashion the circumstances in which 27 Kings of England died, with the conclusion that "to live in this Realm in the Middle Ages was hazardous"[59]. He included in this paper "a few simple statistics....[for] the benefit of those who have been educated in recent times" noting that "These prove nothing and are misleading, but it is customary to shun the medical writings of those who cannot corroborate their story by arithmetic." After two brief introductory paragraphs, the body of the article was in small print, which Barrett explained with the note "Parts of any good article are always printed in small type: the implication being that they are beyond the comprehension of the ordinary doctor"[59].

Barrett was a member of a lighthearted dining club called "The Sette of Odd Volumes". This club was founded in 1878 to discuss books and literature, although by Barrett's day it was devoted to "mutual admiration and the entertainment of guests"[78]. In 1965 he addressed the club on its annual Ladies Night, beginning in the following way.

"Rule XVIII states that: "No O.V. [Odd Volume] shall talk, unasked, on any subject he understands." The opusculum that I shall present accords with this directive exactly, for I shall discuss "after-dinner speaking" - to which I am unaccustomed! Now I expect that those of you who are in the know be surprised that his Oddship did not choose one of his two professional speakers to address you this evening. And, in passing, we may register for our own edifications, that there are five or six people in this room wondering who is the other man"[78].

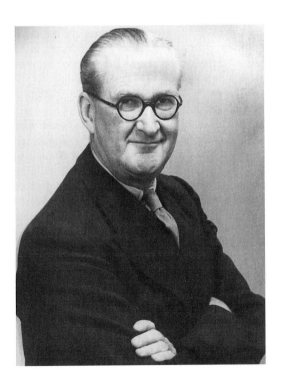

Figure 5. Norman Barrett in 1958, aged about 55.

LATER YEARS

Barrett's scientific cynicism was unaltered by elevation to high office. Lord Richardson noted that "Norman Barrett was indeed always a "character", who nevertheless managed to give little or no offence to his innumerable admirers and the honored band of his friends. This was from no lack of provocation but depended on his essential kindliness, and because the great debunker could laugh at himself even when the Senior Surgeon and surrounded by honor. Shortly before he retired he was going up in one of the lifts to Simon Ward, together with a young nurse who had pressed the button for the third floor. He said to her: "Nurse, you should walk at your age. It would help to keep your figure." As the lift slowed down she replied: "Sir, when I am your age and have your figure, I shall." This story made lunch in the staff room that day very easy to digest. It got there, of course, through the man who enjoyed it most"[9].

After retiring from clinical work at age 65, Barrett continued with his official duties for several more years, acted as medical consultant for a friend's business, and sat on industrial injury tribunals. His chief non-medical interest became tending his garden at Old Palace Place, but he also read a lot, biographies especially, and he made further trips to the United States and elsewhere. Barrett was by nature very critical of his own efforts, and there were periods in his retirement when he seemed unsatisfied with his achievements.

Barrett was diagnosed with Parkinson's disease at age 61. The physical effects of his disease were never severe, but Barrett found the impairment depressing nonetheless, and he noted that among the worse aspects was anxiety about future deterioration. Barrett was intolerant of the new wonder drug L-dopa, which was a great disappointment to him. In his 70's his health deteriorated further, and after three months in St. Thomas's Hospital for treatment of breathlessness he died of a stroke on 8 January 1979, aged 75 years. He remained alert until the end, and he was attended in his last illness and at his funeral, held at St Martin-in-the-Fields, by a host of friends and colleagues, including a roll-call of the distinguished British surgeons of the time.

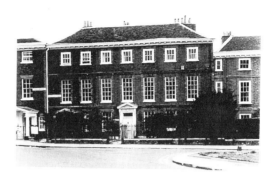

Figure 6. The Barrett's home "Old Palace Place" in Richmond Green London.

13. NORMAN BARRETT AND THE TERM "BARRETT'S ESOPHAGUS"

As this book attests, Barrett's epithelium has become the subject of intensive clinical and biological study. It has been suggested in recent years that Barrett's esophagus should be renamed "the columnar lined esophagus"[112]. The use of eponymns in medicine can be criticized since they generally give little information about the condition they refer to, they often incorrectly immortalize physicians who were not the first to describe the conditions which bear their name, and later studies may demonstrate that the named person's description was at least partly incorrect. These three criticisms can be fairly made regarding Barrett's work and the term "Barrett's esophagus".

The author is nevertheless in favor of retaining Barrett's name, at least for some years more. The term "Barrett's" is recognized readily by those in non-gastrointestinal fields, whereas alternative terms would likely require the explanation when speaking with other health professionals that one is referring to the condition previously known as Barrett's esophagus. Moreover, the single term "Barrett's esophagus" can encompass all the subgroups of columnar metaplasia found in the region of the distal esophagus and gastroesophageal junction, although the clinical importance of each of these different subgroups is currently uncertain.

The use of eponymous terms reminds the medical and scientific communities of the historical and personal aspects of medical progress, aspects that seem increasingly neglected. In this case, the term "Barrett's" is a reminder for the medical community in general of the life and achievements of this outstanding surgical investigator, named the "doyen of esophageal surgery" by Ellis and Olsen in the dedication of their volume on achalasia[113]. Barrett's legacy is contained in his publications, in the continuing strength of the journal *Thorax*, in the thoracic unit at St. Thomas' Hospital that he founded, and in his influence on many surgeons in many countries. W. Spencer Payne observed in his obituary for Barrett that "To write of the essence of an eminent but deceased pioneer thoracic surgeon poses particular problems to one who is of a later surgical generation. Although the perfunctory listing of achievements and honors is at hand for us today, the unique quality and style of the man are best known to his generation"[10]. For the present author, who is at least one surgical generation further removed from his subject, a satisfactory portrayal of Norman Barrett seems even more difficult. Nevertheless, this biographical sketch is presented in the hope that, whether or not his name continues to be attached to the condition he described, the character and achievements of this medical pioneer will continue to be recognized.

The author spent a very pleasant weekend at the home in England of Julia and David Gough, Norman Barrett's daughter and son-in-law. He is very grateful for the hospitality and information he received on this occasion, and for permission to reproduce the illustrations shown. Hugh Barrett from Narrabri, New South Wales, Australia was helpful with information about NRB's Australian relatives. The author also appreciates the information provided by the following former friends and colleagues of Barrett: Dame Cicely Saunders, Sir Ronald H.R. Belsey, F. Henry Ellis Jr., Sir Norman Browse, Ian McInnes, Reginald S.A. Lord. The following archivists and librarians were very helpful: Miss Glen F-Jones (Royal College of Surgeons, London), Catriona Sinclair (St Thomas's Hospital, London) Claire Cross (Wellcome Institute for the History of Medicine, London), Mrs P. Hatfield (Eton College, Windsor), Jonathan Smith (Trinity College, Cambridge), Jane Oliver (Royal Australasian College of Surgeons, Melbourne), and Alison Pilger (Research School of Social Sciences, The Australian National University, Canberra).

REFERENCES

1. Power D, Le Fanu WR. Norman Barrett. In Power D, Le Fanu WR (eds). Lives of the Fellows of the Royal College of Surgeons of England 1930-1951. London:Royal College of Surgeons of England;1953:53-4.
2. Obituary. Sir James Barrett Lancet 1945;1:485.
3. Obituary. Sir James Barrett. Med J Aust 1945;2:58-61.
4. Obituary. Sir James Barrett. Br Med J 1945;1:572.
5. Murray-Smith S. Sir James William Barrett. In Nairn B SG (ed). Australian Dictionary of Biography Vol.7 1891-1939. Melbourne:Melbourne University Press;1979:186-9.
6. Barrett NR. The contribution of Australians to medical knowledge. Medical History 1967;11:321-333.
7. Obituary. NR Barrett CBE MChir FRCS. Ann Roy Coll Surg Engl 1979;61:414-5.
8. Obituaries. Norman R Barrett OBE, MA, MChir, FRCS. Brit Med J 1979;1:203, 280, 420, 903.
9. Obituaries. Norman R Barrett, CBE, MA, MChir, FRCS. St Thomas's Hosp Gaz 1979;77:53-55.
10. Payne WS. Norman Rupert Barrett, CBE, FRCS, M Chir (1903-1979). Bull Am Coll Chest Physicians 1979;18:8-10.
11. Barrett NR. Wealth, power and philanthropy. John Davison Rockefeller. St Thomas's Hosp Gaz 1960;58:33-40.
12. Editors. Thorax 1975;30:8.
13. Barrett NR. Publish or perish. J Thorac Cardiovasc Surg 1962;44:167-79.
14. Cornelius EH, Taylor SF. Norman Barrett. In Cornelius EH, Taylor SF (eds). Lives of the Fellows of he Royal College of Surgeons of England 1974-1982. London:Royal College of Surgeons of England;1988:19-20.
15. Obituary. Norman R. Barrett. The Times . 1979. Ref Type:Newspaper
16. Barrett NR. Benign stricture in the lower esophagus. J Thorac Cardiovasc Surg 1962;43:703-715.
17. Saunders C. Preface. In Saunders C. (ed). The Management of Terminal Malignant Disease. London:Edward Arnold Publishers.;1978.
18. Barrett NR, Thomas D. Pulmonary hydatid disease. Br J Tuberc 1944;38:39-95.
19. Barrett NR, Barnard WG. Some unusual thoracic tumours. Br J Surg 1945;32:447-57.
20. Barrett NR, Bond LT. Serum treatment of Hodgkin's disease, with account of 4 cases treated. Lancet 1933;2:855-7.
21. Barrett NR, Daley R. Method of increasing lung blood supply in cyanotic congenital heart disease. Br Med J 1949;1:699-702.
22. Barrett NR, Franklin RH. Concerning the unfavourable late results of certain operations performed in the treatment of cardiospasm. Br J Surg 1949;37:194-202.
23. Barrett NR, Franklin RH. Non-malignant affections of esophagus. Tr Med Soc London (1948-1950) 1951;66:382-98.
24. Barrett NR, Hickie JB. Cor triatrium. Thorax 1957;12:24-7.
25. Barrett NR, Hoyle C. Case of haemoptysis. Br J Tuberc. Br J Tuberc 1942;36:172-7.

26. Barrett NR, Thomas D. Massive surgical emphysema during the course of general anaesthesia. Br Med J 1944;2:692-3.

27. Barrett NR, Thomas D. Pulmonary hydatid disease. Br J Surg 1952;40:222-4.

28. Barrett NR, Tomlinson RH. "Adenoma" of trachea and bronchi. St Thomas's Hosp Rep 1952;8:5-19.

29. Barrett NR, Tubbs OS. Operations for infection of the pleura. Tubercle 1962;43(suppl):95-101.

30. Barrett NR, Wheaton CEW. The pathology, diagnosis, and treatment of congenital diaphragmatic hernia in infants. Br J Surg 1933;21:420-33.

31. Barrett NR. Diverticula of the thoracic esophagus;report of a case in which the diverticulum was successfully resected. Lancet 1933;1:1009-11.

32. Barrett NR. Some points in the diagnosis and treatment of injuries to menisci of knee-joint. St Thomas's Hosp Gaz 1934;34:355-359, 390-7.

33. Barrett NR. Treatment of post-operative retention of urine. Lancet 1934;2:1046-7.

34. Barrett NR. Bilocular stomach due to hernia of small bowel through transverse mesocolon. Br J Surg 1935;23:469-74.

35. Barrett NR. In praise of Mayo Clinic;some impressions informally set down. St Thomas's Hosp Gaz 1936;35:264-9.

36. Barrett NR. Diversion of urine above bladder. St Thomas's Hosp Gaz 1936;35:314-25.

37. Barrett NR. Decompression of intestine by naso-duodenal suction. St Thomas's Hosp Rep 1936;1:78-96.

38. Barrett NR. Two cases of endothelioma of pleura. Br J Surg 1938;26:314-9.

39. Barrett NR. Putrid lung abscess;review of recent work. St Thomas's Hosp Rep 1938;3:139-77.

40. Barrett NR. Examination of sputum for malignant cells and particles of malignant growth. J Thorac Surg 1938;8:169-83.

41. Barrett NR. Tuberculosis of chest wall. Tubercle 1939;20:445-59.

42. Barrett NR. Discussion on chest injuries. Proc R Soc Med 1940;34:91-4.

43. Barrett NR. Fibroma of esophagus;report of a case. J Thorac Surg 1940;9:672-8.

44. Barrett NR. Effects and management of tubes used to drain pleural cavity. Br J Tuberc 1942;36:62-80.

45. Barrett NR. Lung abscess;pathology and diagnosis of certain types. Lancet 1944;2:647-51.

46. Barrett NR. Right retroperitoneal diaphragmatic hernia. Br J Surg 1945;32:421-5.

47. Barrett NR. Haemothorax;notes and observations. Lancet 1945;1:103-6.

48. Barrett NR. Spontaneous perforation of the esophagus. Review of the literature and report of three new cases. Thorax 1946;1:48-70.

49. Barrett NR. Tribute to John Snow M.D., London 1813-1858. Bull Hist Med 1946;19:517-35.

50. Barrett NR. Report of a case of spontaneous perforation of the esophagus successfully treated by operation. Br J Surg 1947;35:218.

51. Barrett NR. The treatment of pulmonary hydatid disease. Thorax 1947;2:21-57.

52. Barrett NR. Advances in thoracic surgery. Practitioner 1947;159:741-3.

53. Barrett NR. Removal of simple univesicular pulmonary hydatid cyst. Lancet 1949;2:234.

54. Barrett NR. "Observables" at Royal College of Surgeons;Frere Jacques. Ann Roy Coll Surg Engl 1949;5:275-81.

55. Barrett NR. Discussion on treatment of achalasia of the cardia. Proc R Soc Med 1950;43:421-5.

56. Barrett NR. Foreign bodies in ·the cardiovascular system. Br J Surg 1950;37:416-45.

57. Barrett NR. Chronic peptic ulcer of the esophagus and "esophagitis". Br J Surg 1950;38:175-82.

58. Barrett NR. Esophageal and intestinal obstructions;comparison. Practitioner 1950;165:517-27.

59. Barrett NR. A Paper of No Value. St Thomas's Hosp Gaz 1951;49:156-60.

60. Barrett NR. Achalasia:thoughts concerning aetiology;otolaryngology lecture. Ann Roy Coll Surg Engl 1953;12:391-402.

61. Barrett NR. Hiatus hernia;a review of some controversial points. Br J Surg 1954;42:231-43.

62. Barrett NR. Treatment of acute empyema. Ann Roy Coll Surg Engl 1954;15:25-33.

63. Barrett NR. Primary tumours of rib. Br J Surg 1955;43:113-32.

64. Barrett NR. Surgery of aortic valve. Br Med Bull 1955;11:213-4.

65. Barrett NR. Discussion on unusual aspects of esophageal disease;perforations of the esophagus and of the pharynx. Proc R Soc Med 1956;49:529-36.

66. Barrett NR. The lower esophagus lined by columnar epithelium. Surgery 1957;41:881-94.

67. Barrett NR. Idiopathic mediastinal fibrosis. Br J Surg 1958;46:207-18.

68. Barrett NR. Benign stricture of the lower esophagus. Proc R Soc Med 1960;53:399-402.

69. Barrett NR. The anatomy and pathology of multiple hydatid cysts in the thorax. Ann Roy Coll Surg Engl 1960;26:362-79.

70. Barrett NR. Early treatment of stove-in-chest. Lancet 1960;1:293-6.

71. Barrett NR. Hiatus hernia. Br Med J 1960;2:247-52.

72. Barrett NR. Advances in thoracic surgery. Practitioner 1960;185:548-56.

73. Barrett NR. Thoughts about Henry VIII. St Thomas's Hosp Gaz 1960;58:3-8.

74. Barrett NR. Achalasia of the cardia:reflections upon a clinical study of over 100 cases. Br Med J 1964;1:1140.

75. Barrett NR. Benign smooth muscle tumours of the esophagus. Thorax 1964;19:185-94.

76. Barrett NR. Association of esophageal and pulmonary diseases. Postgrad Med 1964;36:470-4.

77. Barrett NR. Elephants, Anthrax and a Nightingale. St Thomas's Hosp Gaz 1965;63:98-101.

78. Barrett NR. After-dinner speaking. St Thomas's Hosp Gaz 1965.

79. Barrett NR. Sir Astley Cooper and the thymus. Guys Hospital Reports 1968;117:207-12.

80. Barrett NR. Do higher diplomas hinder progress? Proc R Soc Med 1969;62:1067-9.

81. Barrett NR. The pleura:with special reference to fibrothorax. Thorax 1970;25:515-24.

82. Barrett NR. King Henry the Eighth. Ann Roy Coll Surg Engl 1973;52:216-233.

83. Bowes RK, Barrett NR. Use of vital staining and wet films in diagnosis of lesions of cervix. Surg Gynec Obstet 1934;60:1072-6.

84. Dudgeon LS, Barrett NR. Examination of fresh tissues by the wet-film method. Br J Surg 1934;22:4-22.

85. Lichter I. Surgery of pulmonary hydatid cyst - the Barrett technique. Thorax 1972;27:529-34.

86. Olsen AM, Clagett OT. Spontaneous rupture of the esophagus. Postgrad Med 1947;2:417-21.

87. Maingot R. Extramucous esophagocardiomyotomy in cardiospasm. Postgrad Med J 1944;20:278-82.

88. Hurt R. The History of Cardiothoracic Surgery from Early Times. Carnforth:Parthenon Publishing Group;1997.

89. Ravitch MM. Discussion. J Thorac Surg 1958;36:460.
90. Ocshner A, DeBakey M. Surgical considerations of achalasia. Arch Surg 1940;41:1146-83.
91. Clagett OT, Moersch HJ, Fischer A. Esophagogastrostomy in the treatment of cardiospasm. Surg Gynec Obstet 1945;81:440-5.
92. Kay EB. Surgical treatment of cardiospasm. Ann Surg 1948;127:34-9.
93. Okike N, Payne WS, Neufeld DM, Bernatz PE, Pairolero PC, Sanderson DR. Esophagomyotomy versus forceful dilatation for achalasia of the esophagus:results in 899 patients. Ann Thorac Surg 1979;28:119-25.
94. Ellis FHJr, Gibb SP, Crozier RE. Esophagomyotomy for achalasia of the esophagus. Ann Surg 1980;192:157-61.
95. Heller E. Extramukose cardiaplastik beim chronischen cardiospasmus ut dilatation des esophagus. Mitt Grenz Med Chir 1914;27:141-9.
96. Allison PR. Peptic ulcer of the esophagus. J Thorac Surg 1946;15:308-17.
97. Allison PR. Peptic ulcer of the esophagus. Thorax 1948;3:20-42.
98. Keith A. On the origin and nature of hernia. Br J Surg 1924;11:455-75.
99. Knaggs RL. On diaphragmatic hernia of the stomach and on torsion of the small omentum and volvulus of the stomach in association with it. Lancet 1904;2:358-64.
100. .Allison PR, Johnstone AS, Royce GB. Short esophagus with simple peptic ulceration. J Thorac Surg 1942;12:432-57.
101. Allison PR, Johnstone AS. The esophagus lined with gastric mucous membrane. Thorax 1953;8:87-101.
102. Lyall A. Chronic peptic ulcer of the esophagus:a report of eight cases. Br J Surg 1937;24:534-547.
103. Lortat-Jacob JL. L'endo-brachy-oesophage. Ann Chir 1957;11:1247-55.
104. Lortat-Jacob JL. What is the definition of Barrett's esophagus? In Guili R MR (ed). Benign Lesions of the Esophagus and Cancer. Answers to 210 Questions. Berlin:Springer-Verlag;1989:619-20.
105. Smith-Lortat-Jacob M. Cinq observations d'ulcere peptique de l'oesophage. These pour le Doctorat de Medicine, Paris 1950.
106. Bosher LHJr, Taylor FH. Heterotopic gastric mucosa in the esophagus with ulceration and stricture formation. J Thorac Surg 1951;21:306-12.
107. Ismail T, Bancewicz J, Barlow J. Yield pressure, anatomy of the cardia and gastro-esophageal reflux. British Journal of Surgery 1995;82:943-47.
108. Zaninotto G, DeMeester TR, Schwizer W, Johansson KE, Cheng SC. The lower esophageal sphincter in health and disease. American Journal of Surgery 1988;155:104-11.
109. Lord RV, Maranzara A, Gee C, Groshen S, DeMeester TR, Peters JH, Oberg S, Gastal O, Bremner CC. Risk factors for gastresophageal reflux disease. Gastroenterology 2000;118:1267.
110. Hayward J. The lower end of the esophagus. Thorax 1961;16:36-55.
111. Bremner CG, Lynch VP, Ellis FH Jr. Barrett's esophagus:Congenital or acquired? An experimental study of esophageal mucosal regeneration in the dog. Surgery 1970;68:209-16.
112. Spechler SJ. The columnar-lined esophagus. History, terminology, and clinical issues. Gastro Clin Nth Am 1997;26:455-66.
113. Ellis FHJr, Olsen AM. Achalasia of the esophagus. WB Saunders;1969.

1.1 ANATOMY AND EMBRYOLOGY OF THE ESOPHAGUS

D. Liebermann – Meffert

1. SURGICAL ANATOMY

1.1 GENERAL ASPECTS

The esophagus is a midline structure lying in front of the spine. It descends through three compartments: the neck, the chest, and the abdomen. This progression has led to the classical anatomical division into cervical, thoracic, and abdominal segments. In order to subdivide the esophagus more suitable for clinicians and physiologists two concepts have been recently developed (Fig.1). Diamant[8] stresses functional aspects; he distinguishes between the esophageal body and the two sphincters. The other proposal, by Siewert et al [52], refers to onco-surgical concepts and distinguishes between the proximal and distal esophagus, using the tracheal bifurcation as partition. The latter integrates the features of embryological development, in particular the differently orientated pathways of lymphatic drainage (see section Embryology, this volume).

Joining the pharynx, the esophagus commences at the cricoid cartilage opposite of the sixth cervical vertebra (Fig.1).

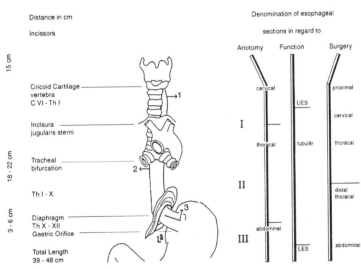

Figure 1. Classic division of the esophagus and its topographic relationship to the cervical (C) and thoracic (Th) vertebrae. The approximate length of each segment is given, and the three deviations of the esophagus are shown. (UES = upper esophageal sphincter, LES = lower esophageal sphincter). More recently, the esophagus has been subdivided for clinical reasons according to its different functions by Diamant (1989). Similarly, Siewert proposed a subdivision of the thoracic esophagus at the level of the tracheal bifurcation for planning treatment strategies in patients with esophageal cancer (1990), and based this concept upon the pathways of lymphatic tumor spread and to the embryological development of the lymphatic system.

It passes into the chest at the level of the sternal notch and travels within the chest cavity on the anterior plane of the posterior mediastinum. Between the thoracic inlet and the diaphragm, it remains in close relationship with the spine. It ends at the esophagogastric junction, opposite the twelfth thoracic vertebra. Three minor deviations are present along its trajectory. The first one is toward the left at the base of the neck (Fig.1). This position facilitates the surgical approach to the esophagus from the left for intestino-cervical anastomoses after esophagectomy[38,39,47]. The second deviation is observed at the level of the seventh thoracic vertebra where the esophagus turns slightly to the right of the spine. On radiological evaluation, however, the esophageal axis is virtually straight. Vascular anomalies or mediastinal masses, may displace, bow or indent the esophagus; any distortion of its axis, however, strongly suggests mediastinal invasion and retraction by tumors, i.e. malignancy[2]. Having turned left to the spine, the esophagogastric junction (cardia) is positioned lateral to the xiphoid process of the sternum which causes the third deviation. At this point, the fundus and the proximal stomach show anterolateral to the body of the vertebrae: the greater curvature and the cranial pole of the adjacent spleen face the posterior

17

H.W. Tilanus and S.E.A. Attwood (eds.), Barrett's Esophagus, 17–30.
© 2001 *Kluwer Academic Publishers. Printed in the Netherlands.*

subdiaphragmatic space and the anterior gastric wall faces towards lateral. This geographic peculiarity is badly displayed in standard anatomy textbooks, but is excellently obtained from computed tomographic studies [57]. This knowledge is relevant for the interpretation of pressure measurement data of the LES[55].

The esophagus, defined as the distance between the cricoid cartilage and the gastric orifice, ranges in the adult from 22 to 28 cm, of which 3 to 6 cm are located in the abdomen [13,32]. To identify and mark the cricoid cartilage is rather difficult. For practical reasons, clinicians therefore measure the length of the esophagus by including the oropharynx and pharynx. They use the incisors as the direct landmark during endoscopic procedures. In regard to the length that surgeons require for esophageal replacement within the thorax, the shortest route between the cricoid cartilage and the celiac axis was shown to be in the posterior mediastinum (30 cm). The retrosternal route (32 cm) and the subcutaneous route (34 cm) to reach the neck proved to be longer.[45]

At rest, the esophagus is collapsed. Forming a soft muscular tube, it is flat in the upper and middle parts and rounded in the lower segment. Adjacent organs, structures such as the aortic arch, the left main bronchus and muscles like the diaphragm narrow the tube by compression. Most apparent, however, are the two muscular constrictions: the upper and the lower esophageal sphincters. They can be identified by means of manometry at the esophageal opening, 14 to 16 cm distant from the incisors, and at the entrance into the stomach, 40 to 45 cm distant from the incisors (Fig.1). Between the thoracic inlet and the tracheal bifurcation lie the paired mediastinal pleura, the lungs and their hilus. On the right are the subclavian artery and the azygos vein which arches over the right pricipal bronchus to end in the superior vena cava. Surgical access to a safe removal of the esophagus and lymphadenectomy for cancer preferably is through the right chest, where the azygos vein must usually be divided before the esophagus can be dissected free. Just above the arch of the azygos vein at a level of T4 - T5 crosses the primarily right side positioned thoracic duct behind the esophagus. Structures on the left of the esophagus are the aortic arch and the aorta which subsequently turns to the midline towards posterior behind the esophagus. In front of the esophagus are the lung hilum and the heart. Both vagi accompany the esophagus while it passes through the hiatus at the level of the tenth thoracic vertebra.

The esophagus, both proximally and distally, is stabilized by bony, cartilaginous, or membranous structures. At the cranial end, the exterior esophageal musculature firmly inserts into the cricoid cartilage[40]. From the neck down to the tracheal bifurcation numerous delicate membranes anchor the esophagus to the trachea, pleura, praevertebral fascia, and surrounding tissue of the posterior mediastinum[38,39]. The membranes consist of collagen and elastic fibers, are stretchable to some extent, and accumulate around the tracheal bifurcation[39a]. While most membranes may easily be torn, pull through dissection of the esophagus may eventually cause tears to the connected structures, because some individuals may possess membranes of up to 700 μm thickness[39b]. This feature is unpredictable. Mediastinoscopic membrane dissection close to the wall instead of blunt transhiatal pull-through esophagectomy appears to be advisable for the upper half of the esophagus in order to reduce the risk of tracheopleural tears and chylothorax[4,38,39].

Bounded by the two diaphragmatic crura the distal esophagus traverses the diaphragm through the esophageal hiatus (Fig.2).

Phreno-Esophageal Membrane

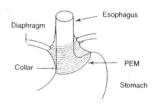

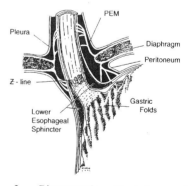

Figure 2. Diagrammatic illustration of the phrenoesophageal membrane (PEM). Viewed from the left lateral aspect. Figure 2a shows that the upper component of the PEM inserts into the muscle tissue of the terminal esophagus, that the lower component of the membrane inserts into the gastric fundus and that the PEM wraps the esophagogastric junction with a wide membranous collar. Figure 2b shows the tissue organization and the supporting structures at the esophagogastric junction. The esophagus is opened alongside the greater and lesser curvatures, the luminal aspect is displayed. The fiber elements that attach the phrenoesophageal membrane into the muscle wall of the terminal esophagus are shown. (Courtesy of Dr Owen Korn, Munich and Santiago di Chile.

The upper component of the left crus of the diaphragm may consist of membranous tissue rather than a significant muscular mass[39,58]. The subdiaphragmatic and the endothoracic aponeuroses blend at the central margin of the diaphragm to constitute the phrenoesophageal membrane (Fig.3), (Laimer's ligament or Allison's membrane). Intraoperatively, this structure can easily be recognized by a well defined lower edge and slightly yellow color, even in case of severe peri-esophagitis. Equal proportions of elastic and collagenous fiber elements, guarantee sufficient pliability to the membrane. Owing to its origin from a fascia, the phrenoesophageal membrane in general is relatively strong. Having split into two sheets (Fig.3), one sheet extends 2 to 4 cm upward through the hiatus, where its fibers traverse the esophageal musculature to insert into the submucosa [12]. The other sheet passes down across the cardia to the level of the gastric fundus to blend into the gastric serosa, the gastrohepatic ligament, and the dorsal gastric mesentery. Alongside the junction between the esophagus and stomach, the phrenoesophageal membrane is clearly separated from the esophageal musculature by interposition of loose connective tissue. At this point the membrane wraps the cardia as by a wide collar (Fig.3). This structural organization allows the terminal esophagus and the junction to move in relationship to the diaphragm and to "slip through the hiatus like in a tendon sheath"[17].

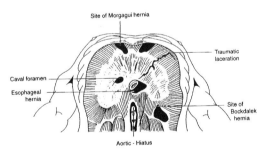

Figure 3. Diagram of the diaphragm. The location of the esophagus in topographical relation to the aorta and vena cava, to the esophageal hiatus and to the most common sites of hernia formation are viewed from the caudal aspect.

The esophagus has neither mesentery nor serosal coating. This and the position within the mediastinum being completely wrapped into loose connective tissue, allows extensive transverse and longitudinal mobility. Respiration induces cranio-caudal movement over several millimeters, and swallows result

in excursions over as much as the height of one vertebral body[9]. Because of this specific feature the esophagus may easily be subjected surgically to blunt stripping from the mediastinum[2,15,34,47]. Ventral to the cervical esophagus lies in direct locoregional contact the flat fibrous membrane of the trachea. The development of an esophagorespiratory fistula either following esophagectomy or irradiation in this preformed weak area is a catastrophic problem for both patient and physician.

1.2 TISSUE STRUCTURES OF THE ESOPHAGUS

The overall tissue structure of the esophagus parallels the basic organization of the digestive tract (Fig.4). It comprises an external fibrous layer (tunica adventitia), a muscular layer (tunica muscularis), a submucous layer (tela submucosa), and an internal mucous layer (tunica mucosa). The *tunica adventitia,* a thin layer composed of loose connective tissue, connects the esophagus with adjacent structures. It contains small vessels, lymphatic channels, and nerve fibers. The *tunica muscularis* is composed of two complete muscle coats, the fibers of which are differently orientated (Fig.5).

1.2.1 Esophageal Body
The fibers of the outer muscle layer parallel the longitudinal axis of the esophagus, while those of the underlying inner layer run in the horizontal axis. The longitudinal layer originates from the small tendon at the dorsal plane of the cricoid cartilage[40]. The bundles are long and course straight down the esophagus to cross the gastric inlet, where the majority of the fibers change their arrangement[32] (Fig.5). The circular layer commences at the level of the cricoid cartilage and continues the cricopharyngeus muscle[32,40]. In their descent, the fibers form imperfect circles with overlapping ends.

1.2.2 Upper esophageal sphincter
This sphincter terminates the pharynx. It is a zone of elevated pressure, 2 to 4 cm in length [59] and marks the entrance into the esophagus. The high pressure may mainly result from the effect of the cricopharyngeus muscle, which loops around the hypopharynx and inserts into the cricoid processes. It is not a true sphincter in the anatomical definition, but in conjunction with the "bony" plane of the cricoid cartilage, the cricopharyngeus muscle behaves like one [11,37,60]. The architecture accounts for the asymmetric pressure profile in manometric measurements [59].

Esophagus   Z - line   Stomach

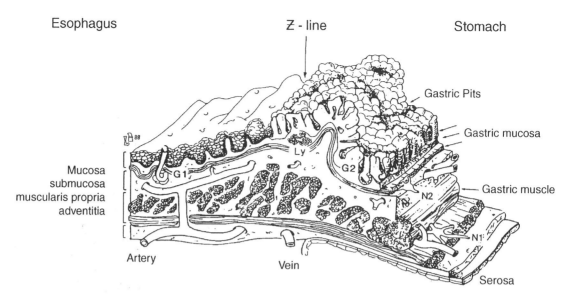

Figure 4. Architecture of the wall at the esophagogastric junction. The tunica muscularis is constituted of both a longitudinal and a circular layer. (G1=esophageal glands, G2=gastric glands, Ly=lymph vessels, N1=myenteric plexus, N2=submucous nerve plexus)

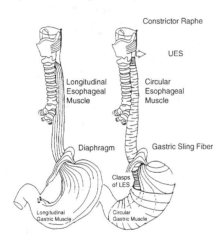

Figure 5. Architecture of the longitudinal and circular muscle layers across the esophagus, stomach, and the respective junctions (UEA=upper esophageal spincter, LES=lower esophageal sphincter). From Liebermann-Meffert D. in: Orringer M, Zuidema G: Shackelfords Surgery of the alimentary tract. The esophagus Vol.1: Philadelphia, Saunders 2000 (by permission)

1.2.3 Lower esophageal sphincter

This sphincter terminates the esophagus. Manometrically, there is a zone of elevated pressure, 3 to 5 cm in length, immediately above the junction of the esophagus with the stomach. In this segment, the muscle behaves differently than the muscle above and below [48,51]. Approximately three centimeter above the junction with the stomach, the muscle fibers increase in number. This causes a stepwise thickening of the inner musculature[32,38]. Coincidentally, the muscle fibers rearrange: as shown in Figure 5 the bundles on the lesser curvature side retain their orientation and form short muscle clasps, whereas those on the greater curvature side change to become the oblique gastric sling fibers. It has been

discussed that the myotomy for achalasia should preferably be performed at place between the muscle claps and sling fibers in order to preserve sphincter competence[3,38,39b]. No doubt is that the high pressure zone correlates with the thickened asymmetrically arranged musculature at the site of the gastric orifice (Fig.6)[27,32,33,55,60]. Partial or total myectomy reduced significantly the specific sphincter pressure values of this muscle arrangement as recorded on manometry [3,49,51,59]. No effect on the pressure values of the sphincter at all was produced by dissection of neither the diaphragm nor the phrenoesophageal membrane[33].

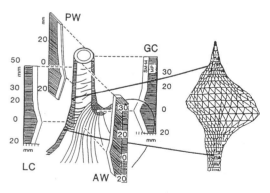

Figure 6. Schematic drawing showing the correlation between radial muscle thickness (left) and three-dimensional manometric pressure image (right) at the human gastroesophageal junction. Muscle thickness across the gastroesophageal junction at the posterior gastric wall. (PW), greater curvature (GC), anterior gastric wall (AW) and lesser curvature (LC) is shown in mm. Radial pressures at the gastroesophageal junction (in mmHg) are plotted around an axis representing atmospheric pressure. Note the marked radial and axial asymmetry of both the muscular thickness and the manometric pressure profile. From Liebermann-Meffert D. In: Fuchs KH, Stein HJ, Thiede A. Gastrointestinale Funktionsstörungen. Berlin, Heidelberg. New York, Springer 1997 (ref. 39, with permission)

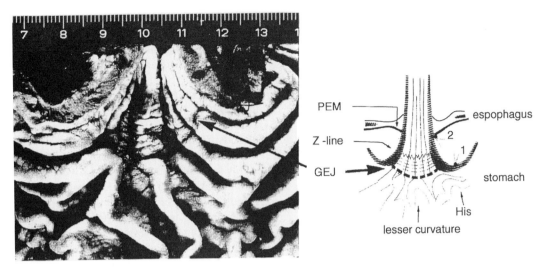

Figure 7. Specimen opened along the greater curve side shows the entire mucosal lumen of the esophagogastric junction (EGJ). The longitudinal esophageal folds, the transverse rippled folds across the EGJ, the large gastric folds, and the thickened muscle of the LES are seen. (1=angle of HIS, 2=lower leaf of the pre-esophageal membrane (PEM). From Liebermann-Meffert D et al, Gastroenterology. Ref. 32)

The *tela submucosa* connects the muscular coat and the mucosa. It contains elastic and collagenous fibers, a meshwork of blood vessels, numerous lymph vessels, nerves, and mucous glands. The deep esophageal glands are small branching glands of a mixed type, and their ducts pierce the muscularis mucosa. The *tunica mucosa* is made up of the muscularis mucosae, the tunica propria, and a stratified squamous non-keratinized epithelium (Fig.4). In the contracted state the muscularis mucosa forms the folds of the mucosa. These long folds follow the longitudinal axis of the esophagus. At the end of the esophagus there are in addition small transversal rippled folds [7,10,32]. These folds disappear when the esophageal lumen becomes expanded. The fibrous tunica propria projects into the epithelium, thus forming the papillae. It contains small lymph vessels, located exclusively on the border adjoining the submucosa, occasional mononuclear cells, clusters of inflammatory cells, and lymphocytes. In the distal esophagus, prevail focal superficial (mucous) glands that resemble cardiac glands.

Clinically, the epithelial lining of the tube, the surface of the esophageal mucosa is reddish in color in its cranial portion and becomes paler toward the lower third of the esophagus. The esophageal mucosa can be easily distinguished from the dark-red mamillated gastric mucosa by its greyish-pink smooth surface. The transition of the squamous epithelium to the columnar epithelium represents the mucosal junction between the esophagus and the stomach and is an objectively recognizable reference point for the endoscopist[50]. The squamous epithelium of the esophagus is stratified, consisting of several layers of polygonal cells that vary greatly in shape. The cells are bound to each other by desmosomes [58]. The layer is 300-400 μm thick. The most superficial cells are flattened squames which overlay one another[58]. Though flattened and degenerating, the cells of the superficial stratum retain their nuclei, a feature known for cells at moist epithelial surfaces. The gastric columnar epithelium consists of glandular cylindrical cells; they are taller than their diameter and set together to form a palisade-like layer. The junction is characterized by an irregularly shaped, abrupt demarcation line, called Z line. Islands of columnar epithelium, however, are often seen in the squamous mucosa of the distal esophagus above the junction even if no inflammatory alteration is present [50]. The same is true for squamous epithelium present in the gastric mucosa below the junction line. The serrated line is located most often shortly above the gastric orifice, i.e. the muscular LES. Any proximal extension of a gastric-like or intestinal-type columnar epithelium is considered as pathologic. It may be attributed to long-lasting gastroesophageal reflux and impairment of clearance which causes chronic severe esophageal mucosal and submucosal damage[22,50].

1.3 STRUCTURES SUPPLYING THE ESOPHAGEAL WALL

1.3.1 Arterial Supply

The author has shown that there are three principal arterial sources to the esophagus (Fig.8)[34,35]. In the neck, small branches deriving from the upper superior and the inferior thyroid arteries supply the cervical esophagus. A group of three to five tracheobronchial arteries arise from the concavity of the aortic arch to give rise to esophageal tributaries. One or two proper esophageal arteries may arise from the anterior wall of the thoracic aorta[34]. At the esophagogastric junction, the left gastric artery gives off up to eleven larger ascending branches for the anterior wall and the right face of the lower esophagus[34,35] (Fig.8).

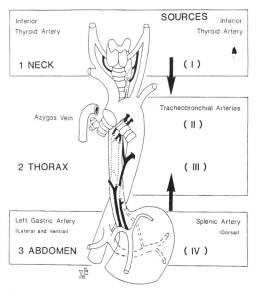

Figure 8. Diagram of the extravisceral sources of arterial blood supply to the esophagus, intramural anastomoses (dotted line) and topographic relationship of the azygos vein to the esophagus and tracheal bifurcation.

Several larger vessels deriving from the splenic artery regularly supply the posterior esophageal wall and parts of the greater curvature. The branches run upward through the diaphragmatic hiatus prior to entering the esophageal wall. Since the branches of the principal vessels anastomose within the submucosa, it is difficult to determine the proportion and percentage of blood distributed from each individual artery[34].

The major arteries divide at some distance from the esophageal wall into minute branches. It appears that such small tributaries, when torn, will have the benefit of contractile hemostasis. Previous claims that essential nutritional vessels arise from the intercostal arteries or phrenic arteries or directly from the aorta were not confirmed[34]. The evident continuity of the vessels and the rich anastomosing intramural vascularity[1,34] explain why, on the one side, the mobilized esophagus retains an excellent blood supply over a long distance and why, on the other side, ligation of the left gastric artery when using a gastric substitute after esophagectomy most of the time this does not compromise the surgical anastomosis[36]. The extremely small caliber of

the nutritional vessels may also explain the failure of esophagointestinal anastomosis by any mechanical damage to the microvascular circulation.

The blunt pull-trough esophagectomy without thoracotomy for esophageal cancer proposed 1913 by Denk[7] and 1935 by Grey-Turner[15] has recently found a number of advocates[2,34,47,52]. The procedure appears relatively safe and involves moderate blood losses provided that it is undertaken near to the esophagus. When hemorrhage occurred after stripping of the esophagus, it was mostly from the site of malignant tumor adhesion, and in particular from injury to the azygos vein.

1.3.2 Venous Drainage

The most comprehensive macroscopic description of esophageal venous drainage presumably has been presented by Butler.[5] The intraesophageal veins include minute subepithelial plexus in the lamina propria mucosae. It drains into the submucous plexus that unite to form small communicating veins [1], which are arranged predominantly in the longitudinal axis[56]. After penetrating the muscle coats they form the extramural veins at the surface of the esophagus[1,5,56] which empty into the locally corresponding large vessels: the inferior and superior thyroid veins, jugular veins, the azygos and hemiazygos veins, the gastric and the splenic veins.

It might be of clinical interest that a specialized venous arrangement[5,56], prevails at the terminal esophagus. It has been suggested that these venous anastomoses possibly constitute a communication between the azygos and the portal system providing bidirectional flow[56].

1.3.3 Lymphatic Drainage

Presumably due to the considerable technical difficulty in identifying the minute channels both in vivo and post mortem, the anatomical knowledge of the lymphatic system of the esophagus is still extremely poor and previous accounts have not so far been substantiated [38,39]. Nevertheless one may accept that initial lymphatic capillaries commence exclusively in the region between the mucosa and submucosa to form longitudinally arranged collecting channels and plexuses in the submucosa[29,38]. At intervals, the plexuses give off branches to the collecting subadventitial and surface trunks [29]. Contrary to the veins in the esophagus, the lymphatic vessels all possess valves.

The lymphatic trunks at the surface of the esophagus commonly empty into the regional lymph nodes.

The concept that lymph flows in the submucosal channels more readily longitudinally than through the few transverse connections in the muscle, lymph nodes is supported by the clinical observation that initial tumor spread follows the longitudinal axis of the esophagus within the submucosa rather than extending in a circular manner. Paucity of lymphatics within the lamina mucosa, and the abundance of submucosal lymphatic channels[29,38,39] may explain why intramural cancer spreads predominantly within this layer. Unappreciated malignant mucosal lesions may be accompanied by extensive tumor spread underneath an intact mucosa, and tumor cells may follow the lymphatic channels for a considerably long distance before they pass the muscular coat to empty into the lymph nodes. Tumor free margin at the resection line, as confirmed by the anatomical point of view, does not guarantee radical tumor removal. This feature may be consistent with the relatively high postoperative recurrence rate at the resection line, including satellite tumors and metastasis in the submucosa far distant from the primary tumor[2,52], even if the margins at the resection line had been previously tumor free.

Tiny lymph nodes of diameters less than one millimeter can be detected microscopically in the tracheoesophageal groove of healthy individuals. Lymph nodes which are occasionally large are concentrated at the tracheal bifurcation, the celiac axis and the venous angle in the neck[38]. As they usually contained black coal particles; they were related presumably to drainage of the trachea and/or the lungs. The classical chain of large lymph nodes surrounding the esophagus, however, as it is described in textbooks and illustrated by Netter[44] could not be substantiated under healthy conditions. This observation coincides with the report of Wirth and Frommhold[61] who found mediastinal lymph nodes in only 5 per cent of 500 normal lymphograms.

From clinical observations in cancer patients [2,28,38,52] the suggestion may be deducted that lymph from above the carina flows towards cranial into the thoracic duct or subclavian lymph trunks, whereas lymph from below the carina flows mainly towards the cysterna chyli via lower mediastinal, left gastric and celiac lymph nodes (Fig.9). This includes in particular the terminal esophagus. Flow may, however, change under pathological conditions [29,38]. In case that lymph vessels are blocked because of tumor invasion and dilated, the valves become incompetent and the flow reversed[62]. This explains the retrograde, unexpected spread in some of the malignant tumors.

LYMPHATIC DRAINAGE

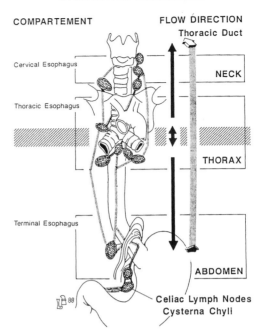

Figure 9. Diagram of the lymphatic pathways in the esophageal wall. The suggested pattern of lymph flow is shown and explains the expected local and distal spread of tumor cells. The embryological development and the presence and alignment of valves suggest this pattern of lymph flow, although it has never been substantiated experimentally.

1.3.4 Thoracic duct

The thoracic duct commences at the proximal end of the cysterna chyli, which is about the twelfth thoracic vertebra and passes the diaphragm upwards through the aortic foramen. It then ascends through the posterior mediastinum between the aorta on its left, the azygos vein on its right aspect, and left dorsal to the esophagus. The great number of anatomical variations[58,61,62], close local relationship of the flimsy thoracic duct to the esophagus and trachea accounts to the occasional injury during esophagectomy and cervical anastomosis causing chylothorax[47].

1.3.5 Innervation

The esophagus is innervated by the visceral (splanchnic) component of the autonomic nervous system. It consists of two parts, the sympathetic and the parasympathetic systems, which exert antagonistic influences on the viscera. According to the classical description the sympathetic nerve supply is through the cervical and thoracic sympathetic chain, which runs downward lateral to the spine. Interconnecting with fibers of the parasympathetic cervical and thoracic plexus, the sympathetic nervous system also uses the vagus nerve as a carrier for some of its fibers [58]. The vagus nerve is the tenth cranial nerve.

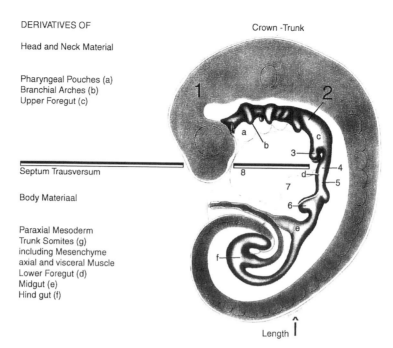

DERIVATIVES OF

Head and Neck Material

Pharyngeal Pouches (a)
Branchial Arches (b)
Upper Foregut (c)

Septum Trausversum

Body Materiaal

Paraxial Mesoderm
Trunk Somites (g)
including Mesenchyme
axial and visceral Muscle
Lower Foregut (d)
Midgut (e)
Hind gut (f)

Crown -Trunk

Length

Figure 10. Half-schematic sagittal section through the body of a 28-day-old human embryo which shows the formation of the foregut, midgut and hindgut. The horizontal line at the left marks the boundary between the branchial derivatives and those of the somites. (After Hinrichsen, KV. In Hinrichsen KV (ed) Human Embryology. Lehrbuch und Atlas der vorgeburtlichen Entwicklung des Menschen. Berlin, Springer-Verlag 1990:516 (with permission).

As thick trunks the right and left vagi descend bilateral. The right inferior laryngeal (recurrent) nerve (RLN) leaves the vagus to turn toward dorsal around the subclavian artery. The left RLN leaves its vagus and circles around the aortic arch. On both sides the RLNs ascend as slack cords that sinuously pass upwards towards the neck[40] to supply the proximal esophagus, trachea and larynx.

More distal the vagal trunks separate into the coarse network of the anterior and posterior esophageal plexuses. Before they cross the diaphragm through the esophageal hiatus, these plexuses join again to form the anterior and posterior abdominal vagus nerves. The anterior branch shows a number of anatomic variants and is usually found on the anterior esophageal wall, where it is visible below the phrenoesophageal membrane. The posterior vagus nerve is usually at some distance from the esophagus and to its right.

The fine structure of the esophageal innervation is composed of a dense network of nerve fibers containing numerous groups of ganglia. The ganglia are located either between the longitudinal and the circular muscle layers (Auerbach's plexus) or in the submucosa (Meissner's plexus).

The ganglia of Auerbach's plexus are scattered, with a variable number of cells, within the entire esophagus. However, the concentration of the ganglion cells is greatest in the terminal

esophagus and at the gastroesophageal junction[10,44,58].

2. ORGANOGENESIS OF THE HUMAN ESOPHAGUS

The information presented in the following text is based upon investigations of the author[30,31] and upon literature of embryology[6,14,16,19,42,53].

2.1 THE FOREGUT AND ITS DERIVATIVES

The digestive tube derives from two germ layers, the endoderm and the mesoderm. The primitive gut forms during the fourth week of gestation[16] and early divides into the foregut, the midgut, and the hindgut (Fig.10). Initially, the human foregut is a uniform tube. It then gives rise to vaults out of which develop the pharynx and its derivatives, the esophagus, the trachea and lungs, the stomach and duodenum including the choledochal duct, the liver, the biliary system, and the pancreas (Fig.10).

The larynx and the trachea derive from the cranial part of the foregut, i.e. from the endodermal lining of the laryngotracheal sacculation, and from the surrounding mesenchyme which originates from the fourth and sixth pairs of bronchial arches. Connective tissues, cartilages, muscles, blood, and lymphatic vessels derive from the splanchnic mesoderm at the ventral plane of the foregut, respectively, into which subsequently the lower respiratory system expands. The primordium of the lower respiratory system is marked by the sacculation of a ventral diverticulum of the foregut (Fig.10). The "tracheal bud", which also shapes the tracheoesophageal groove[16,25,43], represents the primitive trachea and the lungs[54] (Fig.10). It rapidly elongates downward and bifurcates into two lateral protrusions, the lung buds. While elongating, the tracheal tube immediately approaches the esophagus but at no time fuses with it[26,63]. By the end of the seventh week, distinct rings of cartilage appear within the tracheal tube. This knowledge obtained from recent studies[25,26] contradicts the classical concept initiated 1887 by His[20]. He had claimed that the trachea became separated from the esophagus by the formation of a septum which he thought was due to lateral folding that "pinched off" the primitive foregut.

The esophagus is initially very short. It extends from the tracheal groove to the distinct fusiform dilation of the foregut which is to become the stomach. Shortly after the appearance of the tracheal bud, the primitive esophagus lengthens rapidly. The lengthening is caused by the extensive growth of the cranial embryonic tissues on the one hand, and its unbending from the pericardium on the other [43,46]. The erection of the head and neck of the embryo relative to the stable organs such as the heart, cardia, pylorus and vessels stalk position, is responsible for the classical claim that organs migrate upward or downward. In reality, when different embryological serial sections are compared, the extention of the distal esophagus becomes more pronounced than that of the proximal and middle parts. Through the additional rapid growth of its wall at that period, the esophagus reaches the definite topographic relationships with its surrounding structures by the end of the seventh week (18 to 22 mm crown-rump length). The primitive stomach, appears dorsal and caudal to the septum transversum (Fig.10). The location of the later cardia and of the pylorus is already definitely tied up in place by the celiac and pancreatic vessel stalks. Changes through growth of parts of the gastric wall[6,30] mislead to claim positional changes of the stomach[30]. In reality, there is no evidence of any esophageal or gastric mechanical rotation [6,31].

But, as the embryo grows, the left posterior-lateral side of the primitive stomach enlarges progressively to shape the greater curvature [6,31,38]. This temporary asymmetrical

enlargement is caused by an increased local mitotic activity within the wall of the greater curvature. Excessive growth processes occurring in particular in the area of the future gastric fundus[6] delineate the initially ill defined gastroesophageal junction (Fig.11) [32,43,46]. Individual variations in the height of the fundus and the acuteness of the angle of His (cardiac angle) persist during the subsequent fetal period.

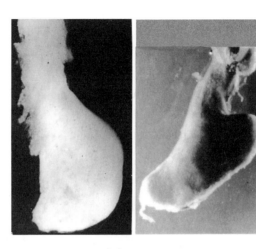

Figure 11. Macroscopic aspect of human stomachs of 8 and 22 mm crown-rump length. Due to localized cell proliferation the greater curvature undergoes an extensive growth during the 5 to 25 mm stages, which will also form the gastric fundus, the cardiac angulation, and the esophagogastric junction. Growth processes will mainly occur at the free margin of the stomach, at the greater curvature. (from the collection of the author)

2.2 EARLY ANCHORING STRUCTURES

The caudal part of the foregut, midgut and hindgut are suspended in the peritoneal cavity by the dorsal mesentery, which derives from the dorsal body mesenchyma. The cranial part of the foregut, instead, is bounded by the broad mesenchymal mass of embryonic connective tissue extending between sternum and spine which forms the primitive ventral and dorsal mediastinum. Caudally, the ventral part of the primitive esophagus and trachea is bounded by the septum transversum. This is a transverse mesenchymal plate separating the primordium of the heart from the liver. Tissue bulges appearing at the lateral body wall will develop mesentery-like folds that later become membranes. The free ends of these membranes fuse with the mesoderm ventral and dorsal to the primitive esophagus, and with the septum transversum. Supported by the rapid growth of the liver, the partitions will become the diaphragm (Fig.12)[38] which separates the pleural and peritoneal cavities. The phrenoesophageal membrane that holds the esophagus in place within its diaphragmatic hiatus (Fig.12) differentiates after the esophageal muscle has developed at 15 mm crown-rump length.

By the end of the embryonic period, in the early ninth week, the definite shapes of all the main organ systems have been established. The external appearance of the organs is now less affected by further development. During the following fetal period around the ninth week maturation of the various tissues and organs takes place.

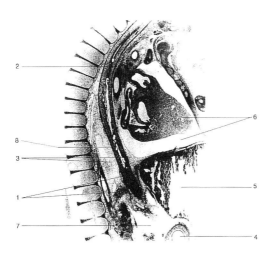

Figure 12. Sagittal section trough the esophagus of a 15 mm crown-rump human embryo. The figure shows: 1=diaphragm, 2=esophagus, 3=phrenoesophageal membrane, 4=stomach, 5=liver, 6=heart and pleural cavity, 7=abdominal cavity, 8=vacuoles in the mucosa. (Courtesy of Fernandez de Sandos MD, Madrid).

2.3 GENESIS OF TISSUE STRUCTURES

The *tunica muscularis* of the esophagus originates from myoblasts in the mesoderm that surrounds the primitive gut. The myoblasts derive from the mesenchymal cells. Muscle tissue appears as a ring-shaped condensation of elongated nuclei in the 8 to 10 mm crown-rump embryo (Fig.13) within the not yet differentiated mesenchyme (embryonic connective tissue) on the outer aspect of the esophageal lumen. This concerns first the circular and shortly later the longitudinal muscle. The muscle formation occurs prior to that of the stomach. The circular and the longitudinal muscle layers are developed and

form a complete sheet around the esophagus at the 20 mm crown-rump stage[38]. By the 24 mm crown-rump stage, the muscularis mucosa becomes apparent, and it is well defined in the 65 mm crown-rump stage[54]. Two muscle types are now recognizable: striated skeletal muscle in the upper esophagus and smooth muscle in the middle and lower esophagus[38]. Macroscopic muscle bundles of the esophagus appear in the 76 to 90 mm crown-heel long fetus[46]. The fiber arrangement of the muscle layers in the esophagus and at the esophagogastric junction is similar to that seen in the adult[31,32].

The *tunica mucosa* differentiates from the endoderm in the 2.5 mm crown-rump length embryo (third week of gestation). The foregut becomes lined by two or three layers of pseudostratified columnar epithelium. This layer is uniformly thick along the entire esophagus and lies within undifferentiated mesenchymal cells (Fig.13). The pseudostratified aspect of the mucosa lasts until the 12 to 13 mm crown-rump stage[23,43] when the mucosa becomes multilayered and thicker owing to cell proliferation Subsequently, at 12 mm crown-rump length, tiny, thin walled vacuoles commence to appear in the basal level of the epithelium (Fig.14). The significance of the vacuolization is unknown. Large dark cells appear in the basal epithelial cell layer of the 30 to 40 mm crown-rump embryo. The stratified columnar epithelium is generally four cells deep. The basal epithelial cells project toward the lumen to become ciliated columnar cells. These cells progress from the middle third of the esophagus towards a cranial and caudal direction. Ciliated cells line the entire mucosa of the esophagus of the 60 mm crown-rump embryo, except for the upper and lower ends. At this location the epithelium further on constitutes of one single layer of large columnar cells[6,24,38,46] occasionally containing mucin-bearing cells (Goblet cells!). It has been observed that during the replacement of the epithelium, islets of ciliated cells actually developed epithelium[6,41]. The stratified squamous epithelium appears in the 90 to 130 mm fetus. Again, this epithelium appears in the middle third of the esophagus and migrates cranially and caudally until the squamous epithelium has progressively and almost completely replaced the ciliated columnar epithelium in the 250 mm fetus. Some patches of ciliated columnar cells occasionally remain until after birth. They may also be found in the proximal esophagus near the upper esophageal sphincter[38]. The sequence of the process described is illustrated in figure 15.

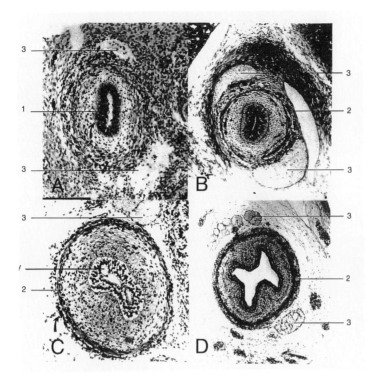

Figure 13. Transverse section through the esophagus in embryos of 8.5 (A), 12.5 mm (B), 20 mm (C) and 40 mm (D) crown rump length. The mucosal epithelium lining the lumen (1) is stratified columnar in the 8.5 mm crown-rump embryo to become vacuolized (V) between 12.5 and 20 mm crown-rump and multilayered columnar in the 40 mm crown-rump stage. The tissue surrounding the mucosal epithelium consists mainly of in undifferentiated mesenchyme in the 8.5 mm crown-rump embryo. Differentiation of the inner muscle coat is marked by the cell condensation around the mucosal ring seen in A (2). Pale areas of neutral cells as precursors of the recurrent laryngeal nerves are seen exterior to the foregut tube (3). In the 12 mm and 20 mm crown-rump stages, the inner muscular layer is further advanced. The outer longitudinal muscle layer and the muscularis mucosae, however, can only be identified at 40 mm crown-rump length. During this development, the extrinsic innervation, in particular the recurrent laryngeal nerve, has become of conspicuous size (3). The development changes of the luminal diameter and shape of the esophagus are seen. (A, B and D from the collection of Liebermann-Meffert D. In: Orringer M, Zuidema GD (eds). The Esophagus, Shackelford's Surgery of the Alimentary tract. Philadelphia, Saunders 2000 (with permission). C from Enterline H and Thompson J. Pathology of the Esophagus. Heidelberg, Springer 1984 (with permission).

The first superficial acini containing glands have been observed during the 160 mm stage. These glands are numerous in the esophagus of 210 mm fetuses and are mostly located at the level of the cricoid cartilage and at the lower end of the esophagus[6,23,46]. During the last 3 months of gestation, the downgrowth of the surface epithelium begins to generate submucosal glands. The development of the mucosa shapes the esophageal lumen. The cell proliferation and the appearance of the vacuoles within the 10 and 21 mm crown-rump stages transform the initially slit-like (Fig.13a) or elliptic lumen. It becomes narrow (Fig.12), asymmetric, and finally bizarre (Fig.13b). This phenomenon is most prominent at the level of the tracheal bifurcation, and caused by cell proliferation. As proliferation and vacuolization progress, this narrows the entire esophageal lumen which may mislead to the speculation of solid occlusion[38]. With the disappearance of the vacuoles at the crown-rump length of 30-40 mm the esophageal lumen widens. Due to the asymmetrical growth within the tissue of the submucosa four to five

large folds develop (Fig.13). These folds parallel the longitudinal axis of the esophagus and constitute the definite configuration of the esophageal lumen.

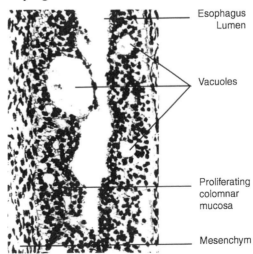

Figure 14. Transverse section through the upper esophagus of a 12.5 mm crown-rump embryo above the level of the developing tracheal bifurcation with narrowing of the lumen due to cell proliferation and formation of vacuoles (from collection Liebermann-Meffert D).

PRENATAL DEVELOPMENT OF THE MUCOSA IN THE HUMAN ESOPHAGUS

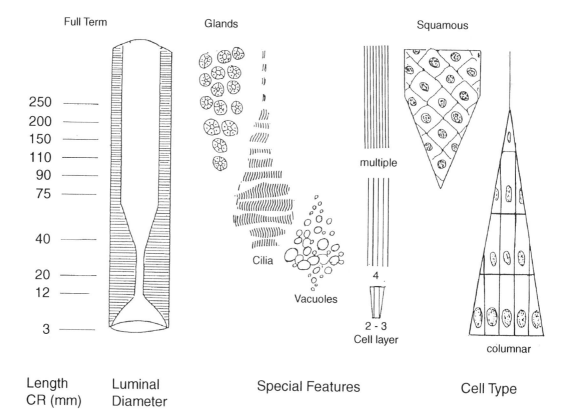

Figure 15. Scheme illustrating the prenatal development and changes of the mucosa found in the human esophagus.

2.4 VASCULARIZATION OF THE FOREGUT

The vessels are formed in the early somite embryo in the somatopleuric mesenchyme of the body wall. The major source of arterial supply to the proximal esophagus is located in the mesenchyme of the fourth to the sixth pharyngeal arches that partly encircles the pharynx and will irrigate the upper and middle foregut, as well as the lung buds. One other major source develops in the mesenchyme around the primitive midgut, where the initially paired dorsal aortae fuse caudally to form one single midline vessel. The visceral vessels of the infradiaphragmatic aorta fuse to form the celiac axis which gives off tributaries to the lower portion of the foregut and to the superior and inferior mesenteric arteries [38].

A number of changes will alter the primitive vascular pattern to result in establishment of the definitive arterial pattern. In this context one must remember that the esophagus derives from two different tissue sources: the head and neck material and the body mesenchyme. This origin results in the formation of two areas that develop simultaneously while keeping a common delimitation which is at the level of the tracheal bifurcation [38]. Vessels deriving from the branchial region continue to irrigate

towards distal, whereas the vessels deriving from the celiac axis contribute the vascular supply to the esophagus to irrigate towards cranial.

Venous and lymphatic drainage follows the same bi-directional pattern but in a reverse flow direction. This orientation will never change later, neither in the fetal nor in the adult life.

The lymphatic system appears concurrently with the venous system, two weeks after the cardiovascular system. Lymph sacculations develop in the jugular region, and definitive lymph vessels are identified in the 11-mm crown-rump embryo during the sixth week, supplying the foregut and the trachea [14,42].

2.5 INNERVATION DEVELOPMENT OF THE FOREGUT

The vagus nerve is formed by the early fusion of nerves from the last three branchial arches. Large efferent and afferent general components are distributed to the whole foregut [19,21].

In the authors material the two vagal trunks can be identified in the 8.5-mm crown-rump embryo [31] (Figure 13a). The inferior laryngeal (recurrent) nerves, are prominent at the 12- to 20-mm stage. Both vagal nerves and the recurrent laryngeal nerves adopt their definite position alongside the esophagus at the early stage when the embryonal body straightens (Figure 13a-d) Neuroblasts from the peri-esophageal plexus seem to enter the esophageal wall at the same period early in the development[38]. The neuroblasts will form a complete peri-esophageal network at the outer plane of the circular muscle layer of the esophagus before the longitudinal muscle differentiates. In the 40-mm crown-rump embryo, several nerve bundles cover the esophagus. By the time the embryo reaches 65 mm, the peri-esophageal plexus consists of large, interlacing vagal bundles. The myenteric plexus is identifiable in the 10-week-old fetus[18,19]. The ganglion cells are not positively identifiable but are represented by numerous pale areas located in the myenteric plexus. The number of cells, their size, and the nerve density peak at the sixteenth to twentieth weeks of gestation [21]. Sparse submucosal nerve fibers can be discerned in the 35-mm crown-rump embryo. These fibers become the submucosal plexus. According to Hewer [18], this plexus is not well developed until the 67-mm stage, but it is complete in the 80-mm fetus. In the 90-mm fetus, the submucosal plexus is extensive and consists of fine nerve fibers and ganglia. The innervation of the muscularis mucosa is particular rich in the fetus of 140-mm crown-heel length.

REFERENCES

1. Aharinejad S, Böck P, Lametschwandtner A. Scanning electron microscopy of esophageal microvasculature in human infants and rabbits. Anat. Embryol 1992;186:33-40

2. Akiyama H. Surgery for carcinoma of the esophagus. Curr Probl Surg 1980;17:53-120.

3. Bombeck CT, Nyhus LM, Donahue PhE. How far should the myotomy extend on the stomach? In Giuli, R, McCallum RW, Skinner DB (eds). Primary motility disorders of the esophagus. Paris London, Libbey Eurotext 1991:455-6.

4. Bumm R, Hölscher AH, Feussner H, et al. Endodissection of the thoracic esophagus. Ann Surg 1993; 218:97-104.

5. Butler H. The veins of the esophagus. Thorax 1951; 6:276-96.

6. Dankmeijer J, Miete M. Sur le développement de l'estomac. Acta Anat (Basel) 1961;47:384-5.

7. Denk W. Zur Radikaloperation des Oesophaguskarzinoms. Z Chir 1913;40:1065-8.

8. Diamant NE. Physiology of esophageal motor function. Gastroent Clin North Am 1989;18:179-94.

9. Dodds WJ, Stewart, ET, Hodges D et al. Movement of the feline esophagus associated with respiration and peristalsis. J Clin Invest 1983;52:1-13.

10. Eckardt VF, LeCompte PM. Esophageal ganglia and smooth muscle in the elderly. Dig Dis Sci 1978;23:443-8.

11. Ekberg O, Lindström C. The upper esophageal sphincter area. Acta Radiol 1987;28:173-6.

12. Eliska O. Phreno-oesophageal membrane and its role in the development of hiatal hernia. Acta Anat 1973 (Basel): 86;137-50.

13. Enterline H, Thompson JJ. Pathology of the Esophagus. NewYork, Springer, 1984.

14. Gaudecker B von. Lymphatische Organe. In; Hinrichsen, K.V. (ed.). Human Embryologie. Lehrbuch und Atlas der vorgeburtlichen Entwicklung des Menschen. Berlin, Springer, 1990:340.

15. Grey-Turner G. Carcinoma of the esophagus;The question of its treatment by surgery. Lancet 1936;18:130-4.

16. Hamilton WJ, Mossman HW. Hamilton, Boyd, and Mossman's Human Embryology; Prenatal Development of Form and Function. 4th Ed. Macmillan, London, 1978.

17. Hayek HV. Die Kardia und der Hiatus Oesophagus des Zwerchfells. Z Anat Entwickl Gesch. 1933;100:218-55.

18. Hewer E. Development of nerve endings in the foetus. J Anat (Lond.) 1934;69:369-79.

19. Hinrichsen, KV. a) Intestinaltrakt, b) peripheres Nervensystem, c) Venen. In;Hinrichsen, K.V. (ed.). Human Embryologie. Lehrbuch und Atlas der vorgeburtlichen Entwicklung des Menschen. Berlin, Springer, 1990, 516, 449, 305.

20. His W. Zur Bildungsgeschichte der Lungen beim menschlichen Embryo Arch Anat Entwickl Gesch 1887;17:89-106.

21. Hitchcock RJI, Pemble MJ, Bishop AE et al. Quantitative study of the development and maturation of human esophageal innervation. J Anat 1992;180:175-80.

22. Ismail-Beigi F, Horton PF, Pope CE. Histological consequences of gastroesophageal reflux in man. Gastroenterology, 1970;58:163-74.

23. Johns BAE. Developmental changes in the esophageal epithelium in man. J Anat (Lond) 1952;86:431-42.

24. Johnson FD. The development of the mucous membrane of the esophagus, stomach, and small intestine in the human embryo. Am J Anat 1910;10:521-59.

25. Kluth D, Habenicht R. Tne embryology of usual and unusual types of esophageal atresia. Pediatr Surg Int 1987;2:223-7.

26. Kluth D, Steding G, Seidl W. The embryology of foregut malformations. J Pediatr Surg, 1987;22:389-93.

27. Korn, O, Stein HJ, Richter TH et al. Gastroesophageal sphincter; a model. Dis Esoph 1997;10:105-9.

28. Lam KH, Cheung HC, Wong, J et al. The present state of surgical treatment of carcinoma of the esophagus. J R Coll Surg Edinb 1982; 27:315-26.

29. Lehnert TH, Erlandson A, Decosse JJ. Lymph and blood capillaries of the human gastric mucosa. A morphologic basis for metastasis in early gastric carcinoma. Gastroenterology 1985;89:939-50.

30. Liebermann-Meffert D. Die Muskelarchitektur der Magenwand des menschlichen Foeten im Vergleich zum Aufbau der Magenwand des Erwachsenen. Morph Jb1966:108;391-400.

31. Liebermann-Meffert D. Form und Lageentwicklung des menschlichen Magens und seiner Mesenterien. Acta Anat (Basel) 1969;72:376-410.

32. Liebermann-Meffert D, Allgöwer M, Schmid P, et al. Muscular equivalent of the lower esophageal sphincter. Gastroenterology 1979;76:31-8.

33. Liebermann-Meffert D, Heberer M, Allgöwer M. The muscular counterpart of the lower esophageal sphincter. In DeMeester TR, and Skinner, DB (eds.). Esophageal Disorders;Pathology and Therapy. New York, Raven Press, 1985.

34. Liebermann-Meffert D, Lüscher U, Neff U, et al. Esophagectomy without thoracotomy; Is there a risk of intramediastinal bleeding. A study on blood supply of the esophagus. Ann Surg 1987;206:184-92.

35. Liebermann-Meffert D, Siewert J.R. Arterial anatomy of the esophagus. A review of literature with brief comments on clinical aspects. Gullet 1992;2:3-10.

36. Liebermann-Meffert D, Meier R, Siewert JR. Vascular anatomy of the gastric tube used for esophageal reconstruction. Ann Thorac Surg 1992;54:1110-5.

37. Liebermann-Meffert D. The pharyngoesophageal segment; Anatomy and innervation. Dis Esoph 1995;8:242-51.

38. Liebermann-Meffert D, Duranceau A, Stein, HJ. Anatomy and Embryology. In Orringer, M.B., and Zuidema, G.D. (eds);Shackelford's Surgery of the Alimentary Tract. The Esophagus, Vol I, 5th edition. Philadelphia London Toronto Sydney Tokyo, Saunders, 2000.

39. Liebermann-Meffert D. Funktionsstörungen des pharyngo-ösophagealen Übergangs;a) Funktionelle und chirurgisch orientierte Anatomie, b) Mobilitätsstörungen des tubulären Ösophagus. In; Fuchs KH, Stein HJ, Thiede, A (eds). Gastrointestinale Funktionsstörungen, Diagnose, Operationsindikation, Therapie. Berlin Heidelberg New York, Springer, 1997.

40. Liebermann-Meffert D, Walbrun B, Hiebert CA. et al. Recurrent and Superior Laryngeal Nerves – A new Look With Implications for the Esophageal Surgeon Ann Thorac Surg 1999;67:212-6.

41. Menard D, Arsenault P. Maturation of human fetal esophagus maintained in organ culture. Anat Rec 1987;217:348-54.

42. Moore KL. The Developing Human; Clinically Oriented Embryology, 4th ed. Philadelphia, W.B. Saunders, 1988.

43. Mueller-Botha GS. Organogenesis and growth of the gastroesophageal region in man. Anat Rec 1959;133:219-39.

44. Netter FH. The Ciba Collection of Medical Illustrations, Vol. 3. Digestive System. Part 1;Upper Digestive Tract. New York, Ciba Pharmaceutical Embassy, 1971.

45. Ngan SYF, Wong J. Lengths of different routes for esophageal replacement. J Thorac Cardiovasc Surg 1986;91:790-4.

46. Neumann J. Die Metaplasie des foetalen Oesophagusepithels Fortschr Med 1897:15;366-9.

47. Orringer MB, Orringer JS. Esophagectomy without thoracotomy; A dangerous operation? J Thorac Cardiovasc Surg 1983;85:72-80.

48. Preiksaitis HG, Tremblay L, Diamant NE. Regional differences in the in vitro behaviour of muscle fibers from the human lower esophageal sphincter. J Gastrointest Motility 1991;3:195-201.

49. Samuelson SL, Bombeck CT, Nyhus LM. Lower esophageal sphincter competence; Anatomic-physiologic correlation. In DeMeester, TR, and Skinner, DB (eds.). Esophageal Disorders. Pathophysiology and Therapy. New York, Raven Press, 1985.

50. Savary M, Miller G. The Esophagus. Handbook and Atlas of Endoscopy Solothurn, Gassmann, 1978.

51. Siewert JR, Jennewein HM, and Waldeck, F.;Experimentelle Un-tersuchungen zur Funktion des unteren Oesophagussphinkters nach Intrathorakalverlagerung, Myotomie und zirkulärer Myektomie. Bruns Beitr Klin Chir 1973;22:818-28.

52. Siewert JR, Liebermann-Meffert D, Fekete F, et al.. Oesophaguscarcinom. In Siewert JR, Harder F, Allgöwer M, et al. (eds). Chirurgische Gastroenterologie, Band 2, 2. Auflage, Berlin Heidelberg New York, Springer, 1990.

53. Skandalakis JE, Gray, SW (eds.). Embryology for Surgeons;The Embryological Basis for the Treatment of Congenital Anomalies, 2nd ed. Baltimore, Williams & Wilkins, 1994.

54. Smith EI. The early development of the trachea and esophagus in relation to atresia of the esophagus and tracheoesophageal fistula. Contr Embryol Carneg Instn 1957;36;41-57.

55. Stein HJ, Liebermann-Meffert D, DeMeester TR, et al. Threedimensional pressure image and muscular structure of the human lower esophageal sphincter. Surgery 1995;117:692-8.

56. Vianna A, Hayes PC, Moscoso G, et.al. Normal venous circulation of the gastroesophageal junction. A route of understanding varices. Gastroenterology 1987;93:876-89.

57. Wegener OH. Whole Body Computerized Tomography. Basel, Karger, 1983.

58. Williams PL, Warwick R. Gray's Anatomy. Edinburgh, Churchill Livingstone, 1980.

59. Winans CS. Manometric asymmetry of the lower esophageal high pressure zone. Gastroenterology 1972; 62:830-1.

60. Winans CS. The pharyngoesophageal closure mechanism; A manometric study. Gastroenterology 1972;63:768-77.

61. Wirth W, Frommhold H. Der Ductus thoracicus und seine Variationen. Lymphographische Studie. Fortschr Roentgenstr 1970;112:450-9.

62. Zschiesche W. Kompensationsmechanismen des menschlichen Ductus thoracicus bei Lymphabflußstörungen. Fortschr Med 11963;81:869-72.

63   Zwa-Tun HA. The tracheo-esophageal septum – fact or fantasy ? Acta Anat. (Basel)1982:114:1-21.

1.2 CELL BIOLOGY OF THE ESOPHAGEAL EPITHELIUM

Stephen E.A. Attwood and Clive D. Morris

1. INTRODUCTION

The aim of this chapter is to provide readers with a basic background of the biology of the esophageal epithelium, its structure, function, growth regulation and repair mechanisms. The epithelial and non-epithelial components of the esophageal lining are discussed in detail along with a discussion on the control of epithelial proliferation by growth factors and the contributions of hormones such as gastrin. How these features are altered to protect the epithelium from injury by reflux of gastro-duodenal juices is then discussed and the concept of epithelial metaplasia is introduced. The reasons why the normal epithelium transforms into a glandular epithelium (Barrett's esophagus) in some patients is not fully understood, but a knowledge of the normal control mechanisms of growth and differentiation should provide a platform from which new hypotheses of Barrett's may be found. The impetus to discovering the cause of Barrett's esophagus is its intimate link with the first step in the development of adenocarcinoma. While much scientific endeavor concerns how and why the Barrett's epithelium becomes malignant, with the hope that these changes can be predicted or prevented, there is just as much potential benefit to be derived from an understanding of the initial changes from the normal squamous epithelium to a glandular mucosa. The current understanding of the generation of Barrett's esophagus will therefore be discussed. The progression from metaplasia to dysplasia and adenocarcinoma is covered in chapter 3.3.

2. THE NORMAL ESOPHAGEAL EPITHELIUM

The epithelium is a non-keratinized stratified squamous epithelium, supported by the lamina propria, and submucosa, containing the esophageal glands. It is generally held that the stratified squamous epithelium is able to withstand wear and tear, and is therefore relatively resistant to the abrasive contact with food.

2.1 EMBRYOLOGY

In order to understand the structure of the normal epithelium and the abnormalities that may be seen, it is helpful to have an understanding of the fundamental embryology of the esophagus. During embryonic development, the endodermal lining of the esophagus proliferates rapidly, to nearly obliterate the esophageal lumen by the 8th week of gestation[1]. A single esophageal lumen is reformed by the 10th week, leaving a superficial layer of ciliated columnar cells. From the 4th month to birth, these ciliated cells are replaced by stratified squamous epithelium, beginning in the middle of the esophagus and extending caudally and cranially. Residual islands of columnar cells remain to form esophageal glands, predominantly in the proximal and distal esophagus[2].

2.2.1 Esophageal inlet patches

During the process of developing a stratified squamous epithelium, occasionally areas of columnar mucosa remain. These patches of columnar mucosa can be seen in approximately 4-10% of patients undergoing upper GI endoscopy[3,4]. Though they can occur throughout the length of the esophagus, they are commonest in the upper segment. They vary in size from a few millimeters to a circumferential area. Clinically they are usually asymptomatic, but they may contain chief and parietal cells and show a local fall in pH on tetragastrin stimulation[5]. These patches have generally been considered to be heterotopic gastric mucosa, but have been shown to contain glucagon immunoreactive cells[6] which are found only in the early stages of embryonic life and not in the adult human stomach, suggesting these patches are an embryonic remnant. They are not related to reflux injury, have no malignant potential and show different immunohistochemical characteristics to Barrett's metaplasia and are therefore thought to be unrelated. They can

H.W. Tilanus and S.E.A. Attwood (eds.), Barrett's Esophagus, 31–49.
© 2001 *Kluwer Academic Publishers. Printed in the Netherlands.*

however be associated with complications such as ulceration, bleeding and stricture formation[7].

2.2 EPITHELIAL CELLS

On light and electron microscopic appearances, the mature esophageal squamous epithelium can be divided into three layers with differing characteristics[8]. These are the *basal, prickle cell* and *functional* layers. The basal layer of cells lies on a thin basement membrane, which represents the line of separation between the epithelium and underlying connective tissue. The membrane is approximately 0.1-2µ in thickness and comprises a thin basal lamina and a network of reticular fibrils[9]. The basement membrane is supported by a relatively thick layer of interwoven collagenous and elastic fibrils called the lamina propria[9]. It invaginates the epithelium as tall narrow papillae, always being separated from the epithelium by the basement membrane.

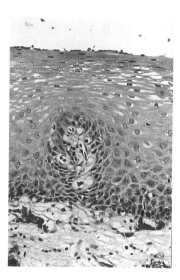

Figure 1. H&E section demonstrating the 3 layers of the normal squamous epithelium. (a) Basal layer, (b) Prickle cell layer, (c) Functional cell layer.

2.2.1 Basal layer (cell division-proliferation)
This easily recognized layer, which normally accounts for 10-15% of the epithelial thickness, is composed of basophilic cells, oblong or cuboidal in shape with central nuclei. This layer is primarily concerned with cellular regeneration to replenish the superficial layers from which cells are lost by desquamation. It is the layer where cell division takes place and scattered mitoses can therefore be seen along the basement membrane[8]. It is in this layer that the stem cells of the esophageal epithelium reside. It is believed that the stem cells with their unlimited capacity

for cell-division and capability for altered differentiation produce a generation of daughter cells, each capable of limited division to produce terminally differentiated cells[10]. In the squamous epithelium of the skin, stem cells can be shown to de-differentiate to form hair follicles[11] and that stem cells within sweat glands and hair follicles can re-form a squamous epithelium if it is damaged[12]. These reports support the idea that these cells are pluripotential and may have the capacity to form Barrett's epithelium (see later). On electron microscopy the cell surfaces are thrown into many processes, which aid in cell adhesion via desmosomes[13]. As this is the only part of the epithelium where cell division takes place, the differentiation of the cells is also determined here.

2.2.2 Prickle cell layer (cell maturation and adhesion)
Superficial to the basal layer lies the prickle cell and then the functional cell layers, which are often difficult to distinguish from each other on H&E staining of paraffin wax sections. They are more readily differentiated on viewing slides of plastic embedded sections where the wider spaces between the prickle cells can be clearly seen[8]. As the cells mature and migrate superficially through the layer, they become larger and gradually begin to flatten. The cells contain abundant glycogen[14], which is stored for use in the more superficial cell layers, remote from the capillary network. Scattered small, neutral fat droplets are seen within this layer[14] and are thought to be related to changes in metabolism between the different layers[8].

2.2.3 Functional cell layer (barrier)
Cells within this layer are flattened with their long axis parallel to the luminal surface. The superficial cells in this layer stain poorly due to loss of cytoplasm and contain basophilic granules representing clumped organelles. On scanning electron microscopy the surface can be seen to be thrown into a complex pattern of microplicas with occasional holes in the surface[8]. The edges of the most superficial cell often overlap[13]. These surface cells are eventually lost from the surface by desquamation. There is little space between the cells in the deeper aspects of this layer, creating a functional barrier between the luminal content and the remainder of the epithelium. The cells of the functional layer also contain glycogen, which is utilized for energy and accounts for the staining seen on Lugol's iodine application during endoscopy. The neutral

fat droplets are greatly increased in this layer, possibly due to changes in metabolism caused by harsh luminal contents[14].

2.3 CELL JUNCTIONS

Parts of the cell membranes are modified to provide attachment to neighboring cells, and usually lie adjacent to a similar area on the apposing cell. In the esophageal epithelium there are a number of different junction types, namely tight junctions, gap junctions, desmosomes and hemi-desmosomes[13]. In tight junctions the outer leaflets of the apposing cell membranes are fused and become a single leaflet with a thickness equal to that of one outer leaflet[15]. They are thought to represent barriers to large molecules that try to cross the epithelium via an intercellular route. In the esophagus they are rare in the uninflamed state but are seen more frequently in the inflamed epithelium[13]. In gap junctions the cell membranes are closely apposed and represent areas of low electrical resistance for propagation of electrical impulses[15]. They are also preferential sites for molecular transport between cells[15]. They are infrequently seen in the basal layer, being much commoner in the prickle cell layer[13]. Desmosomes are distinct plaques at the cell surface[15]. They are paired with a similar area on an apposing cell forming a button like structure in the full desmosome, but occasionally hemi-desmosomes occur where the apposing plaque is absent. Desmosomes occur throughout the epithelium particularly in the intermediate layers, but are also seen joining the overlapping cell edges in the functional cell layer[13]. Hemi-desmosomes are seen in the basal layer towards the lamina propria[13].

2.4 NON-EPITHELIAL CELLS

The esophagus contains cells similar to those of the gut-associated-lymphoid-system. Langerhans cells and T-cells lie within the epithelium, while the lamina propria contains a population of T-cells and B-lymphocytes[16].

2.4.1 Langerhans cells
Langerhans cells are antigen presenting cells of the lymphoid dendritic family[17], and were first discovered in the human esophagus by Al-Yassin in 1975[16]. They share the same ultrastructural morphology as Langerhans cells in other stratified squamous epithelia[17]. They are almost exclusively interspersed between epithelial cells, present in the suprabasal area, along the papillae of the lamina propria but rarely in the basal layer or below[16]. Their function is controversial but it is thought that they may ingest and express foreign antigen on their surface along with major histocompatibility complex (MHC) antigens to activate specific T-cells[17], which lie in close proximity. It has been suggested that disorders in their function may play a part in the infections seen in HIV and papilloma virus infections[17].

2.4.2 Inflammatory cells
Lymphocytes are associated with the esophageal epithelium. Within the epithelium, T-lymphocytes are predominantly of the CD8 suppressor/cytotoxic type, while those of the lamina propria are mainly CD4 helper/inducer phenotype[17]. Small numbers of neutrophils are occasionally seen in the non-inflamed epithelium, but are usually seen in greatly increased numbers in gastro-esophageal reflux disease and infectious disorders[18].

Eosinophils are seen in the epithelium in children but are relatively rare in the adult esophagus, even in the presence of reflux disease[19]. Significantly elevated levels have been found in some patients with a clinical picture of intermittent severe dysphagia and chest pain, but with no evidence of gastro-esophageal reflux on pH testing. There is frequently a history of hypersensitivity or asthma and an elevated peripheral eosinophil count is sometimes found[19,20]. This condition of eosinophilic esophagitis should be remembered in the differential diagnosis of dysphagia as the patients often respond well to treatment with the leukotriene receptor antagonist, *Montelukast*. The typical histology seen in esophageal biopsies is shown in Figure 2.

2.4.3 Argyrophil cells
Argyrophil cells are occasionally seen in the basal layer, being reported in 4 to 36% of autopsy cases[21,22]. These represent melanoblasts[21] and endocrine cells[22]. Melanoblasts, first reported by De-la-Pava[21] have been implicated in the rare development of malignant melanoma, a rare tumor accounting for less than 0.1% of all primary esophageal neoplasms[23].

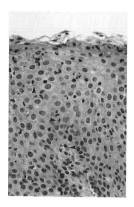

Figure 2. H&E section of esophageal epithelium in patient with esophageal eosinophilia. The eosinophilic infiltration (arrows) is clearly seen.

2.5 ESOPHAGEAL GLANDS

Approximately 700 – 800 submucosal glands are present in the adult human esophagus [8]. They are arranged in straight rows, cranially to caudally and lie within the submucosal connective tissue. Each is composed of a number of lobules containing mucous and serous secreting cells and is similar in structure to the salivary glands[24]. The mucous cells are pyramidal and contain numerous pale secretory granules, which displace the organelles to the periphery. The secretory granules in the serous secreting cells are more electron dense[24]. Large epithelial cells packed with mitochondria named oncocytes are also seen within the glands[24]. The final cell type seen within the acini are contractile myo-epithelial cells[24]. They are anchored to the secretory cells and the underlying basement membrane and aid in the expulsion of secretions. The acini are connected to the lumen by a straight duct lined by a flattened cuboidal epithelium that becomes stratified as it approaches the lumen.

3. EPITHELIAL CELL PROLIFERATION, DIVISION AND ADHESION

Cell proliferative activity appears to follow a diurnal pattern with maximal mitotic activity seen in the early diurnal phase and a trough in the early nocturnal phase[25,26]. The average cell turnover time in the normal squamous epithelium is 7.5 days[27]. However this pattern can be changed and the rate of cell turnover increased particularly in response to epithelial injury such as in gastro-esophageal reflux disease (GERD)[28].

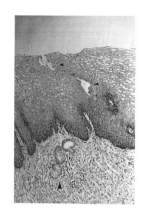

Figure 3: H&E section of the esophageal epithelium demonstrating a sub-mucosal gland

3.1 GROWTH FACTORS

3.1.1 Epidermal growth factor (EGF)

EGF is an acid-stable 53 amino acid peptide chain produced in salivary and esophageal mucous glands[29], which has a role in the maintenance of epithelial integrity. It interacts with the EGF-receptor, an integral plasma membrane glycoprotein with intracellular tyrosine kinase activity, leading to activation of a number of systems including adenyl-cyclase and phospholipase A2. The result is an increase in cell proliferation[29,30]. The EGF-receptor can also be activated by TGF-α, amphiregulin and β-cellulin[29]. There is some evidence that the combined growth factor and receptor may be internalized and the complex then exerts its effect within the cell, which in turn may lead to modulation of the signal by down-regulation and de-sensitization of the EGF-receptor[29]. Esophageal squamous cells are known to have between 20,000 and 200,000 EGF receptors on each cell[31], immunostaining being strong in the basal and prickle layers of the epithelium, with expression decreasing superficially[32]. Their expression is increased in the presence of reflux injury and may therefore be involved in the increased proliferation seen in the inflamed epithelium[32].

Exposure of the esophageal mucosa to acid leads to an increased salivary output of EGF along with bicarbonate and PGE2 by a mechanism involving pH dependent chemoreceptors and the autonomic nervous system[29]. Loss of this protective mechanism leads to increased mucosal damage by acid, and decreased levels of salivary EGF have been correlated with increasing levels of esophageal tissue damage and Barrett's metaplasia [33]. Salivary EGF release has also been shown to be increased by Pentagastrin infusion and decreased by somatostatin[29].

The esophageal epithelium itself secretes EGF[34] along with mucous and PGE2 from the esophageal glands. EGF has also been detected in the capillary endothelium of the esophageal papillae and basal layers[29] though its source is unknown. The quantity of EGF released directly from the healthy esophageal epithelium is significantly higher than that from the salivary glands, being 11 and 4.5 times higher than the corresponding output from the salivary glands under basal and stimulated conditions respectively[35]. However, esophageal production is profoundly inhibited by mucosal exposure to acid[29], which increases the relative importance of salivary EGF secretion.

3.1.2 Other growth factors

Gastrin is a peptide hormone important in the regulation of growth in the GI mucosa. Fully processed gastrin activates the CCK-B receptor in the gastric mucosa and is important in the maintenance of the mucosa and acid secretion[36]. Gastrin has also been shown to increase cell division in gastric cancer cell lines[37], and to be important in the cell proliferation seen within the normal stomach in response to a meal[38]. Both completely and incompletely processed forms of gastrin have been shown to increase cell proliferation in the gastro-intestinal mucosa[39], but as only completely processed gastrin activates the CCK-B receptor, other receptor pathways must also be involved. Gastrin is also important in the control of differentiation in the stomach. Koh *et al* showed a reduction in parietal and ECL cells and an increase in mucous neck cells in the stomachs of gastrin deficient mice[39]. There was no change in proliferation indices suggesting this to be a true effect on differentiation. Less is currently known about the effects of gastrin in the esophageal epithelium. Recently it has been shown that the mitotic rate and bromodeoxyuridine labeling is increased in the rat esophageal epithelium in response to exogenous gastrin[40]. Gastric fundectomy or omeprazole therapy produced similar results, implying gastrin to be the responsible trophic factor. Whether gastrin has any effects in modulating differentiation in the esophagus is unknown.

Insulin like growth factors (IGF) are known to be potent proliferation stimulants in many tissues around the body. Six high affinity binding proteins that exist in most tissues tightly regulate their actions. In esophageal cell lines, IGF has been shown to increase cell proliferation as detected by tritiated thymidine incorporation by between 50 and 100% and is likely to be involved in the repair of esophageal epithelial damage[41].

3.2 CELL ADHESION

An understanding of cell adhesion is important when trying to assess the dissociation of cells as they take on malignant potential. These molecules are also known to play an important role in the development and homeostasis of all tissues[42]. Three main families of adhesion molecules have been demonstrated within the epithelium. They are the integrins, cadherins and CEA type molecules[43].

The integrins are a closely related group of transmembrane receptors that mediate interactions between cells and the extra-cellular matrix, and are therefore thought to play a role in cell differentiation[42]. Unlike the other adhesion molecules, which are composed of single sub-units the integrins are heterodimers of α and β chains and are grouped according to the β chain type[42]. Each group has a principle ligand to which they can bind, such as the structural glycoproteins collagen, laminin and fibronectin[42]. Different integrins can interact with different areas on the same ligand and cells express integrins of differing types. This may be one of the ways that cells can control their trafficking to certain areas of the body[42]. All integrin groups have been shown to have maximal expression in the esophageal epithelial basal layers with little or no expression in the superficial layer[43].

The cadherins are a family of calcium dependent transmembrane glycoproteins, with over a dozen different sub-types identified[44]. They play a vital role in cell-cell adhesion, by interacting in a homophilic manner with molecules of a similar group on other cells[44]. There are subtle changes in their membranous expression on cells of different layers of the epithelium. In the basal layers there is co-expression of E- and P-cadherins, but as the cells migrate superficially there is loss of P-cadherin[45], while E-cadherin is preserved and expression increases[43,45]. Individual cadherins appear to co-operate to form a linear cell adhesion zipper-like arrangement between cells[46]. Dynamic associations with cytoplasmic proteins named catenins anchor the cadherins to the cell cytoskeleton, enabling secure cell adhesion[46]. Regulation of these catenins can modulate the function of the adhesion molecule[46].

The third group of adhesion molecules is the CEA-like proteins. They are members of the immunoglobulin superfamily[42] and are different to the other groups in that they are able to bind to another molecule of the same type or to a completely different ligand i.e. have some features of integrins and cadherins[43]. Dobson and colleagues demonstrated membrane expression in the esophagus superficial to the basal layer only with expression increasing towards the esophageal lumen as the cells matured[43].

Cell adhesion obviously has to be modulated within the esophageal epithelium. In the basal layers the cells must adhere to the basement membrane, forming a secure connection with other cells as they mature and leave the basal zone, culminating in cell shedding superficially with its obligatory loss of cell-cell adhesion. The alterations in expression of each of the 3 adhesion molecule types described above undoubtedly play a part in these changes, though they are likely to be modulated from within the cells by the catenins in the overall control of adhesion.

4.   EPITHELIAL DEFENSE AGAINST LUMINAL CONTENT

The normal esophageal epithelium is regularly exposed to refluxed gastric contents during transient relaxation of the lower esophageal sphincter. This exposure is sensed by the nervous system, leading to esophageal peristalsis and saliva production, which are triggered via an autonomic reflex action. This removes the majority of the acid and the saliva has a buffering effect, thereby minimizing the damage. These mechanisms are fully discussed in the later GERD section of the book. Epithelial defenses are required to protect the esophagus until the acid is fully neutralized. The normal squamous lining of the esophagus has been shown to resist acid damage for considerable periods. Salo et al showed that continuous acid perfusion of the rabbit esophagus for 3.5h often resulted in no gross or histologic damage [47]. As the 'normal' human esophagus is regularly exposed to acid reflux without some inherent tissue resistance everyone would develop esophagitis. The defense mechanisms present can be divided in to three types – pre-epithelial, epithelial and post-epithelial.

4.1 PRE-EPITHELIAL DEFENCES

The pre-epithelial defenses of the esophagus are poorly developed in comparison to the stomach and duodenum. Mucous and serous cells have been demonstrated within the submucosal gland acini. The mucous cells containing neutral, sialated and sulphated mucins[24]. Carbonic anhydrase activity has also been demonstrated within the acini, and is involved in bicarbonate secretion into the esophageal lumen[48]. However there is no well-defined mucous layer, and the surface cells are unable to secrete bicarbonate to contribute to the unstirred water layer. These factors lead to a much lower lumen-surface pH gradient than is seen in the stomach and duodenum[49].

The burden of defense against acid must therefore be assumed by epithelial factors, which can be divided into physical and functional components.

4.2 EPITHELIAL DEFENSES

4.2.1 Physical aspects
Physical defenses include the cell membranes and intercellular junctions. Cell membranes become more prominent as the cells mature and migrate superficially within the epithelium[14], and cell edges may overlap. In animals tight junctions and intercellular glycoconjugates have been demonstrated between cells and afford protection from luminal contents[50]. It has been suggested that the junctions may help to retain the glycoconjugate between the cells, forming a paracellular barrier. Human esophageal intercellular spaces have also been shown to contain glycoconjugates, and there is evidence that it is secreted by cells in the basal and prickle cell layers[51]. Electron microscopy studies have demonstrated many types of cell junction within the epithelium (See above) and there seems to be an increase in tight junctions, which may represent attempts at adaptation to the luminal content.

4.2.2. Functional aspects
Functional components of resistance involve the ability of the cells to buffer and expel H^+ ions. Buffering is accomplished by intracellular proteins, phosphates and bicarbonate. The squamous cells have been shown to have

carbonic anhydrase activity[48], which decreases towards the lumen. This is thought to be involved in intra/extracellular pH maintenance, and not to contribute to luminal bicarbonate secretion[48]. When the buffering systems begin to saturate, and the intracellular pH begins to fall, H^+ ions are extruded from the cell by transport mechanisms including a Na^+/H^+ exchanger and a Na^+ dependent $Cl^-/HCO3^-$ exchanger, with the Na^+/H^+ exchanger having the dominant role[52].

4.3 POST-EPITHELIAL DEFENSES

Post-epithelial defenses are principally mediated by blood flow, which removes H+ and CO2 while delivering nutrients, oxygen and bicarbonate. This supply of HCO3- has been shown to aid protection against luminal acid exposure, with the main locus of its action being the inter-cellular space[53]. It is postulated that this prevents cell damage by maintaining a more physiologic intra-epithelial pH[53]. The defense mechanisms described above are able to protect the esophageal mucosa against 'normal' gastro-esophageal reflux in the majority of people. However in some individuals these mechanisms become overwhelmed, either because of an alteration in the volume or constituents of the refluxate, a decreased ability to clear the refluxed material or as is usually the case, a combination of these factors. (See GERD chapter later in book).

5. INJURY

Injury to the esophageal epithelium appears to be important in the regulation of epithelial differentiation and the subsequent formation of Barrett's esophagus, though the exact mechanism for this control is currently unknown. The exact agent in the refluxed juice that is responsible for the tissue injury in esophagitis and Barrett's esophagus has been the subject of intense research. It was originally attributed to acid but more recently duodenal juices have also been found to be important. Much of our present knowledge of acid induced injury is based on the animal studies of Johnson and Harmon, which demonstrated injury to the esophagus by H^+ ions only at pH<2[54].Greater damage was caused by pepsin in association with acid at pH>2. Others have demonstrated a link between severity of reflux and the extent of tissue damage by showing a greater degree of acid reflux in

patients with complications of GERD such as stricture and Barrett's metaplasia[55].

The realization that acid was not the exclusive injurious agent came from reports of esophagitis occurring in patients with achlorhydria[56] and after total gastrectomy[57]. The role of duodenal juice in the etiology of esophageal injury is controversial and the subject of many studies. Attwood et al showed that acid reflux is similar in patients with and without complications of Barrett's esophagus[58]. In this study those with complications had greater exposure to an alkaline pH environment and a correlation between an alkaline pH and duodenal juices was inferred. The presence of duodenal contents was not conclusive, as other mechanisms of increasing the pH may have been involved. However recent studies with the optical Bilitec probe that directly measures bilirubin have shown an important role for duodenal content[59] and are discussed in detail in Chapter 2.3. This duodeno-esophageal reflux has been shown to increase esophageal epithelial proliferation in the rat[60], and an increased incidence of esophageal carcinoma has been seen in the same model with a shift towards adenocarcinoma[61]. Further animal studies have shown that bile acids can damage the esophageal epithelium with the damage being dependent on the bile acid conjugation and the pH of the refluxate. Harmon et al [62] showed increased damage by conjugated bile acids at low pH, whereas at higher pH damage was caused by unconjugated forms. Kauer et al showed a relationship between the degree of duodenal reflux and esophageal damage[63], and that the majority of this reflux occurred in the pH range 4–7. Trypsin at pH 7.5 also causes severe mucosal damage, but is inactivated by acid, whereas lysolecithin, formed by the action of pancreatic phospholipase on biliary lecithin has been shown to disrupt the epithelium when associated with acid[64]. There is therefore an obvious synergism between gastric and duodenal contents in the pathogenesis of esophageal damage. The injurious effects of acid and duodenal juice may be enhanced by foods and drugs consumed. The direct effects of ingested material include direct pill injury due to K^+ supplements and possibly NSAID's and acidic foodstuffs such as white wine. Indirectly, the materials may enhance injury such as iron supplementation which can increase free radical formation and tissue damage[65] or offer protection such as NSAID's (see below). Foodstuffs such as fat may also indirectly aggravate reflux injury by

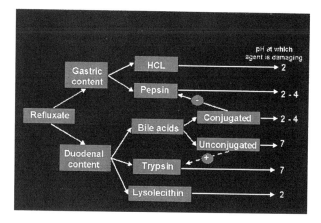

Figure 4. The injurious constituents of the refluxed juice and the pH at which they are most damaging.

decreasing lower esophageal pressure sphincter pressure increasing time of exposure to noxious agents or by changing the nature of juices refluxed from the duodenum. This latter effect is known to be involved in colonic injury, where elevated bile acid concentrations have been detected in patients with tumors[66], this possibly being related to ingestion of a high fat diet[67]. Indeed certain dietary fatty acids (carbon chain higher than 11) have been shown to have a particularly strong effect on CCK secretion and bile production[68]. Further evidence for the interaction between bile acids and the mucosa comes from the work of Garewal et al who have shown an increase in apoptosis in normal intestinal epithelium goblet cells when exposed to bile acids[69]. However in patients with intestinal neoplasia, this bile acid induced apoptosis was reduced implying a failure to remove cells damaged by the bile. As the Barrett's segment also comprises intestinal type epithelium, the same factors may be involved here.

5.1 MECHANISMS OF INJURY

The mechanism of epithelial injury by pepsin and trypsin is obviously related to their proteolytic properties. They increase cell detachment from the epithelium possibly by disrupting cell surface adhesion molecules and intercellular glycoproteins[64].
The mediation of H+ injury is more complex with a number of theories being proposed. Orlando et al showed a disruption of the Na^+/K^+ ATPase pump leading to cell volume disruption and cell death[70], while Snow et al found pH dependent alterations in K^+ and Cl^- conductance had a similar effect[71].

The mechanism for damage by bile acids is not fully understood. One theory is that they disrupt cell membranes by a detergent action on the lipid components. This has been demonstrated in the stomach in animal studies[72], however mucosal disruption has been shown in the rabbit esophagus at bile acid concentrations below those required for phospholipid solubilization[73]. A more favored hypothesis suggests that the unionized bile acids (conjugated forms at acidic pH, unconjugated forms at higher pH) are able to enter the cells via the cell membrane due to their lipophilic state[73]. They are then accumulated within the cells as they become ionized[74], leading to disordered cellular function and damage[73].
Studies have shown reactive oxygen metabolites to be implicated in esophageal tissue damage in animals and humans[75,76]. Wetscher et al showed increased oxidative stress in esophagitis, with the highest levels in Barrett's patients[75]. They also found a decreasing level of endogenous superoxide dismutase (SOD), an important free radical scavenger with increasing degree of tissue damage. Naya et al supported an important role for superoxide ions produced by inflammatory cells in acid induced injury in animal studies and showed that giving exogenous SOD before and during acid exposure could significantly reduce the tissue injury[76]. The induction of inflammation and tissue injury could also be successfully prevented by administration of Ketotifen, a Non Steroidal Anti-Inflammatory (NSAID) drug[76]. The evidence for the beneficial effects of anti-inflammatory medication in the esophagus is further supported by the work of Taha et al who showed decreased histological evidence of esophageal inflammation in patients taking long term NSAID's[77]. From this data it is suggested that cases of esophageal ulceration due

to NSAID's are likely to be due to the direct effects on the mucosa in patients where tablets become adherent to the mucosa. Interestingly, significantly reduced rates of esophageal carcinoma have also been reported in patients taking long term NSAID or aspirin medication[78] and the concept of using NSAID's to prevent tissue injury and neoplasia in the esophagus is being investigated.

5.2 CONSEQUENCES OF INJURY

If gastric or duodenal mucosa is damaged, there is a process of rapid repair (less than 1 hr) by restitution[78,79], where cells surrounding the damage migrate into the defect using the basement membrane as a framework. This is aided by prostaglandin release that increases bicarbonate and mucus secretion and local blood flow. These mechanisms do not seem to take place in the squamous esophageal mucosa where the defect in the epithelium is repaired more slowly, by cell replication and gradual migration into the defect in a similar manner to that seen in the skin[80]. Increased proliferation is evident by the basal cell hyperplasia with thickness more than 15% of the epithelium[28,80]. This is accompanied by increased papillary height, with papillae extending more than two thirds of the thickness of the epithelium[80]. Together, they produce a classical histological appearance in reflux disease, which is often associated with other evidence of inflammation such as neutrophil and eosinophil infiltration[18]. The increased proliferation is at least partly mediated by epidermal growth factor or similar ligands, as increased expression of the EGF receptor has being demonstrated in the inflamed esophagus[32].

Occasionally, early damage is indicated by the presence of large vacuolated cells, in which structural protein breakdown has been demonstrated. These are referred to as 'balloon cells' due to their histological appearance[81]

6. BARRETT'S ESOPHAGUS

How the esophageal squamous epithelium transforms into an intestinal type mucosa is one of the great mysteries of Barrett's esophagus. The precise definition of what constitutes Barrett's esophagus is discussed in Chapter 3.1 along with controversies in diagnosis. Tileston first described the resemblance of the mucosa surrounding 'peptic ulcers of the esophagus' to gastric mucosa in 1906[82], but the original

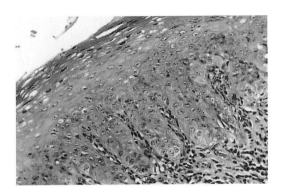

Figure 5: H&E section demonstrating the changes characteristically seen in gastro-esophageal reflux disease. Note the increased basal zone thickness and elongated papillae.

description is often credited to Norman Barrett, who erroneously described ulceration in a congenitally short esophagus with an intra-thoracic tubular stomach in 1950[83]. His name however has become synonymous with the condition. Despite occasional reports in children [84] the consensus of opinion has now moved away from a congenital to an acquired etiology.

The high prevalence of Barrett's in patients with severe GERD, its mid to later-life age of diagnosis and the evidence from the animal models of Bremner[85] and others provide fairly conclusive evidence of an acquired theory. The importance of severity of reflux in generating Barrett's is illustrated by Robertson et al who demonstrated a greater degree of reflux in Barrett's patients than in those with esophagitis only[55].

The condition is now known to be due to replacement of the normal squamous lining of the lower esophagus by metaplastic columnar-type mucosa, and it is now believed that this acid-resistant mucosa develops to protect the esophagus against the acid attack in patients with severe reflux.

6.1 EPITHELIAL TYPES WITHIN THE METAPLASTIC SEGMENT

On routine H&E staining of the columnar lined lower esophagus, 3 main epithelial types can be seen [86]:
1. Junctional type mucosa resembling the gastric cardiac epithelium with mucous-secreting cells lining the surface and pits.

2. Gastric Fundic type epithelium with mucous cells on the surface, with chief and parietal cells in the deeper parts of the glands
3. Specialized epithelium with a villous structure lined by columnar and goblet cells.

The columnar epithelium may resemble gastric mucosa with mainly neutral mucin expression or intestinal metaplasia (IM) which is characterized by a change in morphology to a small-intestinal phenotype and a change from neutral to acid mucin production. These acid mucins can be further sub-divided into sialomucins and sulphomucins. The presence of fully formed goblet cells containing acid mucins within the intestinal metaplasia is universally accepted to represent specialized intestinal metaplasia (SIM), while some would consider the presence of acid mucins in any columnar cells to be part of the spectrum of SIM[87]. A current hypothesis is a progressive theory of evolution where the changes begin at a microscopic level at the squamo-columnar junction (SCJ). This initially comprises a change from neutral to acid mucin production and eventually the formation of fully formed goblet cells. This may gradually evolve into a macroscopic columnar segment that lengthens until an adequate section of the esophagus is protected. This occurs in approximately 10% of patients undergoing endoscopy for GERD[88]. It is now generally held that the extent of the Barrett's specialized epithelium correlates with the severity of reflux [89]. The progressive theory is further supported by the fact that IM detected at the SCJ increases with the patients age and that a spectrum of disease is seen throughout the population. A study from our own institute[87] looking at the gastro-esophageal junction during routine endoscopy in a general medical open access clinic found long segment Barrett's change in 4% of patients and short-segment change in 7%. Of the remaining patients with a macroscopically normal gastro-esophageal junction, 17.5% had microscopic IM while 69.5% had evidence of acid mucins on special stains (Figure 6).

6.2 TIME SCALE FOR METAPLASTIC DEVELOPMENT

The time scale over which a long segment Barrett's esophagus develops is currently unknown but has been reported to occur within 10years of resection of the gastro-esophageal junction[90]. Once formed the segment length remains relatively static, with variation in length

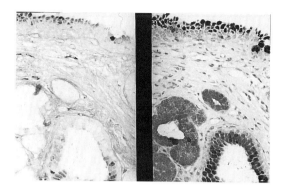

Figure 6. The spectrum of change in mucin production.
Figure 6a. High iron Diamine/Alcian blue and Alcian blue/Periodic acid Schiff stains demonstrating acid mucin Sulphomucins and neutral mucins acid mucins within columnar cells.

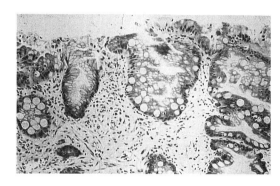

Figure 6b. H&E stain demonstrating fully formed goblet cells in complete intestinal metaplasia.

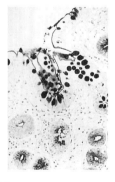

Figure 6c. Alcian blue/Periodic Acid Schiff stain demonstrating neutral mucins and intestinal type acid mucins in intestinal metaplasia with Goblet cells.

of less than 1cm/yr in the majority of patients[91]. Following the control of reflux by medical or surgical methods, complete reformation of the squamous lining has been reported[92] but is rare. However a considerable proportion of patients may develop squamous 'islands' within the columnar segment[93,94]. These observations

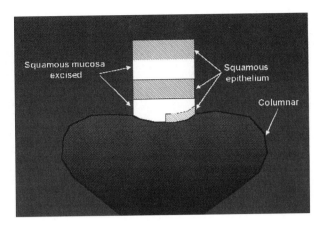

Figure 7. Lower esophageal mucosal rings denuded by Gillen et al[96] to investigate the mechanisms of re-epithalialization (with permission).

suggest the cell type in Barrett's esophagus is not fixed, and varies in relation to its local environment. There is no definite evidence that the disease does progress from one part of the spectrum to another as we have described and an alternative hypothesis for Barrett's metaplasia is the instantaneous field change theory. This implies that in response to the reflux injury the epithelium undergoes a metaplasia to form a long segment immediately, with the length of the segment depending on the severity of the insult.

6.3 MECHANISM OF COLUMNARISATION

The exact mechanism for replacement of the epithelial lining is unknown but there are currently three theories.

6.3.1 Creeping Substitution
Bremner and colleagues[85] removed a ring of squamous mucosa from the lower esophagus of dogs and showed that in the presence of acid hypersecretion or reflux, the defect was replaced by columnar mucosa. In the absence of an increased acid exposure, squamous epithelium regenerated. They postulated that the columnar replacement was by 'creeping substitution' of the gastric mucosa. Further work from the same group suggesting that metaplasia in response to reflux begins in the cardia[95] would appear to support this theory.

6.3.2 Stem cell theories
There is however evidence that the columnar epithelium may arise from the squamous epithelium itself. Gillen and co-workers also removed mucosal rings from the lower esophagus of dogs but left intervening squamous

mucosal rings between the denuded areas[96] (Figure 7). In the absence of reflux, squamous epithelium regenerated, but in the presence of acid or acid/bile reflux the denuded rings were replaced with columnar mucosa suggesting replacement by an intrinsic cell source as the gastric epithelium could not 'creep' over the squamous rings. They further disproved the creeping replacement theory by showing the new mucosa had different mucin staining characteristics to that of the cardiac epithelium. They postulated that stem cells were stimulated to differentiate into columnar cells by their exposure to the refluxate due to mucosal injury. Li et al[97] showed that regenerating columnar and squamous cells were in continuity with the ducts of esophageal glands, supporting the idea of a multipotential stem cell located within these submucosal glands, these being responsible for controlling the differentiation of the esophageal lining. The third and currently favored hypothesis of Barrett's development is that of alterations in differentiation of stem cells lying within the epithelium itself. In response to reflux there is an increased thickness of the proliferating basal zone and increased size of the papillae. Jankowski et al proposed that during reflux injury the functional stem cells of the basal zone near the tip of the papillae are relatively superficial and are therefore susceptible to refluxed or ingested mutagens within the lumen [98]. Surface cell sloughing due to reflux injury aggravates this. If the reflux is controlled, squamous regrowth may occur but if reflux continues and the depth of injury increases, the stem cells may undergo columnar metaplasia to form a surface more resistant to acid injury[98] (Figure 8).

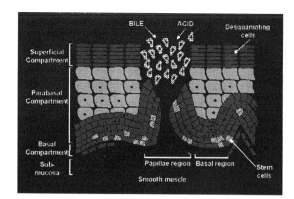 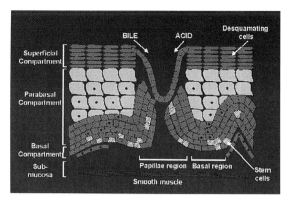

Figure 8. Mechanism of stem cell damage and subsequent columnar re-epithelialization proposed by Jankowski *et al*[8]. (a) damage to superficial stem cells near tip of papillae, (b) columnar development for subsequent protection (with permission).

This theory would explain why not all reflux patients develop Barrett's and why it is those with the most severe reflux that do. If duodenal juice is combined with the acid reflux then intestinal metaplasia may result to protect against these duodenal contents, as this is the cell type normally found protecting the intestine from this insult. This could explain the association of bile reflux with complications of Barrett's such as neoplastic progression.

Shields demonstrated a range of cells within the Barrett's mucosa by scanning electron microscopy[99]. In addition to normal gastric and intestinal type glands they found a cell type that had microvilli (a feature of glandular cells) and intercellular ridges (a feature of squamous epithelia) supporting the idea of a stem cell that can differentiate into squamous or glandular mucosa. The cell type was not found in any biopsies from patients without Barrett's change. The surface characteristics of this cell are the same as those of the metaplastic cells in the uterine cervix, a common site of metaplasia[99].

Feurle showed the presence of glucagon and neurotensin-immunoreactive cells which are not present in adult gastric mucosa within the Barrett's epithelium[6], suggesting the epithelium must arise from an immature multipotent stem cell. Rindi et *al* supported the theory of a pluripotential stem cell within the epithelium and concluded that they were capable of both gastric and intestinal type glandular differentiation[100], while Banner et *al* showed tumors arising within Barrett's mucosa can show multidirectional differentiation[101]. The heterogeneous mosaic of metaplastic phenotypes seen in Barrett's esophagus would also support this theory. The reason behind this heterogeneity is not fully

understood, but may be in part related to the composition of the refluxate. There may also be a genetic control as clonal divergence in chromosomes 5,8,9,12,17 and 18 has been described in benign Barrett's epithelium[102,103]. Genotypic changes have also been demonstrated in areas of carcinoma, dysplasia and surrounding metaplasia but not in distant metaplasia, suggesting the emergence of a clonal population leading to dysplasia and cancer[104]. These cytogenetic changes have been shown to precede the development of neoplasia in Barrett's epithelium[105]. This clonal evolution in Barrett's is also supported by the work of Reid and co-workers who showed a gradual accumulation of flow-cytometrically detected abnormalities as patients progressed from benign appearances to malignancy[106].

6.4 GENETIC CONSIDERATIONS

Though there is persuasive evidence for an acquired aetiology in Barrett's esophagus, there may well be a genetic predisposition. Romero *et al*. showed that parents and siblings of patients with Barrett's adenocarcinoma had reflux symptoms twice as often as controls (their spouses)[107]. No increase was found in relatives of patients with uncomplicated esophagitis. Others have confirmed a familial clustering of reflux symptoms[108]. Families with multiple members who have Barrett's esophagus have been reported[109] but the incidence of affected relatives of Barrett's patients is currently unknown. A genetic predisposition to gastro-esophageal reflux could have an important bearing on patients management following the findings of Lagergren et *al* who demonstrated an increased risk of adenocarcinoma in those patients with symptomatic reflux[110]. A full account is given elsewhere in this book.

6.5 CONTROL OF PROLIFERATION AND DIFFERENTIATION

The degree of differentiation and proliferation in the Barrett's epithelium may be partly controlled by the timing of the reflux episodes. Fitzgerald, in a tissue culture model showed that continuous acid exposure led to increased villin expression suggesting a differentiated cell type[111]. The constant acid also led to decreased cell proliferation. In contrast, pulsed acid led to increased cell proliferation with no effect on cell differentiation. In a follow-up study the same group showed that these effects may be mediated via changes in the intra-cellular pH mediated by the Na^+/H^+ exchanger[112], and blocking this exchanger could abolish that the proliferation induced by acid pulses. How the changes in intracellular pH lead to increased proliferation is not fully understood. It is suggested that on recovery from the cell acidification caused by an acid pulse there is a period of 'alkaline overshoot', which may stimulate cells to move from G0/G1 to the S phase of the cell cycle, leading to proliferation[112].

The degree of proliferation in the Barrett's mucosa has been extensively researched. Increased proportions of proliferating cells have been shown in benign Barrett's compared to normal gastric mucosa, but with a similar localization of cells to the naturally occurring proliferative zones[113,114]. Gray et al demonstrated variable proliferation in different cell types within the Barrett's epithelium by PCNA detection, with proliferation being greater in specialized cells compared to junctional or gastric types[115]. Gulizia et al showed this increased proliferation also occurred in microscopic SIM[116]. Epithelial hyper-proliferation is known to precede esophageal neoplasia in experimental models[117], and the greater proportion of cells in cycle, that are particularly susceptible to mutagens may help explain the association between SIM and malignancy.

Low rates of apoptosis have been found in Barrett's tissue compared to adjacent squamous epithelium[118], though this low apoptosis may be due to decreased cell injury, as the cell type is more resistant to the reflux insult. It has been suggested that the progression to dysplasia may be a result of a failure of apoptosis[119], though some have documented increasing apoptosis in higher degrees of dysplasia[120,121]. However, differences in bcl-2, bcl-x and bax, proteins that regulate apoptosis have been found in varying degrees of dysplasia[119,121] suggesting that the control of apoptosis may be altered in dysplastic change, though their exact roles and control mechanisms remain to be elucidated. Elevated levels of COX-2, the rate limiting enzyme in the production of prostaglandins have been found in Barrett's esophagus[122] and data from our own institution shows significant further elevations in dysplasia and adenocarcinoma. There is some evidence that COX-2 expression can be increased by exposure of the esophageal epithelium to bile acids[123] and that epithelial cells with increased levels of COX-2 have alterations in cellular adhesion and apoptosis[124].

Cell adhesion molecules such as the cadherins play an essential role in the induction and maintenance of cell differentiation[42], and a link has been suggested between their expression and the clinicopathological manifestations of cancer[125]. Similar levels of E-cadherin expression are seen in esophagitis and normal esophagus with lower levels in Barrett's epithelium falling further in adenocarcinoma[125]. Others have found preserved expression in metaplastic mucosa with reduced and disorganized expression in dysplastic tissues[126].

6.6 GROWTH FACTORS AND ONCOGENES IN BARRETT'S ESOPHAGUS

We have discussed the role of growth factors in the esophageal epithelium in section 3.1. How they behave when the differentiation changes to intestinal type epithelium is not known. A role for epidermal growth factor (EGF) in Barrett's metaplasia has been sought by a number of investigators. Gray demonstrated decreased salivary EGF levels in patients with Barrett's esophagus compared to esophagitis and control groups, suggesting this may impair the repair of reflux damage and encourage columnarisation[33]. Tissue EGF levels has been shown to be similar in all types of Barrett's metaplasia with no variation in the progression to adenocarcinoma [127]. TGFα is part of the same family as EGF, sharing a high affinity for the EGF receptor, production of mitogenic responses in EGF sensitive cells and a similar primary structure. The studies by Jankowski found elevated levels of TGFα in intestinal-type metaplasia compared to gastric-type[128]. The expression was further increased in dysplasia and adenocarcinoma[128].

The level of the EGF receptor is found to be elevated in intestinal type metaplasia compared to the levels seen in gastric-type Barrett's and gastric mucosa, which show similar expression [128]. A correlation has also been shown between the level of EGFR expression and the presence of dysplasia and adenocarcinoma arising in Barrett's epithelium[128]. How these alterations relate to the induction and progression of Barrett's epithelium is not clear and is currently the subject of intense investigation. Elevated levels of TGFα and EGF alone do not appear to increase neoplastic progression, but increased density of EGFR expression may account for their effects in some tissues[129]. Over-expression of TGFα should down regulate EGFR expression [130], therefore the increased levels of TGFα and EGFR seen in the studies of Jankowski may represent a loss of the normal negative feedback loop leading to the increased proliferation and progression to dysplasia seen in intestinal metaplasia. A number of mechanisms have been proposed for how the over-expression of TGFα and EGFR could lead to mitogenesis and oncogenesis. Co-expression of TGFα, EGF and EGFR is associated with *autocrine* growth regulation in some tissues[133], that is the TGFα activates the EGFR on the same cell. A similar finding has been made involving IGF and the EGF receptor [134]. Alternatively TGFα could activate the EGFR on nearby cells (*paracrine mechanisms*) [135]. Binding of membrane bound TGFα to EGF receptors on other cells may also promote cell proliferation by modulation of cell-cell adhesion[136]

The C-erbB-2 proto-oncogene, which is located on chromosome 7 bears considerable sequence homology with the EGF receptor and has similar tyrosine kinase activity. Its expression appears to be variable in Barrett's epithelium. Kim *et al* showed absent expression in benign samples with only a modest rise seen in dysplasia and neoplasia [131], while others have demonstrated expression in up to 60% of benign cases, rising to 73% in cancer[132].

A further factor may be the role of gut hormones. Alkalization of the gastric antrum as occurs in DGER can cause increased production of gastrin by the parietal G cells. Gastrin has a number of effects on the GI tract and has been implicated in the development of intestinal neoplasia[137]. As

Barrett's mucosa contains areas of intestinal metaplasia, then it may behave in a similar fashion in response to gastrin. However to date gastrin has only been shown to be mitogenic and not mutagenic, that is it stimulates proliferation[138] but has not been shown to induce carcinogenesis, and is therefore most likely to act as a growth promoter. Interestingly despite the raised gastrin levels and high acid secretion seen in patients with Zollinger-Ellison syndrome there appears to be no increase in the prevalence of Barrett's metaplasia[139].

The colonic adenoma-carcinoma sequence proposed by Vogelstein[140] is now widely accepted and there is growing evidence that the development of Barrett's metaplasia and neoplasia follows a similar sequence. In both Barrett's esophagus and colon cancer loss of the 5q and 17p alleles leads to deletions of the sequences encoding the adenomatous polyposis coli (APC) and p53 genes. However in colon cancer the loss of APC precedes the p53 loss whereas in Barrett's esophagus there is evidence that the opposite occurs[141].

The p53 gene is a putative tumor suppressor gene located on the short arm of chromosome 17 encoding for a 53 kDa nuclear phosphoprotein involved in the control of the cell cycle[142]. Mutation of this gene appears to be a common mutation in a variety of human cancers[142]. Quantitative studies have mainly relied upon protein level elevations as a surrogate marker for mutations. Ramel found p53 protein expression in 5% of benign Barrett's rising to 15% in LGD, 43% in HGD and 53% in adenocarcinoma[142]. Higher rates of expression have been found in other studies with Kim *et al* finding increased expression in 36% of patients without dysplasia rising to 90% with invasive cancer[131]. Both of these studies suggest an early role in the metaplasia-dysplasia-cancer sequence, though it is not possible to predict future progression to dysplasia and cancer by p53 detection. Also not all p53 mutations will produce excess protein or an increase in the half-life. Single monoclonal antibodies may not detect all mutations and a negative immunostain may still be accompanied by loss of p53 function, especially in stop-codon mutations. Therefore results have to be viewed with caution. The APC gene on chromosome 5q codes for a protein that is involved in the regulation of cell growth and death. It is a tumor suppressor gene, and germ-line mutation of one copy of the gene with subsequent somatic loss of the second copy causes the inherited familial adenomatous polyposis (FAP) syndrome[143]. APC abnormalities are rare in benign Barrett's epithelium and low-grade dysplasia [144] but rise to approximately 60% in carcinoma, indicating that these abnormalities are likely to be involved late in the metaplasia-dysplasia sequence. The APC abnormalities are always associated with a p53 mutation[141].

A full account of the progression of metaplasia to dysplasia and cancer and the factors involved can be found in Chapters 3.3 and 3.4.

6.7 INFLAMMATION IN THE BARRETT'S SEGMENT

The degree of inflammation within the Barrett's segment is variable. Fitzgerald et al showed 68% of cases to have little macroscopic inflammation, but on microscopic examination to have a more significant degree with T cell, neutrophil and eosinophil infiltration which correlated with the degree of inflammation[145]. They further showed that the histopathological inflammation increased proximally in the Barrett's segment and this was associated with elevated IL-8 pro-inflammatory cytokine levels[146]. This proximal part of the Barrett's segment is known to be the area with the greatest risk of complications such as stricture formation.

Recently the presence of inflammation and SIM in the gastric cardia has been related to GERD[95]. Mendes et al have demonstrated a common pattern of intestinal-type differentiation, namely sucrase-isomaltase and crypt-cell antigen expression in adenocarcinoma of the cardia, esophagus and IM in Barrett's and cardiac mucosa[147]. It was not found in normal esophagus, esophageal submucosal glands or gastric mucosa suggesting a stem cell origin and specific pathway for this pathology. It has also added weight to the growing consensus that adenocarcinoma of the esophagus and of the cardia is one entity.

As we have seen, the normal epithelium has many mechanisms to protect itself against injury from luminal chemicals, but these can be overcome by excess exposure to gastric and duodenal juices. This rapidly results in inflammation, tissue destruction and in most cases, regeneration. However the epithelium in some patients with severe injury can undergo metaplasia to form a more resistant defense, a process that is influenced by environmental and genetic factors. The exact role of each of these factors is yet to be determined but will undoubtedly hold the key to prevention of adenocarcinoma in the esophagus.

REFERENCES

1. Schridde H. Uber die epithelproliferationen in der embryonalen menschlichen speiserohre. Virchows Arch 1908;191:79.
2. Gray S, Skandalakis J. The esophagus, in Embryology for surgeons, S Gray, Editor. 1972, WB Saunders: Philadelphia.
3. Jabbari M, Goresky CA, Lough J, Yaffe C, Daly D, Cote C. The inlet patch: heterotopic gastric mucosa in the upper esophagus. Gastroenterology 1985;89(2):352-6.
4. Borhan Manesh F, Farnum JB. Incidence of heterotopic gastric mucosa in the upper oesophagus. Gut 1991;32(9): 968-72.
5. Nakajima H, Munakata A, Sasaki Y, Yoshida Y. pH profile of esophagus in patients with inlet patch of heterotopic gastric mucosa after tetragastrin stimulation. an endoscopic approach. Dig Dis Sci 1993;38(10):1915-9.
6. Feurle GE, Helmstaedter V, Buehring A, Bettendorf U, Eckardt VF. Distinct immunohistochemical findings in columnar epithelium of esophageal inlet patch and of Barrett's esophagus. Dig Dis Sci 1990; 35(1):86-92.
7. Galan AR, Katzka DA, Castell DO. Acid secretion from an esophageal inlet patch demonstrated by ambulatory pH monitoring. Gastroenterology 1998; 115(6):1574-6.
8. Hopwood D, The oesophageal lining, in Gastrointestinal and oesophageal pathology, R Whitehead, Editor. 1989, Churchil Livingstone:1-12.
9. Rhodin J, Epithelia, in Histology. A Text and Atlas. 1977, Oxford University Press: New York. 65.
10. Watt F. Epidermal stem cells: markers, patterning and the control of stem cell fate. Phil Trans R Soc Lond, 1998. 353:831-7.
11. Reynolds AJ, Jahoda CA. Cultured dermal papilla cells induce follicle formation and hair growth by transdifferentiation of an adult epidermis. Development 1992;115(2): 587-93.
12. Miller SJ, Burke EM, Rader MD, Coulombe PA, Lavker RM. Re-epithelialization of porcine skin by the sweat apparatus. J Invest Dermatol 1998;110(1):13-9.
13. Logan KR, Hopwood D, Milne G. Cellular junctions in human oesophageal epithelium. J Pathol 1978;126(3):157-63.
14. Hopwood D, Logan KR, Bouchier IA. The electron microscopy of normal human oesophageal epithelium. Virchows Arch B Cell Pathol 1978;26(4):345-58.
15. Rhodin J, Cells and organelles, in Histology. A Text and Atlas. 1977, Oxford University Press: New York. 10-63.
16. Yassin TM, Toner PG. Langerhans cells in the human oesophagus. J Anat 1976;122(2):435-45.

17. Terris B, Potet F. Structure and role of Langerhans' cells in the human oesophageal epithelium. Digestion 1995; 56 Suppl 1:9-14.

18. Eastwood GL. Histologic changes in gastroesophageal reflux. J Clin Gastroenterol 1986; 8 Suppl 1:45-51.

19. Attwood SE, Smyrk TC, Demeester TR, Jones JB. Esophageal eosinophilia with dysphagia. A distinct clinicopathologic syndrome. Dig Dis Sci 1992; 38(1):109-16.

20. Borda F, Jimenez FJ, Martinez Penuela JM, Echarri A, Martin Granizo I, Aznarez R. Eosinophilic esophagitis: an underdiagnosed entity? Rev Esp Enferm Dig 1996;88(10):701-4.

21. De-la-Pava S, Nigogosyan G, Pickren J, Cabrera A. Melanosis of the esophagus. Cancer 1963;16: 48-50.

22. Tateishi R, Taniguchi H, Wada A, Horai T, Taniguchi K. Argyrophil cells and melanocytes in esophageal mucosa. Arch Pathol 1974; 98(2):87-9.

23. Stranks GJ, Mathai JT, Rowe Jones DC. Primary malignant melanoma of the oesophagus: case report and review of surgical pathology. Gut 1991; 32(7):828-30.

24. Hopwood D, Coghill G, Sanders DS. Human oesophageal submucosal glands. Their detection mucin, enzyme and secretory protein content. Histochemistry 1986; 86(1):107-12.

25. Attwood S, Bradley C, Dworkin R, McGahan I, Tufferey. Circadian rhythm of mitotic activity in the oesophageal epithelium of the rat (Abstract). Irish J Med Science 1978;147(9):330.

26. Burns ER, Scheving LE, Fawcett DF, Gibbs WM, Galatzan RE. Circadian influence on the frequency of labeled mitoses method in the stratified squamous epithelium of the mouse esophagus and tongue. Anat Rec 1976; 184(3):265-73.

27. Karam SM. Lineage commitment and maturation of epithelial cells in the gut. Front Biosci 1999; 4: D286-98.

28. Livstone EM, Sheahan DG, Behar J. Studies of esophageal epithelial cell proliferation in patients with reflux esophagitis. Gastroenterology 1977; 73(6):1315-9.

29. Marcinkiewicz M, Grabowska SZ, Czyzewska E. Role of epidermal growth factor (EGF) in oesophageal mucosal integrity. Curr Med Res Opin 1998; 14(3):145-53.

30. Jimenez P, Lanas A, Piazuelo E, Esteva F. Effect of growth factors and prostaglandin E2 on restitution and proliferation of rabbit esophageal epithelial cells. Dig Dis Sci 1998;43(10):2309-16.

31. Tuchman D, Dutta S, Vengurlekar S, Gottal R, Bidani J, Dutta D. Reduction of salivary epidermal growth factor (EGF) secretion and alteration in the EGF receptor expression in esophageal mucosa in pediatric patients with reflux esophagitis. Gastroenterology 1992;102: A182.

32. Jankowski J, Murphy S, Coghill G, Grant A, Wormsley KG, Sanders DS, Kerr M, Hopwood D. Epidermal growth factor receptors in the esophagus. Gut 1992;33(4):439-43.

33. Gray MR, Donnelly RJ, Kingsnorth AN. Role of salivary epidermal growth factor in the pathogenesis of Barrett's columnar lined oesophagus. Br J Surg 1991;78(12): 1461-6.

34. Sarosiek J, Hetzel DP, Yu Z, Piascik R, Li L, Rourk RM, McCallum RW. Evidence on secretion of epidermal growth factor by the esophageal mucosa in humans. Am J Gastroenterol 1993;88(7): 1081-7.

35. Li L, Yu Z, Piascik R, Hetzel DP, Rourk RM, Namiot Z, Sarosiek J, McCallum RW. Effect of esophageal intraluminal mechanical and chemical stressors on salivary epidermal growth factor in humans. Am J Gastroenterol 1993;88(10):1749-55.

36. Dockray G. Gastrin and gastric epithelial physiology. Journal of Physiology 1999;518(2):315-24.

37. Iwase K, Evers BM, Hellmich MR, Guo YS, Higashide S, Kim HJ, Townsend CM, Jr. Regulation of growth of human gastric cancer by gastrin and glycine-extended progastrin. Gastroenterology 1997;113(3):782-90.

38. Ohning GV, Wong HC, Lloyd KC, Walsh JH. Gastrin mediates the gastric mucosal proliferative response to feeding. Am J Physiol 1996;271(3 Pt 1):G470-6.

39. Koh TJ, Goldenring JR, Ito S, Mashimo H, Kopin AS, Varro A, Dockray GJ, Wang TC. Gastrin deficiency results in altered gastric differentiation and decreased colonic proliferation in mice. Gastroenterology 1997;113(3):1015-25.

40. Van Nieuwenhove Y, De Backer T, Chen D, Hakanson R, Willems G. Gastrin stimulates epithelial cell proliferation in the oesophagus of rats. Virchows Arch 1998;432(4):371-5.

41. Tchorzewski MT, Qureshi FG, Duncan MD, Duncan KL, Saini N, Harmon JW. Role of insulin-like growth factor-I in esophageal mucosal healing processes. J Lab Clin Med 1998;132(2):134-41.

42. Hynes RO, Lander AD. Contact and adhesive specificities in the associations, migrations and targetting of cells and axons. Cell 1992;68: 303-22.

43. Dobson H, Pignatelli M, Hopwood D, C DA. Cell adhesion molecules in oesophageal epithelium. Gut 1994;35(10):1343-47.

44. Takeichi M. Cadherins: a molecular family important in selective cell-cell adhesion. Annu Rev Biochem 1990;59:237-52.

45. Sanders DS, Bruton R, Darnton SJ, Casson AG, Hanson I, Williams HK, Jankowski J. Sequential changes in cadherin-catenin expression associated with the progression and heterogeneity of primary oesophageal squamous carcinoma. Int J Cancer 1998;79(6):573-9.

46. Aberle H, Schwartz H, Kemler R. Cadherin-catenin complex: protein interactions and their implications for cadherin function. J Cell Biochem 1996;61(4):514-23.

47. Salo J, Kivilaakso E. Role of luminal H+ in the pathogenesis of experimental esophagitis. Surgery 1982; 92(1):61-8.

48. Christie K, Thomson C, Morley S, Anderson J, Hopwood D. Carbonic anhydrase is present in human oesophageal epithelium and submucosal glands. Histochem J 1995;27(8):587-90.

49. Orlando RC. Esophageal epithelial defense against acid injury. J Clin Gastroenterol 1991;13 Suppl 2:S1-5.

50. Orlando RC, Lacy ER, Tobey NA, Cowart K. Barriers to paracellular permeability in rabbit esophageal epithelium. Gastroenterology 1992;102(3):910-23.

51. Hopwood D, Milne G, Jankowski J, Howat K, Johnston D, Wormsley KG. Secretory and absorptive activity of oesophageal epithelium: evidence of circulating mucosubstances. Histochem J 1994;26(1):41-9.

52. Layden TJ, Schmidt L, Agnone L, Lisitza P, Brewer J, Goldstein JL. Rabbit esophageal cell cytoplasmic pH regulation: role of Na(+)-H+ antiport and Na(+)-dependent HCO3- transport systems. Am J Physiol 1992;263(3 Pt 1):G407-13.

53. Tobey NA, Powell DW, Schreiner VJ, Orlando RC. Serosal bicarbonate protects against acid injury to rabbit esophagus. Gastroenterology 1989;96(6):1466-77.

54. Johnson LF, Harmon JW. Experimental esophagitis in a rabbit model. Clinical relevance. J Clin Gastroenterol 1986;(8) Suppl 126-44.

55. Robertson D, Aldersley M, Shepherd H, Smith CL. Patterns of acid reflux in complicated oesophagitis. Gut 1987;28(11):1484-8.

56. Palmer E. Subacute erosive ('peptic') oesophagitis associated with achlorhydria. N Engl J Med 1960;262:929.

57. Helsingen N. Oesophagitis following total gastrectomy. Acta Churgica Scandinavica 1959;118:190-201.

58. Attwood SE, Ball CS, Barlow AP, Jenkinson L, Norris TL, Watson A. Role of intragastric and intraoesophageal alkalinisation in the genesis of complications in Barrett's columnar lined lower oesophagus. Gut 1993;34(1):11-5.

59. Champion G, Richter JE, Vaezi MF, Singh S, Alexander R. Duodenogastroesophageal reflux: Relationship to pH and importance in Barrett's esophagus. Gastroenterology 1994;107(3):747-54.

60. Attwood S, Smyrk T, Marcus J, Murphy B, Steele P, DeMeester T, Mirvish S, Hinder R. Effect of duodenal juice on DNA index and cell proliferation in a model of oesophageal carcinogenesis. Br J Surgery 1991;78(6):754.

61. Attwood SE, Smyrk TC, DeMeester TR, Mirvish SS, Stein HJ, Hinder RA. Duodenoesophageal reflux and the development of esophageal adenocarcinoma in rats. Surgery 1992;111(5):503-10.

62. Harmon JW, Johnson LF, Maydonovitch CL. Effects of acid and bile salts on the rabbit esophageal mucosa. Dig Dis Sci 1981;26(1):65-72.

63. Kauer WK, Peters JH, DeMeester TR, Ireland AP, Bremner CG, Hagen JA. Mixed reflux of gastric and duodenal juices is more harmful to the esophagus than gastric juice alone. The need for surgical therapy re-emphasized. Ann Surg 1995;222(4):525-31.

64. Salo JA, Lehto VP, Kivilaakso E. Morphological alterations in experimental esophagitis. Light microscopic and scanning and transmission electron microscopic study. Dig Dis Sci 1983;28(5): 440-8.

65. Goldstein SR, Yang GY, Curtis SK, Reuhl KR, Liu BC, Mirvish SS, Newmark HL, Yang CS. Development of esophageal metaplasia and adenocarcinoma in a rat surgical model without the use of a carcinogen. Carcinogenesis 1997;18(11):2265-70.

66. Stadler J, Yeung KS, Furrer R, Marcon N, Himal HS, Bruce WR. Proliferative activity of rectal mucosa and soluble fecal bile acids in patients with normal colons and in patients with colonic polyps or cancer. Cancer Lett 1988;38(3):315-20.

67. Stadler J, Stern HS, Yeung KS, McGuire V, Furrer R, Marcon N, Bruce WR. Effect of high fat consumption on cell proliferation activity of colorectal mucosa and on soluble faecal bile acids. Gut 1988;29(10):1326-31.

68. McLaughlin J, Grazia Luca M, Jones MN, M DA, Dockray GJ, Thompson DG. Fatty acid chain length determines cholecystokinin secretion and effect on human gastric motility. Gastroenterology 1999;116(1):46-53.

69. Garewal H, Bernstein H, Bernstein C, Sampliner R, Payne C. Reduced bile acid-induced apoptosis in "normal" colorectal mucosa: a potential biological marker for cancer risk. Cancer Res 1996; 56(7)1480-3.

70. Orlando RC, Bryson JC, Powell DW. Mechanisms of H+ injury in rabbit esophageal epithelium. Am J Physiol 1984;246(6 Pt 1)G718-24.

71. Snow JC, Goldstein JL, Schmidt LN, Lisitza P, Layden TJ. Rabbit esophageal cells show regulatory volume decrease: ionic basis and effect of pH. Gastroenterology 1993;105(1):102-10.

72. Thomas AJ, Nahrwold DL, Rose RC. Detergent action of sodium taurocholate on rat gastric mucosa. Biochim Biophys Acta 1972; 282(1):210-3.

73. Schweitzer EJ, Harmon JW, Bass BL, Batzri S. Bile acid efflux precedes mucosal barrier disruption in the rabbit esophagus. Am J Physiol 1984;247(5 Pt 1):G480-5.

74. Batzri S, Harmon JW, Schweitzer EJ, Toles R. Bile acid accumulation in gastric mucosal cells. Proc Soc Exp Biol Med 1991;197(4):393-9.

75. Wetscher GJ, Hinder RA, Bagchi D, Hinder PR, Bagchi M, Perdikis G, McGinn T. Reflux esophagitis in humans is mediated by oxygen-derived free radicals. Am J Surg 1995;170(6):552-6.

76. Naya MJ, Pereboom D, Ortego J, Alda JO, Lanas A. Superoxide anions produced by inflammatory cells play an important part in the pathogenesis of acid and pepsin induced oesophagitis in rabbits. Gut 1997;40(2): 175-81.

77. Taha AS, Dahill S, Nakshabendi I, Lee FD, Sturrock RD, Russell RI. Oesophageal histology in long term users of non-steroidal anti-inflammatory drugs. J Clin Pathol 1994; 47(8):705-8.

78. Silen W, Gastric mucosal defense and repair, in Physiology of the gastrointestinal tract, L Johnson, J Christensen,E Jacobsen, Editors. 1987, Raven Press: New York;1055.

79. Feil W, Wenzl E, Vattay P. Repair of rabbit duodenal mucosa after acid injury in vivo and in vitro. Gastroenterology 1973; 92:1973-86.

80. Ismail-Beigi F, Horton P, Pope CI. Histological consequences of gastroesophageal reflux in man. Gastroenterology 1970; 58:163-74.

81. Jessurun J, Yardley JH, Giardiello FM, Hamilton SR. Intracytoplasmic plasma proteins in distended esophageal squamous cells (balloon cells). Mod Pathol 1988; 1(3):175-81.

82. Tileston W. Peptic ulcer of the esophagus. Am J Med Sci 1906;132:240-65.

83. Barrett N. Chronic peptic ulcer of the oesophagus and oesophagitis. Br J Surg 1950;38:175-82.

84. Hassall E, Dimmick JE, Magee JF. Adenocarcinoma in childhood Barrett's esophagus: case documentation and the need for surveillance in children. Am J Gastroenterol 1993;88(2):282-8.

85. Bremner CG, Lynch VP, Ellis FH, Jr. Barrett's esophagus: congenital or acquired? An experimental study of esophageal mucosal regeneration in the dog. Surgery, 1970;68(1):209-16.

86. Lapertosa G, Baracchini P, Fulcheri E. Mucin histochemical analysis in the interpretation of Barrett's esophagus. Results of a multicenter study. The Operative Group for the Study of Esophageal Precancer. Am J Clin Pathol 1992;98(1):61-6.

87. Byrne JP, Bhatnagar S, Hamid B, Armstrong GR, Attwood SE. Comparative study of intestinal metaplasia and mucin staining at the cardia and esophagogastric junction in 225 symptomatic patients presenting for diagnostic open-access gastroscopy. Am J Gastroenterol 1995;94(1):98-103.

88. GOSPE. Barrett's esophagus: epidemiological and clinical results of a multicentric survey. Gruppo Operativo per lo Studio delle Precancerosi dell'Esofago (GOSPE). Int J Cancer 1991;48(3):364-8.

89. Oberg S, DeMeester TR, Peters JH, Hagen JA, Nigro JJ, DeMeester SR, Theisen J, Campos GM, Crookes PF. The extent of Barrett's esophagus depends on the status of the lower esophageal sphincter and the degree

of esophageal acid exposure. J Thorac Cardiovasc Surg 1999;117(3):572-80.

90. Hamilton S, Yardley J. Regeneration of cardiac type mucosa and acquisition of Barrett mucosa after esophagogastrostomy. Gastroenterology 1977; 72:669-75.

91. Sampliner RE, Garewal HS, Fennerty MB, Aickin M. Lack of impact of therapy on extent of Barrett's esophagus in 67 patients. Dig Dis Sci 1990;35(1):93-6.

92. Attwood SE, Barlow AP, Norris TL, Watson A. Barrett's oesophagus: effect of antireflux surgery on symptom control and development of complications. Br J Surg 1992;79(10):1050-3.

93. Sampliner RE. Effect of up to 3 years of high-dose lansoprazole on Barrett's esophagus [see comments]. Am J Gastroenterol 1994;89(10):1844-8.

94. Sagar PM, Ackroyd R, Hosie KB, Patterson JE, Stoddard CJ, Kingsnorth AN. Regression and progression of Barrett's oesophagus after antireflux surgery. Br J Surg 1995; 82(6):806-10.

95. Oberg S, Peters JH, DeMeester TR, Chandrasoma P, Hagen JA, Ireland AP, Ritter MP, Mason RJ, Crookes P, Bremner CG. Inflammation and specialized intestinal metaplasia of cardiac mucosa is a manifestation of gastroesophageal reflux disease. Ann Surg 1997;226(4):522-30.

96. Gillen P, Keeling P, Byrne PJ, West AB, Hennessy TP. Experimental columnar metaplasia in the canine oesophagus. Br J Surg 1988;75(2):113-5.

97. Li H, Walsh TN, O'Dowd G, Gillen P, Byrne PJ, Hennessy TP. Mechanisms of columnar metaplasia and squamous regeneration in experimental Barrett's esophagus. Surgery 1994; 115(2):176-81.

98. Jankowski J, Wright N, Meltzer S, Triadafilopoulos G, Geboes K, Casson A, Kerr D, Young L. Molecular evolution of the Metaplasia-Dysplasia-Adenocarcinoma sequence in the esophagus. Am J Pathol 1999;154:965-73.

99. Shields HM, Sawhney RA, Zwas F, Boch JA, Kim S, Goran D, Antonioli DA. Scanning electron microscopy of the human esophagus: application to Barrett's esophagus, a precancerous lesion. Microsc Res Tech 1995;31(3):248-56.

100. Rindi G, Bishop AE, Daly MJ, Isaacs P, Lee FI, Polak JM. A mixed pattern of endocrine cells in metaplastic Barrett's oesophagus. Evidence that the epithelium derives from a pluripotential stem cell. Histochemistry 1987;87(4):377-83.

101. Banner BF, Memoli VA, Warren WH, Gould VE. Carcinoma with multidirectional differentiation arising in Barrett's esophagus. Ultrastruct Pathol 1983;4(2-3):205-17.

102. Mackay C, Stuart R, Going J, Baxter J, Keith W. Interphase cytogenetics of non-dysplastic Barrett's esophagus. Gastroenterology 1997;112:A607.

103. Wu TT, Watanabe T, Heitmiller R, Zahurak M, Forastiere AA, Hamilton SR. Genetic alterations in Barrett esophagus and adenocarcinomas of the esophagus and esophagogastric junction region. Am J Pathol 1998;153(1):287-94.

104. Zhuang Z, Vortmeyer AO, Mark EJ, Odze R, Emmert Buck MR, Merino MJ, Moon H, Liotta LA, Duray PH. Barrett's esophagus: metaplastic cells with loss of heterozygosity at the APC gene locus are clonal precursors to invasive adenocarcinoma. Cancer Res 1996;56(9):1961-4.

105. Raskind WH, Norwood T, Levine DS, Haggitt RC, Rabinovitch PS, Reid BJ. Persistent clonal areas and clonal expansion in Barrett's esophagus. Cancer Res 1992;52(10):2946-50.

106. Reid BJ, Haggitt RC, Rubin CE, Rabinovitch PS. Barrett's esophagus. Correlation between flow cytometry and histology in detection of patients at risk for adenocarcinoma. Gastroenterology 1987;93(1):1-11.

107. Romero Y, Cameron AJ, Locke GR, 3rd, Schaid DJ, Slezak JM, Branch CD, Melton LJ, 3rd. Familial aggregation of gastroesophageal reflux in patients with Barrett's esophagus and esophageal adenocarcinoma. Gastroenterology 1997;113(5):1449-56.

108. Trudgill NJ, Kapur KC, Riley SA. Familial clustering of reflux symptoms [see comments]. Am J Gastroenterol 1999;94(5):1172-8.

109. Jochem VJ, Fuerst PA, Fromkes JJ. Familial Barrett's esophagus associated with adenocarcinoma. Gastroenterology 1992;102(4 Pt 1):1400-2.

110. Lagergren J, Bergstrom R, Lindgren A, Nyren O. Symptomatic gastroesophageal reflux as a risk factor for esophageal adenocarcinoma [see comments]. N Engl J Med 1999;340(11)825-31.

111. Fitzgerald RC, Omary MB, Triadafilopoulos G. Dynamic effects of acid on Barrett's esophagus. An ex vivo proliferation and differentiation model. J Clin Invest 1996; 98(9):2120-8.

112. Fitzgerald RC, Omary MB, Triadafilopoulos G. Altered sodium-hydrogen exchange activity is a mechanism for acid-induced hyperproliferation in Barrett's esophagus. Am J Physiol 1998;275(1 Pt 1):G47-55.

113. Hong MK, Laskin WB, Herman BE, Johnston MH, Vargo JJ, Steinberg SM, Allegra CJ, Johnston PG. Expansion of the Ki-67 proliferative compartment correlates with degree of dysplasia in Barrett's esophagus. Cancer 1995;75(2):423-9.

114. Reid BJ, Sanchez CA, Blount PL, Levine DS. Barrett's esophagus: cell cycle abnormalities in advancing stages of neoplastic progression. Gastroenterology 1993;105(1) 119-29.

115. Gray MR, Hall PA, Nash J, Ansari B, Lane DP, Kingsnorth AN. Epithelial proliferation in Barrett's esophagus by proliferating cell nuclear antigen immunolocalization. Gastroenterology 1992;103(6):1769-76.

116. Gulizia JM, Wang H, Antonioli D, Spechler SJ, Zeroogian J, Goyal R, Shahsafaei A, Chen YY, Odze RD. Proliferative characteristics of intestinalized mucosa in the distal esophagus and gastroesophageal junction (short-segment Barrett's esophagus): a case control study. Hum Pathol 1999;30(4):412-8.

117. Craddock VM, Driver HE. Sequential histological studies of rat oesophagus during the rapid initiation of cancer by repeated injection of N-methyl-N-benzylnitrosamine. Carcinogenesis 1987; 8(8):1129-32.

118. Wetscher GJ, Schwelberger H, Unger A, Offner FA, Profanter C, Glaser K, Klingler A, Gadenstaetter M, Klinger P. Reflux-induced apoptosis of the esophageal mucosa is inhibited in Barrett's epithelium. Am J Surg 1998;176(6):569-73.

119. Katada N, Hinder RA, Smyrk TC, Hirabayashi N, Perdikis G, Lund RJ, Woodward T, Klingler PJ. Apoptosis is inhibited early in the dysplasia-carcinoma sequence of Barrett esophagus. Arch Surg, 1997;132(7):728-33.

120. Lauwers GY, Kandemir O, Kubilis PS, Scott GV. Cellular kinetics in Barrett's epithelium carcinogenic sequence: roles of apoptosis, bcl-2 protein, and cellular proliferation. Mod Pathol 1997;10(12):1201-8.

121. Soslow RA, Remotti H, Baergen RN, Altorki NK. Suppression of apoptosis does not foster neoplastic

growth in Barrett's esophagus. Mod Pathol 1999;12(3):239-50.

122. Wilson KT, Fu S, Ramanujam KS, Meltzer SJ. Increased expression of inducible nitric oxide synthase and cyclooxygenase-2 in Barrett's esophagus and associated adenocarcinomas. Cancer Res 1998;58(14):2929-34.

123. Katada N, Hinder RA, Smyrk TC, Hiki Y, Kakita A. Duodenoesophageal reflux induces apoptosis in rat esophageal epithelium. Dig Dis Sci 1999;44(2):301-10.

124. Tsujii M, DuBois RN. Alterations in cellular adhesion and apoptosis in epithelial cells overexpressing prostaglandin endoperoxide synthase 2. Cell 1995;83(3): 493-501.

125. Swami S, Kumble S, Triadafilopoulos G. E-cadherin expression in gastroesophageal reflux disease, Barrett's esophagus, and esophageal adenocarcinoma: an immunohistochemical and immunoblot study. Am J Gastroenterol 1995;90(10):1808-13.

126. Bongiorno PF, al Kasspooles M, Lee SW, Rachwal WJ, Moore JH, Whyte RI, Orringer MB, Beer DG. E-cadherin expression in primary and metastatic thoracic neoplasms and in Barrett's oesophagus. Br J Cancer 1995;71(1):166-72.

127. Jankowski J, McMenemin R, Hopwood D, Penston J, Wormsley KG. Abnormal expression of growth regulatory factors in Barrett's oesophagus. Clin Sci Colch 1991;81(5):663-8.

128. Jankowski J, Hopwood D, Wormsley KG. Flow-cytometric analysis of growth-regulatory peptides and their receptors in Barrett's oesophagus and oesophageal adenocarcinoma. Scand J Gastroenterol 1992;27(2):147-54.

129. Gullick WJ. Prevalence of aberrant expression of the epidermal growth factor receptor in human cancers. Br Med Bull 1991;47(1):87-98.

130. Lai WH, Cameron PH, Wada I, Doherty JJd, Kay DG, Posner BI, Bergeron JJ. Ligand-mediated internalization, recycling, and downregulation of the epidermal growth factor receptor in vivo. J Cell Biol 1989;109(6 Pt 1):2741-9.

131. Kim R, Clarke MR, Melhem MF, Young MA, Vanbibber MM, Safatle Ribeiro AV, Ribeiro U, Jr., Reynolds JC. Expression of p53, PCNA, and C-erbB-2 in Barrett's metaplasia and adenocarcinoma. Dig Dis Sci 1997;42(12):2453-62.

132. Jankowski J, Coghill G, Hopwood D, Wormsley KG. Oncogenes and onco-suppressor gene in adenocarcinoma of the oesophagus. Gut 1992;33(8):1033-8.

133. Markowitz SD, Molkentin K, Gerbic C, Jackson J, Stellato T, Willson JK. Growth stimulation by coexpression of transforming growth factor-alpha and epidermal growth factor-receptor in normal and adenomatous human colon epithelium. J Clin Invest 1990;86(1):356-62.

134. Carbrijan T, Pacarizi H, Levanat S, al e. Autocrine tumour growth regulation by the insulin growth factor 1 (IGF 1) and the epidermal growth factor (EGF). Prog Cancer Res Ther 1988;35:227-30.

135. Sandgren EP, Luetteke NC, Palmiter RD, Brinster RL, Lee DC. Overexpression of TGF alpha in transgenic mice: induction of epithelial hyperplasia, pancreatic metaplasia, and carcinoma of the breast. Cell 1990;61(6):1121-35.

136. Anklesaria P, Teixido J, Laiho M, Pierce JH, Greenberger JS, Massague J. Cell-cell adhesion mediated by binding of membrane-anchored transforming growth factor alpha to epidermal growth factor receptors promotes cell proliferation. Proc Natl Acad Sci U S A 1990;87(9): 3289-93.

137. Thorburn CM, Friedman GD, Dickinson CJ, Vogelman JH, Orentreich N, Parsonnet J. Gastrin and colorectal cancer: a prospective study. Gastroenterology 1998;115(2):275-80.

138. Karaki Y, Shimazaki K, Okamoto M, Ookami H, Fujimaki M. Effect of endogenous hypergastrinemia on carcinogenesis in the rat esophagus. Surg Today 1996;26(1):5-11.

139. Strader DB, Benjamin SB, Orbuch M, Lubensky TA, Gibril F, Weber C, Fishbeyn VA, Jensen RT, Metz DC. Esophageal function and occurrence of Barrett's esophagus in Zollinger-Ellison syndrome. Digestion 1995;56(5):347-56.

140. Fearon ER, Vogelstein B. A genetic model for colorectal tumorigenesis. Cell 1990;61(5):759-67.

141. Blount PL, Meltzer SJ, Yin J, Huang Y, Krasna MJ, Reid BJ. Clonal ordering of 17p and 5q allelic losses in Barrett dysplasia and adenocarcinoma. Proc Natl Acad Sci U S A 1993;90(8):3221-5.

142. Ramel S, Reid BJ, Sanchez CA, Blount PL, Levine DS, Neshat K, Haggitt RC, Dean PJ, Thor K, Rabinovitch PS. Evaluation of p53 protein expression in Barrett's esophagus by two-parameter flow cytometry. Gastroenterology 1992;102(4 Pt 1):1220-8.

143. Gryfe R, Swallow C, Bapat B, Redston M, Gallinger S, Couture J. Molecular biology of colorectal cancer. Curr Probl Cancer 1997;21(5):233-300.

144. Gonzalez MV, Artimez ML, Rodrigo L, Lopez Larrea C, Menendez MJ, Alvarez V, Perez R, Fresno MF, Perez MJ, Sampedro A, Coto E. Mutation analysis of the p53, APC, and p16 genes in the Barrett's oesophagus, dysplasia, and adenocarcinoma. J Clin Pathol 1997;50(3):212-7.

145. Fitzgerald R, Onwuegbusi B, Saeed I, Burnham W, Farthing M. Characterisation of the inflammatory response in Barrett's oesophagus: implications for the disease pathogenesis and complications. Gastroenterology 1999;116(4):A158.

146. Fitzgerald R, Onwuegbusi B, Saeed I, Burnham W, Farthing M. Differential degree of inflammation and cytokine expression in distal compared with proximal Barrett's oesophagus may explain site specific complications. Gastroenterology 1999;116(4): A402.

147. Mendes de Almeida JC, Chaves P, Pereira AD, Altorki NK. Is Barrett's esophagus the precursor of most adenocarcinomas of the esophagus and cardia? A biochemical study. Ann Surg 1997;226(6): 725-33.

1.3   NORMAL PHYSIOLOGY OF THE ESOPHAGUS

Piero M.A. Fisichella and Marco G. Patti

1.   INTRODUCTION

The esophagus is a muscular tube that extends from the level of the 6th cervical vertebra to the 11th thoracic vertebra. *Anatomically*, three different regions can be identified: the cervical esophagus, the thoracic esophagus and the abdominal esophagus. *Functionally*, the esophagus can be divided in 3 areas: the upper esophageal sphincter (UES), the esophageal body, and the lower esophageal sphincter (LES). The coordinated activity of these 3 areas is essential to ensure propulsion of the alimentary bolus from the pharynx into the stomach. In addition, each sphincter has a key role in controlling reflux from the stomach into the esophagus (LES), and from the esophagus into the pharynx and the airway (UES).

2. UPPER ESOPHAGEAL SPHINCTER

The UES is located at the level of C6-C7, and it is considered the upper border of the esophagus. It is composed of the cricopharyngeus muscle, the inferior constrictors of the pharynx, and the cervical esophagus[1]. Embryologically these muscles derive from the branchial clefts and, therefore, differ from the somatic striated muscles present anywhere in the human body[2]. The cricopharyngeus muscle is innervated by the following nerves: (a) the vagus nerve with its branches (pharyngo-esophageal, superior laryngeal nerve and inferior laryngeal nerve); (b) the glossopharyngeal nerve; and (c) the cervical sympathetics. Only the pharyngo-esophageal and the superior laryngeal nerve provide motor fibers. The glossopharyngeal nerve provides sensory fibers. No functional innervation by the inferior laryngeal nerve has been identified[3]. The UES is tonically contracted at rest, secondary to the vagal activity of the nucleus ambiguus[4]. Because of the slit-like configuration of the sphincter, the pressure recorded by esophageal manometry is higher in the antero-posterior axis (100 mmHg) than in the lateral axis (50 mmHg). When a swallow occurs, the action of the mylohyoid, styloglossus, hyoglossus muscles displaces the cricoid and the hyoid bone upward and anteriorly, forcing the bolus into the pharynx. The soft palate is pulled upward, closing the posterior nares. The epiglottis moves backward to close the larynx, therefore avoiding passage of food into the tracheobronchial tree. Respiration temporarily ceases, and the UES relaxes, thus opening the esophageal inlet. As soon as the bolus reaches the esophagus, the UES pressure is promptly reestablished (Fig. 1).

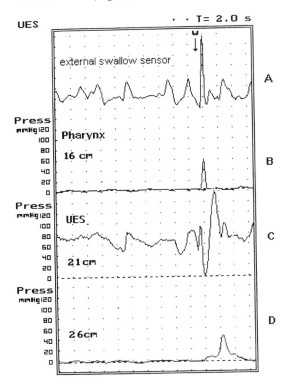

Figure 1. Upper esophageal sphincter.
A.   External swallow sensor
B.   Pharyngeal contraction
C.   Resting UES pressure and relaxation
D.   Peristaltic wave 5 cm below UES

The resting tone of the UES is also important to protect the tracheobronchial tree, as the sphincter is the last barrier to aspiration of gastric refluxate. It has been shown that UES pressure is increased by a decrease in intraluminal pH or by intraluminal distension[5,6]. Patients with respiratory symptoms due to aspiration of gastric contents often have a panesophageal motor disorder characterized by a hypotensive LES, abnormal esophageal peristalsis, and a hypotensive UES[7].

51

H.W. Tilanus and S.E.A. Attwood (eds.), Barrett's Esophagus, 51–55.
© 2001 *Kluwer Academic Publishers. Printed in the Netherlands.*

2. ESOPHAGEAL BODY

The esophageal body is a muscular tube limited by the UES superiorly and by the LES inferiorly. The musculature of the esophageal body is composed by striated muscle proximally and by smooth muscle distally. The muscle fibers progressively blend in the middle esophagus. The fibers are organized in an inner circular layer and an outer longitudinal layer. A nerve network, the *myenteric plexus of Auerbach*, is located between the longitudinal and the circular muscle layers. A second nerve network, *Meissner's plexus*, is located between the muscularis mucosa and the circular muscle layer. The striated muscle is controlled by excitatory vagal innervation only, with the entire control located in the Swallowing Center in the medulla. The vagus also controls the smooth muscle, but the vagal fibers synapse on the neurons of the Auerbach plexus rather than directly at the neuromuscular junction. In addition, vagal stimulation can either excite or inhibit the esophageal smooth muscle. Sympathectomy of the esophagus has no effect on peristalsis. The smooth muscle has also an intrinsic control regulated by the myenteric plexus[8]. Two main types of neurons are present within the myenteric plexus: (1) excitatory neurons, which control contraction of the longitudinal and circular muscle layers through cholinergic receptors; and (2) inhibitory neurons which control mainly the circular layer through non-adrenergic, non-cholinergic (NANC) neurotransmitters, such as vasoactive intestinal polypeptide (VIP) and nitric oxide (NO)[9,10].

Unlike the sphincters, the esophageal body has no motor activity in the resting state. When the food passes through the UES, a contraction wave (*primary peristalsis*) is initiated in the upper esophagus and progresses distally towards the stomach. Each peristaltic wave travels at a speed of about 3-4 cm/second, and reaches a peak amplitude of about 100 mmHg in the distal esophagus (Fig. 2).

While primary peristalsis is initiated by swallowing, secondary peristalsis results from stimulation of sensory receptors in the esophageal body, either by food non-completely cleared by the primary peristalsis or by gastroesophageal reflux. These waves begin at the site of the stimulation and move distally[11]. Tertiary waves are non-propulsive contractions, which can occur at any level in the esophagus and have no physiologic function.

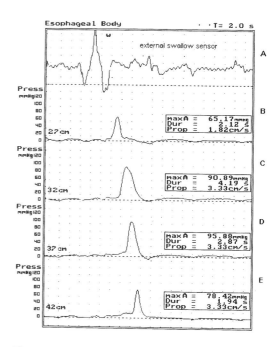

Figure 2. Esophageal peristalsis. Esophageal peristalsis was recorded using 4 sensors, positioned at 18 cm (B), 13 cm (C), 8 cm (D) and 3 cm (E) above the upper border of the LES. A. External swallow sensor.

They are seen often in patients with primary esophageal motility disorders and in elderly patients.

Some abnormalities of esophageal peristalsis are well characterized and constitute the *Primary Esophageal Motility Disorders* (achalasia, diffuse esophageal spasm, nutcracker esophagus, hypertensive LES)[11]. In other patients, however, esophageal manometry shows low amplitude of peristalsis, abnormal morphology (triple peaks) or propagation of the peristaltic waves (simultaneous contractions). These abnormalities are usually referred to as *Non Specific Esophageal Motility Disorders* (NSEMD), and they are seen particularly in patients with gastroesophageal reflux disease (GERD). NSEMD may play a role in symptoms experienced by the patients, but also in the clearance of refluxed gastric contents. About 30% of patients with GERD experience dysphagia in the absence of an esophageal stricture. This form of dysphagia is referred to as *Non Obstructive Dysphagia*, and is due to abnormalities of the peristalsis (simultaneous contractions) present during swallowing of food. As these abnormalities are present at the time of a meal, ambulatory rather than stationary esophageal manometry is the ideal test to identify their presence, as it records about 1000 swallows over a 24-hour period[13]. Interestingly, control of the abnormal reflux by a fundoplication effectively resolves this symptoms as well as heartburn and regurgitation[14].

Esophageal peristalsis is also a key determinant of esophageal acid clearance. It has been shown that patients with esophagitis often have abnormal esophageal peristalsis, and that peristaltic dysfunction prolongs esophageal acid clearance. Kahrilas and colleagues studied the effect of peristaltic dysfunction on volume clearance by simultaneous videofluoroscopic and manometric recording[15]. They showed that hypotensive peristalsis ($\leq$ 25 mm Hg in the distal esophagus; $\leq$ 12 mm Hg in the proximal esophagus) was associated with incomplete volume clearance. We found that patients with impaired peristalsis were exposed to more proximal extent of the gastric refluxate (*high gastroesophageal reflux*) and that acid clearance was slower both in the distal and proximal esophagus[16]. In addition, they had a higher incidence of respiratory symptoms probably due to aspiration of gastric contents into the tracheobronchial tree. Recently the term of *Ineffective Esophageal Peristalsis* has been used to indicate abnormal peristalsis characterized by distal esophageal amplitude of less than 30 mmHg and/or more than 30% simultaneous waves[17,18]. Patients with Barrett's esophagus often have very poor peristalsis, suggesting that there is an inverse relationship between the effectiveness of peristalsis and the degree of mucosal injury observed at endoscopy[19]. Therefore, Barrett's metaplasia could be considered an "end stage form of GERD", probably due to fibrosis of the esophageal wall secondary to the continuous exposure to gastric contents[20]. The quality of peristalsis (as determined by esophageal manometry) should be taken into consideration when planning surgical therapy, as a partial fundoplication should probably be used whenever the "pump" action of the esophageal body is severely compromised such in patients with ineffective esophageal peristalsis.

3. LOWER ESOPHAGEAL SPHINCTER

The sphincter mechanism at the level of gastroesophageal junction plays a key role in allowing passage of food from the esophageal body into the stomach, and in controlling reflux of gastric contents into the esophagus. The sphincter mechanism has two components: an *intrinsic* component, made up by the smooth muscle of the LES, and an *extrinsic* component provided by the right crus of the diaphragm[8].

4. INTRINSIC SPHINCTER

The LES is a tonically contracted segment of smooth muscle, about 3 to 4 cm long. The sphincter has a normal resting pressure ranging between 15 and 24 mm Hg; three-dimensional mapping has shown slight asymmetry of the pressure profile, although less than what is seen in the UES[22]. At the time of a swallow the LES relaxes for 5 to 10 seconds to allow passage of food from the esophagus into the stomach and then regains its resting tone (Fig. 3).

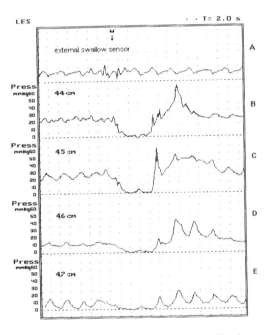

Figure 3. Lower esophageal sphincter. A "staggered" catheter is used to measure LES pressure and relaxation. Four sensor are located at 90° angles, and at 1 cm distance from each other (B, C, D, E). The distance (44 to 47 cm) is measured from the nostrils. Each tracing shows the resting LES pressure and its relaxation in response to swallowing (W).

The resting tone of the sphincter depends mainly on the intrinsic myogenic activity, as it persists even after neural input is abolished by treatment with the neurotoxin tetrodotoxin[23]. Similar to the stomach and the small bowel, during the fasting state the LES shows a cyclic phasic contractile activity which is synchronous with phases II and III of the interdigestive motor complex[24,25]. This is probably regulated by motilin, which acts on the LES by preganglionic stimulation of cholinergic nerves[26].

The relaxation of the sphincter is due to the interplay of excitatory substances such as acetylcholine and substance P, and inhibitory non-adrenergic, non-cholinergic neuro-transmitters such as nitric oxide and vasoactive intestinal polypeptide[27-29]. This balance is lost in achalasia because of the lack of the inhibitory component, resulting in a hypertensive LES, which relaxes only partially in response to swallowing[30].

In addition to its length and resting pressure[31-33], the LES is characterized by its tendency to relax periodically and independently from swallowing[34-37]. These periodic relaxations are called *transient lower esophageal sphincter relaxations* to distinguish them from relaxations due to swallowing. The factors responsible for transient LES relaxation are unknown, but post-prandial gastric distension probably plays an important role[38,39]. Transient LES relaxation accounts for the small amount of physiologic gastroesophageal reflux present in any individual, and is also the most common cause of reflux in patients with GERD[35]. Decrease in length and/or pressure of the LES is responsible for abnormal reflux in the remaining patients[31-33]. Overall, it is thought that while transient LES relaxation is the most common mechanism of reflux in volunteers and patients with either absent of mild esophagitis, the prevalence of a mechanically defective sphincter (hypotensive and short) would increase in patients with severe esophagitis[34]. A Nissen fundoplication controls gastroesophageal reflux by correcting the functional and mechanical abnormalities of the LES. It has been shown in fact, that a 360° fundoplication not only increases the length and resting pressure of the LES, but it also decreases the frequency and extent of transient LES relaxation[40].

5. EXTRINSIC SPHINCTER

The diaphragm has a synergistic role with the LES, as it increases LES pressure. While the end-expiratory resting pressure recorded during esophageal manometry is due to the intrinsic component of the LES, the oscillations in LES pressure are due to contractions of the diaphragm[41]. The increase in pressure is proportional to the force of the diaphragmatic contraction as measured by electromyography, varying from 10 to 20 mm Hg during quite inspiration to 50 to 100 mm Hg with deep inspiration[42,43]. This *pinchcock* action of the diaphragm is particularly important as it protects against reflux caused by sudden increases of intra-abdominal pressure such as with coughing or bending[42]. The synergistic action of the diaphragm is lost when a sliding hiatal hernia is present, as the gastroesophageal junction is displaced above the diaphragm. While in the absence of a hiatal hernia esophageal manometry records the presence of only one high-pressure zone, a "double hump" can be observed in the tracing in the presence of a large hernia: the first increase in pressure is due to the action of the crus on the gastric wall, and the second to the LES resting pressure. In patients with GERD, hiatal hernia size affects LES function, esophageal acid exposure, and the degree of mucosal injury. Patti and colleagues showed that patients with either a small hiatal hernia or without hiatal hernia had similar abnormalities of LES function and acid clearance. Instead, in patients with larger hernias the LES was shorter and weaker, the amount of reflux was greater, and acid clearance was less efficient. Consequently, the degree of esophagitis was worse in patients with a large hiatal hernia[44].

REFERENCES

1.   Lang IM, Shaker R. Anatomy and physiology of the upper esophageal sphincter. Am. J. Med. 1997;103 (5A):50S-55S.
2.   Pope CE II. The esophagus for the nonesophagologist. Am. J. Med. 1997;103:19S-22S.
3.   Medda BK, Lang IM, Dodds WJ, Christl M, Kern M, Hogan WJ, Shaker R. Correlations of electrical and contractile activities of the cricopharyngeus muscle in the cat. Am. J. Physiol. 1997;273:G470-G479.
4.   Castell DO. Anatomy and physiology of the esophagus and its sphincters. In:Castell DO, Richter JE, Boag

Dalton C (Eds):Esophageal motility testing. New York, Elsevier Science, 1987, 13-27.
5.   Gerhardt DC, Shuck TJ, Bordeaux RA, Winship DH. Upper esophageal sphincter:response to volume, osmotic and acid stimuli. Gastroenterology 1978;75:268-74.
6.   Enzmann DR, Harrell GS, Zboralske FF. Upper esophageal responses to intraluminal distention in man. Gastroenterology 1977;72:1292-8.
7.   Patti MG, Debas HT, Pellegrini CA. Esophageal manometry and 24 hour pH monitoring in the diagnosis

of pulmonary aspiration secondary to gastroesophageal reflux. Am. J. Surg. 1992;163:401-6.

8. Patti MG, Gantert W, Way LW. Surgery of the esophagus. Anatomy and physiology. Surg. Clin. North Am. 1997;77:959-70.

9. Preiksaitis HG, Tremblay L, Diamant NE. Nitric oxide mediates inhibitory nerve effects in human esophagus and lower esophageal sphincter. Dig. Dis. Sci. 1994;39:770-5.

10. Singaram C, Sengupta A, Sugarbaker DJ, Goyal RK. Peptidergic innervation of the human esophageal smooth muscle. Gastroenterology 1991;101(5):1256-63.

11. Kahrilas PJ. Functional anatomy and physiology of the esophagus. In Castell DO (Ed):The Esophagus. Boston, Little & Brown Co., 1992, 1-27.

12. Patti MG, Way LW. Evaluation and treatment of primary esophageal motility disorders. West. J. Med. 1997;166:263-9.

13. Triadafilopoulos T. Nonobstructive dysphagia in reflux esophagitis. Am. J. gastroenterol. 1989;84:614-8.

14. Patti MG, Feo CV, De Pinto M, Arverito M, Tong J, Gantert W, Tyrrell D, Way LW. Results of laparoscopic antireflux surgery for dysphagia and gastroesophageal reflux disease. Am. J. Surg. 1998;176:564-8.

15. Kahrilas PJ, Dodds WJ, Hogan WJ. Effect of peristaltic dysfunction on esophageal volume clearance. Gastroenterology 1988;994:73-80.

16. Patti MG, Debas HT, Pellegrini CA. Clinical and functional characterisation of high gastroesophageal reflux. Am. J. Surg. 1993;165:163-8.

17. Leite LP, Johnston BT, Barrett J, Castell JA, Castell DO. Ineffective esophageal motility (IEM):the primary finding in patients with non-specific esophageal motility disorders. Dig. Dis. Sci. 1997;42:1859-65.

18. Fouad YM, Katz PO, Hatlebackk JG, Castell DO. Ineffective esophageal motility:the most common motility abnormality in patients with GERD-associated respiratory symptoms. Am. J. Gastroenterol. 1999;94:1464-7.

19. Stein HJ, Barlow AP, DeMeester TR, Hinder RA. Complications of gastroesophageal reflux disease. Role of the lower esophageal sphincter, esophageal acid and acid/alkaline exposure, and duodenogastric reflux. Ann. Surg. 1992;216:35-43.

20. Stein HJ, Hoeft S, DeMeester TR. Functional foregut abnormalities in Barrett's esophagus. J. Thorac. Cardiovasc. Surg. 1993;105:107-11.

21. Patti MG, Arcerito M, Feo CV, De Pinto M, Tong J, Gantert W, Tyrrell D, Way LW. Analysis of operations for GERD. The important elements must be identified. Arch. Surg. 1998;133:600-7.

22. Stein HJ, Liebermann-Meffert D, DeMeester TR, Siewert JR. Three-dimensional pressure image and muscular structure of the human LES. Surgery 1995;117:692-8.

23. Goyal RK, Rattan S. Genesis of basal sphincter pressure. Effect of tetrodotoxin on the lower esophageal sphincter. Gastroenterology 1976;71:62-7.

24. Dent J, Dodds WJ, Skiguchi T. et al. Interdigestive phasic contractions of the human lower esophageal sphincter. Gastroenterology 1983;84:453-60.

25. Holloway RH, Blank E, Takahashi J et al. Variability of the lower esophageal sphincter pressure in the fasted unanesthetized opossum. Am. J. Physiol. 1985;248:398-406.

26. Holloway RH, Blank E, Takahashi J et al. Motilin:A mechanism incorporating the opossum lower esophageal sphincter into the migrating motor complex. Gastroenterology 1985;89:507-15.

27. Aggestrup S, Uddman R, Jensen SL, Hakanson R, Sundler F, Schaffalitzky de Muckadell O. Emson P. Regulatory peptides in lower esophageal sphincter of pig and man. Dig. Dis. Sci. 1986;31:1370-5.

28. Dodds WJ, Dent J, Hogan WJ, Arndorfer RC. Effect of atropine on esophageal motor function in humans. Am. J. Physiol. 1981;240:G290-G296.

29. Boulant J, Fioramonti J, Dapoigny M, Bommelaer G, Bueno L. Cholecystokinin and nitric oxide in transient lower esophageal sphincter relaxation to gastric distention in dogs. Gastroenterology 1994;107:1059-66.

30. Aggestrup S, Uddman R, Sundler F, Fahrenkrug J, Hakanson R, Sorensen HR, Hambraeus G. Lack of vasoactive intestinal polypeptide nerves in esophageal achalasia. Gastroenterology 1983;84:924-7.

31. Bonavina L, Evander A, DeMeester TR, Walther B, Cheng SC, Palazzo L, Concannon JL. Length of the distal esophageal sphincter and competency of the cardia. Am. J. Surg. 1986;151:25-34.

32. O'Sullivan GC, DeMeester TR, Joelsson BE, Smith RB, Blough RR, Johnson LF, Skinner DB. The interaction of the LES pressure and length of sphincter in the abdomen as determinants of gastroesophageal competence. Am. J. Surg. 1982;143:40-7.

33. Zaninotto G, DeMeester TR, Schwizer W, Johansonn KE, Cheng SC. The lower esophageal sphincter in health and disease. Am. J. Surg. 1988;155:104-11.

34. Dent J, Hollaway RH, Toouli J, Dodds WJ. Mechanisms of lower esophageal sphincter incompetence in patients with symptomatic gastroesophageal reflux. Gut 1988;29:1020-8.

35. Dodds GK, Egide MS. Mechanisms of gastroesophageal reflux in patients with reflux esophagitis. N. Engl. J. Med. 1982;307:1547-52.

36. Mittal RK, McCallum RW. Characteristics and frequency of transient relaxations of the lower esophageal sphincter in patients with reflux esophagitis. Gastroenterology 1988;95:593-9.

37. Schoeman MN, Tippett MD, Akkermans LMA, Dent J, Hollaway RH. Mechanisms of gastroesophageal reflux in ambulant healthy human subjects. Gastroenterology 1995;108:83-91.

38. Hollaway RH, Hongo M, Berger K, McCallum RW. Gastric distention:A mechanism for postprandial gastroesophageal reflux. Gastroenterology 1985;89:779-84.

39. Hollaway RH, Kocyan P, Dent J. Provocation of transient lower esophageal sphincter relaxations by meals in patients with symptomatic gastroesophageal reflux. Dig. Dis. Sci. 1001;36:1034-9.

40. Ireland AC, Holloway RH, Toouli J, Dent J. Mechanisms underlying the antireflux action of fundoplication. Gut 1993;34:303-8.

41. Boyle JT, Altsculer SM, Nixon TE, Tuchman DN, Pack AI, Cohen S. Role of the diaphragm in the genesis of lower esophageal sphincter pressure in the cat. Gastroenterology 1985;88:723-30.

42. Mittal RK, Rochester DF, McCallum RW. Effect of the diaphragmatic contraction on lower esophageal sphincter pressure in man. Gut 1987;28:1564-8.

43. Mittal RK, Rochester DF, McCallum RW. Electrical and mechanical activity in the human LES during diaphragmatic contraction. J. Clin. Invest. 1988;81:1182-9.

44. Patti MG, Goldberg H, Arcerito M, Bortolasi L, Tong J, Way LW. Hiatal hernia size affects lower esophageal sphincter function, esophageal acid exposure, and the degree of mucosal injury. Am. J. Surg. 1996;171:182-6.

1.4 PATHOPHYSIOLOGY OF GASTRO-ESOPHAGEAL REFLUX DISEASE

André J.P.M. Smout

1. INTRODUCTION

Barrett's esophagus, defined as the presence of columnar metaplastic epithelium in the distal tubular esophagus over a length of more than 2 to 3 centimeter, is usually considered a complication of long-standing gastro-esophageal reflux disease (GERD) [1-9].
The arguments in favor of this concept are numerous. In dogs, induction of excessive gastro-esophageal reflux by means of surgical destruction of the gastro-esophageal junction leads to replacement of squamous esophageal epithelium by columnar epithelium [10]. In man, numerous studies using 24-hour ambulatory esophageal pH measurements have shown that patients with Barrett's esophagus have an increased esophageal acid exposure when compared to controls or to patients with mild reflux disease [1,11-16]. Patients with Barrett's esophagus and patients with severe esophagitis have similar levels of esophageal acid exposure [15,16]. It is unclear whether patients with Barrett's esophagus and complications thereof, such as ulceration or stricture, have esophageal acid exposures which are similar to those found in uncomplicated Barrett's esophagus and in severe esophagitis [3,4,13]. In one study the increase in total reflux time found in patients with Barrett's esophagus was found not to be caused by more frequent reflux episodes, but rather by an increase in the duration of the reflux episodes, resulting in a significantly increased number of reflux periods lasting longer than 5 minutes [13]. In another study, however, an increased number of periods with a duration of longer than 5 minutes was only found in the supine position [11], whereas our own observations indicate that both an increased incidence and a prolonged duration of reflux episodes are responsible for the excessive acid exposure in patients with Barrett's esophagus.
Thus, the available information indicates that Barrett's esophagus is associated with abnormal esophageal acid exposure, but the differences in acid exposure between severe esophagitis, uncomplicated and complicated Barrett's esophagus, if any, are small.
The pathophysiological processes that lead to increased esophageal acid exposure in Barrett's esophagus have not been the subject of many studies. However, if one accepts that Barrett's

esophagus is a manifestation of GERD, the numerous studies on the pathophysiology of GERD may also be considered relevant to Barrett's esophagus. This is the view that was taken in this chapter, which will focus on the pathophysiology of the lower esophageal sphincter and adjacent structures. In addition, some of the other mechanisms involved in the pathophysiology of GERD will be summarized. The role of the nature of the refluxate will be discussed in more detail elsewhere in this book.

2. COMPONENTS OF THE ANTI-REFLUX BARRIER

The key factor in the pathogenesis of GERD and Barrett's esophagus is a defective anti-reflux barrier at the esophagogastric junction. This barrier is composed of at least two structures: the lower esophageal sphincter (LES) and the crural diaphragm. According to traditional teaching, a third factor is formed by the anatomical configuration of the gastric cardia in the form of a relatively sharp angle between the distal esophagus and the gastric fundus, the angle of His (Figure 1).

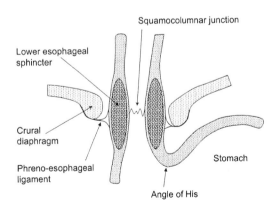

Figure 1. Anatomy of normal esophagogastric junction. The LES is surrounded by the right diaphragmatic crus. The distal esophagus is attached to the crus by means of the phreno-esophageal ligaments.

Under normal circumstances, i.e. in the absence of a hiatus hernia, the right crus of the diaphragm surrounds the LES and these two structures act in synergy. To a certain extent this configuration can be compared with that of the

H.W. Tilanus and S.E.A. Attwood (eds.), Barrett's Esophagus, 57–70.

internal and external anal sphincters. Over the years several swings of opinion on the role of each of these three components of the anti-reflux barrier (LES, diaphragm and angle of His) have taken place. Relatively little new information on the angle of His has become available in the last decennium. In contrast, new investigational techniques such as prolonged manometry have yielded important new insights about the function of the LES and the crural diaphragm.

3. TECHNIQUES FOR EVALUATION OF THE ANTIREFLUX BARRIER IN MAN

There are several investigational techniques with which information about the antireflux barrier in living human beings can be obtained. None of these techniques by itself provides a complete picture and all available techniques have obvious limitations.

Radiography and endoscopy provide information about the position of the esophagogastric junction with respect to the diaphragm. In other words, these techniques are suitable for demonstration of a hiatus hernia. Otherwise, radiography and endoscopy have little or nothing to offer in the assessment of the function of the antireflux barrier. Some radiologists believe that the ability to provoke gastro-esophageal reflux during a radiographic study of the esophagus is of clinical value, but there is no evidence to support this view. Radiological studies have been found to detect reflux in only 30% of GERD patients with pathological reflux as measured by 24-hour pH recording[17]. The same can be said about the belief maintained by some endoscopists that LES function can be assessed by endoscopic observation of the "tightness" with which the sphincter surrounds the endoscope.

Gastro-esophageal reflux can be quantified by radionuclide studies, in which reflux is monitored after ingestion of radioactively labeled material (e.g. acidified water). Various provocation maneuvers can be carried out. Although the technique is non-invasive and involves minimal radiation exposure, its value for the detection of reflux has been questioned because of its low sensitivity[18]. Furthermore, scintigraphy does not provide direct information about the function of the LES and crural diaphragm, but, at best, allows assessment of the consequences of a weakened barrier.

Ambulatory 24-hour esophageal pH monitoring is considered by many as the gold standard for the assessment of gastro-esophageal reflux. Obviously this technique is of less value when

gastric acidity is diminished (by use of acid secretion inhibitors, after meals and after partial gastrectomy or vagotomy). As discussed for scintigraphy, pH monitoring does not provide information about the function of the antireflux barrier as such.

Beyond doubt, manometry is the most important technique for evaluation of LES and diaphragmatic contributions to the antireflux barrier. Manometry can either be performed by water-perfused tube assemblies connected to external pressure transducers or by solid-state catheters in which microtransducers are incorporated.

All conventional manometric techniques share the disadvantage that movements of the sphincteric complex with respect to the transducers, in particular during breathing and swallowing, render prolonged monitoring of the intraluminal pressure within the high pressure zone difficult, if not impossible. To overcome this problem, specialized sensors have been developed. The perfused sleeve sensor developed by Dent is generally considered to be the best device for prolonged sphincter recording. The sensor consists of a membrane under which the perfusion fluid flows. As a consequence, the perfused sleeve measures the highest pressure exerted on any point of the membrane[19]. Other, non-perfused, sphinctometer devices record the mean pressure of all pressures exerted on the membrane[20], which is considered a serious disadvantage. When non-specialized manometric catheters are used, basal sphincter pressure is usually measured with the so-called stationary pull-through technique. During this procedure the catheter is withdrawn at regular time intervals over distances of 0.5-1 cm. This technique allows us to assess the length of the sphincter, the length of the intra-abdominal and intrathoracic segments, basal sphincter pressure and swallow-related relaxations of the sphincter (Figure 2). During the stationary pull-through maneuver one typically sees an increase in the amplitude of the respiration-associated phasic pressure variations when the measuring port is in the high-pressure zone. These are brought about by contractions of the crural diaphragm. Approximately at the midpoint of the high-pressure zone the polarity of these phasic pressure variations changes. In the distal part of the high-pressure zone inspiration is associated with an increase in pressure, in the proximal part inspiration gives rise to a pressure decrease. The point at which polarity changes is called the 'pressure inversion point' (Figure 2). This point marks the boundary between the intra-

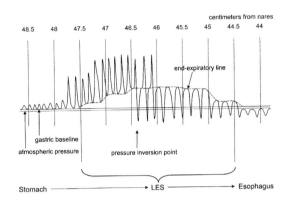

Figure 2. Manometric signal recorded during a stationary pull-through maneuver (schematic). The catheter is withdrawn in steps of 0.5 cm. When the pressure sensor enters the high-pressure zone the amplitude of the respiration-associated peaks increases. At about the midpoint of the sphincter the polarity of the respiratory peaks changes (pressure inversion point), indicating transition from the intra-abdominal to the intrathoracic part of the sphincter.

abdominal and intrathoracic parts of the sphincter. Basal sphincter pressure is measured with respect to intragastric pressure. This can be done in three ways. Most commonly the end-expiratory points in the pressure curve are used (Figure 2), but end-inspiratory and mid-inspiratory pressures can also be taken. The end-expiratory sphincter pressure is thought to represent tonic LES pressure. Alternatively, one may use the so-called rapid pull-through technique to measure sphincter pressure. In this technique the catheter is rapidly pulled through the gastro-esophageal junction during an episode of halted respiration, preferably using a mechanical puller device. This technique does not allow determination of the pressure inversion point, the intra-abdominal and intrathoracic parts and sphincter relaxations. For these reasons, the technique is not used in many laboratories. It should be noted that all manometric techniques measure a pressure within the esophagogastric junction which is the resultant of the LES and the surrounding diaphragmatic crus. Almost without exception the term 'LES pressure' is used to denote the tonic pressure measured in the high-pressure zone, as if there were no contribution of the diaphragm to this pressure. As will be discussed later, even in the presence of a hiatus hernia, when the diaphragmatic crus no longer surrounds the LES, the contributions of the LES and the diaphragm to manometric readings can usually not be separated. However, in order to

avoid further confusion, in this chapter the *pars pro toto* term 'LES pressure' will be used as it is in the literature. The puritanists among the readers may read it as 'end-expiratory basal pressure in the high-pressure zone at the esophagogastric junction'.

4. THE LOWER ESOPHAGEAL SPHINCTER

This sphincter is characterized anatomically and manometrically as a 3 to 4-cm long zone of specialized smooth muscle which maintains a tonic activity. The endexpiratory pressure in the sphincter is 8-20 mmHg above the endexpiratory gastric pressure. If a pressure barrier were not present, reflux would occur with many of the inspiratory movements, since intra-abdominal pressure rises and intrathoracic pressure falls with each inspiration. Under normal circumstances, i.e. in the absence of columnar metaplasia, the highest pressure is found at the squamo-columnar junction[21]. In man, the major component of neurogenic control of tonic LES pressure is mediated by cholinergic nerves, since basal LES pressure can be reduced by 70% by atropine[22]. The LES is kept in place by the phreno-esophageal ligament which forms a sheath around the esophagus, anchoring its most distal end to the diaphragm (Figure 1). Nevertheless, during respiratory movements minor variations in the position of the LES occur: during inspiration the LES slides upwards with respect to the hiatus. Under normal circumstances the distal 2 centimeters of the LES lie below the hiatus and therefore within the abdominal cavity (Figure 1). It is thought that during abdominal straining this segment of the sphincter is exposed to intra-abdominal pressure and, as a consequence, the LES pressure is augmented. The hypothesis that a sufficiently long intra-abdominal segment of the sphincter is of importance in preventing gastro-esophageal reflux has gained popularity, in particular among surgeons. For many years, a chronically decreased basal LES pressure was considered to be the most important factor in the pathogenesis of GERD. This view could only be maintained by ignoring the existence of a considerable overlap in LES pressure between patients with GERD and normal subjects[23]. Although, on average, LES pressure is significantly decreased in patients with severe or complicated reflux disease, many healthy individuals without GERD have a low LES pressure and patients with milder forms of GERD often have normal LES pressure [23-25]. Controversy still exists as to whether lowered

LES tone is the cause or the result of chronic reflux. In laboratory animals the induction of esophagitis leads to a decrease in LES pressure, suggesting that the hypotension of the LES found in GERD may be secondary to the mucosal inflammation[26]. On the other hand, studies in humans have shown that healing of reflux esophagitis is not associated with a significant improvement of LES pressure[25,27,28]. However, the latter observations do not disprove the hypothesis that LES malfunction in GERD is secondary to the inflammation since the damage may have been irreversible. In contrast to popular belief, the pressure in the LES is far from stable and considerable minute-to-minute variations in LES pressure occur. Using prolonged manometry with a sleeve sensor, large variations related to the interdigestive migrating motor complex (MMC) were found[29,30], the LES pressure being lowest during phase I (motor quiescence) and highest during phase III (activity front) of the MMC. This participation of the LES in the MMC has been thought to prevent reflux during late phase II and phase III[29]. However, others have reported that in the fasting state reflux episodes are significantly more frequent during presence of phase II and phase III in the antrum. As many as 95% of the nocturnal reflux episodes are associated with interdigestive gastric motor activity[31]. It is as yet unclear whether impaired LES involvement in the MMC plays a role in the pathogenesis of GERD. About two decades ago studies using prolonged LES pressure monitoring revealed that both in GERD patients and in healthy subjects spontaneous transient relaxations of the LES (TLESRs) are the most prevalent mechanism of gastro-esophageal reflux[32]. This discovery caused a major shift in our view on the role of the LES in the pathophysiology of GERD, from a static towards a more dynamic one.

5. TRANSIENT LES RELAXATIONS

Transient LES relaxations (TLESRs) occur spontaneously, i.e. they are not preceded by a swallow. These "inappropriate" relaxations last longer (10-45 sec) than swallow-associated relaxations (5-8 sec) and often are deeper (i.e. nadir pressure is lower) than swallow-induced relaxations (Figure 3). TLESRs constitute the mechanism through which gas can escape from the stomach during the process of belching. To some extent they serve as the safety valve of the stomach. It has been shown that distension of the proximal stomach, by inflation of a balloon, by free air or gas or by a meal, is the most

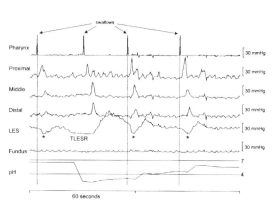

Figure 3. Transient LES relaxation, recorded with a perfused Dent sleeve. Note that the TLESR is not swallow-induced and that it lasts considerably longer than the swallow-associated relaxations (indicated with *).

important trigger for TLESR induction[33,34].
By dividing the canine stomach in different compartments, it was shown that the cardiac region of the stomach is the most sensitive part[35]. In addition to TLESRs so-called swallow-associated prolonged LES relaxations can be distinguished. The latter fulfill all of the criteria for TLESRs but they are preceded by a swallow. (Figure 4)

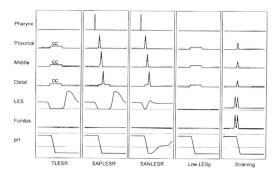

Figure 4. Scheme of the 5 most common reflux mechanisms. A TLESR is a deep and prolonged relaxation that is not associated with a swallow. A swallow-associated prolonged LES relaxation (SAP LESR) probably constitutes a TLESR that is incidentally associated with a swallow. Reflux can also occur during a swallow-associated normal LES relaxation (SAN LESR) during periods with low LES pressure (Low LESp) and during straining which increases intra-abdominal pressure. During prolonged LES relaxations associated with reflux a "common cavity (cc)" phenomenon is usually observed in the esophageal body tracings.

It is felt to be most likely that most of the swallow-associated prolonged LES relaxations are in fact TLESRs, i.e. that the association between the swallow and the prolonged relaxation occurs by chance. TLESRs constitute the single most common mechanism underlying reflux, both in GERD patients and in healthy individuals. Some studies have shown that patients with GERD have an increased incidence of TLESRs[32,36]. However, this could not be confirmed in another study[34]. More importantly, the percentage of TLESRs associated with reflux is higher in patients with reflux disease (60-70%) than in normal subjects (40-60%)[24,37]. Interestingly, the proportion of reflux episodes resulting from TLESRs decreases with increasing severity of reflux disease: in healthy volunteers and in patients without endoscopic evidence of esophagitis, reflux occurs exclusively during TLESRs, whereas in patients with erosive esophagitis about 2/3 of reflux episodes occur by this mechanism[24,32,36,38]. In the latter other reflux mechanisms occur more frequently, such as reflux during a swallow-associated normal LES relaxation, reflux during periods with low LES pressure and reflux during straining (Figure 4)[24,39]. Postprandial gastric distension and TLESR induction is the main mechanism for the postprandial increase in gastro-esophageal reflux seen in health and disease[33]. It has been shown that body position affects gastro-esophageal reflux, the right lateral decubitus position being associated with a greater esophageal acid exposure than the left lateral decubitus position. This phenomenon was found to exist both in healthy volunteers[40] and in patients with GERD[41]. In order to elucidate the mechanism underlying this phenomenon we carried out a study using prolonged LES pressure monitoring[42]. This study in healthy volunteers showed that after a high-fat meal the incidence of TLESRs was 6.5 per hour in the right recumbent position versus 3.2 per hour in the left recumbent position. In addition it was found that TLESRs were associated with reflux more often in the right than in the left position (57.0 versus 22.4%). No effect of body position on pH at the gastric cardia and in the gastric corpus was found. Esophageal acid exposure was significantly higher in the right recumbent position (7.0%) than in the left recumbent position (2.0%) and the incidence of reflux episodes was about 4 times higher in the right recumbent position (3.8 versus 0.9 per hour). The increased incidence of TLESRs in the right recumbent position might be caused by the fact that in this position the subcardiac region is triggered more than in the left lateral position. Experiments with dogs have shown that the subcardiac region is the most sensitive part of the stomach for triggering TLESRs induced by

distension[35]. This hypothesis is in agreement with a fluoroscopic study showing that GERD patients positioned in the right lateral decubitus had barium pooled in the cardiac region, whereas in the left lateral decubitus barium was present in the dependent fundus and the cardiac region was in the air above the barium-air interface[43]. The observation that a higher percentage of TLESRs is associated with reflux in the right recumbent position, could be due to the fact that in the right recumbent position more fluid is available at the esophageal gastric junction, ready to reflux.

6. PHARMACOLOGY OF TLESRs

Vagal cooling abolishes the triggering of TLESRs, suggesting that TLESRs are mediated via a vago-vagal reflex[44]. Splanchnectomy has no effect on the incidence of TLESRs suggesting that orthosympathetic fibers are not involved in the process of TLESRs mediation. It is therefore likely that transient LES relaxations are mediated through tension receptors in the proximal stomach which are activated by gastric distention and that these receptors send signals to brainstem centers via afferent vagal fibers. These vagal afferents terminate in the nucleus tractus solitarius and dorsal motor nucleus of the vagal nerve. The efferent arm of the reflex is probably also in the vagus nerve and it is likely that this arm shares common elements with swallow-induced LES relaxation[45]. Inhibition of the crural diaphragm during TLESRs is most likely also mediated by the vagal nerve, although a recent study suggests the existence of a peripheral inhibitory pathway[46]. Various neurotransmitters appear to be involved in the neuronal reflex that leads to TLESRs. These neurotransmitters and their receptors are localized in the vagal afferent fibers, in the nucleus tractus solitarius and in the dorsal motor nucleus of the vagal nerve. Until today, studies have provided evidence for a role of acetylcholine, cholecystokinine (CCK), gamma-aminobutyric acid (GABA), glutamate, nitric oxide (NO) and opioids[47-51]. Anticholinergic agents, such as atropine, reduce the rate of TLESRs. The site of action of atropine is probably presumably central as the muscarinic antagonist metscopolamine bromide, which does not pass the blood brain barrier, does not reduce the rate of TLESRs[52]. The effect of opioids such as morphine may be located centrally, but it is also possible that a morphine-induced increase in intragastric tone plays a role. Blockade of nitric oxide synthesis, for instance by L-NMMA, inhibits transient

LES relaxations. The site at which nitric oxide plays a role is thought to be either central or at an afferent level. A peripheral effect is considered unlikely because inhibition of NO synthesis does not affect swallow-induced LES relaxation. One of the most exciting discoveries of the past few years is that GABA$_B$-agonists such as baclofen, are important inhibitors of TLESRs. The major site of action of GABA is thought to be central, as a peripherally selective GABA$_B$-agonist was found to have no effect on the rate of TLESRs. Glutamate is an important excitatory neurotransmitter in the central nervous system (nucleus tractus solitarius) and the most likely site of involvement is therefore a central one. Exogenous CCK increases the rate of TLESRs in response to gastric distention[49]. Stimulation of postprandial release of endogenous CCK by administration of cholestyramine increases the incidence of TLESRs[53]. Antagonists of the CCK$_A$ receptor, such as loxiglumide, diminish the incidence of TLESRs by about 40-50%. CCK neurotransmission is most likely to take place at the level of vagal afferent fibers, since intracerebroventricular administration of CCK$_A$ receptor antagonists does not modify the rate of TLESRs, whereas systemic administration does. The above-described knowledge of the neurotransmitters involved in the elicitation of TLESRs has given rise to hope that pharmacological therapy leading to reduction of TLESR incidence is within reach. As described above, morphine, atropine, the CCK$_A$ receptor antagonist loxiglumide, the GABA$_B$ agonist baclofen and the inhibitor of NO synthesis L-NMMA have been shown to reduce TLESR incidence. Because of their side-effects, however, none of these agents fulfils the criteria for a clinically useful drug. Attempts are being made to modify these substances in order to reduce their side-effects.

7. THE CRURAL DIAPHRAGM AND HIATUS HERNIA

In patients with a (sliding) hiatus hernia the two components of the antireflux barrier, i.e. the LES and the crural diaphragm, have become separated (Figure 5). It is unclear how hiatus hernias develop. Some suggest that reflux leads to esophageal shortening and that the stomach is pulled into the thorax by the esophagus. Others believe that there is a congenital or acquired weakness of the phreno-esophageal ligament that is the principal mechanism. Discussions about the role of hiatus hernia in the pathogenesis of GERD have been ongoing for

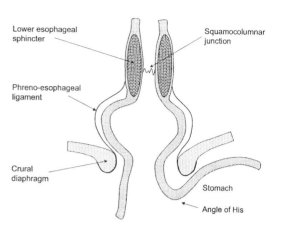

Figure 5. Anatomy of the esophagogastric junction in the presence of a hiatus hernia

several decades and the role ascribed to hiatus hernia has varied considerably over the years. At certain stages hiatus hernia and GERD were virtually considered synonyms, at other stages the role of hiatus hernia in the pathogenesis of reflux disease was almost denied. However, it is an incontrovertible fact that hiatus hernia is overrepresented in reflux disease. Several observations clearly indicate that an association exists between presence of a hiatus hernia, particularly when large, and severe esophagitis and Barrett's esophagus[54-56]. In addition, ambulatory esophageal pH studies have demonstrated that the frequency of gastro-esophageal reflux episodes is higher in GERD patients with hiatal hernia than in patients without[57,58]. However, the relationship between hiatal hernia and gastro-esophageal reflux is not a simple one. In a series of patients who were endoscoped because of dyspeptic symptoms 42% of the patients with hiatal hernia did not have esophagitis. Conversely, only 63% of patients with endoscopically proven reflux esophagitis had hiatal hernia[54]. The mechanisms underlying the association between hiatus hernia and GERD have been subject of a number of studies. Over the years, the impact of dislodgement of the LES from its position within the diaphragmatic crus has been found to be far more complex than initially assumed.

7.1 DECREASED SPHINCTER TONE

One of the earliest thoughts about the mechanisms through which hiatus hernia predisposes to gastro-esophageal reflux has been that presence of hiatus hernia is associated with LES hypotension, in one way or another. Indeed, displacement of the LES from the diaphragmatic hiatus has been found to be associated with a reduction in basal LES pressure[59]. Other manometric observations indicated, however, that basal LES pressure is not decreased in patients with hiatus hernia, as compared to those without[60]. In retrospect, one of the most important factors leading to these discrepant manometric findings is that manometric detection of the diaphragm's contribution to tonic pressure within the esophagogastric junction is extremely difficult, if not impossible, when conventional manometric techniques are used. In patients who have undergone esophagectomy a high pressure zone with superimposed phasic oscillations can still be found at the level of the diaphragm, indicating the diaphragm is capable of contributing to tonic pressure[61]. In patients with a hiatus hernia one would expect to find two distinct tone high-pressure zones; a distal zone generated by the diaphragm and a proximal zone generated by the LES. In practice this phenomenon is observed extremely rarely during a conventional manometric study. The reasons for this inability of conventional manometry probably include the axial movements caused by respiration and swallowing and the fact that the hiatal sack may act as a compartment in which 'common cavity' pressures may be measured.

A recent study by Kahrilas and coworkers finally yielded more robust information on the contribution of the crural diaphragm to the pressure measured within the high-pressure zone at the esophagogastric junction[62]. In their study the investigators used concurrent fluoroscopy and manometry to map the characteristics of the gastro-esophageal junction. The squamocolumnar junction and the intragastric margin of the gastro-esophageal junction were marked with endoscopically placed radio-opaque clips. With these specialized manometric techniques Kahrilas and colleagues were able to show the presence of two distinct high-pressure zones in patients with hiatus hernia, whereas subjects without hiatus hernia had only one high-pressure zone with a higher amplitude[62]. The distal pressure segment in the hiatus hernia patients was shown to be caused by extrinsic compression by the hiatal canal (Figure 6). Algebraic summing of the proximal and distal pressure zones resulted in a pressure profile that was similar to that found in subjects without hiatus hernia.

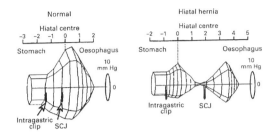

Figure 6. Mean pressure profiles (wireframe representations) of the gastro-esophageal junction in normal subjects (left) and patients with hiatus hernia (right). In patients with hiatus hernia the high pressure zone at the junction has two discrete segments, one attributable to the LES, the other to the compression within the hiatal canal. From Kahrilas PJ et al (ref.62), with permission.

7.2 INSPIRATION-ASSOCIATED REFLUX

In the absence of a hiatal hernia the right diaphragmatic crus surrounds the LES. With each inspiration the crural diaphragm contracts, thereby increasing the pressure within the sphincter complex at moments when reflux would be facilitated by an increase in abdominal pressure and a decrease in intrathoracic pressure. Manometrically, this contribution can be recognized as phasic pressure oscillations superimposed on the tonic pressure. These oscillations may reach values of 50-150 mmHg with deep inspiration. In case of presence of a hiatus hernia one would expect to see these phasic pressure oscillations at a site distal to the LES, but in conventional manometric studies they are still superimposed upon the LES pressure in most patients. Even the pressure inversion point, believed to represent the transition from the abdominal part of the sphincter to the thoracic part, is still in the LES in most cases. In other words, displacement of the LES to a position above the diaphragm is not associated with a complete loss of a manometrically intra-abdominal part of the LES. This is believed to be due to the fact that the phreno-esophageal ligament remains attached to both the sphincter and the diaphragmatic hiatus, thereby creating an extension of the abdominal cavity that surrounds the hiatus hernia (Figure 4). Nevertheless, evidence for an impaired protection against inspiration-associated reflux in hiatus hernia patients has been found. In a combined fluoroscopic-manometric study it was observed that in patients with a small reducible hiatus hernia antegrade flow of barium suspension emptied from the esophagus ceased during inspiration[63]. During expiration the crus relaxed and antegrade flow resumed. During the same or a subsequent inspiration barium trapped in the hiatal sac was found to reflux into the esophagus frequently. This occurred only when the pressure in the hiatal sac exceeded the LES pressure[63]. Thus, in patients with hiatus hernia the inspiration-associated contraction of the diaphragmatic crus counteracts rather than reinforces the function of the antireflux barrier.

7.3 SWALLOW-ASSOCIATED REFLUX

Animal studies and human studies employing electromyographic techniques have shown that the diaphragmatic crus partially relaxes in response to swallowing, allowing food boluses to pass[60]. In patients with hiatus hernia this crural relaxation takes place at the wrong site, i.e. distal to the LES, but this is an abnormality that is not likely to promote reflux. However, swallow-associated reflux does occur more commonly in patients with a hiatus hernia, especially in patients in whom a large hiatal hernia is present that does not reduce between swallows. Using videofluoroscopy combined with manometry Kahrilas and coworkers found that retention of swallowed barium suspension in the hiatal sac occurred frequently. During a subsequent swallow retrograde flow from the hiatal sac to the esophagus can occur immediately after the onset of the swallow-associated LES relaxation[63]. Esophageal clearance of the refluxed material was also found to be more disturbed in patients with a nonreducing hiatal hernia than in those without[63].

7.4 STRAINING-ASSOCIATED REFLUX

Animal studies and human studies employing electromyographic techniques have shown that the diaphragmatic crus contracts in response to increased intra-abdominal pressure[60]. In addition, intra-abdominal pressure is passively transmitted to the LES, due to the fact that the distal end of the sphincter is in the abdominal cavity. These two phenomena act in concert as protective mechanisms against reflux that might occur during straining.
Presence of a hiatus hernia is associated with a diminished augmentation of LES pressure during straining[62].

7.5 TLESR-ASSOCIATED REFLUX

Recently evidence was presented that presence of a hiatus hernia is associated with a decreased triggering threshold for TLESRs[64]. Eight normal subjects and 15 patients with GERD (8 with and 7 without hiatus hernia) were studied. Acid reflux and LES pressure were monitored for 2 hours during intragastric air infusion. It was found that air infusion increased the incidence of TLESRs in all three groups (controls, nonhernia patients and hernia patients), but the increase in frequency was most pronounced in the hiatus hernia group (4.0, 4.5 and 9.5/hour, respectively)[64].

In another recent manometric study we further investigated the dynamics of the LES underlying increased esophageal acid exposure in patients with hiatus hernia[65]. Twelve GERD patients with and 10 GERD patients without hiatus hernia were studied for 24 hours. Combined esophageal pH- and manometric recordings of pharynx, LES and stomach were performed using a multiple-lumen assembly incorporating a Dent sleeve connected to a portable water-perfused manometric system and pH glass electrode. The study confirmed that patients with hiatus hernia have a higher esophageal acid exposure and higher incidence of reflux episodes than those without. Basal LES pressure, incidence of TLESRs and the proportion of TLESRs associated with acid reflux were comparable in both groups of patients. Both patient groups had an equal number of reflux episodes associated with TLESRs and swallow-associated prolonged LES relaxations. However, the distribution of the mechanisms underlying the individual reflux episodes was found to be dependent on the presence or absence of hiatus hernia. Whereas in patients without hiatus hernia most reflux episodes were caused by TLESR and swallow-associated prolonged LES relaxation (60.2% and 17.6%, respectively), in patients with hiatus hernia a more heterogeneous pattern of motor mechanisms was responsible for acid reflux. In the latter group, TLESR accounted for 32.8%, low LES pressure for 22.5%, straining during LES pressure < 0.4 kPa (3 mmHg) for 15.5% and swallow-associated normal LES relaxation for 13.8% of the reflux episodes. As shown in Figure 7 the increased number of reflux episodes in patients with hiatus hernia was accounted for by an increased number of reflux episodes caused by swallow-associated normal LES relaxations, low LES pressure and both straining and deep inspiration during LES pressure < 3 mmHg. The incidences of reflux episodes associated with both TLESRs and swallow-associated prolonged LES relaxations were similar in patients with and without hiatus hernia. The above-described findings underline the importance of the crural diaphragm in the prevention of gastro-esophageal reflux during periods with low LES pressure. They are in accordance with the observation that during prolonged complete LES relaxations induced by pharyngeal stimulation with water no reflux occurs, whereas the only difference between these LES relaxations and TLESRs is the absence of a simultaneous inhibition of the crural diaphragm[66].

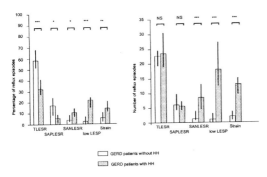

□ GERD patients without HH
▨ GERD patients with HH

Figure 7. Contribution of the various reflux mechanisms to reflux in reflux patients with and without hiatus hernia. In patients with hiatus hernia the percentage of reflux episodes caused by TLESRs is lower (left panel), but the absolute number (right panel) of TLESR-associated reflux episodes is equal to that in patients without hiatus hernia. In the hiatus hernia patients additional reflux mechanisms (in particular low LES pressure and straining) are responsible for the excess reflux. From Van Herwaarden MA et al. 2000 (ref. 65), with permission.

8. THE ANGLE OF His

At the entrance of the esophagus into the stomach a relatively sharp angle is present on the greater curvature (Figure 1). It has been proposed that the angle of His acts as a flap valve that contributes to the competence of the gastro-esophageal anti-reflux barrier[67]. It is further thought that surgical procedures that sharpen the angle augment the anti-reflux effect. Whereas during the 1950s and 1960s the main focus of attention in GERD was on the angle of His, this feature appears to have been dropped from consideration in later years. The possibility that an obtuse angle of His is often associated with a sliding hiatus hernia appears not to have been studied in any detail. It is not unlikely that the anatomy of the esophagogastric junction will receive renewed attention in the near future.

9. ESOPHAGEAL CLEARANCE

About half of the patients with reflux disease have prolonged acid clearance times, both in the controlled setting of the acid clearance test, as well as in the non-controlled but more physiological setting of ambulatory pH monitoring. Under normal circumstances esophageal acid clearance occurs as a two-step process. In the initial step most of the reflux volume is cleared rapidly, by one or two peristaltic contractions. The remaining acid is neutralized more slowly by swallowed saliva[68,69]. Thus, both abnormal esophageal peristalsis and abnormal saliva production could play a role in the pathogenesis of GERD. An increased incidence of weak and failed peristaltic contractions in patients with esophagitis has been reported repeatedly. The prevalence of peristaltic dysfunction was found to increase with the increasing severity of esophagitis, in the sense that 25% of individuals with mild esophagitis and 50% of patients with severe esophagitis have peristaltic dysfunction[23]. In patients with low-grade esophagitis, the esophageal motor response to reflux may be normal, whereas abnormal responses are found almost invariably in high-grade esophagitis [70,71]. One of the factors involved in abnormal peristalsis in reflux disease is parasympathetic nerve dysfunction, which correlates well with parameters of esophageal transit and peristalsis[72]. There is still some debate as to whether the abnormal peristalsis found in patients with GERD is a primary abnormality, or the consequence of repeated acid injury. Several studies have addressed this question by comparing esophageal contractile activity and LES function before and after healing of esophagitis. In none of the studies reported until now healing of esophagitis was found to improve esophageal peristalsis[25,28,73,74]. In a recent study, however, the aboral traction force generated by graded intraluminal distension was found to be improved after healing of esophagitis[74]. At night esophageal acid clearance is prolonged. Normally reflux occurring during sleep is associated with arousal and an increased swallowing rate. When arousal does not take place, clearance times are markedly increased, leading to damage to the esophageal mucosa [75,76]. There is little evidence that impaired saliva production or abnormal composition of the saliva plays an important role in the pathogenesis of reflux esophagitis[77]. In contrast, both in healthy controls and in patients with reflux esophagitis, saliva flow increases two- to four-fold when heartburn is induced by esophageal acid perfusion[78]. When acid infusion does not lead to heartburn, salivary flow is affected to a smaller extent[78]. The increased saliva production that accompanies heartburn may act as an endogenous antacid that serves as a protective response to symptomatic gastro-esophageal reflux. When increased saliva flow in response to heartburn (or another gastrointestinal symptom) is perceived by the patient, it is referred to as "water brash". Until recently no data were available about the proximal extent of the intra-esophageal refluxate in various patient groups with reflux disease. With the introduction of the multichannel Ion Sensitive Field Effect Transistor (ISFET) pH-catheter, 24-hour ambulatory pH measurement at up to 6 different esophageal levels has become feasible. In a study in GERD patients without esophagitis, with low-grade esophagitis, with severe esophagitis and patients with Barrett's esophagus we have found that both distal an proximal esophageal acid exposure increased with increasing mucosal damage (Figure 8).

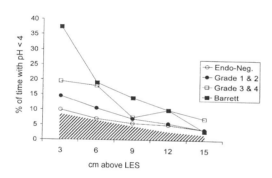

Figure 8. Esophageal acid exposure at 3,6,9,12 and 15 cm above the LES in patients with Barrett's esophagus, severe esophagitis, mild esophagitis and endoscopy-negative reflux disease. The shaded area indicates the normal range.

The differences in acid exposure times were most pronounced in the supine period. In patients with Barrett's esophagus, who had the most severe acid exposure and the most proximal extent of the refluxate, the length of the Barrett's segment was correlated to supine acid exposure at 15 centimeters from the distal esophageal sphincter (r = 0.58, p < 0.03). It is unclear to which extent the proximal extent of refluxate is dependent on saliva production, esophageal peristalsis and volume of the refluxed material.

10. RESISTANCE OF ESOPHAGEAL MUCOSA

The correlation between esophageal acid exposure, as measured with 24-hour pH monitoring, and the severity of reflux esophagitis is poor[79-81]. It is therefore thought that abnormalities in the defensive capacity of the esophageal mucosa play a role in the pathogenesis of reflux esophagitis. Esophageal epithelial cells have at least three ion exchangers that regulate intracellular pH in response to acidification or alkalinization[82]. In rabbits serosal bicarbonate ions play a role in the esophageal protection against acid-induced damage[83]. It is unclear, however, whether this mechanism is also effective in man. Intrinsic bicarbonate secretion from submucous glands in the esophageal mucosa has been identified in some mammals, including man. These glands have been shown to produce up to two-thirds of the bicarbonate measured in the esophagi of healthy subjects[84]. It is now clear that salivary and esophageal bicarbonate secretion are responsible for episodes of alkalization of the esophagus as observed during pH monitoring[85]. These episodes should, therefore, not be interpreted as "alkaline reflux". In addition to these factors, variations in the blood supply to the esophagus appear to play a role in the maintenance of esophageal mucosal integrity. It has been shown that the esophageal blood supply can increase in response to exposure to luminal acid[86].

11. ABNORMAL COMPOSITION OF REFLUXATE

Patients with GERD do not have a significant increase in basal, meal-stimulated or maximal gastric acid or pepsin secretion and the severity of reflux esophagitis is not related to gastric acid output[87]. These observations contradict the notion that GERD, in general, is due to abnormal acid secretion. This does not rule out the possibility that enhanced gastric acid secretion might play a role in the development of Barrett's esophagus. The results of one study suggest that gastric hypersecretion is a factor in the pathogenesis of Barrett's esophagus[87]. However, in other, more recent studies no evidence for this hypothesis could be found. Patients with Barrett's esophagus were found to have gastric acid secretion rates and intragastric pH profiles that are similar to those found in patients with esophagitis[89,90].

A much debated topic in the pathophysiology of GERD in general and Barrett's esophagus in particular is the role of duodenogastro-esophageal reflux. It has been shown that bile salts can cause esophageal mucosal injury, independently of acid, whereas the presence of bile salts can also enhance the damaging effect of the hydrogen ion[91]. Trypsin is also capable of inducing esophageal injury, in a dose-dependent manner[92].

Since the component of duodenal juice that is most harmful to the esophageal mucosa is bile salts, the most appropriate assessment of duodenal gastric reflux would consist of measurement of intra-esophageal bile acid concentration. However, this is technically difficult. In the few studies that used this technique the concentrations of bile acids and trypsin in the esophagus were found to be too low to cause significant damage[93,94], and esophageal bile acid concentrations were found not to be different among normal subjects, patients with esophagitis and patients with Barrett's esophagus[93].

In most human studies on duodenogastric reflux bilirubin is used as a green marker of bile, and bile reflux is assessed by means of measurement of intraluminal light absorption. The validation of the latter technique has been questioned and the technique has not yet found widespread acceptance by all experts in the field[95]. Using the bilirubin probe technology Champion et al. found higher intra-esophageal bilirubin concentrations in patients with Barrett's esophagus than in those with esophagitis and higher bilirubin concentrations in patients with esophagitis than in normal controls[12]. Interestingly, the same group of investigators also studied a group of patients who had undergone gastrectomy and showed that these had similar esophageal bilirubin concentrations to those with Barrett's esophagus, suggesting that duodenogastric reflux in the absence of gastric acid does not lead to development of Barrett's esophagus. In another study it was shown that with increasing severity of GERD (from grade 0 to Barrett's esophagus with complications) the degree of mucosal damage is as strongly correlated with acid as with duodenal reflux[96]. The available evidence indicates therefore, that in patients with an intact stomach, reflux of duodenal contents does not play an important pathophysiological role. Bilirubin, bile acids and trypsin can reach the esophagus, but their presence in the esophagus reflects the presence of gastric contents.

In other words, acid and "bile" reflux usually are parallel phenomena and there is no evidence for a specific composition of the refluxate in patients with severe forms of GERD, including Barrett's esophagus.

It has been thought that episodes with intra-esophageal pH between 7 and 8 constitute a distinguishing factor between patients with GERD with and without complications[1], and the assumption was made that "alkaline reflux" was identical to duodenogastro-esophageal reflux. It is now clear, however, that alkalization of the esophagus should not be considered evidence of duodenogastric reflux. With the use of simultaneous pH recording in the distal esophagus and stomach, no correlation was found between periods with high intragastric pH and high intra-esophageal pH[85,97]. Furthermore it has been found that time with esophageal pH > 7 and esophageal bilirubin concentrations correlate poorly[12]. It has become clear that most episodes of esophageal alkalization are caused by saliva production and local bicarbonate secretion in the distal esophagus[85].

12. DELAYED GASTRIC EMPTYING AND ALTERED INTRAGASTRIC DISTRIBUTION

It has been reported that 41% of GERD patients have delayed gastric emptying of a solid-liquid meal[98]. This observation supports the hypothesis that delayed gastric emptying facilitates reflux through the presence of greater postprandial gastric volumes and through an increasing frequency and duration of transient LES relaxations induced by gastric distension[33]. However, evidence that this sequence of events actually occurs, is lacking. In fact, other, more recent studies have shown that gastric emptying in patients with GERD is often normal or even rapid [99,100]. Thus, the available data indicate that delayed gastric emptying is unlikely to be a major factor in the pathogenesis of GERD. However, it may not be wise to apply this general statement to individual patients, since markedly delayed gastric emptying is encountered occasionally in GERD.

Recently, it was found that the accommodation response of the proximal stomach to a meal is prolonged in GERD patients and that emptying from the proximal stomach is delayed in these patients[101]. These observations suggest that in GERD patients more food is stored in the proximal stomach for a longer period of time. This would explain why postprandial reflux episodes occur more frequently in GERD than in health, whereas the incidence of TLESRs is not markedly different between these two groups.

REFERENCES

1. Bremner RM, Crookes PF, DeMeester TR, Peters JH, Stein HJ. Concentration of refluxed acid and esophageal mucosal injury. Am J Surg 1992;164:522-7

2. Pera M, Trastek VF, Pairolero PC, Cardesa A, Allen MS, Deschamps C. Barrett's disease: Pathophysiology of metaplasia and adenocarcinoma. Ann Thorac Surg 1993; 56:1191-7

3. Attwood SEA, Ball CS, Jenkinson L, Norris TL, Watson A. Role of intragastric and intraeosophageal alkalinisation in the genesis of complications in Barrett's columnar lined lower oesophagus. Gut 1993;34:11-5

4. Vaezi MF, Richter JE. Synergism of acid and duodenogastro-esophageal reflux in complicated Barrett's esophagus. Surgery 1995;117:699-704

5. Cameron AJ, Lomboy CT. Barrett's esophagus: Age, prevalence, and extent of columnar epithelium. Gastroenterology 1992; 103:1241-5

6. Fass J, Silny J, Braun J, Heindrichs U, Dreuw B, Schumpelick V et al. Measuring esophageal motility with a new intraluminal impedance device. Scand J Gastroenterol 1994; 29:693-702

7. Hassall E. Barrett's esophagus: Congenital or acquired? Am J Gastroenterol 1993;88:819-24

8. Fahmy N, King JF. Barrett's esophagus: An acquired condition with genetic predisposition. Am J Gastroenterol 1993;88:1262-6

9. Winters C, Spurling TJ, Chobanian SJ, Curtis DJ, Esposito RL, Hacker JF et al. Barrett's Esophagus. A prevalent, occult complication of gastro-esophageal reflux disease. Gastroenterology 1987;92:118-24

10. Gillen P, Keeling P, Byrne PJ, West AB, Hennessy TPJ. Experimental columnar metaplasia in the canine oesophagus. Br J Surg 1988;75:113-5.

11. Robertson DAF, Aldersley MA, Shepherd H, Lloyd RS, Smith CL. H2 antagonists in the treatment of reflux oesophagitis: can physiological studies predict the response? Gut 1987;28:946-9

12. Champion G, Richter JE, Vaezi MF, Singh S, Alexander R. Duodenogastro-esophageal reflux: relationship to pH and importance in Barrett's esophagus. Gastroenterology 1994;107:747-54

13. Gillen P, Keeling P, Byrne PJ, Hennessy TPJ. Barrett's oesophagus: pH profile. Br J Surg 1987;74:774-6.

14. Sing P, Taylor R, Colin-Jones DG. Esophageal motor dysfunction and acid exposure in reflux esophagitis are more severe if Barrett's metaplasia is present. Am J Gastroenterol 1994;89:349-56.

15. Neumann CS, Cooper BT. 24 Hour ambulatory oesophageal pH monitoring in uncomplicated Barrett's oesophagus. Gut 1994;35:1352-5.

16. Parrilla P, Ortiz A, Martinez de Haro LF, Aguayo JL, Ramirez P. Evaluation of the magnitude of gsatro-oesophageal reflux in Barrett's oesophagus. Gut 1990;31:964-7.

17. Ott DJ. Gastro-esophageal reflux: what is the role of barium studies? Am J Roentgenol 1994;162:627-9.

18. Ott DJ. Gastro-esophageal reflux disease. R Clin N Am 1994;92:1147-66.

19. Dent J, Chir B. A new technique for continuous sphincter pressure measurement. Gastroenterology 1976; 1:263-7.

20. Gotley DC, Barham CP, Miller R, et al. The sphinctometer: a new device for measurement of lower oesophageal sphincter function. Br J Surg 1991;78:933-5.

21. Talley NJ. Review article: 5-hydroxytryptamine agonists and antagonists in the modulation of gastrointestinal motility and sensation: clinical implications. Aliment Pharmacol Ther 1992;6:273-89

22. Gotley DC, Barham CP, Miller R, Arnold R, Alderson D. The sphinctometer: a new device for measurement of lower oesophageal sphincter function. Br J Surg 1991;78:933-5.

23. Kahrilas PJ, Dodds WJ, Hogan WJ, Kern M, Arndorfer RC, Reece A. Esophageal peristaltic dysfunction in peptic esophagitis. Gastroenterology 1986; 91:897-4.

24. Dent J, Holloway RH, Toouli J, Dodds WJ. Mechanisms of lower oesophageal sphincter incompetence in patients with symptomatic gastrooesophageal reflux. Gut 1988;29:1020-8.

25. Timmer R, Breumelhof R, Nadorp JHSM, Smout AJPM. Oesophageal motility and gastro-oesophageal reflux before and after healing of reflux oesophagitis. A study using 24 hour amulatory ph and pressure monitoring. Gut 1994; 35:1519-22.

26. Eastwood GL, Castell DO, Higgs RH. Experimental eophagitis in cats impairs lower esophagal sphincter pressure. Gastroenterology 1975;69:146-53.

27. Katz PO, Knuff TE, Benjamin S.B., Castell D.O. Abnormal esophageal pressures in reflux esophagitis: cause or effect? Am J Gastroenterol 1986;81:44-6.

28. Eckardt VF. Does healing of esophagitis improve esophageal motor function? Dig Dis Sci 1988;33:161-5.

29. Dent J, Dodds WJ, Sekiguchi T, Hogan WJ, Arndorfer RC. Interdigestive phasic contractions of the human lower esophageal sphincter. Gastroenterology 1983;84:453-60.

30. Smout AJPM, Bogaard JW, van Hattum J, Akkermans LMA. Effects of cimetidine and ranitidine on interdigestive and postprandial lower esophageal sphincter pressure and plasma gastrin levels in normal subjects. Gastroenterology 1985;88:557-63.

31. Gill RC, Kellow JE, Wingate DL. Gastro-oesophageal reflux and the migrating motor complex. Gut 1987;28:929-34.

32. Dodds WJ, Dent J, Hogan WJ, Helm JF, Hauser R, Patel GK et al. Mechanisms of gastro-esophageal reflux in patients with reflux esophagitis. New Engl J Med 1982;307:1547-52.

33. Holloway RH, Hongo M, Berger K, McCallum RW. Gastric distension: a mechanism for postprandial gastro-esophageal reflux. Gastroenterology 1985;89:779-84.

34. Holloway RH, Kocyan P, Dent J. Provocation of transient lower esophageal sphincter relaxations by meals in patients with symptomatic gastro-esophageal reflux. Dig Dis Sci 1991;36:1034-9.

35. Franzi SJ, Martin CJ, Cox MR, Dent J. Response of canine lower esophageal sphincter to gastric distension. Am J Physiol 1990;259:G380-5.

36. Mittal RK, McCallum RW. Characteristics and frequency of transient relaxations of the lower esophageal sphincter in patients with reflux esophagitis. Gastroenterology 1988;95:593-9.

37. Penagini R, Schoeman MN, Dent J, Tippett MD, Holloway RH. Motor events underlying gastro-oesophageal reflux in ambulant patients with reflux oesophagitis. J Neurogastroenterol Mot 1996;8:131-41.

38. Schoeman MN, Tippett MD, Akkermans LMA, Dent J, Holloway RH. Mechanisms of gastro-esophageal reflux in ambulant healthy human subjects. Gastroenterology 1995;108:83-91.

39. van Herwaarden MA, Samsom M, Van Nispen CHM, Verlinden M, Smout AJPM. The effect of motilin agonist ABT-229 on gastro-oesophageal reflux: oesophageal motility and lower oesophageal sphincter characteristics in GERD patients. Aliment Pharmacol Ther 2000;14:453-62.

40. Katz LC, Just R, Castell DO. Body position affects recumbent postprandial reflux. J Clin Gastroenterol 1994;18:280-3.

41. Khoury RM, Camacho-Lobato L, Katz PO, Mohiuddin MA, Castell DO. Influence of spontaneous sleep positions on nighttime recumbent reflux in patients with gastro-esophageal reflux disease. Am J Gastroenterol 1999;94:2069-73.

42. Van Herwaarden MA, Katzka DA, Smout AJ, Samsom M, Gideon M, Castell D. Effect of different recumbent positions on postprandial gastro-esophageal reflux in normal subjects. Am J Gastroenterol 2000;95:2731-6.

43. Shay SS, Conwell DL, Mehindru V, Hertz B. The effect of posture on gastro-esophageal reflux event frequency and composition during fasting. Am J Gastroenterol 1996;91:54-60.

44. Martin CJ, Patrikios J, Dent J. Abolition of gas reflux and transient lowr esophageal sphincter relaxation by vagal blockade in the dog. Gastroenterology 1986;91:890-6.

45. Holloway RH, Wyman JB, Dent J. Failure of transient lower oesophageal sphincter relaxation in response to gastric distension in patients with achalasia: evidence for neural mediation of transient lower oesophageal sphincter relaxations. Gut 1989;30:762-7.

46. Liu J, Yamamoto Y, Schirmer BD, Ross RA, Mittal RK. Evidence for a peripheral mechanism of esophagocrural diaphragm inhibitory reflex in cats. Am J Physiol 2000;278:G281-8.

47. Staunton E, Smid SD, Dent J, Blackshawm L.A. Triggering of transient LES relaxations in ferrets: role of sympathetic pathways and effects of baclofen. Am J Physiol 2000; 79:G157-62.

48. Lidums I, Checklin H, Mittal RK, Holloway RH. Effect of atropine on gastro-oesophageal reflux and transient lower oesophageal sphincter relaxations in patients with gastro-oesophageal reflux disease. Gut 1998; 3:12-16.

49. Boulant J, Mathieu S, D'Amato M, Abergel A, Dapoigny M, Bommelaer G. Cholecystokinin in transient lower esophageal sphincter relaxation due to gastric distension in man. Gut 1997; 40:575-81.

50. Boulant J, Fioramonti J, Dapoigny M, Bommelaer G, Bueno L. Cholecystokinin and nitric oxide in transient lower esophageal sphincter relaxation to gastric distension in dogs. Gastroenterology 1994; 107:1059-66.

51. Penagini R, Bianchi PA. Effect of morphine on gastro-esophageal reflux and transient lower esophageal sphincter relaxation. Gastroenterology 1997; 13:409-14.

52. Fang JC, Sarosiek I, Yamamoto Y, Liu J, Mittal RK. Cholinergic blockade inhibits gastro-oesophageal reflux and transient lower oesophageal sphincter relaxation through a central mechanism. Gut 1999;44:603-7.

53. Clave P, Gonzalez A, Moreno A, Lopez R, Farre A, Cusso X et al. Endogenous cholecystokinin enhances postprandial gastro-esophageal reflux in humans through extrasphincteric receptors. Gastroenterol 1998; 15:597-604.

54. Berstad A, Weberg R, Larsen IF, Hoel B, Hauer-Jensen M. Relationship of hiatus hernia to reflux oesophagitis: A prospective study of coincidence, using endoscopy. Scand J Gastroenterol 1986;21:55-8.

55. Patti MG, Goldberg HI, Arcerito M, Bortolasi L, Tong J, Way LW. Hiatal hernia size affects lower esophageal sphincter function, esophageal acid exposure, and the degree of mucosal injury. Am J Surg 1996; 71:182-6.

56. Cameron AJ. Barrett's esophagus: prevalence and size of hiatal hernia. Am J Gastroenterol 1999;94:2054-9.

57. Ott DJ, Glauser SJ, Ledbetter MS, Chen MY, Koufman JA, Gelfand DW. Association of hiatal hernia and gastro-esophageal reflux: correlation between presence and size of hiatal hernia and 24-hour pH monitoring of the esophagus. Am J Roentgenol 1995; 65:557-9

58. DeMeester TR, Lafontaine E, Joelsson BE, Skinner DB, Ryan JW, O'Sullivan GC et al. Relationship of a hiatal hernia to the function of the body of the esophagus and the gastro-esophageal junction. J Thorac Cardiovasc Surg 1981;82:547-58.

59. Cohen S, Harris LD. Does hiatus hernia affect competence of the esophageal sphincter? N Engl J Med 1971;284:1053-6.

60. Mittal RK, Rochester DF, McCallum RW. Effect of the diaphragmatic contraction on lower oesophageal sphincter pressure in man. Gut 1987;28:1564-8.

61. Klein WA, Parkman HP, Dempsey DT, Fisher RS. Sphincterlike thoracoabdominal high pressure zone after esophagogastrectomy. Gastroenterology 1993;105:1362-9.

62. Kahrilas PJ, Lin S, Chen J, Manka M. The effect of hiatus hernia on gastro-oesophageal junction pressure. Gut 1999; 44:476-82.

63. Sloan S, Kahrilas PJ. Impairment of esophageal emptying with hiatal hernia. Gastroenterology 1991;100:596-605.

64. Kahrilas PJ, Shi G, Manka M, Joehl RJ. Increased frequency of transient lower esophageal sphincter relaxation induced by gastric distention in reflux patients with hiatal hernia. Gastroenterology 2000;118:688-95.

65. Van Herwaarden MA, Samsom M, Smout AJ. Excess gastro-esophageal reflux in patients with hiatus hernia is caused by mechanisms other than transient LES relaxations. Gastroenterology 2000;119:1439-46.

66. Mittal RK, Chiareli C, Liu J, Shaker R. Characteristics of lower esophageal sphincter relaxation induced by pharyngeal stimulation with minute amounts of water. Gastroenterology 1996; 111:378-84.

67. Thor KB, Hill LD, Mercer DD, Kozarek RD. Reappraisal of the flap valve mechanism in the gastro-esophageal junction. A study of new valvuloplasty procedure in cadavers. Acta Clin Scand 1987;153:25-8.

68. Helm JF, Dodds WJ, Pelc LR, Palmer DW, Hogan WJ, Teeter BC. Effect of esophageal emptying and saliva on clearance of acid from the esophagus. New Engl J Med 1984; 310:284-8.

69. Shaker R, Kahrilas PJ, Dodds WJ, Hogan WJ. Oesophageal clearance of small amounts of equal or less than one millilitre of acid. Gut 1992;33:7-10.

70. Timmer R, Breumelhof R, Nadorp JHSM, Smout AJPM. Oesophageal motor response to reflux is not impaired in reflux oesophagitis. Gut 1993;34:317-20.

71. Timmer R, Breumelhof R, Nadorp JHSM, Smout AJPM. Ambulatory esophageal pressure and pH monitoring in patients with high-grade reflux esophagitis. Dig Dis Sci 1994; 9:2084-9.

72. Cunningham KM, Horowitz M, Riddell PS, Maddern GJ, Myers JC, Holloway RH et al. Relations among autonomic nerve dysfunction, oesophageal motility, and gastric emptying in gastro-oesophageal reflux disease. Gut 1991;32:1436-40.

73. Allen ML, McIntosh DL, Robinson MG. Healing or amelioration of esophagitis does not result in increased lower esophageal sphincter or esophageal contractile pressure. Am J Gastroenterol 1990;85:1331-4.

74. Williams D, Thompson DG, Heggi L, O'Hanrahan T, Bancewicz J. Esophageal clearance function following treatment of esophagitis. Gastroenterology 1994;196:108-16.

75. Orr WC, Johnson LF, Robinson MG. Effect of sleep on swallowing, esophageal peristalsis, and acid clearance. Gastroenterology 1984;86:814-9.

76. Sondheimer JM. Clearance of spontaneous gastro-esophageal reflux in awake and sleeping infants. Gastroenterology 1989; 7:821-6.

77. Sonnenberg A, Steinkamp U, Weise A, Berges W, Wienbeck M, Rohner HG et al. Salivary secretion in reflux esophagitis. Gastroenterology 1982;83:889-95.

78. Helm JF, Dodds WJ, Hogan WJ. Salivary response to esophageal acid in normal subjects and patients with reflux esophagitis. Gastroenterology 1987;93:1393-7.

79. Schindlbeck NE, Heinrich C, König A, Dendorfer A, Pace F, Müller-Lissner SA. Optimal thresholds, sensitivity, and specificity of long-term pH-metry for the detection of gastro-esophageal reflux disease. Gastroenterology 1987;93:85-90.

80. Mattioli S, Pilotti V, Spangaro M, Grigioni WF, Zannoli R, Felice V et al. Reliability of 24-hour home esophageal pH monitoring in diagnosis of gastro-esophageal reflux. Dig Dis Sci 1989;34:71-8.

81. Howard PJ, Maher L, Heading RC. Symptomatic gastro-oesophageal reflux, abnormal oesophageal acid exposure, and mucosal acid sensitivity are three separate, though related, aspects of gastro-oesophageal reflux disease. Gut 1991;32:128-32.

82. Tobey NA, Reddy SP, Khalbuss WE, Silvers SM, Cragoe EJ, Orlando RC. Na+ -dependent and -independent Cl- /HCO3- exchangers in cultured rabbit esophageal epithelial cells. Gastroenterology 1993;104:185-95.

83. Tobey NA, Powell DW, Schreiner VJ, Orlando RC. Serosal bicarbonate protects against acid injury to rabbit esophagus. Gastroenterology 1989;96:1466-77.

84. Brown CM, Snowdon CF, Slee B, Rees WDW. Measurement of bicarbonate output from the intact human oesophagus. Gut 1993;34:872-80.

85. Singh S, Bradley LA, Richter JE. Determinants of oesophageal "alkaline" ph environment in controls and patients with gastrooesophageal reflux disease. Gut 1993;34:309-16.

86. Hollwarth ME, Smith M, Kvietys PR, Granger DN. Esophageal blood flow in the cat. Normal distribution and effects of acid perfusion. Gastroenterology 1986;90:622-7.

87. Hirschowitz BI. A critical analysis, with appropriate controls, of gastric acid and pepsin secretion in clinical esophagitis. Gastroenterology 1991;101:1149-58.

88. Mulholland MW, Reid BJ, Levine DS, Rubin CE. Elevated gastric acid secretion in patients with Barrett's metaplastic epithelium. Dig Dis Sci 1989;34:1329-34.

89. Hirschowitz BI. Gastric acid and pepsin secretion in patients with Barrett's esophagus and appropriate controls. Dig Dis Sci 1996;41:1384-91.

90. Savarino V, Mela GS, Zentilin P, Mele MR, Mansi C, Remagnino C et al. Time pattern of gastric acidity in Barrett's esophagus. Dig Dis Sci 1996; 41:1379-83.

91. Hopwood D, Bateson MC, Milne G, Bouchier IAD. Effects of the bile acids and hydrogen ion on the fine structure of oesophageal epithelium. Gut 1981;22:306-11.

92. Lillemoe KD, Johnson LF, Harmon JW. Alkaline esophagitis: A comparison of the ability of components of gastroduodenal contents to injure the rabbit esophagus. Gastroenterology 1983;85:621-8.

93. Gotley DC, Morgan AP, Ball D, Owen RW, Cooper MJ. Composition of gastro-oesophageal refluxate. Gut 1991;32:1093-9.

94. Mittal RK, Reuben A, Whitney JO, McCallum RW. Do bile acids reflux into the esophagus? Gastroenterology 1987;92:371-5.

95. Ostrow JD. Bilitec to quantitate duodenogastric reflux: is it valid? Gastroenterology 1995;108:1332-4.

96. Vaezi MF, Richter JE. Role of acid and duodenogastro-esophageal reflux in gastro-esophageal reflux disease. Gastroenterology 1996;111:1192-9.

97. Mattioli S, Pilotti V, Felice V, Lazzari A, Zannoli R, Bacchi ML et al. Ambulatory 24-hr pH monitoring of esophagus, fundus, and antrum. A new technique for simultaneous study of gastro-esophageal and duodenogastric reflux. Dig Dis Sci 1990;35:929-38.

98. McCallum RW, Berkowitz DM, Lerner E. Gastric emptying in patients with gastro-esophageal reflux. Gastroenterology 1981;80:285-91.

99. Johnson DA, Winters C, Drane WE, Cattau EL, Karvelis KC, Silverman ED et al. Solid-phase gastric emptying in patients with Barrett's esophagus. Dig Dis Sci 1986;31:1217-20.

100. Shay SS, Eggli D, McDonald C, Johnson LF. Gastric emptying of solid food in patients with gastro-esophageal reflux. Gastroenterology 1987;92:459-65.

101. Penagini R, Hebbard G, Horowitz M, Dent J, Bermingham H, Jones K et al. Motor function of the proximal stomach and visceral perception in gastro-oesophageal reflux disease. Gut 1998;42:251-7.

2.1 THE NATURAL HISTORY OF GASTRO-ESOPHAGEAL REFLUX DISEASE

Brian T. Johnston and Andrew H.G. Love[†]

1. INTRODUCTION

The natural history of gastro-esophageal reflux disease (GERD) has been poorly understood for many years. This is because different papers have used a variety of definitions for GERD. Older studies relied on the radiological diagnosis of a hiatus hernia as evidence of GERD. Other studies have been inconsistent in their definition of esophagitis. Recent papers have addressed these issues and we now have follow-up data on (i) patients with symptoms alone, (ii) patients with symptoms and excessive acid reflux on esophageal pH monitoring and (iii) patients with erosive esophagitis. The natural history of GERD in these groups of patients will be reviewed in this chapter. Two other important issues will be addressed. Firstly, the influence of GERD on quality of life (QoL) and secondly, the impact of proton pump inhibitors (PPIs) on disease progression in GERD.

2. THEORIES: STATIC OR PROGRESSIVE

2.1 PROGRESSIVE

Intuitively, it appears logical that ongoing reflux of acid and stomach/duodenal contents into the esophagus will progressively cause worsening damage. What began with mild heartburn may end up with esophagitis complicated by stricturing. This is the traditional, progressive, theory of GERD (Figure 1a). The strongest evidence in its favor comes from the recent publication by Lagergren et al[1]. In a case control study, the authors were able to demonstrate a titratable relationship between the frequency, severity and duration of reflux symptoms and development of esophageal adenocarcinoma (Figure 2). This progression theory is supported by other publications demonstrating that the complications of GERD, namely strictures, haemorrhage and Barrett's Esophagus occur at an older age and after a longer duration of symptoms[2,3].

2.2 STATIC

The static theory of GERD suggests that each individual have a pre-determined response to acid reflux (Figure 1b). This response is not

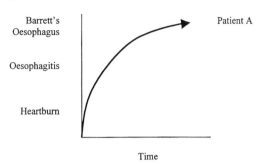

Figure 1a. The progressive model of GERD envisages patients progressing to increasingly severe GERD with the passage of time

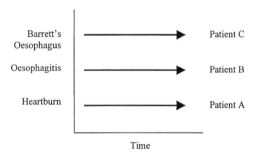

Figure 1b. The static model views each patient as having a pre-determined level of GERD severity which does not change with time.

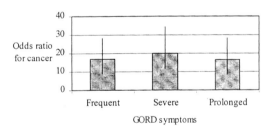

Figure 2: The odds ratios for developing esophageal adenocarcinoma. Frequent = symptoms >x3/week, Severe = >4 points on scale, Duration = symptoms >20 years. Adapted from Lagergren et al [1].

progressive. Rather, the patient rapidly reaches a steady-state, whether that is symptoms alone or Barrett's Esophagus. The degree of GERD is influenced in a multifactorial manner by both genes and environment. The paper by Cameron et al on the follow-up of Barrett's Esophagus is used as supporting evidence[4]. Over a 7 year period there was no change in length of Barrett's segment (8.3 +/- 0.8cm v. 8.3 +/- 0.8cm). Similarly, in canine models, Barrett's Esophagus develops rapidly to full length over a 2-6 month period[5,6]. Evidence of a genetic component in GERD is increasingly emerging with familial clustering or genetic

H.W. Tilanus and S.E.A. Attwood (eds.), Barrett's Esophagus, 71–80.

TABLE 1: Prevalence of heartburn (1976-1997)

Study	No. subjects	Heartburn frequency		
		Daily	Weekly	Monthly
Nebel et al (66)	385	7%	21%	36%
Thompson et al (67)	301	4%	10%	21%
Anonymous (13)	1023	3%	10%	21%
Ruth et al (68)	407	3%	---	25%
Locke et al (11)	1511		20%	

linkage being demonstrated for simple GERD[7], childhood GERD[8,9] and Barrett's Esophagus[10]. Evidence of genetic links does not conclusively indicate a static as opposed to a progressive natural history for GERD. It does, however, emphasize that environmental issues, such as ongoing acid exposure, are not the sole determinants of disease manifestation. Distinguishing between these two theories is important. Each has different implications regarding the need for follow-up and long-term treatment. If the disease is static and each individual is pre-programmed, no long-term therapy or further investigations are required for the patient who initially has symptoms alone. Alternatively, if there is progression, simple heartburn may ultimately develop into complicated esophagitis.

3. PREVALENCE DATA

The prevalence of reflux symptoms has been remarkably consistent in various studies conducted in Europe and North America (Table 1). The symptom prevalence does not appear to have altered over the 3 decades covered by the studies. The paper by Locke III et al also demonstrated that the proportion of the population experiencing reflux symptoms does not increase with age (Figure 3)[11]. If anything, the specific symptom of heartburn may decrease with age.

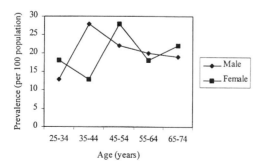

Figure 3: The age- and sex- specific prevalence rates of weekly heartburn or acid regurgitation per 100 of the population. Adapted from Locke et al [11].

Symptoms are persistent, 60% reporting a >5 year history and 40% having experienced the symptoms for >10 years. Despite the persistence of their symptoms, only ¼-1/3 of sufferers consults their family doctor[12,13]. One study found that only 5.4% patients had attended a doctor in the last 12 months[11]. The vast majority was self-medicating. Data on disease incidence are more scarce. Brunnen et al surveyed the incidence of complicated esophagitis (ulcers/stricture) in Scotland over the period 1951-67[14]. They reported an incidence of 4.5/100,000 for new presentation with esophageal strictures or ulcers. From these data, they estimated that the incidence of simple esophagitis would be 86/100,000. The incidence of complicated esophagitis was age dependent, increasing with older age. Two decades later, a study from Sweden demonstrated remarkably similar incidences: esophagitis 120/100,000, complications (esophageal ulcer/stricture) 5.6/100,000[15]. Once again complications were noted to be age-dependent. To summarize the prevalence data on GERD, symptoms are persistent but do not increase in frequency with age. By contrast, complications of GERD do increase with age[3] (Figure 4).

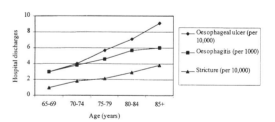

Figure 4: Esophageal diagnoses listed on discharge from hospital. Data are annual rates per 10,000 living population (per 1000 in case of esophagitis). Adapted from Sonnenberg et al[3].

4. THE NATURAL HISTORY OF GERD – A HISTORICAL PERSPECTIVE

Older studies have limited application to current practice because their definition of GERD largely centered on the radiological diagnosis of a hiatus hernia. This can be illustrated by the title of one of the studies, 'The hiatus hernia-esophagitis-esophageal

stricture complex'[16]. However, this study by Palmer and that by Rex at al[17] are of some relevance: they are large studies, they followed their patients for up to 20 years and they reflect the natural history of GERD in the pre-H2 receptor antagonist (H2RA) era - both studies began in the 1940s. Rex et al followed up 365 patients who had a diagnosis of hiatus hernia made 10 years previously[17]. Of 301 patients with a simple sliding hiatus hernia, 60% were asymptomatic. This was irrespective of the presence or absence of esophagitis in those examined endoscopically (62% v. 56%). Sixteen of the 301 patients had bleeding or anemia. These 16 had a poorer outcome. Fifty-eight patients had a shortened esophagus in addition to the hiatus hernia. Among these patients, only 38% were asymptomatic at 10 years. Nine of these shortened-esophagus patients had esophageal strictures at diagnosis. Seven had ongoing symptoms requiring repeated dilatation. Palmer followed a personal series of 1011 GERD patients for between one and 20 years[16]. Endoscopic diagnosis of esophagitis (included hyperemia) was made in 413 patients. Of 142 patients with simple esophagitis, 15% became worse, 20% remained the same, 17% improved and in 35% it disappeared. Overall, 52% were improved or cured. This was similar to Rex et al's results for simple hiatus hernia. Forty-five (10.9%) of the esophagitis patients also had a stricture. All of these required recurrent dilatation. Significant bleeding from esophagitis or an esophageal ulcer was reported in 76/1011 patients (7.5%). These patients required an average transfusion of >3l blood (one patient was transfused 45l!). Two lessons can be learned from this historical review. Firstly, a large number of mild cases were included since >50% improved with what would be regarded nowadays as simple, conservative measures. Secondly, there was a significant subgroup of patients who did badly. These patients were characterized by a shortened esophagus, stricturing and bleeding. Generally, they did not improve. Those with strictures continued to need dilatation; those who bled required large volume transfusions.

5. THE CURRENT NATURAL HISTORY OF GERD

As mentioned in the previous section, the vast majority of GERD sufferers self-medicate. Of those who do present to their family doctor, most are managed without referral to secondary or tertiary care and without the need for further investigation. This has been described as the part of the GERD iceberg that lies below the surface. Although it comprises the bulk of GERD patients, little research has been done in this area[18]. By contrast, we have a much greater knowledge of the natural history of patients whose reflux symptoms have been sufficiently severe as to merit referral to hospital and investigation. On the basis of investigations, it is possible to divide these patients into three groups: those with erosive esophagitis, those without esophagitis but with increased esophageal acid exposure on pH monitoring and those with typical symptoms but normal endoscopy and pH monitoring. Studies of consecutive patients suggest a breakdown of 40-50% esophagitis, 20-30% positive pH monitoring and 30-40% symptoms only (Figure 5)[19,20]. The following sections will analyze the natural history of these three groups.

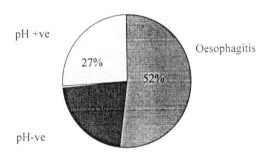

Figure 5: The breakdown of GERD patients referred to secondary care. The three groups are: patients with symptoms alone, patients with symptoms and excessive acid reflux on esophageal pH monitoring and patients with erosive esophagitis. Adapted from DeMeester et al[19].

5.1 SYMPTOMS ALONE

What happens to symptom-only GERD patients? Can they truly be categorized as refluxers? How do they fit into the category of non-erosive reflux disease (NERD)? In attempting to address these issues we have followed up patients in all three groups who had previously been well investigated by endoscopy, biopsy and esophageal pH monitoring[21]. Of 32 symptom-only patients followed-up for 3-5 years, 10 (31%) had progressed to either an abnormal tracing on esophageal pH monitoring or erosive esophagitis (Figure 6). Twelve (37%) continued to need daily acid suppression (H2RA/PPI) (Figure 7). Symptom-only patients can be further sub-divided into those whose symptoms correlate with brief episodes of acid reflux on pH monitoring (positive Symptom Index) and those whose symptoms do not correlate (negative Symptom Index) (Figure 8). Patients with a positive Symptom

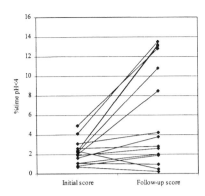

Figure 6: Results of esophageal pH monitoring on follow-up after 3-5 years among patients who initially had both normal endoscopy and normal pH monitoring. Adapted from McDougall et al[21].

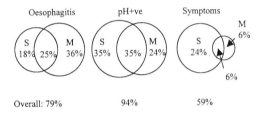

Figure 7: Percentage of patients with ongoing frequent symptoms (S) or taking daily medication (M) or both 4 years after initial presentation. Adapted from McDougall et al[21].

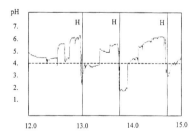

Figure 8: A three-hour sample of esophageal pH monitoring. All three episodes of heartburn (H) correlate with drops in pH below pH4. The Symptom Index = 100%[33].

Index are referred to as having a 'sensitive esophagus'. Such patients respond well to PPIs in the short term [22]. However, 4-6 year follow-up demonstrated a similar ongoing requirement for daily acid suppression among sensitive esophagus patients as patients who have abnormal levels of acid reflux (52% V. 56%) and a similar persistence of symptoms (87% v. 79%)[23]. One study, based in primary care, demonstrated a relapse rate of 75% after 6 months off therapy among 123 NERD patients[24]. This compared with a relapse rate of 90% in 145 patients with esophagitis. Although relapse is higher among patients with erosive esophagitis, many NERD patients also demonstrate an ongoing need for acid suppression. This is especially true if their

symptoms had not been completely relieved on initial therapy[25].

5.2 INCREASED ESOPHAGEAL ACID EXPOSURE (PH+VE)

Approximately 25% of patients presenting to secondary care with reflux symptoms will have raised levels of esophageal acid exposure on pH monitoring despite a normal endoscopy. Many of these patients have esophageal acid exposure equivalent to those who do have esophagitis at endoscopy. Yet their mucosa remains intact. What happens to such patients on follow-up? Do they inevitably progress to esophagitis? Our prospective study of 17 such patients demonstrated that 16 (94%) continued to have frequent symptoms or require daily H2RA/PPI therapy or both after 3-5 years[21]. Four (24%) progressed to develop esophagitis. Yet esophageal pH results were unchanged (%time pH<4, 9.5% (7.4-17.1%) v. 8.7% (4.9-12.6%). Pace et al showed similar progression to esophagitis in 5/33 (15%) patients over a six month period[26]. Nineteen (58%) continued to be symptomatic but 14 (42%) remained asymptomatic off therapy. Interestingly, these 14 had been rendered asymptomatic simply with antacids and prokinetics. The degree of reflux on pH monitoring did not predict ongoing symptoms or development of esophagitis. A better overall outcome for these patients with excessive acid reflux on pH monitoring was demonstrated in a study of such 117 patients (32% also had esophagitis)[27]. On follow-up after three years, only 35 (30%) were either on daily therapy (20 on H2RAs, 3 on PPIs) or had undergone fundoplication[12]. However, only 13/117 (11%) was asymptomatic off therapy. The authors speculated that the low incidence of maintenance therapy did not reflect a more benign disease process but rather physician reluctance to prescribe expensive medication. Increased acid reflux during the supine period was predictive of a worse outcome. The presence or grade of esophagitis was not.

5.3 ESOPHAGITIS

There are many good studies on the short term outcome of esophagitis after stopping therapy. Patients who have required a PPI to heal their erosive esophagitis will almost universally (>80%) relapse within 12 months of stopping therapy (Figure 9)[28,29]. However, even within the diagnosis of esophagitis there would appear to be a variety of responses. Poynard et al were able to maintain 76% patients in remission at six months on <1 antacid sachet per day[30].

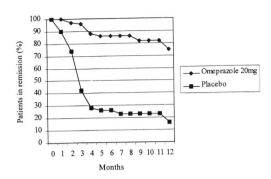

Figure 9: Endoscopic relapse of esophagitis after initial healing with omeprazole. Omeprazole 20mg daily was significantly better than placebo at preventing relapse (p<0.001). Adapted from Bate et al[29].

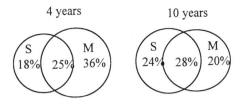

Overall: 79%   71%

Figure 10: Percentage of esophagitis patients with ongoing frequent symptoms (S) or taking daily medication (M) or both 4 and 10 years after initial presentation. Adapted from McDougall et al [21,33].

At initial endoscopy 57% of the 1030 patients had grade I esophagitis and 42% a higher grade. All had been healed by H2RAs or PPIs. Even among patients with Grade III esophagitis remission was maintained in 56%. Similarly, a three and six year follow-up found 1/3 of esophagitis patients either asymptomatic or requiring only antacids[31]. These authors speculated that aggressive use of lifestyle measures was the key to their results and that such advice is often neglected by more medication-based protocols. At the other end of the esophagitis spectrum, Klinkenberg-Knol et al reported their experience of omeprazole among patients whose esophagitis had been resistant to H2RA therapy[32]. Although 100% were healed by omeprazole 40mg, 40 (47%) relapsed on maintenance therapy of omeprazole 20mg daily. Relapsers were maintained on 40mg daily and 7/40 (18%) had a further relapse and required 60mg daily. This group included 9 who had been hospitalized with esophageal bleeding and 28 with esophageal strictures. Three to five year follow-up of patients with erosive esophagitis noted ongoing severe symptoms in 50%[21]. This was despite 61% of patients remaining on daily H2RA/PPI. Overall, 79% were either on daily H2RA/PPI therapy or continued to have frequent symptoms or both. The long term nature of the ongoing symptoms and dependence on daily acid suppression was confirmed in a 10 year follow-up of esophagitis patients[33]. One hundred and one patients were contacted a mean of 11 years after their initial endoscopic diagnosis of esophagitis. Seventy-one percent continued to have frequent symptoms or require daily acid suppression (Figure 10). The most extensive data on follow-up of esophagitis come from a paper by Ollyo et al[34]. Their review of 701 patients suggests that in 46% the initial episode

is isolated without recurrence. Recurrence to a same or lesser grade of esophagitis was noted in 31% and progression to a worse grade in 26%. These data are hard to interpret because the period of follow-up varied from one month to 27 years and no information is provided regarding treatment during this period. Perhaps the key message is that ¼ progressed to more severe esophagitis.

5.4 COMPLICATIONS

5.4.1 Stricture
Review of the two historical series quoted above reveals a stricture rate of 10.9% among esophagitis patients[16] and 11% among 109 GERD patients who underwent endoscopy[17]. This is consistent with the estimate of 4-20% in a previous publication[35]. Ollyo at al reported the development of either stenosis or ulceration in 9% in their long term follow-up[34] and an earlier abstract suggested progression to stricturing in 8% over just 12 months[36]. A much lower prevalence of esophageal stricturing was suggested by a review of nearly 4000 patients with esophagitis[37]. Only 1.2% of these patients had an esophageal stricture.

Although these are not follow-up data, they are supported by a 10 year follow-up of 101 patients in whom only 2 (2%) developed esophageal stricturing[33]. Stricture patients are older than control subjects with simple GERD and have a longer duration of heartburn[2]. When assessed manometrically, their lower esophageal sphincter (LOS) pressure is lower and they have a higher likelihood of esophageal body dysmotility. The natural history of esophageal strictures can be estimated from a series of 154 patients followed over an eight year period[38]. Approximately half required no further dilatation after the initial restoration of normal swallowing. The other half required repeat dilatations at a median rate of one per year. There were three deaths related to stricturing (two from perforation).

5.4.2 Ulcer/hemorrhage

Historically, hemorrhage and anemia from complicated esophagitis were significant problems, older series quoting rates of 5.3-7.5%[16,17]. These figures were supported in a review, with estimates of 5% and 2% for the development of ulceration and hemorrhage respectively[35].

A recent analysis confirms the high incidence of hemorrhage in esophagitis (8%)[39]. This was primarily among patients with severe esophagitis and often was not preceded by typical reflux symptoms.

5.4.3 Barrett's Esophagus

Barrett's Esophagus is discussed more fully throughout the rest of this book. However, it can be classified as a complication of GERD, as part of the natural history of GERD. In our study, 11% of patients with esophagitis developed Barrett's Esophagus over a 3-5 year follow-up[21]. A similar result of 7.7% of esophagitis patients progressing to Barrett's Esophagus was reported over a mean follow-up of 6.5 years of 582 patients[40]. Follow-up of 210 patients over a 6.5 year period demonstrated progression to Barrett's Esophagus in 20 (9.5%) despite being on PPIs[41]. In contrast, a Finnish study noted a 40% progression from esophagitis to Barrett's Esophagus over 17-22 years[42]. Factors associated with its development include a longer duration of symptoms compared with GERD case controls: 16(1-63) years v. 12(1-53) years[43]. Complicated esophagitis was also associated with developing Barrett's Esophagus: odds ratios, stricture 4.5 (1.9-10.4), ulcer 3.4 (1.3-8.8), hematemesis 3.7 (1.8-7.5). By contrast, the actual length of columnar mucosa does not appear to progress with time[4].

5.4.4 Esophageal adenocarcinoma

This is the most serious complication. For years it had been placed at the pinnacle of the GERD iceberg, only reached by progression through the Barrett's metaplasia-dysplasia-carcinoma sequence.

However, a recent publication has raised the possibility that symptoms alone are a risk factor for esophageal adenocarcinoma, regardless of the presence of Barrett's Esophagus[1]. This issue is dealt with more fully in subsequent sections of the book. However, there have been several editorials and leading articles regarding its implications for the natural history of GERD[44-46].

These emphasize the importance of taking symptoms seriously, even in the absence of Barrett's Esophagus.

6. PROGNOSTIC FACTORS

It is difficult to reach a consensus regarding which factors actually predict a poor prognosis for GERD patients. This is because different studies have produced conflicting results. In part, this may be explained by the small sample size of many studies or their use of only univariate analysis. It can also be explained by differing inclusion/exclusion criteria and differing end-points, e.g. symptomatic relapse, endoscopic relapse, development of complications. Table 2 outlines various factors that have shown significant associations with poor prognosis. It would appear that likelihood of rapid relapse after healing is predicted by grade of esophagitis, duration and dose of medication and failure to render asymptomatic on initial therapy. This fits well with the two contrasting studies quoted above [30,32]. Those patients who were easily healed had a low relapse rate; those who were refractory to initial therapy were more likely to relapse.

Long term outcome also appears dependent upon the severity of esophagitis and greater age of patient. However, it is less clear whether the degree of esophageal acid exposure is also an independent risk factor. It is more likely to simply be a surrogate marker for degree of esophagitis. This is probably also true for manometric parameters such as LOS pressure. The influence of body mass index, gender, smoking and other epidemiological factors remain to be determined.

7. QUALITY OF LIFE

Gastro-esophageal reflux disease does not adversely affect longevity. This was the conclusion reached more than 30 years ago in a series that included six deaths from esophagitis and four peri-operative deaths at the time of fundoplication[14]! Even assessing life expectancy in GERD patients with Barrett's Esophagus, little difference can be demonstrated compared with the general population[47,48]. However, increasingly data are being produced demonstrating the significant morbidity associated with GERD. In particular, research has concentrated on quality of life (QoL) (Figure 11)[49,50]. Studies have demonstrated that GERD can result in an impairment of QoL equivalent to that seen in chronic heart failure[51,52]. This low QoL can be demonstrated in NERD patients as well as those with esophagitis[22,53]. There is no difference between those with normal and abnormal levels of acid reflux on pH monitoring. This low QoL is chronic,

TABLE 2: Factors associated with a worse outcome for GERD patients

Predictive Factors	References
Erosive esophagitis	(25,31,69,70)
Esophageal pH monitoring – ↑%time (total/supine) pH<4	(27,70)
Not asymptomatic after initial therapy	(25,27)
Refractory to initial healing	(25,29,32)
Hiatus hernia	(70)
Reflux on barium meal	(31)
Low LOS pressure	(31)
Older age	(69)
High body mass index (BMI)	(69)
Refractory childhood symptoms	(65)

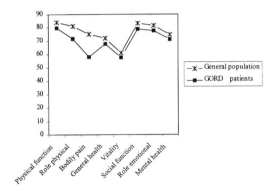

Figure 11: Quality of life scores in GERD patients demonstrating significant (p<0.001) reductions in all aspects of the SF36 survey compared with the general population. Adapted from Revicki et al[50].

persisting even 10 years after the GERD was diagnosed and treatment started[33]. The QoL enjoyed by GERD sufferers can be returned to normal levels by treatment with PPIs[54]. This is true even when symptoms are not fully abolished or esophagitis fully healed [51,43]. Much of the data referred to in this section comes from studies conducted in the secondary and tertiary care setting. It portrays a disease process which appears progressive, which carries the potential of serious complications and markedly impares QoL. However, there are minimal data on the long term outcome of refluxers in the primary care setting. Even less is known of the prognosis of those who self-medicate without ever consulting their family doctor. These individuals comprise the bulk of GERD sufferers. It is likely that the natural history of their GERD is much more benign.

8. THE FUTURE NATURAL HISTORY OF GERD

The natural history of GERD is changing. The widespread use of PPIs has altered the severity of the disease and the frequency of its complications. Proton pump inhibitors can be classed as disease-modifying agents. They have the ability to heal esophagitis and esophageal ulcers refractory to other forms of therapy[28,32]. They have the ability to maintain remission in 100% of patients if used at appropriate doses[41]. They prevent the recurrence of esophageal strictures[41,55,56], something not achieved by H2Ras[57,58]. It therefore seems likely that the increasing use of PPIs will result in fewer patients progressing to stricturing or ulceration. The number of admissions to hospital with these complications will also decline[3]. Recent review of the published data also suggests that these drugs are safe for long term use at the doses currently used[59]. The one area in which PPIs do not appear to modify disease relates to progression of Barrett's Esophagus. During a 6.5-year follow-up, 9.5% of patients developed Barrett's Esophagus despite being on sufficient medication to cure their esophagitis[41]. One of 64 patients with known Barrett's Esophagus also progressed to carcinoma.

Review of studies of patients with Barrett's Esophagus suggests little or no regression of the lesion on PPIs, albeit with some development of squamous islands[60,61]. Two other factors must be added to the lack of impact on Barrett's Esophagus: firstly, the dramatic rise in esophageal adenocarcinoma[62,63] and secondly, the link between symptoms and esophageal adenocarcinoma regardless of the presence of Barrett's Esophagus[1]. These issues suggest that the natural history of GERD may increasingly become that of a premalignant condition. To summarize the future of GERD, it would appear that we will be able to eliminate the benign complications and the associated reduction in QoL. However, this consequently will highlight the degree to which it remains a premalignant condition. We are not yet able to modify this aspect of the disease.

9. CHILDHOOD REFLUX

Gastro-esophageal reflux is a very common problem in infancy. Does it have any relevance to adult GERD? In the vast majority of cases, its natural history is one of spontaneous resolution by two years of age. However, there is evidence of a worse prognosis among those who have an associated hiatus hernia (partial thoracic stomach). Two studies have been performed which between them included 200 children with partial thoracic stomachs and followed them into adulthood [64,65]. The duration of follow-up was 20-40 years and included children diagnosed between 1945 and 1972. Both studies demonstrated a persisting hiatus hernia in 50%. There was a resolution of symptoms in the majority of cases such that the prevalence of reflux symptoms among these patients differed little from the general adult population. However, two issues emerge from the more recent study[65]. Firstly, those who responded poorly as infants had a significantly greater use of antacids as adults suggesting that infantile reflux may have some bearing on adult disease. Secondly, two of the small group of subjects with persisting, severe symptoms agreed to endoscopy and both had Barrett's Esophagus. A third patient with significant symptoms was also known to have developed a stricture. Although this represents a small percentage of all those who experienced infantile GERD, it does suggest that those symptoms persist into adult life merit endoscopy. This has particular significance given the Lagergren data concerning long term reflux symptoms being a risk factor for esophageal adenocarcinoma.

10. CONCLUSIONS

The following conclusions regarding the natural history of GERD can been drawn from a review of the literature:
1. The prevalence of heartburn and acid regurgitation in the community is consistently 15-20%. This has not changed in three decades and is not age dependent.
2. There is evidence to support the progression of GERD with time.
3. If esophagitis is present, GERD will continue to be a relapsing, symptomatic problem for 75%of patients.
4. Quality of life is reduced with GERD and this is a longstanding outcome.
5. Widespread use of proton pump inhibitors is reducing the incidence of complications.
6. The disease-modifying nature of proton pump inhibitors does not seem to hold true for Barrett's Esophagus. This is especially of concern given the increasing incidence of esophageal adenocarcinoma.
7. Childhood reflux is a different disease entity with a more benign natural history. Occasional exceptions with severe symptoms persisting into adulthood merit investigation.

REFERENCES

1. Lagergren J, Bergstrom R, Lindgren A, Nyren O. Symptomatic gastresophageal reflux as a risk factor for esophageal adenocarcinoma. N Engl J Med 1999;340(11):825-31.
2. Ahtaridis G, Snape WJ, Cohen S. Clinical and manometric findings in benign peptic strictures of the esophagus. Digestive Diseases & Sciences 1979;24:858-61.
3. Sonnenberg A, Massey BT, Jacobsen SJ. Hospital discharges resulting from esophagitis among Medicare beneficiaries. Digestive Diseases & Sciences 1994;39(1):183-8.
4. Cameron AJ, Lomboy CT. Barrett's esophagus: age, prevalence, and extent of columnar epithelium. Gastroenterology 1992;103(4):1241-5.
5. Bremner CG, Lynch VP, Ellis FH. Barrett's esophagus: congenital or acquired? An experimental study of esophageal mucosal regeneration in the dog. Surgery 1970;68(1):209-16.
6. Gillen P, Keeling P, Byrne PJ, West AB, Hennessy TP. Experimental columnar metaplasia in the canine esophagus. Br J Surg 1988;75(2):113-5.
7. Trudgill NJ, Kapur KC, Riley SA. Familial clustering of reflux symptoms. Am J Gastroenterol 1999;94(5):1172-8.
8. Hu FZ, Preston RA, Post JC, White GJ, Kikuchi LW, Wang X, Leal SM, Levenstien MA, Ott J, Self TW, et al. Mapping of a gene for severe pediatric gastroesophageal reflux to chromosome 13q14. JAMA 2000;284(3):325-34.
9. Carre IJ, Johnston BT, Thomas PS, Morrison PJ. Familial hiatal hernia in a large five generation family confirming true autosomal dominant inheritance. Gut 1999;45(5):649-52.
10. Romero Y, Cameron AJ, Locke GR, Schaid DJ, Slezak JM, Branch CD, Melton LJ. Familial aggregation of gastroesophageal reflux in patients with Barrett's esophagus and esophageal adenocarcinoma. Gastroenterology 1997;113(5):1449-56.
11. Locke GR, Talley NJ, Fett SL, Zinsmeister AR, Melton LJ. Prevalence and clinical spectrum of gastresophageal reflux: a population-based study in Olmsted County, Minnesota. Gastroenterology 1997;112(5):1448-56.
12. Jones R, Lydeard S. Prevalence of symptoms of dyspepsia in the community. British Medical Journal 1989;298:30-2.
13. Anonymous. A Gallup survey on heartburn across America. Princeton, NJ: The Gallup Organisation Inc.; 1988.
14. Brunnen PL, Karmody AM, Needham CD. Severe peptic esophagitis. Gut 1969;10:831-7.
15. Loof L, Gotell P, Elfberg B. The incidence of reflux esophagitis. A study of endoscopy reports from a

defined catchment area in Sweden. Scandinavian Journal of Gastroenterology 1993;28(2):113-8.

16. Palmer ED. The hiatus hernia - esophagitis - esophageal stricture complex. American Journal of Medicine 1968;44:566-79.

17. Rex JC, Andersen HA, Bartholomew LG, Cain JC. Esophageal hiatal hernia - a 10-year study of medically treated cases. JAMA 1961;178:271-4.

18. Graham DY, Smith JL, Patterson DJ. Why do apparently healthy people use antacid tablets? American Journal of Gastroenterology 1983;78:257-60.

19. De Meester TR, Wang CI, Wernly JA, Pellegrini CA, Little AG, Klementschitsch P, Bermudez G, Johnson LF, Skinner DB. Technique, indications and clinical use of 24 hour esophageal pH monitoring. Journal of Thoracic and Cardiovascular Surgery 1980;79:656-70.

20. Johnston BT, McFarland RJ, Collins JS, Love AH. Symptom index as a marker of gastro-esophageal reflux disease. Br J Surg 1992;79(10):1054-5.

21. McDougall NI, Johnston BT, Collins JS, McFarland RJ, Love AH. Disease progression in gastro-esophageal reflux disease as determined by repeat esophageal pH monitoring and endoscopy 3 to 4.5 years after diagnosis. Eur J Gastroenterol Hepatol 1997;9(12):1161-7.

22. Watson RG, Tham TC, Johnston BT, McDougall NI. Double blind cross-over placebo controlled study of omeprazole in the treatment of patients with reflux symptoms and physiological levels of acid reflux-- the "sensitive esophagus". Gut 1997;40(5):587-90.

23. Trimble KC, Douglas S, Pryde A, Heading RC. Clinical characteristics and natural history of symptomatic but not excess gastrosophageal reflux. Digestive Diseases & Sciences 1995;40(5):1098-104.

24. Carlsson R, Dent J, Watts R, Riley S, Sheikh R, Hatlebakk J, Haug K, de Groot G, van Oudvorst A, Dalvag A, et al. Gastro-esophageal reflux disease in primary care: an international study of different treatment strategies with omeprazole. International GERD Study Group. Eur J Gastroenterol Hepatol 1998;10(2):119-24.

25. Bardhan KD, Muller-Lissner S, Bigard MA, Porro GB, Ponce J, Hosie J, Scott M, Weir DG, Gillon KR, Peacock RA, et al. Symptomatic gastro-esophageal reflux disease: double blind controlled study of intermittent treatment with omeprazole or ranitidine. The European Study Group. Bmj 1999;318(7182):502-7.

26. Pace F, Santalucia F, Bianchi P. Natural history of gastro-esophageal reflux disease without esophagitis. Gut 1991;32:845-8.

27. Schindlbeck NE, Klauser AG, Berghammer G, Londong W, Muller-Lissner SA. Three year follow up of patients with gastroesophageal reflux disease. Gut 1992;33(8):1016-9.

28. Hetzel DJ, Dent J, Reed WD, Narielvala FM, Mackinnon M, McCarthy JH, Mitchell B, Beveridge BR, Laurence BH, Gibson GG. Healing and relapse of severe peptic esophagitis after treatment with omeprazole. Gastroenterology 1988;95(4):903-12.

29. Bate CM, Booth SN, Crowe JP, Mountford RA, Keeling PW, Hepworth-Jones B, Taylor MD, Richardson PD. Omeprazole 10 mg or 20 mg once daily in the prevention of recurrence of reflux esophagitis. Solo Investigator Group. Gut 1995;36(4):492-8.

30. Poynard T. Relapse rate of patients after healing of esophagitis--a prospective study of alginate as self-care treatment for 6 months. French Co-operative Study Group. Aliment Pharmacol Ther 1993;7(4):385-92.

31. Kuster E, Ros E, Toledo-Pimentel V, Pujol A, Bordas JM, Grande L, Pera C. Predictive factors of the long term outcome in gastro-esophageal reflux disease: six year follow up of 107 patients. Gut 1994;35(1):8-14.

32. Klinkenberg-Knol EC, Festen HP, Jansen JB, Lamers CB, Nelis F, Snel P, Luckers A, Dekkers CP, Havu N, Meuwissen SG. Long-term treatment with omeprazole for refractory reflux esophagitis: efficacy and safety. Ann Intern Med 1994;121(3):161-7.

33. McDougall NI, Johnston BT, Kee F, Collins JS, McFarland RJ, Love AH. Natural history of reflux esophagitis: a 10 year follow up of its effect on patient symptomatology and quality of life. Gut 1996;38(4):481-6.

34. Ollyo JB, Monnier P, Fontolliet C, Savary M. The natural history, prevalence and incidence of reflux esophagitis. Gullet 1993;3:3-10.

35. Sonnenberg A. Blum AL, Siewert JR, editors.Refluxtherapie. Berlin: Springer Verlag; 1981;Epidemiologie und Spontanverlauf der Refluxkrankheit. p. 85-106.

36. Lanspa S, Spechler SJ, DeMeester TR, et al. Incidence of esophageal stricture formation in patients with complicated gastresophageal reflux disease (GERD). Gastroenterology 1991;100:A107

37. Ben Rejeb M, Bouche O, Zeitoun P. Study of 47 consecutive patients with peptic esophageal stricture compared with 3880 cases of reflux esophagitis. Dig Dis Sci 1992;37(5):733-6.

38. Patterson DJ, Graham DY, Smith JL, Schwartz JT, Alpert E, Lanza FL, Cain GD. Natural history of benign esophageal stricture treated by dilatation. Gastroenterology 1983;85:346-50.

39. Costa ND, Cadiot G, Merle C, Jolly D, Bouche O, Thiefin G, Zeitoun P. Bleeding reflux esophagitis: a prospective 1-year study in a university hospital. Am J Gastroenterol 2001;96(1):47-51.

40. Brossard E, Monnier P, Ollyo JB, et al. Serious complications - stenosis, ulcer and Barrett's epithelium - develop in 21.6% of adults with erosive reflux esophagitis. Gastroenterology 1991;100:A36

41. Klinkenberg-Knol EC, Nelis F, Dent J, Snel P, Mitchell B, Prichard P, Lloyd D, Havu N, Frame MH, Roman J, et al. Long-term omeprazole treatment in resistant gastresophageal reflux disease: efficacy, safety, and influence on gastric mucosa. Gastroenterology 2000;118(4):661-9.

42. Isolauri J, Luostarinen M, Isolauri E, Reinikainen P, Viljakka M, Keyrilainen O. Natural course of gastresophageal reflux disease: 17-22 year follow-up of 60 patients. American Journal of Gastroenterology 1997;92(1):37-41.

43. Eisen GM, Sandler RS, Murray S, Gottfried M. The relationship between gastresophageal reflux disease and its complications with Barrett's esophagus. American Journal of Gastroenterology 1997;92(1):27-31.

44. Cohen S, Parkman HP. Heartburn--a serious symptom. N Engl J Med 1999;340(11):878-9.

45. Johnston BT. The significance of heartburn. QJM 2000;93(6):321-2.

46. Dent J, Jones R, Kahrilas P, Talley NJ. Management of gastro-esophageal reflux disease in general practice. Bmj 2001;322(7282):344-7.

47. Cameron AJ, Ott BJ, Payne WS. The incidence of adenocarcinoma in columnar-lined (Barrett's) esophagus. N Engl J Med 1985;313(14):857-9.

48. Van d, V, Dees J, Blankensteijn JD, Van Blankenstein M. Adenocarcinoma in Barrett's esophagus: an overrated risk. Gut 1989;30(1):14-8.

49. Johnston BT. Gastresophageal reflux disease and a HAPPI quality of life. Am J Gastroenterol 1999;94(7):1723-4.

50. Revicki DA, Wood M, Maton PN, Sorensen S. The impact of gastresophageal reflux disease on health-related quality of life. Am J Med 1998;104(3):252-8.

51. McDougall NI, Collins JS, McFarland RJ, Watson RG, Love AH. The effect of treating reflux esophagitis with omeprazole on quality of life. Eur J Gastroenterol Hepatol 1998;10(6):459-64.

52. Hunter JG, Trus TL, Branum GD, Waring JP, Wood WC. A physiologic approach to laparoscopic fundoplication for gastresophageal reflux disease. Ann Surg 1996;223(6):673-85.

53. Havelund T, Lind T, Wiklund I, Glise H, Hernqvist H, Lauritsen K, Lundell L, Pedersen SA, Carlsson R, Junghard O, et al. Quality of life in patients with heartburn but without esophagitis: effects of treatment with omeprazole. Am J Gastroenterol 1999;94(7):1782-9.

54. Green J, Venables TL, Bate CM, Duggan S, Powell J. Omeprazole produces a greater improvement in quality of life than placebo, antacid-alginate, ranitidine, cimetidine or cisapride in patients with gastro-esophageal reflux disease. British Journal of Medical Economics 1997;11:121-31.

55. Smith PM, Kerr GD, Cockel R, Ross BA, Bate CM, Brown P, Dronfield MW, Green JR, Hislop WS, Theodossi A. A comparison of omeprazole and ranitidine in the prevention of recurrence of benign esophageal stricture. Restore Investigator Group. Gastroenterology 1994;107(5):1312-8.

56. Jaspersen D, Schwacha H, Schorr W, Brennenstuhl M, Raschka C, Hammar CH. Omeprazole in the treatment of patients with complicated gastro-esophageal reflux disease. J Gastroenterol Hepatol 1996;11(10):900-2.

57. Ferguson R, Dronfield MW, Atkinson M. Cimetidine in treatment of reflux esophagitis with peptic stricture. Br Med J 1979;2(6188):472-4.

58. Marks RD, Richter JE. Peptic strictures of the esophagus. American Journal of Gastroenterology 1993;88(8):1160-73.

59. Armstrong D. Long-term safety and efficacy of omeprazole in gastro-esophageal reflux disease. Lancet 2000;356(9230):610-2.

60. Cooper BT, Neumann CS, Cox MA, Iqbal TH. Continuous treatment with omeprazole 20 mg daily for up to 6 years in Barrett's esophagus. Aliment Pharmacol Ther 1998;12(9):893-7.

61. Peters FT, Ganesh S, Kuipers EJ, Sluiter WJ, Klinkenberg-Knol EC, Lamers CB, Kleibeuker JH. Endoscopic regression of Barrett's esophagus during omeprazole treatment; a randomised double blind study. Gut 1999;45(4):489-94.

62. Devesa SS, Blot WJ, Fraumeni JFJ. Changing patterns in the incidence of esophageal and gastric carcinoma in the United States. Cancer 1998;83(10):2049-53.

63. Bytzer P, Christensen PB, Damkier P, Vinding K, Seersholm N. Adenocarcinoma of the esophagus and Barrett's esophagus: a population- based study. Am J Gastroenterol 1999;94(1):86-91.

64. Astley R, Carre IJ, Langmead-Smith R. A 20-year prospective follow-up of childhood hiatal hernia. Br J Radiol 1977;50(594):400-3.

65. Johnston BT, Carre IJ, Thomas PS, Collins BJ. Twenty to 40 year follow up of infantile hiatal hernia. Gut 1995;36(6):809-12.

66. Nebel OT, Fornes MF, Castell DO. Symptomatic gastresophageal reflux: incidence and precipitating factors. Digestive Diseases 1976;21:953-6.

67. Thompson WG, Heaton KW. Heartburn and globus in apparently healthy people. Can Med Assoc J 1982;126(1):46-8.

68. Ruth M, Mansson I, Sandberg N. The prevalence of symptoms suggestive of esophageal disorders. Scandinavian Journal of Gastroenterology 1991;26:73-81.

69. McDougall NI, Johnston BT, Collins JS, McFarland RJ, Love AH. Three- to 4.5-year prospective study of prognostic indicators in gastro-esophageal reflux disease. Scand J Gastroenterol 1998;33(10):1016-22.

70. Gambitta P, Indriolo A, Colombo P, Grosso C, Pirone Z, Rossi A, Bini M, Zanasi G, Arcidiacono R. Management of patients with gastresophageal reflux disease: A long-term follow-up study. Current Therapeutic Research 1998;59:275-87.

2.2 HELICOBACTER PYLORI AND REFLUX DISEASE

A. Cats and E. J. Kuipers

1. INTRODUCTION

The presence of spiral bacteria on the human gastric mucosa was already described more than one hundred years ago.[1] Nevertheless, the clinical importance of this observation only appeared after Warren and Marshall were able to culture bacteria from gastric biopsy samples in 1982.[2] Initially, this bacterium was named *Campylobacter pyloridis* but, after further identification of its biochemical properties the new genus Helicobacter was introduced and the bacterium was renamed *Helicobacter pylori* (*H. pylori*).[3] It appeared that half of the world's population is colonized with this bacterium, which colonization usually persists lifelong and remains asymptomatic in the majority of cases. However, *H. pylori* colonization is virtually always accompanied by chronic active gastritis, which increases the individual's risk for the development of several gastroduodenal diseases, such as gastric and duodenal ulceration, gastric mucosa-associated lymphoid tissue (MALT) lymphoma, and distal gastric cancer, making it a pathogen of great significance. In particular, it is estimated that approximately 10-20% of *H. pylori*-positive subjects ultimately develops ulcer disease, whereas 1-2% develops adenocarcinoma of the distal stomach. The chances of developing these complications depend upon the genetics and acid output of the host, external factors such as diet, and the characteristics of the bacterial strain. For instance, the chance of developing gastric cancer as a result of *H. pylori* colonization is increased in subjects with the IL-1 haplotype encoding for the most pronounced IL-1 (response to colonization,[4] as well as in those with a high-salt intake, or colonized with more virulent strains. All of these factors are associated with more severely active chronic gastritis and thus increase the risk for permanent mucosal damage with atrophy and intestinal metaplasia.

The recognition that major gastroduodenal disorders such as peptic ulcer disease and gastric cancer are mostly the result of a bacterial infection, the unraveling of underlying pathogenic mechanisms and the determination of treatment strategies together comprise one of the major medical achievements of the past 20 years. Recently, clinicians have nevertheless become increasingly aware that colonization with *H. pylori* may also have beneficial effects for the human host. In this respect, the interest is in particular going to the potential preventive effect of *H. pylori* colonization on the development of gastro-esophageal reflux disease (GERD) and its complications such as Barrett's esophagus and adenocarcinoma of the distal esophagus. If so, this will have a major impact on issues such as screening and treatment of *H. pylori* infections. In this chapter, we will discuss the relation between *H. pylori* and the development as well as the treatment of GERD. For the understanding of the association between *H. pylori*, gastric acidity and potential prevention of GERD, we first focus on the epidemiology and transmission of *H. pylori*, then on microbiological aspects with importance for disease outcome, to continue with the role of *H. pylori* in the development and treatment of GERD.

2. EPIDEMIOLOGY AND TRANSMISSION

H. pylori colonization is very common among humans. In Western countries, the prevalence of this bacterium varies between 30-50%,[5] and in developing countries between 80-90%.[6,7] Most new infections are thought to occur in the first two decades of life. Sero-epidemiological studies in Western countries show a rise of H. pylori prevalence with age.[8] Only 10-20% of those aged less than 30 years is H. pylori-positive. This raises to more than 70% in those over seventy years of age. This phenomenon is largely due to an age-cohort effect, reflecting a decreasing chance of infection in recent decades in the Western societies as a result of changes in the presence of risk factors for acquisition of *H. pylori*.[9,10] These factors include low socio-economic status with clustering of persons in a limited number of rooms, lack of bathing facilities and private water supplies and a low level of education. Thusfar, the exact route of transmission is however unknown. The transmission of *H. pylori* probably occurs from person to person, either feco-oral or oro-oral.[11] No other habitat has so far been found, although the significance of reports of these bacteria in pet

H.W. Tilanus and S.E.A. Attwood (eds.), Barrett's Esophagus, 81–105.

animals as well as in sewage water remains to be clarified.[12] The feco-oral transmission route is supported by the detection of *H. pylori* in human feces, in sewage water and in vegetables fertilized with human fecal material. However, epidemiological studies on the seroprevalence of *H. pylori* show no concordance with the presence of serum-antibodies against hepatitis A, a known feco-orally transmitted infection.[13] Other data

demonstrated the presence of *H. pylori* in saliva and dental plaque, supporting the hypothesis that transmission could be oro-oral.[14,15] Further studies with special emphasis on DNA fingerprints of *H. pylori* should provide greater insight into the route of transmission. Whether *H. pylori* infection is an occupational risk remains an unsolved issue at this moment. Although some authors

TABLE 1. Intragastric barriers and defense mechanisms of *Helicobacter pylori* enabling survival in the stomach.

Barriers	*Type*	*Defense mechanism*
Chemical	Acid	Urease
		Motility
Physical	Mucus flow	Motility
	Mucus viscosity	Adhesion
Biological	Immune response	Antigenic variability
	Nutrients limitation	PMN killing resistance
		Nutrient accumulation factors
		Cytotoxicity and *cagA*

demonstrated a higher seroprevalence of *H. pylori* in gastroenterologists in comparison to matched controls, other studies failed to show such a difference.[15-18] The risk of infection for dentists and endoscopy nurses also does not seem to be increased. Endoscopic transmission of *H. pylori* infection has been observed on several occasions, and has led to more strict cleaning and desinfecting guidelines.[20]

3. PATHOGENIC PROPERTIES AND VIRULENCE FACTORS OF *HELICOBACTER PYLORI*

3.1 VIRULENCE FACTORS INVOLVED IN COLONIZATION

H. pylori is a micro-aerophilic Gram-negative rod. The 3-4 μm long and 0.5-1.0 μm wide organism contains 4-6 unipolar flagella on its outer surface, thus providing the bacterium a remarkable motility in viscous solutions, such as the gastric mucus layer. It normally has a curved- or S-type shape, but spiral and coccoidal forms do occur, the latter phenotype reflecting cell death.[21] The bacterium is an acid-tolerant neutrophil, i.e. the optimal pH for bacterial growth is 7, but it can resist a much lower pH range. Only few bacteria are able to survive the hostile acidic environment of the human stomach. Several mechanisms however allow *H. pylori* to persistently colonize this turbid ecological niche (Table 1). Two important

mechanisms are urease activity and the presence of sheathed flagella on the outer surface of the bacterium, which enable bacterial transfer through the acidic gastric lumen into the viscous epithelial mucus layer.[22] The flagellar filament consists of two different proteins, FlaA and FlaB, which are both essential for motility.[23] Allelic disruption of *flaA* and *flaB*, the genes encoding for the FlaA and FlaB proteins, evoked mutant *H. pylori* strains with reduced motility, that were unable to colonize gnotobiotic piglets.[24] Functional studies revealed that motility is dependent on viscosity and pH.[25-27] Upon entering the stomach, *H. pylori* heads towards the mucus layer which is rich of high-molecular-weight mucins, urea and sodium bicarbonate. After penetrating this viscous layer, adherence of the bacteria to the nearby epithelium is facilitated by formation of bacterial pedestals.[28] Subsequent binding of bacterial adhesins to epithelial cell outer membrane structures such as blood group antigens and extracellular matrix proteins such as collagen, laminin and vitronectin, establishes firm adherence to the epithelial surface.[29-31] The affinity for specific receptor structures presented by different epithelial cells may affect the distribution of *H. pylori*-colonization throughout the stomach. Apart from motility and adhesion, survival in the gastric acid environment is facilitated by enzymatic activity of the bacteria (Table 2). The major enzyme produced by *H. pylori* is urease. Seven genes comprise the urease gene cluster of this bacterium. These genes are homologous to urease-encoding genes from other bacterial species. *UreA* and *ureB* encode for the structural subunits of the enzyme.[32] *UreD, ureE, ureF* and *ureG* are accessory genes encoding proteins that function to insert nickel ions, which are essential for catalytic activity, into the active site of the apo-enzyme.[33] The role of the seventh gene, *ureI*, is unknown. This gene has no homology with other urease clusters and is not essential for urease activity. Urease catalyses the hydrolysis of urea to yield ammonia and carbamate.[5,34] The latter compound spontaneously decomposes to yield another molecule of ammonia and carbonic acid. In solution, the released carbonic acid and the two molecules of

ammonia are in equilibrium with their deprotonated and protonated forms, respectively. The net effect of these reactions is a local neutralization of acid by generating ammonia.[35] The importance of this mechanism was shown in experiments with urease-negative mutants of *H. pylori*. These mutants were incapable to colonize a mouse stomach at physiological pH, but did colonize it during treatment with a proton pump inhibitor.[36,37] The neutralization of acid appears most critical during transmission of infection into a new host. During the initial stage of colonization, achlorhydria has been observed. After establishment of chronic infection, acid production mostly restores and other functions of urease activity become more important. These include the provision

TABLE 2. Enzymatic activity of *H. pylori*, function and mode of action.

Enzyme	Mode of action
Urease	Survival of *H. pylori*, ammonia production
Toxic enzymes	
VacA	Toxic vacuole formation
CagA	Cytotoxic cell reaction
Phospholipase A$_1$, A$_2$ and C	Formation of toxic lysolecithin and
Alcoholdehydrogenase	Acetaldehyde
Proteolytic enzymes	Protein degradation
Antioxydants	Survival in macrophages
Catalase	
Super oxyde dismutase	Inactivation of O$_2$ metabolites
Metabolic enzymes	Metabolism of
Lactate dehydrogenase	Pyruvate to lactate
Pyruvate decarboxylase	Pyruvate to acetaldehyde
Pyruvate dehydrogenase	Pyruvate to acetate
Aldolase	Glucose and pyruvate to acetate
Phosphatase	Phosphatase metabolism and transport
ATPase	Mediator cytotoxicity, energy metabolism
Fumarate reductase	Enables anaerobic respiration
Adenine-guanine-hypoxanthine-	Purine nucleotide synthesis
Phosphoribosyl transferase	

Adapted from [33]

of nitrogen for protein synthesis. Glutamine is formed by the ligation of ammonia to glutamate by catalysis of glutamine-synthetase. For bacteria such as *H. pylori*, this is the only route to incorporate ammonia into amino acids. Urease therefore may play a nutritional key role in bacterial protein synthesis. Whereas ureases of other bacterial species have only been demonstrated within the cytosol, urease-activity in *H. pylori* has *in vitro* been demonstrated to be present both cytosolic as well as on the bacterial surface.[38,39] Moreover, free urease has been

localized by immunohistochemical staining within gastric tissue.[40] It appears that shedding of the protein from the bacterial surface is possible. As a consequence, secretory immunoglobulins may bind to this "soluble"-antigen instead of the bacterium itself. The host defense apparatus may thus be impaired, causing insufficient clearance of the antigen. Ammonium hydroxide, generated by hydrolysis of urea, causes histological damage to the gastric mucosa. The underlying mechanism may be related to a direct cytotoxic effect of generated hydroxide ions or ammonia may impair normal hydrogen ion back diffusion, resulting in epithelium damage.[41,42]

3.2 VIRULENCE FACTORS INVOLVED IN DISEASE ACTIVITY

Epithelial damage plays a key role in the induction of *H. pylori* colonization, as it may enable the bacterium to obtain essential nutrients such as iron. It is however also a key factor in the establishment of disease during long-term colonization, and probably also a factor in the prevention of GERD.

Epithelial damage is not only the result of ammonia production. For instance, Leunk *et al.* described that supernatants of *H. pylori* cultures could induce vacuoles in eukaryotic cells.[43] Further research revealed that expression of the responsible vacuolating cytotoxin A (VacA) occurred in only 50% of *H. pylori* strains,[44] even though the gene encoding for this cytotoxin (*vacA*) was present in all strains. Strains expressing VacA were significantly more often isolated from patients with peptic ulcer disease.[45] Although the presence of VacA-positive *H. pylori* strains also correlated with both atrophic gastritis and gastric carcinoma, this association was less striking.[46,47] Expression of VacA is considered a marker for more virulent strains with higher cytotoxicity. Different alleles were recently described for the *vacA* gene, they differ in their middle regions (two variants: m1 and m2) and signal sequence regions (four variants: s1a, s1b, s1c and s2).[48,49] Although eight genotypes are thus theoretically possible, strains containing *vacA* s2m1 have not been observed. Strains containing s1m1 are high toxin producers, whereas s2m2 are low producers. Patients with peptic ulcer disease are more often infected with strains containing the s1 genotype.[49]

In Western countries, *H. pylori*-positive patients with ulcer disease, atrophic gastritis or distal gastric cancer also differed from *H. pylori*-positive healthy controls with respect to the prevalence of serum-antibodies against another bacterial protein. The presence of antibodies against this 120 kD CagA (Cytotoxin-associated-gene A) protein was observed in 80-90% of patients with these disorders versus only 40-60% in most Western controls.[50-53] Infection with a *cagA*-positive (*cagA*+) strain appeared associated with higher levels of gastric inflammation and greater intramucosal IL-8 production.[53,55] Strains carrying the CagA+ phenotype thus seem to be more virulent than CagA-strains. Unlike the *vacA* gene, the *cagA* gene is not conserved in all *H. pylori* strains. In Western countries *cagA*+ strains are found in around 60% of infected subjects, in developing countries the prevalence of *cagA*+ strains is higher. The *cagA* gene is a 30 kb marker for a pathogenicity island, containing several genes including *picA* and *picB*.[56] Transcription of both these genes is linked to that of *cagA* and lack of transcription of one gene causes lack of transcription of all downstream genes. Mutations in the *cagA* gene preserves the virulence of *cagA*+ *H. pylori* strains, whereas mutations in *picA* or *picB* diminish the cytotoxic activity of the strain. The virulence of cagA+ strains thus essentially depends on expression of *picA* and *picB*. More recently, a novel gene has been identified, transcription of which is induced by contact with epithelium. This *iceA* gene contains two mosaic variations: *iceA1* and *iceA2*.[57] At present the function of this gene is not fully understood. In a recent report an association was found between peptic ulcers and the presence of *iceA1* containing strains.[57] The allelic type of *iceA* is independent of the *cagA* and *vacA* status.

In summary, strains that contain *vacA* s1, *cagA*+ or *iceA1* are considered highly pathogenic and are strongly associated with more severe gastritis and its complications such peptic ulcer disease, whereas type *vacA* s2ms, *cagA*-, *iceA2* are considered less pathogenic. More virulent strains also have a greater effect on acid production and therefore may play a more significant role in GERD as will be discussed below.

4.   *HELICOBACTER PYLORI,* GASTRITIS AND ACID PRODUCTION

4.1 PEPTIC ULCER DIASEASE

Even though virtually all *H. pylori* colonized subjects develop chronic gastric inflammation, most of them do not have any symptoms associated with this condition. A number of *H. pylori*-positive subjects suffer from upper abdominal symptoms. There still exists controversy whether or not these symptoms improve if *H. pylori* is eradicated by multiple drug treatment. Therefore, so-called 'non-ulcer dyspepsia' has not been generally accepted as an indication for *H. pylori* screening and treatment.

The main indication for treatment of *H. pylori* is the occurrence of peptic ulcer disease. This disorder has long been thought to have a multifactorial pathogenesis without a common denominator. A subset of all peptic ulcers is caused by the intake of NSAID's and aspirin, and by rare disorders such as the Zollinger-Ellison syndrome and Crohn's disease. However, 80% of all gastric ulcers and more than 90% of duodenal ulcers were considered to be 'idiopathic'. After the initial isolation of *H. pylori*, it appeared that these ulcers virtually always occurred in the presence of this organism and that its eradication in these patients could significantly affect the ulcer recurrence rate. If a patient presents with a peptic ulcer in either stomach or duodenum, the chance of recurrence after healing is more than 30% in the first year, even with maintenance therapy with acid suppressive drugs. However, after eradication of *H. pylori*, only few patients have recurrent attacks and acid suppressive therapy can be fully withdrawn.[58,59] In developed countries, about ten percent of the persons colonized by *H. pylori* develop gastric or duodenal ulceration. The issue of why colonization with *H. pylori* leads to recurrent peptic ulceration in some individuals, but not in others, has not yet been solved. As mentioned, this is likely related to differences in bacterial strains, but bacterial heterogeneity can not fully explain differences in the occurrence of peptic ulcer disease. Socio-behavioral and genetic host factors also are thought to play a role. Cigarette smoking is a behavioral factor that has been identified to increase the risk of ulcer disease in the presence of *H. pylori*. However, once *H. pylori* is eradicated, persistent smoking does not affect the chance of ulcer recurrence. With respect to genetic factors, only relatively few data are yet available. However, concordance rates for peptic ulceration have been shown to be higher for monozygotic twins than for dizygotic twins[60] and, for reasons unknown, ulcer disease is known to be associated with blood group O and with a non-secretor status of ABO blood group antigens. From observations in a number of chronic mucosal intestinal disorders, in particular inflammatory bowel disease and celiac disease, it has been shown that specific genetic polymorphisms in human cytokine genes correlate with disease outcome. Likewise, a number of studies have focused on the relation between ulcer disease and such genetic polymorphisms of the host. These researchers claimed that ulcer disease is more common among subjects with specific HLA-DQ alleles.[61,62] Finally, epidemiological data suggest that the type of ulcer disease depends on the age at which a subject became colonized with *H. pylori*.

Gastric ulcer disease is probably more common among subjects who became colonized at a very young age, whereas colonization at a later age would be more associated with duodenal ulcer disease.[63] This hypothesis helps to explain geographical differences in the incidence of gastric and duodenal ulcer disease. In countries with a high *H. pylori* prevalence among very young children, gastric ulcer is more common than duodenal ulcer. In contrast, in developed countries with a relatively low prevalence of infection among very young children, duodenal ulcer disease is more common.

Ulcer disease is thus likely to be influenced by bacterial, host and environmental factors. However, irrespective of all these co-factors, recurrence of ulcer disease is rare after eradication of *H. pylori*. As such, *H. pylori* has probably been the most important 'emerging infection' of the past two decades and the recognition of its role in peptic ulcer disease has had a major impact on healthcare worldwide.

4.2 GASTRIC CANCER

Chronic *H. pylori*-induced inflammation can eventually lead to loss of the normal architecture of the gastric mucosa with destruction of gastric glands, and replacement by fibrosis and intestinal metaplastic cells. These conditions, atrophic gastritis and intestinal metaplasia, eventually occur in approximately half of the *H. pylori* colonized population.[64] Subjects with atrophy and intestinal metaplasia of their gastric mucosa have a significantly increased risk for gastric cancer. This risk is estimated to be five- to ninety-fold increased dependent upon the severity of the atrophy and upon the type of metaplasia.[65] Subjects in whom the metaplastic cells resemble epithelial cells of the colon ('type III' intestinal metaplasia) have a higher risk for cancer than those in whom the metaplasia resembles small bowel epithelium ('type I' intestinal metaplasia).[66] In recent years, it has become clear that these conditions are rare in the absence of *H. pylori* colonization.[64] This is not surprising, as they are the result of chronic gastric mucosal inflammation, which is strongly associated with *H. pylori*. Evidence that *H. pylori* can thus, via the sequence of atrophy and metaplasia, cause gastric cancer originates from various studies, in particular from a number of cohort follow-up studies.[67-69] These studies showed that *H. pylori*-positive subjects approximately three to six-fold more often than non-infected controls develop gastric cancer involving the distal stomach. This was supported by other data that showed geographical associations between the prevalence of H. pylori and the incidence of gastric cancer.[70,71] Retrospective studies comparing the prevalence of H. pylori among patients with gastric cancer and controls did not always show the expected higher prevalence of H. pylori among the cancer patients.[72] However, this discrepancy between prospective and retrospective data can be explained by the gradual disappearance of H. pylori colonization during the process of development of atrophic gastritis and intestinal metaplasia.[64,73,74] This explanation is supported by a meta-analysis of prospective data showing that the calculated odds ratio for gastric cancer in the presence of H. pylori becomes close to 9.0 with a longer observation period.[75]

It is estimated on the basis of these findings that H. pylori colonization increases the risk for gastric cancer approximately ten-fold. In 1994, the International Agency for Research on Cancer, a department of the World Health Organization, classified H. pylori a class I carcinogen, which means that the Agency considered the evidence on the relation between H. pylori and gastric cancer conclusive.[72] The lifetime gastric cancer risk among H. pylori-positive subjects is close to one percent. In the developed world, 60% to 80% of gastric cancers are therefore related to the long-term presence of H. pylori. For that reason, large studies have begun to evaluate whether early H. pylori eradication can prevent atrophic gastritis and gastric cancer. Epidemiological calculations suggest that such a strategy can be cost-effective in populations with a high prevalence of H. pylori and a high incidence of gastric cancer.[76] However, the prevention of atrophy and cancer in the general population is not yet an indication for widespread treatment of H. pylori infection as long as the results of prospective studies on this issue are not yet available. This restrictive policy is supported by the shortage of data on potential benefits of H. pylori infection and on the importance of bacterial and host heterogeneity.[77] The incidence of gastric cancer has significantly decreased over the past decades in developed countries. In the US, it decreased in the past 60 years from approximately 30 to 5 cases per 100.000 inhabitants per year. This decrease parallels the decrease in the prevalence of H. pylori, which is related to socio-economic changes. This decrease,

which is still ongoing, will have a significant impact on the incidence of H. pylori associated conditions and on the feasibility of potential population screening and treatment programs.[76]

As with peptic ulcer disease, it needs to be determined why some individuals develop atrophy and cancer in the presence of H. pylori, whereas others do not develop these conditions. It is believed that the risk for atrophy and cancer is associated with the severity of gastritis, in that severe mucosal inflammation will sooner lead to destruction of glands and replacement by fibrosis and/or metaplasia. This hypothesis is supported by the finding that cagA+ strains[54,52] cause more severe inflammation than cagA- strains, and that cagA+ strains are also associated with an approximate two-fold higher risk for atrophic gastritis and gastric cancer.[52,53,78] Another factor that has significant influence on the pattern and severity of gastritis in the presence of H. pylori is acid production. H. pylori may be an acidophil; the optimal pH for survival and growth under physiologic circumstances is probably between 5 and 6. This optimal pH is normally found in the distal or antral part of the stomach, away from the acid-producing parietal cells. This phenomenon helps to explain why H. pylori usually causes antral-predominant gastritis. However, if acid suppression is impaired, for example because of use of acid suppressive drugs or the presence of atrophic gastritis with loss of parietal cells, H. pylori colonization and gastritis increase in the proximal stomach.[79,80] Research involving an animal model suggests that under these circumstances the organisms may also penetrate deeper in the gastric pits.[81] Thus, one hypothesis is that distribution and severity of H. pylori gastritis increase during a reduction of acid secretion and consequently increases the risk for atrophy and cancer. This hypothesis is supported by various cohort studies that show an increased incidence of atrophic gastritis in H. pylori-positive subjects with conditions affecting acid output.[82]

5. HELICOBACTER PYLORI AND THE DEVELOPMENT OF REFLUX DISEASE

The term GERD is used to include all symptoms and mucosal lesions resulting from retrograde flow of gastric contents into the esophagus. GERD has long been considered to occur independent of H. pylori colonization, i.e. to occur with the same

TABLE 3. The prevalence of *Helicobacter pylori* in gastro-esophageal reflux disease

Authors	Study design/Possible bias	Geographic region	No. of GERD patients (% H. pylori-positive)	Mean age ± SD	No. of controls (% H. pylori-positive)	Mean age ± SD	Establishment of H. pylori	Comments
Cheng	Case-control/Selection of controls	USA	11/27 (41)		11/35 (31)		Antral mucosal histology and culture and urease activity	Endoscopic esophagitis. Cohort including 12 patients with duodenal ulcer; cohort age: 61 ± 9
Abbas	Uncontrolled cross-sectional	Pakistan	18/29 (62)	45 (24-80)*			Antral mucosal histology	Endoscopic esophagitis. * median (range)
Liston	Case-control/Selection of cases	UK	28/37 (76)		27/33 (82)		Antral and corpus mucosal histology, urease activity, serology and 13C-UBT	Macroscopic and microscopic reflux esophagitis; PPI therapy excluded. Cohort of elderly patients
Werdmuller	Case-control/Selection of controls	Netherlands	34/118 (29)	62	204/399 (51)	48	Antral mucosal histology and serology in all; urease activity and culture in a non-characterized subgroup	Endoscopic esophagitis. Similar results for 109 patients with hiatal hernia
Newton	Case-control	UK	13/36 (36)	52 (11-78)*	9/25 (36)	54 (13-83)*	Antral and fundus mucosal histology and urease activity	Endoscopic esophagitis. Controls are patients with anemia without endoscopic abnormalities
Csendes	Case-control/Selection of controls	Chile	14/55 (25) a 26/81 (32) b	43 43	38/190 (20)	42	Antral mucosal histology	No previous anti-reflux therapy. a= reflux as determined by 24-hour pH-monitoring, b= erosive esophagitis
Varanasi	Retrospective case-control	USA	35/114 (31)	50 ± 1	168/400 (42)	53 ± 1	Antral and corpus mucosal histology and rapid urease test	Cases consist of endoscopic and/or histologic evidence of esophagitis
Hackelsberger	Matched, retrospective case-control	Germany	50/130 (39)	54 ± 15	89/227 (39)	51 ± 17	Antral and corpus mucosal histology and rapid urease test for cases; 13C-UBT for controls	Cases including unreported number of Barrett's esophagus patients
Vicari	Case-control	USA	30/84 (36)	55 ± 15	26/57 (46)	59 ± 16	Antral and fundus mucosal histology and serology	Exclusion of PPI therapy one month prior to study entry. Patients: (non)erosive GERD by history and endoscopy
Wu	Matched case-control	Hong Kong	33/106 (31)	56 ± 20	73/120 (61)	56 ± 18	Serology. In case of endoscopy: antral urease activity and antral as well as corpus mucosal histology	Cases: symptoms of heartburn improving with acid-suppression or endoscopic esophagitis. Controls: asymptomatic
Manes	Case-control	Italy	40/110 (36) a 57/92 (62) b	55 ± 12 52 ± 13	110/200 (55) c 80/200 (40) d	54 ± 13 54 ± 11	Antral and corpus mucosal histology in a,b,c. Serology in d	a=erosive GERD, b=reflux and regurgitation without endoscopic signs, c=functional dyspepsia, d=healthy blood donors
Öberg	Uncontrolled cross-sectional	Sweden and USA	16/126 (13) a 8/69 (12) b				Antral mucosal histology	a=abnormal acid exposure determined by 24-hour pH-monitoring, b=erosive esophagitis
Koike	Matched case-control	Japan	59/175 (34)	63 ± 1	126/175 (72)	63 ± 1	Antral and corpus mucosal histology, urease activity, serology	Exclusion of PPI and H2RA therapy one months prior to study entry. Additional assessment of atrophic gastritis
Wu	Uncontrolled cross-sectional	China	77/225 (34) a 33/77 (43) b 38/77 (49) c 6/77 (8) d	57 ± 19			Antral and corpus mucosal histology, urease activity	a=all GERD patients, b=non-erosive GERD, c=grade 1+2 Savary-Miller, d=grade 3+4

frequency and severity in *H. pylori*-positive and *H. pylori*-negative subjects. This opinion was based upon cross-sectional observations that the prevalence of *H. pylori* among GERD patients was not higher than among controls.[83] However, the fact that the prevalence of *H. pylori* among cases was actually lower was discarded. This one-sided focus obviously resulted from the many previous studies in which patients with upper gastrointestinal disorders, such as peptic ulcer disease, atrophic gastritis and gastric cancer, always had a higher prevalence of *H. pylori* than healthy controls. Furthermore, because *H. pylori* may lead to increased acid production and disturbed gastric emptying, it was hypothesized that *H. pylori* added these risk factors to GERD development. The higher prevalence of *H. pylori* among cases appeared not the case with GERD. In contrast, further studies and closer observations suggested that *H. pylori* might actually protect against the development of GERD. This slowly emerging concept came from repeated observations of a low prevalence of *H. pylori* among GERD patients, a high incidence of GERD after *H. pylori* eradication, opposing time trends for *H. pylori* versus GERD and its complications, and the recognition of reduced acid production in the presence of *H. pylori* induced corpus gastritis. By now, the potential role of *H. pylori* in the development of GERD is a key issue in the treatment of patients with upper gastrointestinal disorders. The next paragraphs will address the questions whether *H. pylori* influences the prevalence of GERD, whether *H. pylori*-eradication would increase the risk for development of GERD, what underlying mechanisms would explain such phenomena, and finally whether the efficacy of treatment for GERD depends on *H. pylori*.

5.1 EPIDEMIOLOGY OF *HELICOBACTER PYLORI* AND REFLUX DISEASE

Both GERD and *H. pylori* colonization are common phenomena. Their different geographical distribution is a first hint that *H. pylori* may be negatively associated with GERD. The prevalence of heartburn, the cardinal symptom of GERD,[84] ranges from 4% to 45%,[85,86] and the endoscopic presence of esophagitis varies between 5 and 23% with higher prevalences in Western Europe and the United States,[87] and lower prevalences in developing regions such as China and possibly also Africa.[88,89] As for *H. pylori*, serological studies reveal high prevalences in developing regions and lower prevalences in Western countries. For instance, in Africa prevalence rates of *H. pylori* are higher than 80%, whereas in developed countries these rates approximate 40%.[6] A selection of prevalence studies that appeared as full peer-reviewed papers is depicted in table 3. Within both the developing and developed countries, a lower prevalence of *H. pylori* was repeatedly observed among patients with endoscopic signs of GERD compared to controls with normal endoscopic findings. For example, in a Dutch study of 118 patients with reflux esophagitis, 13 patients with Barrett's esophagus, 109 patients with hiatal hernia and 399 patients without abnormal endoscopic findings, Werdmuller and Loffeld evaluated the prevalence of *H. pylori*-colonization by means of serology and gastric biopsy specimens for rapid urease test, histology and/or culture[83]. The prevalence of *H. pylori* was lower in the groups with esophagitis (29%), Barrett's esophagus (23%) and hiatal hernia (34%) compared to the reference group (51%). No difference was found between esophagitis patients with or without hiatal hernia, nor did the presence of *H. pylori* affect the severity of the esophagitis. *H. pylori*-positive patients in the esophagitis and reference groups were about 8 years older than their *H. pylori*-negative counterparts. Concomitant use of acid-suppressive therapy was not evaluated. Another cross-sectional endoscopy-based study also reported a lower prevalence of *H. pylori* in patients with esophagitis (31%) than in controls without esophagitis (42%) resulting in an odds ratio of 0.6 for the development of esophagitis in *H. pylori*-colonized patients.[90] In this study, neither age nor gender affected the prevalence of *H. pylori*. In Asian countries, the same picture was observed. For instance, in a cross-sectional study in a Chinese population, the prevalence of *H. pylori* was lower (31%) among 106 patients with reflux symptoms or endoscopic signs of GERD than among 120 matched controls (61%).[91] GERD patients with concomitant *H. pylori* infection showed more severe gastritis in the antrum than in other parts of the stomach, such as corpus, fundus and cardia.

Other Asian studies showed similar results.[92,93] In a large population-screening study among more than 6000 Japanese subjects, the prevalence of *H. pylori* was 41% among 120 subjects with esophagitis compared to nearly 50% among other tested subjects, corresponding with an odds ratio adjusted for gender and age of 0.7 (95% CI: 0.5-1.0).[93] Apart from a lower prevalence of GERD among *H. pylori*-positives, some also reported that if GERD is present in *H. pylori*-positive subjects, it may be less severe. For instance, in a prospective study of 137 patients with reflux esophagitis, the 88 *H. pylori*-negative patients presented with more severe endoscopically classified esophagitis and a higher prevalence of Barrett's esophagus than the 49 *H. pylori*-positive patients.[94] The study is in concordance with a recent large American study in 289 Barrett's esophagus patients and 217 GERD patients. When Barrett's esophagus patients were sub-grouped according to the degree of dysplasia, *H. pylori* was found to be less prevalent among patients with high-grade dysplasia (14.%) and adenocarcinoma (15%) than among patients with GERD (44.%), Barrett's esophagus alone (35.%) or low-grade dysplasia (36%).[95] An Italian group tested the prevalence of *H. pylori* in 92 patients with symptomatic GERD, 110 patients with erosive GERD and 200 asymptomatic controls.[96] The prevalences of *H. pylori* infection were 62%, 36% and 40%, respectively, corresponding with a significantly lower prevalence of *H. pylori* among patients with erosive compared to non-erosive GERD, but with no difference between controls and erosive GERD. The study is in agreement with a matched case-control study in ethnic Chinese patients with symptomatic or endoscopic signs of GERD.[97] In a group of 225 patients, *H. pylori*-uninfected patients had significantly more severe esophagitis than the infected group.

In contrast to the aforementioned studies, others however did not observe a lower prevalence of *H. pylori* among GERD patients.[98-101] For instance, in a well-designed case-control study from Chile, endoscopy was performed in 236 patients with GERD as confirmed by 24-hour pH monitoring and in 190 controls without a history of gastro-esophageal reflux symptoms.[99] The prevalence of *H. pylori* infection was very similar, i.e. 20-25%, in the 55 patients with endoscopic negative GERD, the 81 patients with erosive esophagitis and the 100 patients with Barrett's esophagus, as well as in the control group. Similar results were obtained from a German case-control study.[101] The prevalence of *H. pylori*-colonization was similar, i.e. 39%, among 130 patients with esophagitis and 227 matched asymptomatic controls, which underwent screening for *H. pylori* by the ^{13}C-urea breath test. These

contrasting results are in part explained by multiple confounding factors such as characterization of the control group and the presence or absence of concurrently administered anti-secretory drugs and NSAID's. Also the criteria for the diagnosis of GERD fluctuate and may cause different outcomes. For instance, questionnaire studies can lead to both over-reporting of non-reflux-related dyspeptic symptoms and under-reporting of atypical reflux-related presentations, such as non-cardiac chest pain. Notwithstanding this, the evaluation of GERD through endoscopy or esophageal pH-metry is very impractical for population-based studies and has limited sensitivity, in particular for lesser degrees of GERD. However, the repeated report of a lower prevalence of *H. pylori* among GERD patients compared to controls rather suggests a protective than a causative role for *H. pylori* against GERD. In a meta-analysis of 26 case-control and cross-sectional studies, several of them being preliminary reports, 562 of 1426 GERD patients were *H. pylori*-positive (39%) compared with 1009 of 2010 control subjects (50%).[102]

These observations have been made against the background of changing time trends in the prevalence of *H. pylori* and the incidence of GERD and GERD complications. As mentioned, the prevalence of *H. pylori* in Western countries has steadily decreased in the past decades as a result of socio-economic changes. This has led to a significant drop in the incidence of *H. pylori*-associated disorders such as peptic ulcer disease and adenocarcinoma of the distal stomach.[103] In the same period however, the incidence of GERD and GERD complications such as Barrett's esophagus and adenocarcinoma of the gastro-esophageal junction has increased four- to seven-fold.[103-105,77] We will elaborate on this topic in the section on *H. pylori* and GERD complications.

5.2 PROPOSED MECHANISMS FOR THE INTERACTION BETWEEN *HELICO-BACTER. PYLORI* AND REFLUX DISEASE

Epidemiological observations gain significance if supported by hypotheses for underlying mechanisms. Reflux disease results from the interaction between acid production, lower esophageal sphincter pressure, esophageal clearance and gastric emptying. *H. pylori* may affect several of these factors. In particular acid production can be affected in *H. pylori*-positive subjects by various mechanisms. Some individuals respond to *H. pylori* colonization with an exaggerated gastrin response, leading to increased acid production and limitation of *H. pylori* gastritis to the gastric emptying.[106] These subjects, making up for an estimated 10-15% of all *H. pylori*-positive subjects, are at risk for duodenal ulcer disease, and theoretically also for reflux disease. In many others however, gastric acid production is impaired due to several factors, including the release of substances such as the VacA protein, which directly inhibits parietal cell function and bacterial urease activity generating large amounts of acid-buffering ammonia. As a result of these factors, *H. pylori* gastritis extends into the gastric corpus where mucosal inflammation further impairs acid production, among others by the generation of interleukin-1, which has a 100-fold stronger acid-suppressive capacity than proton pump inhibitors. Most importantly however, more than 50% of the *H. pylori*-positive subjects eventually develop chronic atrophic gastritis. This results in a loss of parietal cells and thus a further impairment of acid production.[64] These factors which lead to a persistent decrease in acid production can explain why *H. pylori* may protect against GERD.

These hypotheses are supported by observations of inverse associations between GERD and the presence of more severe corpus gastritis or atrophy. El-Serag *et al.* demonstrated a 54% reduced risk for reflux esophagitis compared to controls in subjects with corpus gastritis.[107] The *H. pylori* colonization rate was similar in both groups. The authors concluded that the distribution and severity of *H. pylori*-related gastritis, rather than the mere presence or absence of *H. pylori* might be involved in the pathogenesis of GERD. Also in a matched case-control study in Japan, GERD patients were not only less often colonized with *H. pylori* than controls (34 versus 72%), but in particular had a less severe *H. pylori*-induced atrophic gastritis as classified according to the Updated Sydney system score.[108] Persuasive indirect support for the hypothesis that severe corpus inflammation has a protective effect on reflux disease comes from studies evaluating the prevalence of *H. pylori*-strains harboring the *cagA* gene. Subjects colonized with *cagA*-positive strains generally have more severe gastritis and have an increased risk for development of atrophic gastritis.[52] A Dutch cross-sectional study compared the prevalence of CagA serum antibodies in GERD patients and controls. It

appeared that GERD patients not only had a lower prevalence of *H. pylori*, but that in particular the *cagA*-positive strains were reduced compared to controls.[109] Similar findings were obtained from a Canadian study. Although the prevalence of the *cagA* gene was similar (94-97%) in patients with GERD, non-ulcer dyspepsia, duodenal ulcer, gastric cancer and controls, the CagA antibody was less prevalent in GERD (69%) and non-ulcer dyspepsia (69%) than in those with gastroduodenal pathology (92%).[110] Therefore, these studies support the hypothesis that more severe mucosal inflammation as well as parietal cell loss protect against GERD. These findings were not found in China where 225 GERD patients and their matched controls had the same prevalence of CagA serum antibodies.[97] One has to remark that associations between these antibodies and *H. pylori*-associated diseases are always weaker in Asia than in Western countries as a result of the very high general prevalence (about 90%) of *cagA*-positive strains in Asian countries, whereas in Western countries this equals 60%.[111] Therefore, epidemiological studies strengthen the idea that *H. pylori* protects against GERD development through the induction of atrophic gastritis, the latter being associated with reduced acid production.

5.3 *HELICOBACTER PYLORI* AND GERD COMPLICATIONS

If *H. pylori* gastritis protects against GERD, one would also expect to find a negative correlation between *H. pylori* and GERD complications, in particular Barrett's esophagus and adenocarcinoma of the gastro-esophageal junction. Various authors studied these correlations, but interpretation of the outcome of these studies are complicated by several factors. For example, the numbers of patients studied are often small, Barrett's esophagus patients are frequently included in a further non-specified GERD group and a distinction between gastric- and intestinal type Barrett's epithelium is not always made. In tables 4 and 5 a selection of epidemiological studies concerning the relation between *H. pylori* and both Barrett's esophagus and adenocarcinoma of the gastro-esophageal junction is given. We already mentioned the prospective endoscopical study in which *H. pylori*-negative patients had a higher prevalence of Barrett's esophagus than *H. pylori*-positive GERD patients.[94] Others reported that in particular patients

TABLE 4. Prevalence of Helicobacter pylori in Barrett's esophagus

Authors	Study design	Geographic region	No. of Barrett's esophagus patients (% H. pylori-positive)	Mean age ± SD	No. of controls (% H. pylori-positive)	Mean age ± SD	Establishment of H. pylori	Comments
Paull	Case-control/Selection of controls	USA	10/26 (39)	58 (27-80)*	11/26 (42)	58 (25-79)*	'gastric' mucosal histology	*mean (range)
Abbas	Uncontrolled cross-sectional	Pakistan	14/29 (48)	45 (24-80)*			Antral mucosal histology	Junctional type (57%), gastric fundic type (41%) epithelium; * median (range)
Werdmuller	Case-control/Selection of controls	Netherlands	3/13 (23)		204/399 (51)		Antral mucosal histology and serology in all	
Csendes	Case-control	Chile	20/100 (20)	56	38/190 (20)	42	Antral mucosal histology	No previous anti-reflux therapy
Newton	Case-control	UK	4/16 (25)	68 (40-83)*	9/25 (36)	54 (13-83)*	Antral and fundus mucosal histology and urease activity	Control group of patients with anemia without endoscopic abnormalities. Patients with Barrett's esophagus are significantly older
Vicari	Case-control	USA	15/48 (31)	57 ± 14	26/57 (46)	59 ± 16	Antral and fundus mucosal histology and serology	Including patients on PPI therapy
Öberg	Uncontrolled cross-sectional	Sweden and USA	5/40 (13)				Antral mucosal histology	
Schenk	Case-control	Netherlands	10/49 (20)	60 ± 14	39/88 (44)	60 ± 13	Antral and corpus mucosal histology	Controls are patients with GERD
Weston	Case control/selection of controls	USA	95/289 (33)	62 ± 14	96/217 (44)	61 ± 14	Antral, corpus and cardia mucosal histology	Controls are patients with GERD

TABLE 5. Prevalence of *Helicobacter pylori* in esophageal adenocarcinoma

Authors	Study design	Geographic region	No. of esophageal adenocarcinoma patients (% H. pylori-positive)	Mean age ± SD	No. of controls (% H. pylori-positive)	Mean age ± SD	Establishment of H. pylori	Comments
Vicari	Case-control	USA	7/21 (33)	60 ± 12	26/57 (46)	59 ± 16	Antral and fundus mucosal histology and serology	PPI therapy and esophagectomy (n=12) allowed. Patients: Barrett's esophagus complicated by dyspepsia or adenocarcinoma
Huang	Meta-analysis		90/158 (57)		383/761 (50)		Serology	Cardia carcinoma. OR=1.23 (0.56-2.7)
Hansen	Nested case-control	Norway	?/45		?/228		Serology from serum samples >= 6 years earlier	Adenocarcinoma of gastro-esophageal junction and cardia; esophageal cancers excluded. OR 0.40 (0.20-0.77)
Öberg	Uncontrolled cross-sectional	Sweden and USA	5/37 (14) a 17/77 (22) b				Antral mucosal histology	Adenocarcinoma of a=esophagus and b=gastroesophageal junction

younger than 60 years with Barrett's esophagus had a lower *H. pylori* prevalence than controls, a phenomenon which was not observed among patients with uncomplicated GERD.[112] They concluded that the presence of *H. pylori* might delay the development of Barrett's esophagus. For cardia cancer, an inverse association with *H. pylori* (OR 0.40; 95% CI 0.20-0.77) was demonstrated in a large serologic case-control study nested within a cohort of more than 100.000 inhabitants of Norway.[113] Simultaneously, for non-cardia cancer a positive association (OR 5.15; 95% CI 2.83-9.37) was observed. Earlier, a meta-analysis of 19 cohort and case-control studies has reported a comparable odds ration for non-cardia cancer.[114] This study did not provide evidence that *H. pylori* decreased the risk for cardia cancer, probably due to the paucity of data given on cardia cancer in the studies included in the meta-analysis. Additional support for a protective role of *H. pylori* comes from recent studies comparing the development of adenocarcinomas of the distal esophagus and stomach with the serological presence of CagA.[115-117] Vicari *et al.* prospectively compared the prevalence of CagA serum antibodies in 153 patients with GERD and its sequelae with that in 57 controls, who underwent upper endoscopy for other reasons.[116] There was no difference in the carriage of *cagA*-positive *H. pylori*-strains between controls (46%) and non-erosive GERD patients (41%), but a progressive decrease in the prevalence of antibodies was observed in patients with more severe complications of GERD, such as erosive GERD (31%), Barrett's esophagus (13%) and Barrett's with dysplasia or adenocarcinoma (0%). Likewise, a retrospective study reported that infection with *cagA*-positive strains was associated with a reduced risk for esophageal and cardia adenocarcinomas (OR 0.4; 95% confidence interval 0.2-0.8), whereas the risk for non-cardiac gastric cancer was not affected by *cagA* status.[115] Another sero-epidemiological study found that *H. pylori*, CagA and VacA antibodies were more common in duodenal ulcer patients when compared to esophageal adenocarcinoma and normal mucosa patients.[117] Similarly, gastric adenocarcinoma patients had *H. pylori*-, CagA- and VacA-antibodies more frequently than esophageal adenocarcinoma and normal mucosa patients.[117] Again, these observations are persuasive indirect support for the hypothesis that severe corpus inflammation, being linked to *cagA*-positive organisms, has a protective effect on the entire spectrum of reflux disease through inhibition of acid secretion. The time-trend observations of decreasing *H. pylori* prevalence and increasing incidence of cancer of the gastro-esophageal junction gives additional support for the hypothesis. In Western countries, the incidence of GERD and its complications, including adenocarcinomas of the distal esophagus, have increased four- to seven-fold in the past decades, whereas the prevalence of *H. pylori* infection has decreased.[77,103-105] Blot *et al.*[118] analyzed the incidence of adenocarcinomas of the esophagus and cardia according to gender and race from nine cancer registries accounting for 10% of the United States population. During the period from 1976 to 1987 the increase of annual incidence rates for adenocarcinomas of the esophagus and cardia exceeded that of esophageal squamous cell carcinoma and adenocarcinoma of the distal portion of the stomach by far. Similar trends have been observed in Europe.[119-121] In the Netherlands, the incidence of cancer of the esophagus and gastro-esophageal junction showed a dramatic increase with 34% in the short period from 1989 to 1995. This increase was solely due to an increase of adenocarcinomas, thus changing the pattern of esophageal cancer from largely squamous cell carcinomas of the proximal and mid-esophagus, to an equal incidence of this type of lesion and that of adenocarcinomas of the distal esophagus and the junction. The incidence of distal gastric cancer decreased with 18% during the same period. In Dutch females the incidence of esophageal cancer has now surpassed that of distal gastric cancer. In the United States, the male-female ratio for esophageal adenocarcinomas ranges from 7.6 to 14 and the white-black ratio approximates 3.[118] The higher white-black ratio underscores a possible protective role of *H. pylori*, as the frequency of *H. pylori* colonization in white Americans is lower (34%) than in black Americans (70%).[122] However, the high male-female ratio can not be explained by differences in *H. pylori* colonization between males and females, as this shows a rather equal distribution. At present it remains largely unexplained what other factors may contribute to the high male-female ratio. Thus, both the decrease in the incidence of distal gastric cancer, as well as the increase in the incidence of proximal gastric cancer are thought to be related to the decreasing prevalence of *H. pylori*.

5.4 HELICOBACTER PYLORI-ERADICATION AND GERD DEVELOPMENT

The above-listed epidemiological data tend to support the hypothesis that *H. pylori* prevents against the development of GERD. The next question therefore is whether *H. pylori* eradication increases the risk for subsequent newly development of GERD or deterioration of pre-existing GERD. Labenz and colleagues were the first to report such an increased risk in a German population of 460 former duodenal ulcer patients. Those in whom *H. pylori* had been eradicated, had a significantly higher incidence of GERD within the next three years than those in whom *H. pylori* persisted (26 versus 13%).[123] The risk for the development of GERD was in particular increased in those who had had previous *H. pylori* corpus gastritis. This landmark study led to much debate and further investigations. The issue has many potential serious confounders, such as the fact that patients with reflux disease may have similar symptoms as those with peptic ulcer disease, which in both cases respond to anti-secretory drugs. However, if peptic ulcer disease is treated by a short course of *H. pylori*-eradication followed by cessation of long-term acid suppressive therapy, GERD symptoms may become apparent after *H. pylori* eradication therapy. In case of such persisting symptoms, it is difficult to judge whether this is due to the newly development of GERD following *H. pylori*-eradication or to the unmasking of (pre-existing) GERD following cessation of acid-suppressants. Other studies supported the findings from Labenz *et al*. Among 87 Canadian duodenal ulcer patients followed for one year, the incidence of GERD symptoms as well as endoscopic esophagitis was significantly higher in those in whom *H. pylori* was eradicated (*n*=67) than in those in whom *H. pylori* persisted (37 versus 13%).[124] McColl and colleagues from Scotland also suggested that *H. pylori* eradication in ulcer patients may be associated with a subsequent worsening of reflux symptoms within three years follow-up.[125] In contrast, in an American study with a six month duration no relation was observed between *H. pylori* eradication and the induction of reflux symptoms.[126] Other studies also did not observe a worsening of pre-existent GERD after *H. pylori* eradication in comparison with the follow-up findings in persistently *H. pylori*-positive GERD patients.[127] Additionally, Axon *et al*. observed a similar recurrence rate of esophagitis after withdrawal of proton pump inhibitor (PPI) therapy in *H. pylori*-positive patients independent of achievement of *H. pylori*-eradication.[128] In summary, the issue whether *H. pylori* eradication increases the risk for subsequent development of GERD needs to be further elucidated.

6. THE ROLE OF *HELICOBACTER PYLORI* ON MORPHOLOGICAL CHANGES AT THE GASTRO-ESOPHAGEAL JUNCTION

Currently, a rationale for the increase of adenocarcinomas at the gastro-esophageal junction during recent decades has not been identified. As we discussed before, the decreasing prevalence of *H. pylori* may be related to this increase. Further insight can be gained from studies investigating morphological changes that occur in the areas surrounding the squamo-columnar junction. Studies on *H. pylori* initially concentrated on the type and degree of mucosal damage in the gastric mucosa of the antrum and corpus. In recent years, data on the prevalence of *H. pylori* in areas lining the squamo-columnar junction and on the association between *H. pylori* and the degree of mucosal inflammation and/or presence of intestinal metaplasia in these regions are rapidly accumulating. They may give answers to the question whether *H. pylori*, the effect of acid reflux or both give rise to the histological changes observed in the distal esophagus and proximal part of the stomach of patients with GERD. In addition, they have the potential to detect putative precursor lesions in these areas. In the next paragraphs we will discuss these studies. One has to keep in mind that interpretation of these studies is jeopardized by the lack of universally accepted and clearly reproducible anatomic landmarks identifying the distal esophagus and gastric cardia.[129] For example, endoscopically both the squamo-columnar junction (i.e. the Z-line) and the gastro-esophageal junction are used as a reference point. This may cause a major difference in the site of obtaining biopsy specimens for research, especially in the presence of a sliding hiatal hernia. Furthermore, the histological criteria for cardiac epithelium are not uniform.[129]

6.1 HELICOBACTER PYLORI IN THE ESOPHAGUS

H. pylori has occasionally been detected in both normal and inflamed esophageal squamous cell mucosa.[130-132] In the majority of cases this probably represents contamination by gastric contents during endoscopy.[133] However, *H. pylori* can colonize metaplastic gastric epithelium in the distal esophagus. Several studies reported on the presence of *H. pylori* in biopsy samples of Barrett's esophagus.[102] In a recent report O'Connor reviewed 19 studies that assessed the prevalence of *H. pylori* in 818 patients with Barrett's esophagus. *H. pylori* in Barrett's epithelium was present in 29% of the cases, with a large range of 0 to 88%. In nine studies the presence of *H. pylori* was evaluated in the gastric mucosa as well, and collectively showed a *H. pylori*-positive prevalence of 30% (range 13-63%). Few studies identified the type of Barrett's epithelium in which colonization occurred. It appeared that *H. pylori*-colonization nearly only occurred in the gastric-type epithelium.[134-137] This predilection for gastric-type mucosa is in concordance with the findings that *H. pylori* can colonize heterotopic gastric epithelium elsewhere in the digestive tract, such as in the duodenal bulb, in Meckel's diverticula and the rectum,[138] but is not observed in specimens from these sites if there is no gastric metaplasia.[130]

H. pylori may colonize gastric type epithelium in Barrett's esophagus, which similar to the situation in the stomach appears to be associated with chronic inflammation. In a recent study, the Barrett's esophagus of 19 out of 82 (23%) patients contained *H. pylori*.[137] All these patients exhibited the gastric-type metaplasia. In the *H. pylori*-positive patients esophageal inflammation was more severe than in the *H. pylori*-negative patients. In the distal stomach, such chronic active gastritis forms a risk for the development of progressive lesions of atrophy, metaplasia and dysplasia which cascade can end in the development of an adenocarcinoma. It is unclear whether *H. pylori*-induced inflammation in a Barrett segment would similarly contribute to the development of progressive preneoplastic lesions. This question is difficult to answer, at least with epidemiological data, as *H. pylori* colonization of the stomach appears to play a protective role for GERD and progressive GERD-associated complications including Barrett metaplasia.

Nevertheless, two retrospective studies reported on the prevalence of *H. pylori* in Barrett's esophagus with dysplasia or carcinoma.[139,140] Histological examination of biopsy specimens of 19 dysplastic/malignant and 94 benign cases of Barrett's esophagus found a lower prevalence of *H. pylori* in the first group, respectively 17 versus 34%.[140] In another study, the resection specimens of 19 adenocarcinomas arising in Barrett's esophagus revealed that none of these specimens carried *H. pylori*.[139] Available sections of non-dysplastic Barrett's esophagus and stomach of the same patients were uniformly negative for *H. pylori*. These studies focusing at Barrett epithelium itself confirm the serological data of a lower prevalence of *H. pylori* in patients with progressive dysplastic Barrett lesions. In the distal stomach, *H. pylori* infection is strongly associated with the development of intestinal metaplasia, dysplasia and subsequently adenocarcinoma. In Barrett's esophagus, especially of the intestinal type, the development of esophageal adenocarcinoma resembles this histological cascade of gastric carcinogenesis.

Nevertheless, characterization of intestinal metaplasia by morphology, mucin histochemistry and scanning electron microscopy have all shown fundamental differences between esophageal and gastric intestinal metaplasia.[129]

In conclusion, progressive Barrett lesions are negatively associated with *H. pylori*. In the minority of Barrett's esophagus patients in whom this bacterium is present, it can be associated with local inflammation of the cylindric epithelium. Although this is largely confined to the non-preneoplastic fundic type metaplasia, it has not been excluded that this chronic inflammation might to some extent contribute in the carcinogenesis of pre-existent Barrett lesions.

6.2 *HELICOBACTER PYLORI* AT THE CARDIA

In 1994, Genta *et al.* were the first to report that *H. pylori*-induced inflammation occurred as frequently at the cardia as at other gastric sites, such as the antrum and corpus.[141] In the cardia, colonization with *H. pylori* was identified in 95% of 42 *H. pylori*-infected subjects. The degree of inflammation was higher at both the cardia and antrum compared to the corpus.[141] Hackelsberger *et al.* confirmed these findings in 135 *H. pylori*-positive individuals, although the colonization density and inflammatory responses in the cardia were somewhat lower in the cardia than in the antrum.[142] Furthermore, these authors distinguished a sub-group of 14 patients with erosive esophagitis, in which the density of bacteria was markedly lower in the cardia than in both the antrum and corpus. It was hypothesized that this reduced degree of colonization was the consequence of abnormal acid reflux causing down-regulation of growth of *H. pylori*. The question that arises is whether carditis is the result of *H. pylori*-induced pangastritis or whether other etiological factors, such as gastro-esophageal reflux, are involved. Several studies addressed this question.

In an endoscopic case-control study in 58 GERD patients and 27 controls, neither the prevalence of *H. pylori* (41 versus 48%) nor that of cardia inflammation (40 versus 41%) was found to differ between cases and controls.[143] An interesting finding was that all the controls and 22 of the 23 cases with carditis were colonized with *H. pylori*, suggesting a causative role for *H. pylori* only. This was supported by a study in 116 unselected patients, in which the *H. pylori* prevalence rate increased with greater degrees of cardiac inflammation, and in which there was no association between carditis and clinical or histological evidence of GERD.[144] However, it might be that this is not the whole story, as contradictory results were obtained in two other studies.[145-146] The first focused on the relation between both esophageal acid exposure and motility on the one hand and histologic examination of the gastro-esophageal junction on the other hand.[145] It appeared that the presence of carditis was associated with insufficiency of the lower esophageal sphincter and increased esophageal acid exposure. The prevalence of *H. pylori* was not determined in this study. Secondly, in a case-control study in patients with GERD,[146] carditis was found more often in the cases than in the controls (47 versus 8%). Also *H. pylori* colonization was observed more often in the cases than in the controls (30 versus 13%). In a large cohort of 1053 patients, cardiac inflammation was detected in 75% of the patients.[147] Of the carditis group, 549 had chronic gastritis (70% being *H. pylori*-positive) and 241 had normal histology. The predominant risk factor for carditis was colonization with *H. pylori*, but GERD was an independent risk factor for carditis in individuals with a histologically normal stomach.[147] This may imply that two distinctive types of chronic inflammation of the cardia exist, one in conjunction with chronic *H. pylori*-related gastritis and one with GERD. Another study favors this explanation by demonstrating

active inflammation of the cardia in 25 of 28 (89%) *H. pylori*-positive and in 34 of 68 (50%) *H. pylori*-negative GERD patients.[148] As discussed above, the site of obtaining the biopsy specimens may be equally important. Lembo *et al* described that in 30 patients with GERD the severity of carditis was higher in samples containing both squamous and columnar epithelium than in those containing just columnar epithelium.[149] Although *H. pylori* was present in only four patients, the severity of carditis 1-2 cm below the Z-line was markedly higher in *H. pylori*-positive than *H. pylori*-negative patients, whereas the severity of carditis in samples containing both squamous and columnar epithelium did not differ between both groups. Chronic inflammation promotes the development of intestinal metaplasia.[129] Intestinal metaplasia not only occurs in the esophagus and distal stomach, but also in the gastric cardia. It is not known whether intestinal metaplasia of the cardia and that originating from the other localizations have a common pathogenesis and have a similar intrinsic potential for cancer development. In a previously described study, which excluded patients with Barrett's esophagus, intestinal metaplasia of the cardia was observed in 21% of 135 *H. pylori*-positive individuals.[142] In a subsequent study performed by the same authors, 13% of 315 patients with an endoscopically unremarkable squamo-columnar junction showed intestinal metaplasia of the cardia.[150] In these patients the presence of intestinal metaplasia was associated with increased age, *H. pylori* gastritis (OR 7.85; 95% CI 2.82-21.85) and intestinal metaplasia elsewhere in the stomach (OR 6.96; 95% CI 2.48-19.54). Concerning the latter two associations similar results were obtained by others.[143,151-153] In patients with GERD an association between *H. pylori* and intestinal metaplasia of the cardia is less convincing. In the study by Hackelsberger *et al*.[150] a group of 108 patients with Barrett's esophagus was evaluated as well. In these patients, reflux symptoms (OR 19; 95% CI 6-65), erosive esophagitis (OR 12; 95% CI 3-38), and male sex, but not *H. pylori*-infection were associated with intestinal metaplasia of the cardia. This finding is confirmed by several other studies.[153-155] It suggests that intestinal metaplasia at the cardia and distal esophagus represents two distinct pathogenic mechanisms with different risk factors. In patients with Barrett's esophagus it is the consequence of gastro-esophageal reflux, and in individuals with an unremarkable stomach it is related to the presence *of H. pylori*. In agreement with this concept is the increased frequency of inflammation, intestinal metaplasia and atrophy at the cardia in subjects carrying the more aggressive *cagA+* strains compared to those with *cagA-* strains.[155] Despite the association between *H. pylori* and distal gastric cancer, there is still no evidence that *H. pylori*-colonized patients have an increased risk for cardia cancer. Thus, the clinical relevance of cardiac intestinal metaplasia still has to be elucidated.

7. INTERACTIONS BETWEEN *HELICOBACTER PYLORI* AND ACID SUPPRESSIVE THERAPY

Proton pump inhibitors are very effective for both the initial and maintenance treatment of GERD. Recent evidence suggests that *H. pylori* infection may interact with this treatment, both with respect to efficacy as well as with respect to long-term side effects. As such, colonization with *H. pylori* may not only interfere with the etiology of GERD, but also with its management. The following section will discuss the effect of *H. pylori* on PPIs, as well as the effect of PPIs on *H. pylori*.

7.1 EFFECTS OF *HELICOBACTER PYLORI* ON PROTON PUMP INHIBITORS

7.1.1 H. pylori, PPI s and gastric pH
In 1995, Verdú and colleagues from Switzerland showed that intragastric pH during omeprazole therapy depends on the *H. pylori* status of an individual.[156] They measured the 24-hour intragastric pH in 14 *H. pylori*-negative and 18 *H. pylori*-positive healthy volunteers both during treatment with 20 mg omeprazole and during treatment with placebo. During treatment with placebo, median 24-hour pH values did not differ between *H. pylori*-infected and -uninfected subjects (1.5 versus 1.4). However, during treatment with omeprazole, median 24-hour pH values were higher in *H. pylori*-positive than in *H. pylori*-negative subjects (5.5 versus 4.0). These results were subsequently confirmed in a number of different studies. The same group showed that *H. pylori* eradication resulted in a decrease of 24-hour intragastric pH during omeprazole therapy, whereas the pH during the untreated state did not change.[157] Another paper showed that a similar effect occurred in duodenal ulcer patients.[158] These measurements were performed six to eight weeks after *H. pylori*

eradication. The efficacy of omeprazole in lowering intragastric pH remains permanently decreased after *H. pylori* eradication, as shown by repeated measurements one year after bacterial eradication.[159] The effect of *H. pylori* on drug-induced intragastric acid reduction is not restricted to omeprazole or other PPIs. In another study, 18 *H. pylori*-infected duodenal ulcer patients were treated with 300 mg ranitidine once daily before as well as six to eight weeks after bacterial eradication.[160] Before eradication, the intragastric pH during ranitidine treatment was higher than after eradication. In summary, *H. pylori* infection exaggerates the effect of acid suppressing drugs on intragastric pH. The mechanism underlying this phenomenon remains to be elucidated. Possible explanations include the hypothesis that it is due to bacterial production of ammonia buffering gastric acid, or to a direct effect of bacterial products, such as VacA and the acid inhibitory protein of *H. pylori* on parietal cell function. The most likely explanation is that it is related to the effect of acid suppression on the distribution of *H. pylori* gastritis. *H. pylori* prefers an acidic environment. The distribution of bacterial colonization and that of associated gastritis change depend on acid secretion. Profound acid suppressive therapy changes the usual antral predominant gastritis pattern into a corpus predominant pattern.[79] Inflammation of the corpus mucosa impairs acid production. As such, the increase of corpus gastritis will exaggerate the acid lowering effect of acid suppressive therapy. The magnitude of this phenomenon increases with more profound acid suppression. In case of treatment with 300 mg ranitidine daily, *H. pylori* eradication led to a decrease of the percentage of time per 24 hours during which the intragastric pH was above 4.0 from 39% to 27% . In contrast, this percentage changed from 73 to 38 during treatment with 20 mg omeprazole daily.[159] This difference between mild and profound acid suppression can be explained by the fact that more pronounced acid suppression leads to more severe corpus gastritis in *H. pylori*-infected subjects. An additional explanation could be that the effect of *H. pylori* on proton excretion is independent of acid suppression, but small, and therefore only measurable at higher pH due to its log scale.

7.1.2 H. pylori, PPIs and esophageal pH
Does the effect of *H. pylori* infection on the efficacy of acid suppressive drugs have any

clinical relevance for the management of GERD?

One could hypothesize that *H. pylori*-infected GERD patients require a lower dose of acid suppression than uninfected GERD patients. A large study reported the effects of 40 mg pantozole once daily on healing of esophagitis in 846 patients with grade II–III esophagitis according to the Savary-Miller criteria.[161] After four weeks treatment, healing had occurred significantly more often in the *H. pylori*-positives than in the *H. pylori*-negative patients (87 versus 76%). After eight weeks of treatment, this effect was although smaller still present (96 versus 92%). The authors conclude that *H. pylori* positively contributes to the healing of esophagitis during PPI treatment as a result of the augmenting effect on suppression of gastric acid production.

This effect however appears to have little significance during maintenance treatment. A meta-analysis of three clinical trials focused on disease relapse in 340 GERD patients during 12 months treatment with either ranitidine 300 mg, omeprazole 10 mg or omeprazole 20 mg daily. In each treatment group, the relapse rate was somewhat higher among *H. pylori*-infected patients, but these differences were not significant.[162] In another study, 137 GERD patients were evaluated for 5 years by endoscopy from the start of omeprazole treatment and at annual follow-up during treatment.[163] Omeprazole was started at a dose of 20 mg daily, this dose was increased during follow-up in case of endoscopic or symptomatic relapse with steps of 20 mg. If the required daily dose surpassed 40 mg, the dosing scheme was adjusted to twice daily. Although the *H. pylori*-negative patients at baseline had more symptoms of severe GERD, in particular Barrett's esophagus, there was no difference at all for the dose of omeprazole needed in both groups. The median daily dose in both groups at the end of follow-up was 40 mg (p=0.35).[163] Finally, a large international study in 230 patients also focused on the efficacy of maintenance treatment with omeprazole for GERD. This study also did not observe any association between *H. pylori* status and the relapse rate or required omeprazole dose during 1490 patient years follow-up.[164] In another study, 24-hour esophageal acid exposure was measured in 30 *H. pylori*-negative and 28 *H. pylori*-positive patients with a Barrett's esophagus at baseline and during treatment with either 150 mg ranitidine twice daily or 40 mg omeprazole once daily.[165] It appeared that *H.*

pylori infection did not influence esophageal acid reflux in these patients, nor did it influence the effect of low or profound acid suppression on reflux. Although none of these studies used patients as their own controls by studying them before and after *H. pylori* eradication, they strongly suggest that *H. pylori* status does not affect the efficacy of acid suppressive therapy in the management of GERD. This means that the dose of acid suppression does not have to be titrated upon *H. pylori* status.

7.2 EFFECTS OF PROTON PUMP INHIBITORS ON *HELICOBACTER PYLORI*

7.2.1 PPIs and accelerated development of atrophic gastritis

As mentioned above, *H. pylori* exaggerates the effect of proton pump inhibitors on intragastric pH. On the other hand, proton pump inhibitors also have a significant effect on *H. pylori*. *H. pylori* is an acidophil with an optimum pH, which in the presence of urea, presumably lies around 5.0. Therefore, drugs that affect acid production also affect the intragastric distribution of *H. pylori* and thereby affect *H. pylori*-associated gastritis. Acid suppression induces an increased inflammation of the gastric body mucosa in *H. pylori*-infected subjects.[79,80] This effect occurs at the start of therapy and persists throughout the duration of therapy. The magnitude of the effect depends on the level of acid suppression. It has been observed to a limited extent during H2-blocker therapy,[167] and is more pronounced during intake of PPIs.[79,89] Furthermore, it has been associated with increased epithelial cell proliferation as determined immunohistochemically.[168]

The question is whether the increased severity of corpus gastritis induced by acid suppressive therapy in *H. pylori*-infected patients has any clinical relevance, in particular with respect to the development of atrophic gastritis.[79,82] The latter condition, characterized by a loss of gastric glands,[169] can develop as a result of chronic active gastritis and is associated with an increased gastric cancer risk. Development of atrophic gastritis is usually a slow process. It takes approximately 20 years before one out of every three subjects with chronic gastritis has developed signs of atrophic gastritis. The annual incidence of atrophic gastritis among *H. pylori*-infected subjects varied between 1% and 3% in a number of cohort studies.[64,170-171] These studies all focused on 'healthy' volunteers, i.e. subjects with a presumable normal acid production. In contrast, various cohort studies focusing on patients with a condition that impaired acid production, reported a 3.8-8.7% annual incidence of atrophic gastritis.[82] These studies focused on patients with gastric ulcer disease,[172] duodenal ulcer patients after vagotomy,[173,174] or on patients treated with omeprazole for different indications.[175,176] Although none of these studies specified results according to H. pylori status, the results were rather concordant and contrasted with the 1-3% annual incidence of atrophic gastritis in cohorts of subjects without specific disease or treatment. Nevertheless, there were no direct comparisons of different populations within one study available. It was also unknown whether development of atrophic gastritis in subjects with reduced acid output was also associated with H. pylori, or with other unidentified factors. For these reasons, two populations of GERD patients were prospectively compared.[166] One group of 105 Dutch patients was treated with omeprazole maintenance therapy and another group of 72 Swedish patients was treated with a fundoplication procedure, without any further acid suppression. Both groups were followed for 5 years with endoscopy and gastric biopsy sampling at regular intervals. One pathologist evaluated all the biopsy specimens. Development of atrophic gastritis was rare in the H. pylori-negative patients of both treatment groups. Among the H. pylori-positive patients treated with a fundoplication, the upper limit of the 95% confidence interval (95% CI) for incidence of atrophic gastritis was 2.2%, which is fully in accordance with the findings of previous studies in patients with unsuppressed acid production.[64] In the H. pylori-positive group treated with omeprazole however, the annual incidence of atrophic gastritis was 6.1% (95% CI 3.8-8.8).[64] After 5 years of treatment, atrophy was thus observed in approximately 1 out of every 3 H. pylori-infected patients treated with omeprazole, which is in sharp contrast with the usual 20 years needed for such a prevalence of atrophy to develop. Development of argyrophil cell hyperplasia was also strongly associated with H. pylori and atrophic gastritis.[64] Both atrophic gastritis and argyrophil cell hyperplasia almost remained absent in the group of non-infected patients. Based on these findings and with the above-mentioned background, it was concluded that profound acid suppressive therapy accelerates the natural course of H. pylori gastritis.

7.3 ACCELERATED ATROPHY DEVELOPMENT REFUTED BY OTHER DATA?

This conclusion was seriously debated when other studies were presented which were considered to refute previous findings. Lundell and colleagues from Sweden presented a randomized study of GERD patients treated with either a fundoplication or omeprazole.[177] No significant differences were observed between both groups with respect to the incidence of atrophic gastritis during a follow-up of three years. These findings were interpreted as that the progression to atrophic gastritis in H. pylori-positive subjects does not depend on the level of acid secretion. However, the incidence of atrophic gastritis among the omeprazole treated patients was high (4.2% annually) as in previous PPI studies, whereas the absence of a difference with the findings in the fundoplication group could fully be explained by the lack of discriminative power in this study with limited patient numbers and limited follow-up. In addition, a serious potential confounder was introduced by the fact that all fundoplication patients were treated with omeprazole in the pre-operative phase, which medication was also allowed post-operatively. Some of these patients also underwent a vagotomy. As such, the fundoplication group could not function as a proper control. This is reflected by the finding of a relatively high incidence of atrophic gastritis in this group (2.8%) in comparison to the 1-2% observed in previous Western studies in populations with normal acid production.[82,166] Another negative study suffered from similar flaws. Unpublished data presented at a FDA meeting on this issue (November 1996), described a 1% incidence of atrophic gastritis among 99 H. pylori-infected GERD patients treated with lansoprazole for 15 months. However, the limited size and follow-up of this study led to large confidence limit for the reported incidence. More importantly, the investigators performed a protocol by which histological specimens were stepwise scored by different pathologists in case of abnormalities. This policy is likely to have induced a selection against the diagnosis of atrophy. In another lansoprazole study, the incidence of atrophy in H. pylori-infected subjects was consistent with the observations during omeprazole therapy.[178] In two other studies, Stolte and colleagues from Germany observed no development of atrophic gastritis in two populations with each approximately

60 patients during 12 months treatment with omeprazole for either duodenal ulcer disease or GERD.[179-180] The size of these populations and the limited follow-up did again not allow a firm conclusion about the incidence of atrophic gastritis, but the authors nevertheless proposed that *H. pylori* should be eradicated in patients on PPI maintenance therapy because of the induction of active chronic body gastritis, which in their opinion is a separate risk factor for gastric cancer.

In summary, the cumulative data support the hypothesis that reduction of acid output by pharmaceutical agents or vagotomy induces an increase of corpus gastritis in *H. pylori*-positive patients, which leads to further reduction of acid output because the active inflammation both impairs parietal cell function and accelerates development of corpus atrophy. Because of the latter phenomenon, *H. pylori* eradication has been suggested for younger *H. pylori*-positive patients in need of PPI maintenance therapy for GERD. Such a strategy does not seem to have an effect on the efficacy of such therapy, but long-term prospective studies have to show that it prevents the development of atrophic gastritis.

8. CONCLUSIONS

H. pylori colonization is very common among humans, with individual strains showing clear variations in pathogenetic properties. In particular, strains containing the *cagA* locus are more virulent than strains without this genetic factor. Virtually all *H. pylori*-positive subjects have chronic active gastritis. *H. pylori* colonization and associated gastritis strongly interact with gastric acid production. Some individuals have an antral-predominant gastritis with normal to increased acid production, in others gastritis equally or predominantly affects the corpus which pattern is mostly associated with decreased acid production. The evidence is accumulating that in particular the latter pattern of *H. pylori* colonization protects against GERD. This

hypothesis is supported by the finding of a low *H. pylori* prevalence, in particular of the *cagA*-positive type, in GERD patients and patients with GERD complications. Other support comes from the opposing geographic- and time-trends in the prevalence of *H. pylori* versus GERD, as well as Barrett's esophagus and adenocarcinoma of the gastro-esophageal junction. Finally, some studies have suggested that *H. pylori*-positive patients are after eradication therapy at increased risk for the newly development of GERD. However, this is an issue that still remains to be agreed upon. Based on the hypothesis that *H. pylori* prevents against GERD and its complications, it is expected that the ongoing decrease in *H. pylori* prevalence in Western countries will lead to a further increase in the prevalence of GERD and the incidence of complications such as Barrett's esophagus and adenocarcinoma of the junction.

H. pylori not only plays a role in the etiology of GERD, but also in the treatment of GERD. The presence of *H. pylori* corpus gastritis augments the effects of acid suppressive medication, in particular of proton pump inhibitors. This may have some effect during the initial treatment, where some suggest that *H. pylori*-positive patients show a somewhat quicker healing and symptom reduction than *H. pylori*-negative patients. During maintenance therapy however, *H. pylori* has little effect on the efficacy of PPI therapy and *H. pylori*-positive and -negative patients require similar doses of a PPI. However, in this phase the ongoing profound acid suppression facilitates the persistent presence of a more prominent chronic active body gastritis. This accelerates the progression to gland loss or atrophic gastritis. This effect can be prevented by *H. pylori* eradication in those who need maintenance PPI treatment for GERD. Although the long-term consequences of this phenomenon still have to be elucidated further, *H. pylori* eradication should currently be considered in younger *H. pylori*-positive GERD patients requiring maintenance PPI therapy.

REFERENCES

1. Pel PK. Diseases of the stomach (In Dutch). Amsterdam: De Erven Bohn, 1899.
2. Warren JR, Marshall BJ. Unidentified curved bacilli on gastric epithelium in active chronic gastritis. Lancet, 1983; i, 1273-1275.
3. Goodwin CS, Armstrong JA, Chilvers T, Peters M, Colins MD, Sly L, McConnell W, Harper WES. Transfer of Campylobacter pylori and Campylobacter mustelae to Helicobacter gen. nov. as Helicobacter pylori comb. nov. and Helicobacter mustelae comb.

nov., respectively. Int J Syst Bacteriol, 1989; 39; 397-405.
4. El-Omar EM, Carrington M, Chow WH, McColl KE, Bream JH, Young HA, Herrera J, Lissowska J, Yuan CC, Rothman N, Lanyon G, Martin M, Fraumeni JF, Jr., Rabkin CS. Interleukin-1 polymorphisms associated with increased risk of gastric cancer. Nature, 2000; 404: 398-402.
5. Blaser MJ. Epidemiology and pathophysiology of Campylobacter pylori infections. Rev Inf Dis, 1990; 129: 44-59.

6. Pounder RE, Ng D. The prevalence of Helicobacter pylori infection in different countries. Aliment Pharmacol Ther, 1995; 9: 33-39.

7. Malaty HM, Kim JG, Kim SD, Graham DY. Prevalence of Helicobacter pylori infection in Korean children:inverse relation to socio-economic status despite a uniformly high prevalence of adults. Am J Epidemiol, 1996; 143: 257-262.

8. Mendall MA, Goggin PM, Molineaux N, Levy J, Toosy T, Strachan D, Northfield TC. Childhood living conditions and Helicobacter seropositivity in adult life. Lancet, 1992; 339: 896-897.

9. Kuipers EJ, PeÒa AS, van Kamp G, Uyterlinde AM, Pals G, Pels NFM, Kurz-Pohlmann E, Meuwissen SGM. Seroconversion for Helicobacter pylori. Lancet, 1993; 342: 328-331.

10. Roosendaal R, Kuipers EJ, Meuwissen SGM, van Uffelen CWJ, Vandenbroucke-Grauls CMJE. Helicobacter pylori and the birth-cohort effect:evidence for continuous decrease of infection rates in childhood. Am J Gastroenterol, 1997; 92: 1480-1482.

11. MÈgraud F. Transmission of Helicobacter pylori:faecal-oral versus oral-oral. Aliment Pharmacol Ther, 1995; 9: 85-91.

12. Deltenre M, Koster Ed. How come I've got it? (A review of Helicobacter pylori transmission). Eur J Gastroenterol Hepatol, 2000; 12: 479-482.

13. PÈrez-PÈrez GI, Taylor DN, Bodhidatta L, Wongrichanalai J, Baze WB, Dunn BE, Echeverria PD, Blaser MJ. Seroprevalence of Helicobacter pylori infections in Thailand. J Infect Dis, 1990; 161: 1237-1241.

14. Nguyen AMH, Engstrand L, Genta RM, Graham DY, El-Zaatari FAK. Detection of Helicobacter pylori in dental plaque by reverse transcription-polymerase chain reaction. J Clin Microbiol, 1993; 31: 783-787.

15. Namavar F, Roosendaal R, Kuipers EJ, Groot Pd, Bijl MWvd, PeÒa AS, Graaff Jd. Detection of Helicobacter pylori in stomach, faeces and oral cavity of dyspeptic patients. Eur J Clin Microbiol Infect Dis, 1995; 14: 234-237.

16. Pristautz H, Eherer A, Brezinschek R, Truschnig-Wilders M, Pitritsch W, Schreiber F, Hammer HF, Wenzl H, Hinterleitner T, Reicht G. Prevalence of Helicobacter pylori antibodies in the serum of gastroenterologists in Austria. Endoscopy, 1994; 26: 690-696.

17. Nishikawa J, Kawai H, Takahashi A, Seki T, Yoshikawa N, Akita Y, Mitamura K. Seroprevalence of immunoglobulin G antibodies against Helicobacter pylori among endocopy personnel in Japan. Gastrointest Endosc, 1998; 48: 237-243.

18. Mones J, Martin-de-Argila C, Samitier RS, Gisbert JP, Sainz S, Boixeda D. Prvalence of Helicobacter pylori infectopn in medical professionals in Spain. Eur J Gastroenterol Hepatol, 1999; 11: 239-242.

19. Langenberg W, Raues EAJ, Oudbier JH, Tytgat GNJ. Patient-to-patient transmission of Campylobacter pylori infection by fiberoptic gastroduodenoscopy and biopsy. J Infect Dis, 1990; 161: 507-511.

20. Tytgat GNJ. Endoscopic transmission of Helicobacter pylori. Aliment Pharmacol Ther, 1995; 9: 105-110.

21. Kusters JG, Gerrits MM, van Strijp JA, Vandenbroucke-Grauls CM. Coccoid forms of Helicobacter pylori are the morphological manifestation of cell death. Infect Immun, 1997; 65: 3672-3679.

22. Suerbaum S, Josenhans C, Labigne A. Cloning and genetic characterization of the Helicobacter pylori and Helicobacter mustelae flaB flagellin genes and construction of H. pylori flaA- and flaB-negative mutants by electroporation-mediated allelic exchange. J Bacteriol, 1993; 175: 3278-3288.

23. Josenhans C, Labigne A, Suerbaum S. Comparative ultrastructural and functional studies of Helicobacter pylori and Helicobacter mustulae flagellin mutants:both flagellin subunits, FlaA and FlaB, are necessary for full motility in Helicobacter species. J Bacteriol, 1995; 175; 3278-3288.

24. Eaton K, Suerbaum S, Josenhans C, al e. Colonization of gnotobiotic piglets by Helicobacter pylori deficient in two flagellin genes. Infect Immun, 1996; 64: 2445-2458.

25. Hazell S, Lee A, Brady L, al e. Campylobacter pyloridis and gastritis:association with intercellular spaces and adaptation to an environment of mucus as important factors in colonization of the gastric epithelium. J Infect Dis, 1986; 153: 658-663.

26. Karim Q, Dhir N, Baron J, al e. Urease influences Helicobacter pylori motility at the gastric mucosal surface. Gut, 1997; 37: A19.

27. Worku M, Sidebotham R, Baron J, Misiewicz J, Logan R, Keshavarz T, Karim G. Motility of Helicobacter pylori in a viscous environment. Eur J Gastroenterol Hepatol 1999; 11: 1143-1150.

28. Caselli M, Figura N, Trevisani L, Pazzi P, Guglielmetti P, Bovolenta MR, Stabellini G. Patterns of physical modes of contact between Campylobacter pylori and gastric epithelium:implications about the bacterial pathogenicity. Am J Gastroenterol, 1989; 84: 511-513.

29. BorÈn T, Falk P, Roth KA, Larson G, Normark S. Attachment of Helicobacter pylori to human gastric epithelium mediated by blood group antigens. Science, 1993; 262:1892-1895.

30. Moran AP, Kuusela P, Kosunen TU. Interaction of Helicobacter pylori with extracellular matrix proteins. J Appl Bacteriol, 1993; 75: 184-189.

31. Wadstrom T, Hirmo S, Boren T. Biochemical aspects of Helicobacter pylori colonization of the human gastric mucosa. Aliment Pharmacol Ther, 1996; 10: 17-27.

32. Mobley HLT, Island MD, Hausinger RP. Molecular biology of microbial ureases. Microbiol Rev, 1995; 59: 451-480.

33. Nilius M, Malfertheiner P. Helicobacter pylori enzymes. Alimen Pharmacol Ther, 1996; 10: 65-71.

34. Kim H, Park C, Jang WI, Lee KH, Kwon SO, Robey-Cafferty SS, Ro JY, Lee YB. The gastric juice urea and ammonia levels in patients with Campylobacter pylori. Am J Clin Path, 1990; 94: 187-191.

35. Weeks DL, Eskandari S, Scott DR, Sachs G. A H+-gated urea channel:the link between Helicobacter pylori urease and gastric colonization. Science, 2000; 287: 482-485.

36. Eaton KA, Brooks CL, Morgan DR, Krakowka S. Essential role of urease in pathogenesis of gastritis induced by Helicobacter pylori in gnotobiotic piglets. Infect Immun, 1991; 59: 2470-2475.

37. Eaton KA, Krakowka S. Effect of gastric pH on urease-dependent colonization of gnotobiotic piglets by Helicobacter pylori. Infect Immun, 1994; 62: 3604-3607.

38. Mulrooney SB, Pankratz HS, Hausinger RP. Regulation of gene expression and cellular localization of cloned Klebsiella aerogenes (Klebsiella pneumoniae) urease. J Gen Microbiol, 1989; 135: 1769-1776.

39. Dunn BE, Cambell GP, PÈrez-PÈrez GI, Blaser M. Purification and characterization of urease from Helicobacter pylori. J Biol Chem, 1990; 265: 9464-9469.

40. Mai UEH, Perez-Perez GI, Allen JB, Wahl SM, Blaser MJ, Smith PD. Surface proteins from Helicobacter pylori exhibit chemotactic activity for human leucocytes and are present in gastric mucosa. J Exp Med, 1992; 175: 517-525.

41. Barer MR, Elliott TSJ, Berkeley D, Thomas JE, Eastham EJ. Intracellulair vacuolization caused by urease activity is toxic to human gastric epithelial cells. J Infect Dis, 1990; 161: 1302-1304.

42. Hazell SL, Lee A. Campylobacter pyloridis, urease, hydrogen ion back diffusion and gastric ulcers. Lancet, 1986; ii: 15-17.

43. Leunk RD, Johnson PT, David BC, Kraft WG, Morgan DR. Cytotoxic activity in broth-culture filtrates of Campylobacter pylori. J Med Microbiol, 1988; 26: 93-99.

44. Cover TL, Dooley CP, Blaser MJ. Characterization of and human serologic response to proteins in Helicobacter pylori broth culture supernatants with vacuolizing cytotoxin activity. Infect Immun, 1990; 58: 603-610.

45. Goossens H, Glupczynski Y, Burette A, Lambert JP, Vlaes L, Butzler JP. Role of the vacuolating toxin from Helicobacter pylori in the pathogenesis of duodenal and gastric ulcer. Med Microbiol lett, 1992; 1: 153-159.

46. Blaser MJ, Kobayashi K, Cover TL, Cao P, Feurer ID, PÈrez-PÈrez GI. Helicobacter pylori infection in Japanese patients with adenocarcinoma of the stomach. Int J Cancer, 1993; 55: 799-802.

47. Harai M, Azuma T, Ito S, Kato T, Kohli Y, Fujiki N. High prevalence of neutralizing activity to Helicobacter pylori cytotoxin in serum gastric-carcinoma patients. Int J Cancer, 1994; 55: 799-802.

48. Cover TL, Tummuru MKR, Cao P, Thompson SA, Blaser MJ. Divergence of genetic sequences of the vacuolating cytotoxin among Helicobacter pylori strains. J Biol Chem, 1994; 269: 10566-10573.

49. Atherton JC, Cao P, Peek RM, Tummuru MKR, Blaser MJ, Cover TL. Mosaicism in vacuolating cytotoxin alleles of Helicobacter pylori. J Biol Chem, 1995; 270: 17771-17777.

50. Cover TL, Glupczynski Y, Lage AP, Burette A, Tummuru MK, PÈrez-PÈrez GI, Blaser MJ. Serologic detection of infection with cagA+ Helicobacter pylori strains. J Clin Microbiol, 1995; 33: 1496-1500.

51. Crabtree JE, Wyatt JI, Sobala GM, Miller G, Tompkins DS, Primrose JN, Morgan A. Systemic and mucosal humaoral responses to Helicobacter pylori in gastric cancer. Gut, 1993; 34: 1339-1343.

52. Kuipers EJ, PÈrez-PÈrez GI, Meuwissen SGM, Blaser MJ. Helicobacter pylori and atrophic gastritis;importance of the cagA status. J Natl Cancer Inst, 1995; 87: 1777-1780.

53. Blaser MJ, PÈrez-PÈrez GI, Kleanthous H, Cover TL, Peek RM, Chyou PH, Stemmerman GN, Nomura A. Infection with Helicobacter pylori strains possessing cagA is associated with an increased risk of developing adenocarcinoma of the stomach. Cancer Res, 1995; 55: 2111-2115.

54. Peek RM, Miller GG, Tham KT, PÈrez-PÈrez GI, Zhao XM, Atherton JC, Blaser MJ. Heightened inflammatory response and cytokine expression in vivo to cagA+ Helicobacter pylori strains. Lab Invest, 1995; 73: 760-770.

55. Sharma SA, Tummuru MKR, Miller GG, Blaser MJ. Interleukin-8 response of gastric epithelial cell lines to Helicobacter pylori. Infect Immun, 1995; 63: 1681-1687.

56. Tummuru MKR, Sharma SA, Blaser MJ. Helicobacter cagA, a homolog of the Bordutella pertussis toxin secretion protein, is required for induction of IL-8 in gastric epithelial cells. Mol Microbiol, 1995; 18: 867-876.

57. Peek RM, Thompson SA, Donahue JP, Tham KT, Atherton JC, Blaser MJ, Miller GG. Adherence to gastric epithelial cells induces expression of a novel ulcer-associated H. pylori gene, iceA, that is associated with clinical outcome. Proc Assoc Am Physicians, 1998; 110: 531-544.

58. Rauws EAJ, Tytgat GNJ. Cure of duodenal ulcer associated with eradication of Helicobacter pylori. Lancet, 1990; 335: 1233-1235.

59. Hopkins RJ, Girardi LS, Turney EA. Relationship between anti-Helicobacter pylori eradication and reduced duodenal and gastric ulcer recurrence. Gastroenterology, 1996; 110: 1244-1252.

60. Riccardi VM, Rotter JI. Familial Helicobacter pylori infection. Societal factors, human genetics, and bacterial genetics. Ann Intern Med, 1994; 120: 1043-1045.

61. Beales ILP, Davey NJ, Pusey CD, Lechler RI, Calam J. Long-term sequelae of Helicobacter pylori gastritis. Lancet, 1995; 346: 381-382.

62. Azuma T, Ohtaki Y, Ito Y, Miyaji H, Yamazaki Y, Sato F, Ito S, Kuriyama M, Keida Y, Kohli Y. HLA-DQA gene contributes to the host's response against Helicobacter pylori infection:host's genetic analysis in two areas in Japan with contrasting gastric cancer risks. Gastroenterology, 1996; 110: A54.

63. Blaser MJ, Chyou PH, Nomura A. Age at establishment of Helicobacter pylori infection and gastric carcinoma, gastric ulcer, and duodenal ulcer risk. Cancer Res, 1995; 55: 562-565.

64. Kuipers EJ, Uyterlinde AM, PeÒa AS, Roosendaal R, Pals G, Nelis GF, Festen HPM, Meuwissen SGM. Long term sequelae of Helicobacter pylori gastritis. Lancet, 1995; 345: 1525-1528.

65. Sipponen P, Kekki M, Haapakoski J, Iham‰oki T, Siurala M. Gastric cancer risk in chronic atrophic gastritis:statistical calculations of cross-sectional data. Int J Cancer, 1985; 35: 173-177.

66. Filipe MI, MuÒoz N, Matko I, Kato I, Pompe-Kirn V, Jutersek A, Teuchmann S, Benz M, Prijon T. Intestinal metaplasia types and the risk of gastric cancer:a cohort study in Slovenia. Int J Cancer, 1994; 57: 324-329.

67. Forman D, Newell DG, Fullerton F, Yarnell JWG, Stacey AR, Wald N, Sitas F. Association between infection with Helicobacter pylori and risk of gastric cancer:evidence from a prospective investigation. Br Med J, 1991; 302: 1302-1305.

68. Nomura A, Stemmermann GN, Chyou P, Ikuki K, Perez-Perez GI, Blaser MJ. Helicobacter pylori infection and gastric carcinoma among Japanese Americans in Hawaii. N Engl J Med, 1991; 325: 1132-1136.

69. Parsonnet J, Friedman GD, Vandersteen DP, Chang Y, Vogelman JH, Orentreich N, Sibley RK. Helicobacter pylori infection and the risk of gastric carcinoma. N Engl J Med, 1991; 325: 1127-1131.

70. Forman D, Sitas F, Newell DG, Stacey AR, Boreham J, Peto R, Campbell TC, Li J, Chen J. Geographic association of Helicobacter pylori antibody prevalence and gastric cancer mortality in rural China. Int J Cancer, 1990; 46: 608-11.

71. The Eurogast Study Group. An international association between Helicobacter pylori infection and gastric cancer. Lancet, 1993; 341: 1359-1362.

72. International Agency for Research on Cancer. IARC Monographs on the evaluation of carcinogenic risks to humans, Vol 61, Schistosomes, liver flukes and Helicobacter pylori. Lyon, 1994.

73. Valle J, Kekki M, Sipponen P, Iham‰oki T, Siurala M. Long-term course and consequences of Helicobacter pylori gastritis. Scand J Gastroenterol, 1996; 31: 546-550.

74. Karnes WE, Samloff IM, Siurala M, Kekki M, Sipponen P, Kim SWR, Walsh JH. Positive serum antibody and negative tissue staining for Helicobacter pylori in subjects with atrophic gastritis. Gastroenterology, 1991; 101: 167-174.

75. Forman D, Webb P, Parsonnet J. Helicobacter pylori and gastric cancer. Lancet 1994;343:243-4.

76. Parsonnet J, Harris RA, Hack HM, Owens DK. Modelling cost-effectiveness of Helicobacter pylori screening to prevent gastric cancer:a mandate for clinical trials. Lancet, 1996; 348: 150-154.

77. Blaser MJ. All Helicobacters are not created equal:should all be eliminated? Lancet, 1997; 349: 1020-1022.

78. Parsonnet J, Friedman GD, Orentreich N, Vogelman H. Risk for gastric cancer in people with CagA positive or CagA negative Helicobacter pylori infection. Gut, 1997; 40: 297-301.

79. Kuipers EJ, Uyterlinde AM, PeÒa AS, Hazenberg HJA, Bloemena E, Lindeman J, Klinkenberg-Knol EC, Meuwissen SGM. Increase of Helicobacter pylori

associated corpus gastritis during acid suppressive therapy:Implications for long-term safety. Am J Gastroenterol, 1995; 90: 1401-1406.

80. Logan RPH, Walker MM, Misiewicz JJ, Gummett PA, Karim QN, Baron JH. Changes in the intragastric distribution of Helicobacter pylori during treatment with omeprazole. Gut, 1995; 36: 12-16.

81. Danon SJ, O'Rourke JL, Moss ND, Lee A. The importance of local acid production in the distribution of Helicobacter felis in the mouse stomach. Gastroenterology, 1995; 108: 1386-1395.

82. Kuipers EJ, Lee A, Klinkenberg-Knol EC, Meuwissen SGM. The development of atrophic gastritis - Helicobacter pylori and the effects of acid suppressive therapy. Aliment Pharmacol Ther, 1995; 9: 331-340.

83. Werdmuller BFM, Loffeld RJLF. Helicobacter pylori has no role in the pathogenesis of reflux esophagitis. Dig Dis Sci, 1997; 42:103-105.

84. Klauser AF, Schindlbeck NE, Muller-Lissner SA. Symptoms in gastro-oesophageal reflux disease. Lancet, 1990; 335: 205-208.

85. Nebel O, Fornes M, Castell D. Symptomatic gastroesophageal reflux:incidence and precipitating factors. Am J Dig Dis, 1976; 21: 953-956.

86. Locke GR, Talley NJ, Fett SL, Zinsmeister AR, LJ LJM. Prevalence and clinical spectrum of gastroesophageal reflux:a population-based study in Olmsted County, Minnesota. Gastroenterology, 1997; 112: 1448-1456.

87. Ollyo JB, Monnier P, Fontelliet C, al e. The natural history, prevalence and incidence of reflux esophagitis. Gullet, 1993; 3 (suppl): 3-10.

88. Chang C-S, Poon S-K, Lien H-C, Chen G-H. The incidence of reflux esophagitis among Chinese. Am J Gastroenterol, 1997; 92: 668-671.

89. Ofoegbu RO. Incidence, pattern, and African variations of common benign disorders of the esophagus. Experience from Nigeria. Am J Surg, 1982; 144: 273-276.

90. Varanasi RV, Fantry GT, Wilson KT. Decreased prevalence of Helicobacter pylori infection in gastroesophageal reflux disease. Helicobacter 1998; 3: 188-194.

91. Wu J, Sung J, Ng E, Go M, Chan W, Leung W, Choi C, Chung S. Prevalence and distribution of Helicobacter pylori in gastroesophageal reflux disease:a study from the East. Am J Gastroenterol, 1999; 94: 1790-1794.

92. Mihara H, Haruma K, Kamada K, Klyohira K, Goto T, Sumii M, Tanaka S, Yoshihara M, Sumii K, Kajiyama G. Low prevalence of H. pylori infection in patients with reflux esophagitis. Gut, 1996; 39: A94.

93. Yamaji Y, Maeda S, Ogura K, Okamoto M, Yoshida H, Kawabe T, Shiratori Y. Completely inverse background between reflux esophagitis and gastric cancer in view of serum Helicobacter pylori antibody and pepsinogen. Gastroenterology, 1999; 116: A360.

94. Schenk BE, Kuipers EJ, Klinkenberg-Knol EC, Eskes SA, Meuwissen SGM. Helicobacter pylori and the efficacy of omeprazole for gastroesophageal reflux disease. Am J Gastroenterol, 1999; 94: 884-887.

95. Weston AP, Badr AS, Topalovski M, Cherian R, Dixon A, Hassanein RS. Prospective evaluation of he prevalence of gastric Helicobacter pylori infection in patients with GERD, Barrett's esophagus, Barrett's dysplasia, and Barrett's adenocarcinoma. Am J Gastroenterol, 2000; 95: 387-394.

96. Manes G, Mosca S, Laccetti M, Lioniello M, Balzano A. Helicobacter pylori infection, pattern of gastritis, and symptoms in erosive and nonerosive gastroesophageal reflux disease. Scand J Gastroenterol, 1999; 34: 658-662.

97. Wu JCY, Sung JJY, Chan FKL, Ching JYL, Ng ACW, Go MYY, Wong SKH, Ng EKW, Chung SCS. Helicobacter pylori infection is associated with milder gastro-esophageal reflux disease. Aliment Pharmacol Ther, 2000; 14: 427-432.

98. Newton M, Bryan R, Burnham WR, Kamm MA. Evaluation of Helicobacter pylori in reflux oesophagitis and Barrett's oesophagus. Gut, 1997; 409-413.

99. Csendes A, Smok G, Cerda G, Burdiles P, Mazza D, Csendes P. Prevalence of Helicobacter pylori infection in 190 control subjects and in 26 patients with gastoesophageal reflux, erosive esophagitis or Barrett's esophagus. Dis Esophagus, 1997; 10: 38-42.

100. Öberg S, Peters JH, Nigro JJ, Theisen J, Hagen JA, DeMeester SR, Bremner CG, DeMeester TR. Helicobacter pylori is not associated with the manifestations of gastroesophageal reflux disease. Arch Surg, 1999;134: 722-726.

101. Hackelsberger A, Schultze V, G nther T, Arnim Uv, Manes G, Malfertheiner P. The prevalence of Helicobacter pylorigastritis in patients with reflux oesophagitis:a case-control study. Eur J Gastroenterol Hepatol, 1998; 10: 465-468.

102. O'Connor HJ. Helicobacter pylori and gastro-oesophageal reflux disease - clinical implications and management. Aliment Pharmacol Ther, 1999; 13: 117-127.

103. El-Serag HB, Sonnenberg A. Opposing time trends of peptic ulcer and reflux disease. Gut, 1997; 43: 327-333.

104. Hesketh PJ, Clapp RW, Doos WG, Spechler SJ. The increasing frequency of adenocarcinoma of the esophagus. Cancer, 1989; 64: 526-530.

105. Prach AT, MacDonald TA, Hopwood DA, Johnston DA. Increasing incidence of Barrett's oesophagus:education, enthusiasm, or epidemiology. Lancet, 1997; 350: 933.

106. Gillen D, El-Omar EM, Wirtz AA, Ardill JES, McColl KEL. The acid response to gastrin distinguishes duodenal ulcer patients from Helicobacter pylori-infected healthy subjects. Gastroenterology, 1998; 114: 50-57.

107. El-Serag HB, Sonnenberg A, Jamal MM, Inadomi JM, Crooks LA, Feddersen RM. Corpus gastritis is protective against reflux oesophagitis. Gut, 1999; 45: 181-185.

108. Koike T, Ohara S, Sekine H, Iijima K, Kato K, Shimosegawa T, Toyota T. Helicobacter pylori infection inhibits reflux esophagitis by inducing atrophic gastritis. Am J Gastroenterol, 1999; 94: 3468-3472.

109. Loffeld RJLF, Werdmuller BFM, Kusters JG, PÈrez-PÈrez GI, Blaser MJ, Kuipers EJ. Colonisation with cagA positive H. pylori strains inversely associated with reflux esophagitis and Barrett's oesophagus. Digestion, 2000; in press.

110. Fallone CA, Barkun AN, Gottke MU, Best LM, Loo VG, Zanten SVv, Nguyen T, Lowe A, Fainsilber T, Kouri K, Beech R. Association of Helicobacter pylori genotype with gastroesophageal reflux disease and other upper gastrointestinal diseases. Am J Gastroenterol, 2000; 95: 659-669.

111. Freston JW, Asaka M. Acid-related disorders in the new millennium:European, Japanese and North American perspectives. Eur J Gastroenterol Hepatol, 1998; 10: S1-S40.

112. Kiltz U, Baier J, Hagemann D, Schmidt WE, Adamek RJ. Does the development of Barrett'sesophagus depend on duration of Helicobacter pylori infection? Gastroenterology, 2000; 118: A1256.

113. Hansen S, Melby KK, Aase S, Jellum E, Vollset SE. Helicobacter pylori infection and the risk of cardia cancer and non-cardia gastric cancer. Scand J Gastroenterol, 1999; 34: 353-360.

114. Huang J-Q, Sridhar S, Chen Y, Hunt R. Meta-analysis of the relationship between Helicobacter pylori seropositivity and gastric cancer. Gastroenterology, 1998; 114: 1169-1179.

115. Chow WH, Blaser MJ, Blot WJ, Gammon MD, Vaughan TL, Risch HA, PÈrez-PÈrez GI, Schoenberg JB, Stanford JL, Rotterdam H, West AB, Fraumeni JF. An inverse relation between cagA+ strains of H. pylori

infection and risk of esophageal and gastric cardia adenocarcinoma. Cancer Res, 1998; 58: 588-590.

116. Vicari JJ, Peek RM, Falk GW, Goldblum JR, Easley KA, Schnell J, PÈrez-PÈrez GI, Halter SA, Rice TW, Blaser MJ, Richter JE. The seroprevalence of cagA-positive Helicobacter pylori strains in the spectrum of gastroesophageal reflux disease. Gastroenterology, 1998; 115: 50-57.

117. Grimley CE, Holder RL, Loft DE, Morris A, Nwokolo CU. Helicobacter pylori-associated antibodies in patients with duodenal ulcer, gastric and oesophageal adenocarcinoma. Eur J Gastroenterol Hepatol, 1999; 11: 503-509.

118. Blot WJ, Devesa SS, Kneller RW, Fraumeni JF. Rising incidence of adenocarcinoma of the esophagus and gastric cardia. JAMA, 1991; 265: 1287-1289.

119. MacDonald WC, MacDonald JB. Adenocarcinoma of the esophagus and/or gastric cardia. Cancer, 1987; 60: 1094-1098.

120. Powell J, McConkey CC. Increasing incidence of adenocarcinoma of the gastric cardia and adjacent sites. Br J Cancer, 1990; 62: 440-443.

121. Craanen ME, Dekker W, Blok P, Ferwerda J, Tytgat GN. Time trends in gastric carcinoma:changing patterns of type and location. Am J Gastroenterol, 1992; 87: 572-579.

122. Graham DY, Malaty HM, Evans DG, Evans DJ, Klein PD, Adam E. Epidemiology of Helicobacter pylori in an asymptomatic population in the United States. Effect of age, race, and socio-economic status. Gastroenterology, 1991; 100: 1495-1501.

123. Labenz J, Blum AL, Bayerd'rffer E, Meining A, Stolte M, B'rsch G. Curing Helicobacter pylori infection in patients with duodenal ulcer may provoke reflux esophagitis. Gastroenterology, 1997; 112: 1442-1447.

124. Fallone CA, Barkun AN, Friedman G, Mayrand S, Loo V, Beech R, Joseph L. IsHelicobacter pylori eradication associated with gastro-esophageal reflux disease? Am J Gastroenterol, 2000; 95: 914-920.

125. McColl KE, Dickson A, El-Nujumi A, El-Omar E, Kelman A. Symptomatic benefit 1-3 years after H. pylori eradication in ulcer patients:impact of gastroesophageal reflux disease. Am J Gastroenterol, 2000; 95: 101-105.

126. Vakil N, Hahn B, McSorley D. Recurrent symptoms and gastro-oesophageal reflux disease patients with duodenal ulcer treated for Helicobacter pylori infection. Aliment Pharmacol Ther, 2000; 14: 45-51.

127. Tefera S, Hattlebak JG, Berstad A. The effect of Helicobacter pylori eradication on gastro-oesophageal reflux. Aliment Pharmacol Ther, 1999; 13: 915-920.

128. Axon ATR, Bardhan K, Moayyedi P, Dixon MF, Brown L. Does eradication of Helicobacter pylori influence the recurrence of symptoms in patients with symptomatic gastro-oesophageal reflux disease? - A randomised double blind study. Gastroenterology, 1999; 116: A117.

129. Spechler SJ. The role of gastric carditis in metaplasia and neoplasia at the gastroesophageal junction. Gastroenterology, 1999; 117: 218-228.

130. Walker SJ, Birch PJ, Stewart M, Stoddard CJ, Hart CA, Day DW. Patterns of colonisation of Campylobacter pylori in the oesophagus, stomach and duodenum. Gut, 1989; 30: 1334-1338.

131. Cheng E, Bermanski P, Silversmith M, Valenstein P, Kawanishi H. Prevalence of Campylobacter pylori in esophagitis, gastritis, and duodenal disease. Arch Intern Med, 1989; 149: 1373-1375.

132. Coelho LG, Das SS, Payne A, Karim QN, Baron JH, Walker MM. Campylobacter pylori in esophagus, antrum, and duodenum. A histological and microbiological study. Dig Dis Sci, 1989; 34: 445-448.

133. Fallingborg J, Agnholt J, Moller-Peterson J, Christensen LA, Lomborg S, Sondergaard G, Teglbjaerg PS, Rasmussen SN. Campylobacter pylori in esophagus. Dig Dis Sci, 1989; 34: 1802-1803.

134. Paull G, Yardley J. Gastric and esophageal Campylobacter pylori in patients with Barrett's esophagus. Gastroenterology, 1988; 95: 216-218.

135. Loffeld RJLF, Tije BJt, Arends JW. Prevalence and significance of Helicobacter pylori in patients with Barrett's esophagus. Am J Gastroenterol, 1992; 87: 1598-1600.

136. Abbas Z, Hussainy A, Ibrahim F, Jafri S, Shaikh H, Khan A. Barrett's esophagus and Helicobacter pylori. J Gastroenterol Hepatol, 1995; 10: 331-333.

137. Henihan RDJ, Stuart RC, Nolan N, Gorey TF, Hennessy TPJ, O'Morain CA. Barrett's esophagus and the presence of Helicobacter pylori. Am J Gastroenterol, 1998; 93: 542-546.

138. Cothi GAd, Newbold KM, O'Connor HJ. Campylobacter-like organisms and heterotopic gastric mucosa in Meckel's diverticula. J Clin Pathol, 1989; 42: 132-134.

139. Quddus MR, Henley JD, Sulaiman RA, Palumbo TC, Gnepp DR. Helicobacter pylori infection and adenocarcinoma arising in Barrett's esophagus. Hum Pathol, 1997; 28: 1007-1009.

140. Wright TA, Myskow M, Kingsnorth AN. Helicobacter pylori colonization of Barrett's esophagus and its progression to cancer. Dis Esophagus, 1997; 10: 196-200.

141. Genta RM, Huberman RM, Graham DY. The gastric cardia in Helicobacter pylori infection. Hum Pathol, 1994; 25: 915-919.

142. Hackelsberger A, G,nther T, Schultze V, Labenz J, Roessner A, Malfertheiner P. Prevalence and pattern of Helicobacter pylori gastritis in the gastric cardia. Am J Gastroenterol, 1997; 92: 2220-2224.

143. Goldblum JR, Vicari JJ, Falk GW, Rice TW, Peek RM, Easley K, Richter JE. Inflammation and intestinal metaplasia of the gastric cardia:the role of gastroesophageal reflux and Helicobacter pylori. Gastroenterology, 1998; 114: 633-639.

144. Chen YY, Antonioli DA, Spechler SJ, Zeroogian JM, Goyal RK, Wang HH. Gastroesophageal reflux disease versus Helicobacter pylori infection as the cause of gastric carditis. Mod Pathol, 1998; 11: 950-956.

145. Öberg P, Peters JH, DeMeester TR, Chandrasoma P, Hagen JA, Ireland AP, Ritter MP, Mason RJ, Crookes P, Bremner CG. Inflammation and specialized intestinal metaplasia of the cardiac mucosa is a manifestation of gsatroesophageal reflux disease. Ann Surg, 1997; 226: 522-530.

146. Csendes A, Smok G, Burdiles P, Sagastume H, Rojas J, Puente G, Quezada F, Korn O. 'Carditis':an objective histological marker for pathologic gastroesophageal reflux disease. Dis Esophagus, 1998; 11: 101-105.

147. Voutilainen M, F‰orkkil‰ M, Mecklin J-P, Juhola M, Sipponen P. Chronic inflammation at the gastroesophageal junction (carditis) appears to be a specific finding related to Helicobacter pylori infection and gastroesophageal reflux disease. Am J Gastroenterol, 1999; 94: 3175-3180.

148. Bowrey DJ, Clark GWB, Williams GT. Patterns of gastritis in patients with gastro-esophageal reflux disease. Gut, 1999; 45: 798-803.

149. Lembo T, Ippoliti AF, Ramers C, Weinstein WM. Inflammation of the gastro-esophageal junction (carditis) in patients with symptomatic gastro-esophageal reflux disease:a prospective study. Gut, 1999; 45: 484-488.

150. Hackelsberger A, G,nther T, Schultze V, Manes G, Dominguez-MuÒoz J-E, Roessner A, Malfertheiner P. Intestinal metaplasia at the gastro-esophageal junction:Helicobacter pylori gastritis or gastro-esophageal reflux disease? Gut, 1998; 43: 17-21.

151. Trudgill NJ, Suvara SK, Kapur KC, Riley SA. Intestinal metaplasia at the squamocolumnar junction in patients attending for diagnostic gastroscopy. Gut, 1997; 41: 585-589.

152. Morales TG, Bhattacharyya A, Camargo E, Johnson C, Sampliner RE. Methylene blue staining for intestinal metaplasia of the gastric cardia with follow-

up for dysplasia. Gastrointest Endosc, 1998; 48(1): 26-31.

153. Hirota WK, Loughney TM, Lazas DJ, Maydonovitch CL, Rholl V, Wong RK. Specialized intestinal metaplasia, dysplasia,and cancer of the esophagus and esophagogastric junction:prevalence and clinical data. Gastroenterology, 1999; 116: 277-285.

154. Morales TG, Bhattacharyya A, Johnson C, Sampliner RE. Is Barrett's esophagus associated with intestinal metaplasia of the gastric cardia? Am J Gastroenterol, 1997; 92: 1818-1822.

155. Peek RM, Vaezi MF, Falk GW, Goldblum JR, PÈrez-PÈrez GI, Richter JE, Blaser MJ. Role of Helicobacter pylori cagA+strains and specific host immune responses on the development of premalignant and malignant lesions in the gastric cardia. Int J Cancer, 1999; 82: 520-524.

156. Verd☐ E, Armstrong D, Fraser R, Viani F, Idstrˆm J-P, Cederberg C, Blum AL. Effect of H. pylori status on intragastric pH during treatment with omeprazole. Gut, 1995; 36: 39-43.

157. Verd☐ EF, Armstrong D, Idstrˆm J-P, Labenz J, Stolte M, Dorta G, Bˆrsch G, Blum AL. Effect of curing Helicobacter pylori infection on intragastric pH during treatment with omeprazole. Gut, 1995; 37: 743-748.

158. Labenz J, Tillenburg B, Peitz U, Idstrˆm J-P, Verd☐ EF, Stolte M, Bˆrsch G, Blum AL. Helicobacter pylori augments the pH-increasing effect of omeprazole in patients with duodenal ulcer. Gastroenterology, 1996; 110: 725-732.

159. Labenz J, Tillenburg B, Peitz U, Bˆrsch G, Idstrˆm J-P, Verd☐ E, Stolte M, Blum AL. Efficacy of omeprazole one year after cure of Helicobacter pylori infection in duodenal ulcer patients. Am J Gastroenterol, 1997; 92: 576-581.

160. Labenz J, Tillenburg B, Peitz U, Verd☐ E, Stolte M, Bˆrsch G, Blum AL. Effect of curing Helicobacter pylori infection on intragastric acidity during treatment with ranitidine in patients with duodenal ulcer. Gut, 1997; 41: 33-36.

161. Holtmann G, Cain C, Malfertheiner P. Gastric Helicobacter pylori infection accelerates healing of reflux esophagitis during treatment with the proton pump inhibitor pantoprazole. Gastroenterology, 1999; 117: 11-16.

162. Carlsson R, Bate C, Dent J, Frison L, Gnarpe H, Hallerb‰ck B, Unge P. Does H. pylori influence the response to treatment with acid inhibition in patients with gastroesophageal reflux disease? Scand J Gastroenterol, 1997; 32: 56.

163. Schenk BE, Kuipers EJ, Klinkenberg-Knol EC, Eskes SA, Meuwissen SGM. Helicobacter pylori and the efficacy of omeprazole therapy for gastro-esophageal reflux disease. Am J Gastroenterol, 1997; 94: 884-887.

164. Klinkenberg-Knol EC, Nelis F, Dent J, Snel P, Mitchell B, Prichard P, Lloyd D, Havu N, Frame MH, Roman J, Walan A. Long-term omeprazole treatment in resistant gastroesophageal reflux disease:efficacy, safety and influence on gastric mucosa. Gastroenterology, 2000; 118: 661-669.

165. Peters FTM, Kuipers EJ, Ganesh S, Sluiter WJ, Klinkenberg-Knol EC, Lamers CBHW, Kleibeuker JH. The influence ofHelicobacter pylori on oesophageal acid exposure in GERD during acid suppressive therapy. Aliment Pharmacol Ther, 1999; 13: 921-926.

166. Kuipers EJ, Lundell L, Klinkenberg-Knol EC, Havu N, Festen HPM, Liedman B, Lamers CBHW, Jansen JBMJ, Dalenback J, Snel P, Nelis GF, Meuwissen SGM. Atrophic gastritis and Helicobacter pylori infection in patients with reflux esophagitis treated with

omeprazole or fundoplication. N Engl J Med, 1996; 334: 1018-1022.

167. Stolte M, Bethke B, Blum AL, Sulser E, Stadelmann O. Antacid treatment has a deleterious effect on the severity and activity of gastritis of the corpus mucosa. Ir J Med Sc, 1992; 161: 6.

168. Berstad AE, Hattlebakk JG, Maartman-Moe H, Berstad A, Brandzaeg P. Helicobacter gastritis and epithelial cell proliferation in patients with reflux oesophagitis after treatment with lansoprazole. Gut, 1997; 41: 740-747.

169. Dixon MF, Genta RM, Yardley JH, Correa P. Classification and grading of gastritis. The up-dated Sydney system. Am J Surg Pathol, 1996; 20:1161-1181.

170. Correa P, Haenszel W, Cuello C, Zavala D, Fontham E, Zarama G, Tannenbaum S, Collazos T, Ruiz B. Gastric precancerous process in a high risk population:cohort follow-up. Cancer Res, 1990; 50: 4737-4740.

171. Villako K, Kekki M, Maaroos HI, Sipponen P, Tammur R, Tamm A, Keevallik R. A 12-year follow-up study of chronic gastritis and Helicobacter pylori in a population-based random sample. Scand J Gastroenterol, 1995; 30: 964-967.

172. Maaroos HI, Salupere V, Uibo R, Kekki M, Sipponen P. Seven-year follow-up study of chronic gastritis in gastric ulcer patients. Scand J Gastroenterol, 1985; 20: 198-204.

173. Jönsson K, Ström M, Bodemar G, Norrby K. Histologic changes in the gastroduodenal mucosa after long-term medical treatment with cimetidine or parietal cell vagotomy in patients with juxtapyloric ulcer disease. Scand J Gastroenterol, 1988; 23: 433-441.

174. Peetsalu A, Maaroos HI, Sipponen P, Peetsalu M. Long-term effect of vagotomy on gastric mucosa and Helicobacter pylori in duodenal ulcer patients. Scand J Gastroenterol, 1991; 26: 77-83.

175. Solcia E, Fiocca R, Havu N, Dalv‰ˆg A, Carlsson R. Gastric endocrine cells and gastritis in patients receiving long-term omeprazole treatment. Digestion, 1992; 51: 82-92.

176. Lamberts R, Creutzfeldt W, Str‚ber HG, Brunner G, Solcia E. Long-term omeprazole therapy in peptic ulcer disease:gastrin, endocrine cell growth, and gastritis. Gastroenterology, 1993; 104: 1356-1370.

177. Lundell L, Miettinen P, Myrvold HE, Pedersen SA, Thor K, Andersson A, Hattlebakk J, Havu N, Janatuinen E, Levander K, Liedman B, Nystrˆm P. Lack of effect of acid suppression therapy on gastric atrophy. Gastroenterology, 1999; 117: 319-326.

178. Eissele R, Brunner G, Simon B, Solcia E, Arnold R. Gastric mucosa during treatment with lansoprazole:Helicobacter pylori is a risk factor for argyrophil-cell hyperplasia. Gastroenterology, 1997; 112: 707-717.

179. Meining A, Kiel G, Stolte M. Changes in Helicobacter pylori-induced gastritis in the antrum and corpus during and after 12 months of treatment with ranitidine and lansoprazole in patients with duodenal ulcer disease. Aliment Pharmacol Ther, 1998; 12(8): 735-740.

180. Stolte M, Meining A, Schmitz JM, Alexandridis T, Seifert E. Changes in Helicobacter pylori-induced gastritis in the antrum and corpus during 12 months of treatment with omeprazole and lansoprazole in patients with gastro-oesophageal reflux disease. Aliment Pharmacol Ther, 1998; 12: 247-253.

181. Liston R, Pitt M, Banerjee A. Reflux esophagitis and Helicobacter pylori infection en elderly patients. Postgrad Med J, 1996; 72: 221-223.

2.3 ACID AND BILE IN THE ESOPHAGUS

William J Owen and Robert EK Marshall

1. INTRODUCTION

Heartburn affects 5-10% of the Western population daily. The vast majority of sufferers self-medicate and only a small minority reach the hands of gastroenterologists and undergo endoscopy. Longitudinal studies on those suffering from gastroesophageal reflux disease reveal that 90% still suffer from heartburn even ten years on, but that complications are rare, strictures occurring in 2% and Barrett's esophagus in 1%[1]. Interestingly, reflux symptoms in Barrett's esophagus are often milder than in patients with gastroesophageal reflux disease (GERD) but without Barrett's esophagus, the metaplastic mucosa being less sensitive[2]. The associated impairment of esophageal motility characterized by poor esophageal clearance and lower esophageal sphincter hypotonia may either be secondary to chronic reflux , or represent a primary deficiency. There are no good long-term studies correlating esophageal body motor function and lower esophageal sphincter function with the extent of gastroesophageal reflux and the development of Barrett's esophagus.

2. EVIDENCE FOR ESOPHAGEAL MUCOSAL DAMAGE BY ACID AND BILE

2.1 IN VITRO AND IN VIVO EFFECT OF CONSTITUENTS

In patients with an intact stomach, the acid-pepsin combination is acknowledged as a principal cause of esophageal mucosal damage. However, it has long been known that bile is capable of causing erosive esophagitis in the absence of gastric juice. This may be seen after total gastrectomy[3] and in the presence of pernicious anemia and achlorhydria secondary to atrophic gastritis[4]. The bile constituents available to cause damage include bile salts (unconjugated and taurine or glycine conjugated), lysolecithin (formed when pancreatic phospholipase A hydrolyses the lecithin in bile) and trypsin. These constituents have been studied using either the in vivo rabbit esophagus model, or ex vivo esophageal preparations. The cellular mechanism of damage has been studied by

light and electron microscopy to assess morphological damage, measurement of transmucosal potential difference, and assessment of net flux of H^+, Na^+ and glucose as a measure of mucosal barrier function. The degree of damage has been found to be dependent on pH, concentration, and the combination of constituents present.

The first in vivo isolated esophageal perfusion study was performed by Cross and Wangensteen in 1951[5]. They perfused the cat esophagus with bile, pancreatic juice, a mixture of the two and jejunal juice collected from a dog, as well as human bile. They observed the most severe esophagitis with a mixture of bile and pancreatic juice, pancreatic juice alone causing only minimal changes. Since then, commercially available preparations of bile constituents have been used. In 1972, Henderson et al.[6] reported the effects of instilling bile salts with or without hydrochloric acid (HCl) into the isolated dog esophagus. They found that bile salts alone caused little esophagitis, whereas HCl plus bile salts (particularly taurine conjugates), produced severe esophagitis. The effect of pH was further investigated by Lillemoe et al.[7]. At pH 7.5, trypsin caused severe morphological damage but only minimal disruption of the esophageal mucosal barrier as estimated by H^+, K^+ and glucose flux. Taurodeoxycholic acid (TDCA) caused minimal esophagitis but severe mucosal barrier disruption. Pepsin had no effect at this pH. At pH 2, however, trypsin caused no damage, pepsin caused marked esophagitis and barrier disruption, and TDCA again caused minimal esophagitis but severe mucosal barrier disruption[8]. These experiments reflect the optimum working pH of pepsin and trypsin. Salo et al.[9] observed that pure HCl produced virtually no damage, but in combination with pepsin, taurocholic acid (TCA) or lysolecithin damage occurred. Chaparala et al.[10] made similar observations, noting that without HCl, pepsin and TCA produced little damage. Lillemoe et al.[11] studied the comparative effects of tauroursodeoxycholic acid (TUDCA) and taurochenodeoxycholic acid (TCDCA) on esophageal mucosa at pH 2, and noted significant differences, TUDCA causing significantly less damage. Kivilaakso et al.[12]

H.W. Tilanus and S.E.A. Attwood (eds.), Barrett's Esophagus, 107–120.

found that at pH 3.5, it was the conjugated bile salt TCA which resulted in mucosal damage, whereas at pH 7.4 it was the unconjugated bile salts deoxycholic acid (DCA) and chenodeoxycholic acid (CDCA) causing damage. This reflects the relatively low pKa and high solubility of taurine conjugated bile salts at low pH, and vice versa for unconjugated bile salts. Being precipitated, unconjugated bile salts are not available for mucosal damage at low pH.

Under normal circumstances these constituents appear together, and therefore their synergistic effect has been studied. As early as 1958, Redo et al.[13], using the perfused dog esophagus model, observed that bile alone (at pH 7) produced little esophagitis, but in combination with pancreatic secretions produced severe erosive esophagitis. The addition of bile to gastric juice resulted in a conspicuous diminution of the damage caused by gastric juice alone. Lillemoe et al.[14] investigated the modulatory effect of TDCA on the effects of trypsin and pepsin, and found that at pH 2, TDCA when combined with pepsin reduced the damage caused by pepsin alone. On the other hand, when combined with trypsin at pH 7.5, the damaging effect of trypsin was increased. Salo and Kivilaakso[15] observed that cholic acid had a greater synergistic effect on trypsin at pH 7 than TCA. Tompkins et al.[16,17] studied the effect of different bile acids on the *in vitro* activity of pepsin, and found it to be diminished. The degree of inhibition was inversely proportional to the number of hydroxyl substituents on the bile acid molecule, lithocholic acid being the strongest inhibitor. The fact that, at a given pH, some luminal constituents cause erosive esophagitis and some cause mucosal barrier disruption without morphological damage, suggests that there may be differing mechanisms of damage. It may be expected that the detergent effect of bile salts would result in disruption of the cell surface lipid membrane. However, it appears that the deeper cell layers of the mucosa are damaged first, in the absence of gross histological changes[18,19].

2.2 ANIMAL SURGICAL DIVERSION STUDIES OF ESOPHAGEAL MUCOSAL DAMAGE

The *in vitro* and *in vivo* isolated esophagus studies are not truly physiological, being unrepresentative of the naturally occurring mixture of reflux constituents. They are also performed over a short time period. In addition, the concentrations of reagents used are much higher than are found in the human *in vivo*. When Gotley et al.[20] analyzed the refluxate of patients with GERD, they found the vast majority of bile acid concentrations to be in the range 0-0.6 mM/l, whereas the later animal studies were carried out with bile acid concentrations in the range of 1-20 mM/l, with significant mucosal damage seen at the top of this range. To try to reproduce the *in vivo* situation more closely, surgical diversion studies have been performed. Biliary, pancreatic and gastric secretions, alone or in combination, have been diverted into the stomach and esophagus in order to study their effect on gastric and esophageal mucosal inflammation and neoplastic change.

In 1951, Cross and Wangensteen[5] performed anatomical diversions on dogs to allow bile, pancreatic juice, a mixture of the two, or succus entericus into the esophagus, for a period of 1 to 3 months. All combinations produced severe esophagitis. Lambert[21], in similar procedures on rats, observed that pancreatic juice alone produced more severe esophageal lesions than bile alone, but that when combined, bile augmented the damaging effect of pancreatic juice. These findings were later to be mirrored by Lillemoe et al.[14] with their experiments on the isolated perfused rabbit esophagus. Studies by Moffat and Berkas[22] in 1965 confirmed the corrosive nature of bile. Gillison et al.[23] resected the gastroesophageal junction in monkeys, and produced esophagitis with pure gastric juice or pure bile. They were then able to prevent the esophagitis by performing a Nissen valvuloplasty. A further study by the same authors[24] demonstrated that the esophagitis produced by bile contaminated gastric juice was worse than with gastric juice alone, findings confirmed in a similar study by Henderson et al.[25]. Mud et al.[26] performed a range of control and experimental procedures in rats to produce free esophageal reflux of gastric acid, bile and pancreatic juice, in all combinations. They substantiated their findings by measuring bile acid and trypsin concentrations in the refluxates. They found that it was only in those animals with pancreatic juice reflux, confirmed by high levels of trypsin, that developed esophagitis.

The ability of gastric and duodenal contents to induce esophageal malignancy has been studied. Again using a rat model, Attwood et al.[27] demonstrated a far higher rate of carcinogenesis in animals subjected to a duodenoesophageal anastomosis than those in whom free gastroesophageal reflux had been established. Pera et al.[28], by diverting biliary and pancreatic secretions into the esophagus, once again found higher rates of cancer induction in those rats subjected to free pancreatic reflux. Clark et al.[29] showed that cancer induction by free duodenoesophageal reflux could be increased in the presence of the carcinogen methyl-n-amyl nitrosamine, and that this process was promoted by a high fat diet. Ireland et al.[30] operated on 270 rats to produce esophageal reflux of duodenal contents with or without gastric juice, in the presence of methyl-n-amyl nitrosamine. They found that the presence of gastric juice in refluxed duodenal juice protects against the development of esophageal adenocarcinoma. They argued that profound acid suppression may be detrimental by encouraging esophageal metaplasia and carcinogenesis in patients with duodenogastric reflux (DGR). Wetscher et al.[31] performed similar experiments, without the use of a carcinogen, but introducing the use of omeprazole to induce acid suppression. They also found that DGR-induced growth stimulation of the foregut is potentiated by gastric acid suppression, questioning the chronic use of anti-secretory medication.

3. PATHOGENESIS OF BARRETT'S ESOPHAGUS: ACID OR BILE ?

The role of acid in the pathogenesis of Barrett's esophagus is strongly supported by experimental evidence. In 1970 Bremner et al.[32] denuded the dog lower esophagus of squamous mucosa and showed that in the absence of gastroesophageal reflux, squamous mucosa regenerated, whereas in the presence of acid reflux, regeneration was with columnar mucosa. Gillen et al.[33] demonstrated that columnar re-epithelialisation in the dog esophagus occurred in the presence of acid reflux, acid and bile reflux, but not with bile reflux alone. By denuding rings of esophageal mucosa above squamous mucosa, and thus producing 'squamous barriers', they were also able to conclude that columnar re-epithelialisation may occur from primordial stem cells intrinsic to the esophagus, rather than by proximal migration of cardiac columnar epithelium (Figure 1). Further studies by Seto and Kobori[34] reinforced these findings: rats which underwent gastrectomy and oesophago-jejunostomy, inducing free bile

reflux, were more likely to develop columnar epithelium if they were fed 'acid' water at pH 1.8 than if they were fed water of pH 6.5, although columnar epithelium developed in both groups.

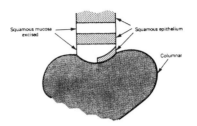

Figure 1 The experimental design of Gillen et al.[33] created 'upper' and 'lower' ring mucosal defects in the esophagus with intervening normal squamous epithelial barrier. Half the squamocolumnar junction was left *in situ* and half excised.

3.1 BARRETT'S ESOPHAGUS AND PREVIOUS GASTRIC SURGERY

Either because of total or partial vagotomy, or anatomical diversion, gastric surgery predisposes the esophagus to lesser amounts of acid reflux and/or greater amounts of duodenal content reflux. It has long been known that duodenal contents are capable of causing erosive esophagitis in the absence of gastric juice[3], and Barrett's esophagus and adenocarcinoma have been shown to develop after total gastrectomy[35]. If bile were to be considered an important factor in the pathogenesis of Barrett's esophagus, it might be speculated that gastric surgery would predispose to the development of Barrett's esophagus and adenocarcinoma. A retrospective study of 22,236 endoscopies by Parrilla et al.[36] found no difference in the prevalence of Barrett's esophagus between those with an intact stomach and those with an operated stomach. They concluded that gastric surgery did not increase the risk of developing Barrett's esophagus. Birgisson et al.[37] compared the frequency of gastric surgery between patients with esophageal squamous carcinoma and adenocarcinoma, and found no difference between the groups. Both these studies suggest that gastric surgery and its associated duodenogastroesophageal reflux do not play a significant role in the development of Barrett's esophagus.

4. ACID REFLUX IN BARRETT'S ESOPHAGUS

4.1 pH MONITORING

Since the seminal 1974 paper by Johnson and DeMeester[38], gastroesophageal acid reflux has been quantified by the use of ambulatory pH monitoring. The relationship between acid reflux and the extent of esophageal mucosal damage was first investigated by Iascone et al.[2]. They found significantly greater acid exposure (pH less than 4) in those patients with Barrett's esophagus (2 cm or more columnar epithelium) when compared to healthy controls and patients with simple esophagitis. Many subsequent studies have been performed looking at this issue, but they are difficult to directly compare because of differing definitions of Barrett's esophagus, inclusion of various grades of esophagitis and relative small numbers in several cases. Nonetheless, the overall impression is of increasing esophageal acid exposure as the degree of mucosal injury worsens, with Barrett's esophagus having the greatest acid exposure[2,39-48]. Barrett's esophagus has been categorized as to whether it is complicated (associated with dysplasia, ulceration or stricture formation) or uncomplicated. Little difference in acid exposure has been found between patients with uncomplicated Barrett's esophagus and erosive esophagitis, implicating perhaps a further aetiological factor[44,49]. Differences in acid exposure between complicated and uncomplicated Barrett's esophagus have also been investigated. Vaezi et al.[43,50] found significantly greater esophageal acid exposure in complicated Barrett's esophagus (22.8% total acid exposure time) compared with uncomplicated Barrett's esophagus (14.7% acid exposure time). However, studies by Gillen et al.[51] and Attwood et al.[52] in slightly larger groups failed to show a difference.

pH monitoring has allowed not only the measurement of total 24 hour acid exposure, but has made it possible to examine the differences in reflux episode characteristics in various grades of mucosal damage. Compared to uncomplicated esophagitis and healthy controls, Barrett's esophagus is associated with the greatest number of individual acid reflux episodes, the greatest average length of reflux episodes, and the greatest number of reflux episodes longer than 5 minutes[44,48,49]. This is in association with a reduced lower esophageal sphincter pressure[44,48] and a reduced amplitude of esophageal body contraction[48].

Initially it was thought that the increased acid reflux of Barrett's esophagus was associated with an increase in gastric acid production[53,54]. However, these are relatively small studies. A more detailed study by Hirschowitz[55], looking at basal and Pentagastrin stimulated gastric acid production, found no difference in Barrett's esophagus when they were compared to controls carefully matched for sex and background gastrointestinal disease. They also found no differences in the pepsin output both in the basal and stimulated state between Barrett's esophagus and their appropriate controls. Further studies by Savarino et al.[56] and Fiorucci et al.[57] have confirmed that gastric acid production in esophagitis and Barrett's esophagus is not increased. The relatively low prevalence of Barrett's esophagus in a series of 92 cases with Zollinger Ellison syndrome (3%) confirmed the absence of any correlation between Barrett's metaplasia and gastric hyper secretion[58].

5. BILE REFLUX IN BARRETT'S ESOPHAGUS

The role of bile and its constituents in esophageal mucosal damage and the pathogenesis of Barrett's esophagus has long been a source of inquiry for several reasons: animal experiments showed its damaging effect, Barrett's esophagus was seen to develop after total gastrectomy, and it was difficult to distinguish between erosive esophagitis and Barrett's esophagus using pH monitoring, suggesting the presence of an aetiological factor other than acid. The mere presence of bile in the stomach or even in the esophagus at endoscopy is not considered reliable evidence for pathological duodenogastric reflux or duodenogastroesophageal reflux (DGER)[59].

Bile reflux has proved difficult to objectively identify and quantify. pH monitoring was first used to identify this 'alkaline' reflux by Pellegrini et al.[60] in 1978. The presence of bile was defined as an esophageal pH greater than 7. This was recognized to be an indirect method of detecting bile, and that an alkaline pH could be caused by saliva, dental infection or pooling of saliva above a stricture. In addition, small amounts of DGER might be masked by gastric acidity, would probably fail to raise the pH above 7, and therefore a pH less than 7 would not exclude DGER.

Nonetheless, several authors have related alkaline exposure time (pH greater than 7) to the extent of esophageal mucosal damage. The conclusions from these studies are mixed: several show no difference in alkaline exposure time between the groups[39,42,43,50,61,62], although Attwood et al.[47,52] have found greater alkaline exposure time in complicated compared to uncomplicated Barrett's esophagus. Attempts have been made to improve the interpretation of esophageal alkaline pH by using combined gastric and esophageal pH monitoring, and temporally relating gastric alkaline pH shifts to esophageal alkaline pH shifts. Again, the assumption being made is that a gastric pH > 4 is due to DGR (although the same caveats apply). While increased alkaline exposure has been shown in both the stomach and the esophagus in patients with complications of Barrett's esophagus[47], and gastric alkaline exposure to be greatest in patients with an esophageal stricture or Barrett's esophagus[40], other investigators have found no such relationships and the technique not to be useful[39,61,62].

Scintagraphy using HIDA to label bile has been widely used to assess DGR. DGER has been found to be increased in erosive esophagitis compared with controls[63]. However, not only it is an insensitive method, it is not ambulatory and measures only a small time window. Aspiration of esophageal contents as a direct method of identifying bile is certainly of interest as a research tool, but has limited clinical applications. In 1988, Johnsson et al.[64] performed combined 24-hour esophageal pH monitoring and aspiration on healthy controls and patients with esophagitis. In the controls they were unable to aspirate any material for analysis. In the esophagitis group, bile salts were present in low concentrations (0-64 μmol/l). There was a mixture of tauro- and glycocholic acids, with undetectable amounts of other conjugated bile acids. These concentrations were similar to those found in the gastric juice of healthy controls, and the authors were unable to draw any conclusions regarding the role of bile salts in esophageal disease. Other studies have shown similarly small amounts of esophageal bile salts in esophagitis patients[65] or no bile salts[66]. Gotley et al.[67] on the other hand, using continuous suction on a slightly smaller (14 Fr) sump tube, detected conjugated bile salts (a range of glycine and taurine conjugated) in only two of 10 controls (maximum 40 μmol/l) but 39 of 45 esophagitis patients (at concentrations of up to

200 μmol/l). It should be noted that they investigated the supine period as well as the upright period. In another study[68] they found that the majority of patients with esophagitis or Barrett's esophagus had undetectable amounts of bile salts in esophageal aspirates, although about 10% of patients in all groups had bile salt concentrations in the range of 100-500 μmol/l. Increasing quantities of pepsin were found in the aspirates of those with the more severe mucosal disease, and they concluded that bile salts appeared in concentrations unlikely to cause mucosal damage, whereas acid and pepsin were more likely to be the factors involved. They also reported a combined pH/aspiration technique, and not only found similarly low levels of bile salts, but also concluded that there was no relationship between an alkaline pH (>7) and the presence of bile salts, bringing into question the validity of pH monitoring as a method of detecting DGER[20]. Iftikhar et al.[69] were able to detect greater quantities of bile salts than other studies, and found significantly greater quantities of bile salts in the esophagus of Barrett's esophagus patients than in esophagitis patients. Most recently, Nehra[70] used an automated esophageal sampling device to aspirate the esophagus in a range of GERD patients. They also observed increased quantities of bile acids in patients with severe esophagitis and Barrett's esophagus (in the range 100-600 μmol/l). Aspiration of gastric contents has provided some important information about the relationship between reflux disease and DGR. Gillen et al.[71] measured both fasting and post-prandial intra-gastric bile acids and found a positive correlation between the amount of bile acids in the post-prandial period and the presence of Barrett's esophagus. This association was more pronounced in cases with complicated Barrett's esophagus. Vaezi and Richter[50] looked at fasting total gastric bile acid concentrations and found significantly higher levels in Barrett's esophagus patients when compared to non-Barrett's esophagus reflux controls. This difference was particularly marked in the complicated Barrett's esophagus cases. While the pattern of increasing DGER with increasing severity of GERD emerges from these studies, they involve a cumbersome, time-consuming and impractical technique which is not suited to routine clinical investigation.

Other methods have been developed for detecting duodenal contents in the esophagus.

Smythe et al.[72] reported on the use of a sodium ion selective electrode. The rationale for use is that the concentration of sodium ions in gastric juice is 5-50 mmol/l, whereas the concentration in bile, pancreatic and duodenal secretions remains constant at around 150 mmol/l. DGER is therefore indicated by a sodium concentration greater than 50 mmol/l. While this technique has the attraction of being ambulatory, it still remains an indirect method of detecting duodenal contents. In addition, it requires acid suppression to avoid interference with hydrogen ions, a major drawback when it is known that omeprazole markedly reduces DGER[73].

5.1   AMBULATORY   BILIRUBIN MONITORING

A direct, ambulatory method of detecting DGER was thus needed to complement pH monitoring. The technique of bilirubin monitoring was first described in 1988[74]. The technique is based on the fact that bile contains pigments with definite light absorption properties (principally bilirubin). Hence a portable, fibreoptic spectrophotometric sensor with the ability to pick up the characteristic wavelength of bilirubin absorption(453 nm) was developed (Bilitec 2000), using bilirubin as a marker for the more harmful constituents of pancreatico-biliary secretions (bile salts, trypsin and lysolecithin). Light passes down a fibreoptic bundle and across a probe tip gap, in which is sampled the refluxate (Fig. 2). The absorption of light at this wavelength equates to the concentration of bilirubin. The bilirubin sensor has been validated by several investigators[42,75-77]. There is a good correlation between absorbance and bilirubin concentration (Fig. 3), although bilirubin absorbance seems to be reduced in acid media by up to 30%[77]. Criticisms of these studies have been made[78], but it is accepted that it is a valid technique for detecting the presence or absence of bilirubin.
In vivo studies of esophageal bile reflux have concentrated on combined pH and bilirubin monitoring across the range of reflux disease severity, from controls to complicated Barrett's esophagus. In 1994 Champion et al.[42] investigated four groups of patients: 12 healthy controls, 13 patients with GERD, 10 patients with Barrett's esophagus and 10 patients who had undergone partial gastrectomy for peptic ulcer disease. The increase in acid reflux across the groups was mirrored by an increase in bilirubin reflux, with very little in healthy

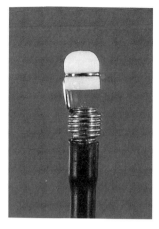

Figure 2. Photograph of the bilirubin sensor. Note the gap between the end of the optical fibres and the white teflon probe tip, within which the refluxate is sampled.

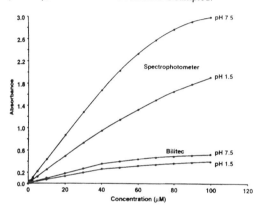

Figure 3.   Titration   curve   comparison   of   the spectrophotometer and Bilitec at pH 7.5 and 1.5 v concentration of bilirubin ditaurate. Note the decrease in absorption in acid media[77].

controls, increasing to a median of 12% total time in GERD patients and 41% total time in Barrett's esophagus patients. As expected, bilirubin reflux was greater than acid reflux in the partial gastrectomy patients (Fig. 4). They also reported no difference in esophageal alkaline exposure time between the groups and no correlation between bilirubin reflux and alkaline exposure, confirming that the term 'alkaline' reflux to describe DGER is a misnomer which should be abandoned. Caldwell et al.[41] and Kauer et al.[79] looked at a similar selection of patients and came to similar conclusions. Vaezi et al.[50] investigated 12 healthy controls, nine patients with uncomplicated Barrett's esophagus and 11 patients with complicated Barrett's esophagus. They found that acid and bilirubin reflux in complicated   Barrett's   esophagus   was significantly greater than in uncomplicated Barrett's esophagus. They also performed gastric aspiration studies on the Barrett's esophagus patients, noting that fasting gastric bile salt concentrations were greater in the complicated Barrett's esophagus patients than the uncomplicated. They suggested that damage caused by the refluxate was secondary to acid and duodenal contents acting in synergism rather than in isolation. The same group also reported the findings of combined 24-hour esophageal pH and bilirubin monitoring in 13 partial gastrectomy patients with symptoms suggestive of chronic DGR[80]. Of the 13 patients, 10 had significant esophageal bilirubin reflux, but only three of these had significant esophageal acid reflux. Symptom episodes were also investigated, and it was found that 65% of these were associated with acid reflux, far more than with bilirubin reflux (although figures for this are not given).

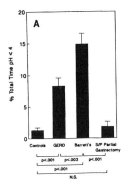

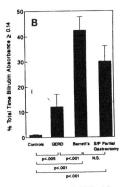

Figure 4. Acid reflux (A) and bilirubin reflux (B) in 4 study populations. Both acid and bilirubin reflux increase with worsening mucosal disease, the greatest in Barrett's esophagus. As expected, bilirubin reflux was significantly increased after partial gastrectomy compared with acid reflux[94].

Interestingly, the only patients with esophagitis on endoscopy were the three with significant acid reflux, and the authors therefore suggested that it was the acid rather than the duodenal contents which was the main culprit in post gastrectomy reflux. In patients with an intact stomach, it therefore seems that the majority either reflux both acid and bile or reflux neither[81]. Isolated bile reflux is an uncommon finding, and when present is rarely associated with significant mucosal damage or reflux symptoms. In contrast, patients who

reflux both acid and bile have a higher prevalence of esophagitis and Barrett's esophagus than patients with isolated acid reflux[82].

Ambulatory bilirubin monitoring is a technique which is not without its drawbacks. Firstly it measures bilirubin rather than the noxious components of bile. However, validation studies suggest that the concentration of bilirubin correlates well with that of bile acids and trypsin[83]. Secondly, validation studies have determined a threshold of 0.14 absorbance units at which bilirubin is said to be present in the refluxate[76]. However, some investigators have used a threshold of 0.2 which makes meaningful comparisons difficult. Thirdly, there is disagreement about whether patients should be allowed an unrestricted diet (with light absorbance at the same wavelength as bilirubin) or a restricted diet which may be less physiological but prevents this interference with bilirubin. Both these last two issues need agreed standards to be set. There is also a tendency for food to clog the probe tip and interfere with light absorption. However, bilirubin monitoring is the best method of ambulatory bile detection available currently.

5.2 THE EFFECT OF OMEPRAZOLE ON ACID AND BILE REFLUX

The profound acid suppression effects of proton pump inhibitors such as omeprazole have long been known and can be objectively studied using pH monitoring. Bilirubin monitoring allows a similar investigation into the effects of omeprazole on bile reflux. This was first studied by Champion et al.[42] in a small number of patients, who found, perhaps unexpectedly, that bilirubin reflux was markedly reduced by omeprazole. Marshall et al.[73] investigated the effect of omeprazole 20 mg bd on 23 patients with Barrett's esophagus, and found that not only was DGER reduced into the normal range in all but one patient, but that DGR was also significantly reduced although to a lesser extent (Fig. 5). Stein et al.[84] compared medical acid suppression with anti-reflux surgery, and again found a reduction in DGER with acid suppression, although the reduction was not as profound as that obtained with anti-reflux surgery. Nonetheless, this is an important finding when one considers that the majority of patients with Barrett's esophagus are treated medically. The reason for this reduction in DGER and DGR is unclear. However, the most likely explanation is that omeprazole causes a significant reduction in the volume of gastric juice available for reflux, and as duodenal contents mix with gastric juice to a greater or lesser extent, there is a smaller volume of gastric contents available for reflux. This hypothesis is supported by the fact that omeprazole has no effect on DGR when the bilirubin probe is placed in the gastric antrum, where the effects of gastric juice volume reduction should be negated[85].

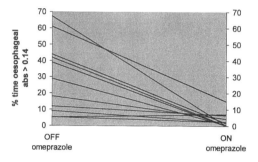

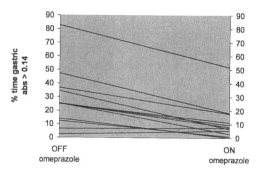

Figure 5. Effect of omeprazole on individual oesophageal and gastric bilirubin values[73].

6. SHORT SEGMENT BARRETT'S ESOPHAGUS AND REFLUX OF ACID AND BILE

The traditional length of columnar mucosa required for the diagnosis of Barrett's esophagus was 3cm. This was introduced to prevent endoscopic overdiagnosis. Iftikhar et al.[86], in a 15 year prospective study, observed that longer lengths of columnar mucosa were associated with significantly greater risk of developing dysplasia. However, the importance of intestinal metaplasia as the pre-malignant marker within the columnar mucosa provoked interest in shorter (less than 3 cm) lengths of columnar mucosa. In 1994 it was

observed by Spechler et al. that intestinal metaplasia was present at the normal appearing squamocolumnar junction in 18% of patients[87]. At a time when adenocarcinoma of the gastroesophageal junction is increasing rapidly[88,89], this has generated further investigations into the pathophysiology of shorter columnar segments.

Weston et al.[90] compared the endoscopic and histological findings in 41 patients with long segment (>2 cm) and 40 patients with short segment (<2 cm) columnar mucosa. There was a similar incidence of hiatus hernia between the two groups. The most striking difference was the absence of dysplasia or carcinoma in short segment Barrett's esophagus, compared to dysplasia in 37% and carcinoma in 10% of long segment Barrett's esophagus. Loughney et al.[91] and Oberg et al.[82] both compared esophageal manometry and 24 hour monitoring in short and long segments of columnar mucosa. Lower esophageal sphincter pressure was lower in the long segment groups[82,91]. Acid exposure times were greater in the long segment groups, although the degree of acid exposure in the short segment groups was still pathological. In addition, there was a trend towards greater bilirubin exposure in long segment compared to short segment Barrett's esophagus[82]. A larger study by Oberg et al.[92] compared 34 patients with intestinal metaplasia confined to the gastroesophageal junction, 44 with intestinal metaplasia in short columnar segments (<3 cm) and 68 with intestinal metaplasia in long columnar segments (>3 cm). They detected decreasing distal esophageal amplitude, increasing number and duration of acid reflux episodes, and increasing acid exposure as the length of intestinalised mucosa increased. They concluded that Barrett's esophagus spreads progressively cranially, with increasing reflux causing weakening of the lower esophageal sphincter, disrupted esophageal body function and progressive intestinalisation over time. Short segment Barrett's esophagus represents part of the disease spectrum.

7. THE TEMPORAL RELATIONSHIP BETWEEN ACID AND BILE IN REFLUX DISEASE

Earlier animal experiments have shown how the extent of mucosal damage is determined not only by the composition of the refluxate but also by the pH. Combined pH and bilirubin monitoring has allowed investigation of the pH at which bile salts and trypsin exist in the esophagus. Trypsin, as expected, causes damage at alkaline pH. Bile salts must be soluble and unionized if they are to enter mucosal cells and cause damage. At pH 7 or more, the vast majority of bile salts are completely ionized and in solution. At pH 2 or less, precipitation occurs and bile salts cannot enter cells. There is, however, a critical pH between 3 and 6 when a mixture of ionized bile salts and lipophilic unionized salt is present. Unionized salts cross the cell membrane, become ionized because of the alkaline intracellular environment, and become trapped. They accumulate, become toxic to the mitochondria, and mucosal damage ensues. Kauer et al.[94] analyzed the esophageal pH during episodes of bilirubin exposure and found that 87% of esophageal bilirubin exposure occurred when the esophageal pH was between 4 and 7 (Fig. 6). For only a tiny amount of time (1.1%) was the esophageal pH greater than 7 (i.e. 'alkaline'). This work was confirmed by Marshall et al.[95]. Not only does this refute the concept of 'alkaline' reflux and the use of pH monitoring to detect bile, but it gives a valuable insight into the damaging potential of bile in Barrett's esophagus, where bile reflux is greatest.

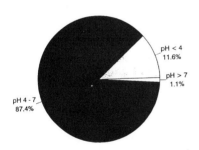

Figure 6. Esophageal luminal pH during periods of bilirubin exposure[94].

In addition to such analysis, combined pH and bilirubin monitoring has allowed 24-hour patterns of acid and bile to be examined (Fig. 7). It is known that reflux in Barrett's esophagus, with its poor esophageal motility and clearance and lower esophageal sphincter hypotonia, is particularly severe in the supine position[95,96]. Savarino et al.[56] showed how gastric acidity was not only no greater in Barrett's esophagus than healthy controls, as previously mentioned, but that the stomach was most acid in the first part of the night, and the pH gradually increased during the night. Marshall et al.[95] performed simultaneous esophageal pH and bilirubin and gastric pH monitoring on 113 subjects with a range of mucosal injury from controls to Barrett's

esophagus. By dividing the supine period into quarters, they showed how the patterns of reflux compare. Acid reflux is greatest in the first half of the night, and declines rapidly as the night progresses. Bile reflux continues, however, throughout the night. The stomach is most acid at the beginning of the night, and gradually becomes more alkaline. Thus the relative pH of the esophagus and stomach is constantly changing, at various times in the night providing the ideal conditions for mucosal damage by the different constituents of reflux (Figs. 8-11).

8. MOTOR AND SENSORY FACTORS ASSOCIATED WITH BARRETT'S ESOPHAGUS

It is apparent from the measurement of lower esophageal sphincter pressure (LESP) that there is a spectrum of gastroesophageal reflux disease, so that in a study by Castell there was a sharp contrast between those suffering from daily heartburn having a mean LESP of 4 mmHg whereas those with heartburn occurring monthly had greater LESP of 12 mm/Hg[97]. An increase prevalence both in the presence and size of hiatal hernia has been found in those with Barrett's esophagus. Furthermore, when reflux inducing provocation maneuvers were used, the combination of a hiatal hernia and a low LESP was particularly associated with a high incidence of reflux[98]. A hypothesis was put forward by Mittal[99] to link some of the factors which are thought to be relevant in the genesis of progressive gastroesophageal reflux disease. The process probably starts with an increased transient lower esophageal sphincter relaxations, leading to increased acid exposure in the lower esophagus, esophageal shortening and fibrosis. This then would have the effect of leading to the formation of a hiatus hernia with stretching of the diaphragmatic sling, thereby weakening the contribution of the diaphragm and further impairing lower esophageal sphincter competence.

Kahrilas[100] has looked at the motor changes in the body of the esophagus in reflux disease. He noted that a peristaltic amplitude of less than 30 mm/Hg was ineffective in clearing a bolus and contractions less than this he termed ineffective peristalsis. With increasing severity of GERD there is not only an increase in the proportion of ineffective peristalsis but also an increase in the proportion of uncoordinated peristalsis, so that the prevalence of "peristaltic dysfunction" is 48% in those with severe esophagitis, 21% with non inflamed GERD and 9% in controls. Other studies have confirmed a progressive reduction not only in the amplitude of distal esophageal contractions but also in the amplitude of the

lower esophageal sphincter pressure in Barrett's esophagus patients as compared to uncomplicated GERD.

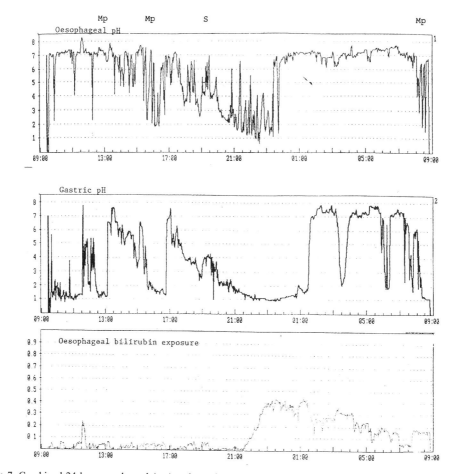

Figure 7. Combined 24 hour esophageal (top) and gastric pH (middle) and esophageal bilirubin (bottom) tracing in a patient with Barrett's esophagus (S=supine, M=meal, p=post-prandial). Note the severe acid reflux in the first half of the night, and gastric alkaline reflux in the second half. Note also the severe supine bilirubin reflux, occurring with both an acid and a normal/alkaline esophagus, and how esophageal bilirubin reflux can occur in the presence of both an acid and alkaline stomach[95].

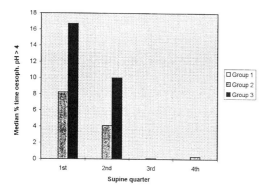

Figure 8. Patterns of acid reflux throughout the night in 3 groups of patients (Group 1: non-erosive GERD; Group 2: erosive GERD; Group 3: Barrett's esophagus). Note how acid reflux is a feature of the first half of the night[95].

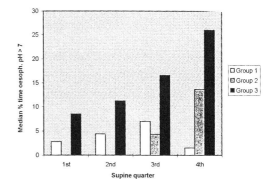

Figure 9. Nocturnal oesophageal alkaline exposure. All 3 groups show a tendency for alkaline exposure to occur towards the end of the night, although this does not represent a significant change[95].

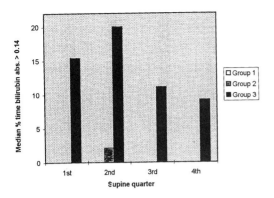

Figure 10. Nocturnal oesophageal bilirubin reflux is principally a feature of Barrett's esophagus(Group 3), where it exists in all quarters of the supine period without a significant change[95].

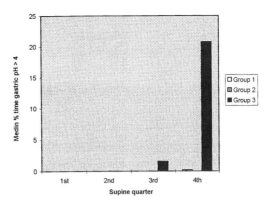

Figure 11. Nocturnal gastric alkaline exposure is a feature of Barrett's esophagus (Group 3) almost exclusively, where it occurs mainly in the last quarter of the night[95]

SUMMARY

It is clinically apparent that Barrett's esophagus is associated with severe, chronic gastroesophageal reflux. Animal experiments have shown how both acid and the individual constituents of bile are capable of causing mucosal injury. Although the *in vivo* evidence suggests a strong role for acid in the pathogenesis, it is likely that acid and bile constituents act synergistically. Studies of acid reflux in to the esophagus show a step-wise increase in acid in the lower esophagus occurring with progressively severe mucosal esophageal disease, the greatest acid reflux occurring in those with Barrett's esophagus complicated by stricture, ulceration or dysplasia. Esophageal bile reflux as measured by ambulatory bilirubin monitoring shows a parallel increase in esophageal bile exposure, and the evidence points to complicated Barrett's esophagus having both the greatest acid and bile exposure. Gastric acid secretion is not increased in Barrett's esophagus patients when compared with non-Barrett's esophagus controls.In addition to severe reflux, Barrett's esophagus is associated with a diminished lower esophageal sphincter pressure and with dysmotility of the body of the esophagus, characterized by both low amplitude contractions and a high proportion of non-peristaltic contractions. The function of the diaphragmatic sphincter is also compromised because of esophageal shortening, with stretching of the left crust of the diaphragm and a tendency to the formation of a hiatus hernia.

REFERENCES

1. McDougall NI, Johnston BT, Kee F. Natural history of reflux esophagitis: a 10 year follow-up of its effects on patients symptomatology and quality of life. Gut 1996;38:481-6.
2. Iascone C, DeMeester TR, Little AG, Skinner DB. Barrett's esophagus: functional assessment, proposed pathogenesis and surgical therapy. Arch Surg 1983;118:543-9.
3. Helsingen N. Esophagitis following total gastrectomy. Acta Chirurgica Scandinavica 1959;118:190-201.
4. Orlando RC, Bozymski EM. Heartburn in pernicious anemia--a consequence of bile reflux. N Eng J Med 1973;289:522-3.
5. Cross FS, Wangensteen OH. Role of bile and pancreatic juice in production of oesophageal erosions and anaemia. Proc Soc Exp Biol Med 1961;77:862-6.
6. Henderson RD, Mugashe F, Jeejeebhoy KN, Cullen J, Szczepanski M, Boszko A, Marryatt G. The role of bile and acid in the production of esophagitis and the motor defect of esophagitis. Ann Thorac Surg 1972;14:465-73.
7. Lillemoe KD, Johnson LF, Harmon JW. Alkaline esophagitis: a comparison of the ability of components of gastroduodenal contents to injure the rabbit esophagus. Gastroenterology 1983;85:621-8.
8. Lillemoe KD, Johnson LF, Harmon JW. Role of the components of the gastroduodenal contents in experimental acid esophagitis. Surgery 1982;92:276-84.
9. Salo J, Kivilaakso E. Role of luminal H+ in the pathogenesis of experimental esophagitis. Surgery 1982;92:61-8.
10. Chaparala RC, Tobey NA, Orlando RC. Effect of HCl, HCl and pepsin or HCl and bile salts on injury to rabbit esophageal epithelium. Gastroenterology 1995;108:A69.
11. Lillemoe KD, Kidder GW, Harmon JW, Gadacz TR, Johnson LF, Bunte RM, Hofmann AF.

Tauroursodeoxycholic acid is less damaging than taurochenodeoxycholic acid to the gastric and esophageal mucosa. Dig Dis Sci 1983;28:359-64.

12. Kivilaakso E, Fromm D, Silen W. Effect of bile salts and related compounds on isolated esophageal mucosa. Surgery 1980;87:280-5.

13. Redo SF, Barnes WA, Ortiz de la Sierra A. Perfusion of the canine oesophagus with secretions of the upper gastrointestinal tract. Ann Surg 1959;149:556-64.

14. Lillemoe KD, Johnson LF, Harmon JW. Taurodeoxycholate modulates the effects of pepsin and trypsin in experimental esophagitis. Surgery 1985;97:662-7.

15. Salo JA, Kivilaakso E. Contribution of trypsin and cholate to the pathogenesis of experimental alkaline reflux esophagitis. Scand J Gastroenterol 1984;19:875-81.

16. Tompkins RK, Chow JF, Clarke JS. Reduction of pepsin activity by bile. A factor favoring ulcer formation after bile-diverting operations. Am J Surg 1972;124:207-11.

17. Tompkins GS, Tompkins RK. Inhibition of pepsin activity by unconjugated bile acids: inverse relation to number of hydroxyl groups. Am J Surg 1982;144:300-1.

18. Kiroff GK, Mukerjhee TM, Dixon B, Devitt PG, Jamieson GG. Morphological changes caused by exposure of rabbit oesophageal mucosa to hydrochloric acid and sodium taurocholate. Aust N Z J Surg 1987;57:119-26.

19. Bateson MC, Hopwood D, Milne G, Bouchier IA. Oesophageal epithelial ultrastructure after incubation with gastrointestinal fluids and their components. J Pathol 1981;133:33-51.

20. Gotley DC, Appleton GV, Cooper MJ. Bile acids and trypsin are unimportant in alkaline esophageal reflux. J Clin Gastroenterol 1992;14:2-7.

21. Lambert R. Relative importance of biliary and pancreatic secretions in the genesis of esophagitis in rats. Am J Dig Dis 1962;11:1026-33.

22. Moffat RC, Berkas EM. Bile esophagitis. Arch Surg 1965;91:963-6.

23. Gillison EW, Kusakari K, Bombeck CT, Nyhus LM. The importance of bile in reflux esophagitis and the success in its prevention by surgical means. Br J Surg 1972;59:794-8.

24. Gillison EW, De Castro VA, Nyhus LM, Kusakari K, Bombeck CT. The significance of bile in reflux esophagitis. Surg Gynecol Obstet 1972;134:419-24.

25. Henderson RD, Mugashe FL, Jeejeebhoy KN, Szczpanski MM, Cullen J, Marryatt G, Boszko A. Synergism of acid and bile salts in the production of experimental esophagitis. Can J Surg 1973;16:12-7.

26. Mud HJ, Kranendonk SE, Obertop H, Van Houten H, Westbroek DL. Active trypsin and reflux esophagitis: an experimental study in rats. Br J Surg 1982;69:269-72.

27. Attwood SE, Smyrk TC, DeMeester TR, Mirvish SS, Stein HJ, Hinder RA. Duodenoesophageal reflux and the development of esophageal adenocarcinoma in rats. Surgery 1992;111:503-10.

28. Pera M, Trastek VF, Carpenter HA, Fernandez PL, Cardesa A, Mohr U, Pairolero PC. Influence of pancreatic and biliary reflux on the development of esophageal carcinoma. Ann Thorac Surg 1993;55:1386-92.

29. Clark GW, Smyrk TC, Mirvish SS, Anselmino M, Yamashita Y, Hinder RA, DeMeester TR, Birt DF. Effect of gastroduodenal juice and dietary fat on the development of Barrett's esophagus and esophageal

30. neoplasia: an experimental rat model. Ann Surg Oncol 1994;1:252-61.

30. Ireland AP, Peters JH, Smyrk TC, DeMeester TR, Clark GW, Mirvish SS, Adrian TE. Gastric juice protects against the development of esophageal adenocarcinoma in the rat. Ann Surg 1996;224:358-71.

31. Wetscher GJ, Hinder RA, Kretchmar D, Stinson R, Perdikis G, Smyrk TC, Klinger PJ, Adrian TE. Duodenogastric reflux causes growth stimulation of foregut mucosa potentiated by gastric acid blockade. Dig Dis Sci 1996;41:2166-73.

32. Bremner CG, Lynch VP, Ellis FH. Barrett's esophagus: congenital or acquired? An experimental study of esophageal mucosal regeneration in the dog. Surgery 1970;68:209-16.

33. Gillen P, Keeling P, Byrne PJ, West AB, Hennessy TP. Experimental columnar metaplasia in the canine oesophagus. Br J Surg 1988;75:113-5.

34. Seto Y, Kobori O. Role of reflux esophagitis and acid in the development of columnar epithelium in the rat oesophagus. Br J Surg 1993;80:467-70.

35. Konishi M, Kato H, Tachimori Y, Watanabe H, Yamaguchi H, Ishikawa T, Itabashi M, Hirota T. Adenocarcinoma in Barrett's oesophagus following total resection of the gastric remnant: a case report. Jpn J Clin Oncol 1992;22:292-6.

36. Parrilla P, Liron-Ruiz R, Martinez de Haro LF, Ortiz A, Molina J, De Andres B. Gastric surgery does not increase the risk of developing Barrett's esophagus. Am J Gastroenterol 1997;92:960-3.

37. Birgisson S, Rice TW, Easley KA, Richter JE. The lack of association between adenocarcinoma of the esophagus and gastric surgery: a retrospective study. Am J Gastro 1997;92:216-21.

38. Johnson LF, DeMeester TR. Twenty-four-hour pH monitoring of the distal esophagus. A quantitative measure of gastroesophageal reflux. Am J Gastroenterol 1974;62:325-32.

39. Iftikhar SY, Ledingham S, Evans D, Yusuf SW, Steele RJC, Atkinson M, Hardcastle JD. Alkaline gastroesophageal reflux: dual pH probe monitoring. Gut 1995;37:465-70.

40. Stein HJ, Barlow AP, DeMeester TR, Hinder RA. Complications of gastroesophageal reflux disease. Role of the lower esophageal sphincter, esophageal acid and acid/alkaline exposure, and duodenogastric reflux. Ann Surg 1992;216:35-43.

41. Caldwell MT, Lawlor P, Byrne PJ, Walsh TN, Hennessy TP. Ambulatory oesophageal bile reflux monitoring in Barrett's oesophagus. Br J Surg 1995;82:657-60.

42. Champion G, Richter JE, Vaezi MF, Singh S, Alexander R. Duodenogastroesophageal reflux: relationship to pH and importance in Barrett's esophagus. Gastroenterology 1994;107:747-54.

43. Vaezi MF, Richter JE. Role of acid and duodenogastroesophageal reflux in gastroesophageal reflux disease. Gastroenterology 1996;111:1192-9.

44. Parrilla P, Ortiz A, Martinez de Haro LF, Aguayo JL, Ramirez P. Evaluation of the magnitude of gastro-oesophageal reflux in Barrett's oesophagus. Gut 1990;31:964-7.

45. Fiorucci S, Santucci L, Farroni F, Pelli MA, Morelli A. Effect of omeprazole on gastroesophageal reflux in Barrett's esophagus. Am J Gastroenterol 1989;84:1263-7.

46. Flook D, Stoddard CJ. Gastro-oesophageal reflux (GOR) in patients with esophagitis or a columnar-lined oesophagus. Gut 1983;24:A1007.

47. Attwood SE, DeMeester TR, Bremner CG, Barlow AP, Hinder RA. Alkaline gastroesophageal reflux:

implications in the development of complications in Barrett's columnar-lined lower esophagus. Surgery 1989;106:764-70.

48. Coenraad M, Masclee AAM, Straathof JWA, Ganesh S, Griffieon G, Lamers CBHW. Is Barrett's esophagus characterised by more pronounced acid reflux than severe esophagitis? Am J Gastroenterol 1998;93:1068-72.

49. Neumann CS, Cooper BT. 24 hour ambulatory oesophageal pH monitoring in uncomplicated Barrett's oesophagus. Gut 1994;35:1352-5.

50. Vaezi MF, Richter JE. Synergism of acid and duodenogastroesophageal reflux in complicated Barrett's esophagus. Surgery 1995;117:699-704.

51. Gillen P, Keeling P, Byrne PJ, Hennessy TP. Barrett's oesophagus: pH profile. Br J Surg 1987;74:774-6.

52. Attwood SE, Ball CS, Barlow AP, Jenkinson L, Norris TL, Watson A. Role of intragastric and intraoesophageal alkalinisation in the genesis of complications in Barrett's columnar lined lower oesophagus. Gut 1993;34:11-5.

53. Mulholland MW, Reid BJ, Levine DS, Rubin CE. Elevated gastric acid secretion in patients with Barrett's metaplastic epithelium. Dig Dis Sci 1989;34:1329-34.

54. Collen MJ, Lewis JH, Benjamin SB. Gastric acid hypersecretion in refractory gastroesophageal reflux disease. Gastroenterology 1990;98:654-61.

55. Hirschowitz BI. Gastric acid and pepsin secretion in patients with Barrett's esophagus and appropriate controls. Dig Dis Sci 1996;41:1384-91.

56. Savarino V, Mela GS, Zentilin P, Mele MR, Mansi C, Remagnino AC, Vigneri S, Malesci A, Belicchi M, Lapertosa G, Celle G. The time pattern of gastric acidity in Barrett's esophagus. Dig Dis Sci 1996;41:1379-83.

57. Fiorucci S, Santucci L, Chiucchiu S, Morelli A. Gastric acidity and gastroesophageal reflux patterns in patients with esophagitis. Gastroenterology 1992;103:855-61.

58. Strader DB, Benjamin SB, Orbuch M, Lubensky TA, Gibril F, Weber C, Fishbeyn VA, Jensen RT, Metz DC. Esophageal function and occurrence of Barrett's esophagus in Zollinger-Ellison syndrome. Digestion 1995;56:347-56.

59. Stein HJ, Smyrk TC, DeMeester TR. Clinical value of endoscopy and histology in the diagnosis of duodenogastric reflux disease. Surgery 1992;112:796-803.

60. Pellegrini CA, DeMeester TR, Wernly JA, Johnson LF, Skinner DB. Alkaline gastroesophageal reflux. Am J Surg 1978;135:177-84.

61. Singh S, Bradley LA, Richter JE. Determinants of oesophageal 'alkaline' pH environment in controls and patients with gastro-oesophageal reflux disease. Gut 1993;34:309-16.

62. Penagini R, Yuen H, Misiewicz JJ, Bianchi PA. Alkaline intra-oesophageal pH and gastro-oesophageal reflux in patients with peptic esophagitis. Scand J Gastroenterol 1988;23:675-8.

63. Da Costa PM, Godinho F, Veiga-Fernandes F. Gastro-oesophageal and bile reflux. Simultaneous quantitative assessment with gastric and gallbladder emptying evaluation: clinical applicability of a new computerized gammagraphic method. Nuc Med Comm 1992;13:817-23.

64. Johnsson F, Joelsson B, Floren CH, Nilsson A. Bile salts in the oesophagus of patients with esophagitis. Scand J Gastroenterol 1988;23:712-6.

65. Smith MR, Buckton GK, Bennett JR. Bile acid levels in stomach and oesophagus of patients with acid gastro-oesophageal reflux. Gut 1990;34:A556.

66. Mittal RK, Reuben A, Whitney JO, McCallum RW. Do bile acids reflux into the esophagus? A study in normal subjects and patients with gastroesophageal reflux disease. Gastroenterology 1987;92:371-5.

67. Gotley DC, Morgan AP, Cooper MJ. Bile acid concentrations in the refluxate of patients with reflux esophagitis. Br J Surg 1988;75:587-90.

68. Gotley DC, Morgan AP, Ball D, Owen RW, Cooper MJ. Composition of gastro-oesophageal refluxate. Gut 1991;32:1093-9.

69. Iftikhar SY, Ledingham S, Steele RJ, Evans DF, Lendrum K, Atkinson M, Hardcastle JD. Bile reflux in columnar-lined Barrett's oesophagus. Ann R Coll Surg 1993;75:411-6.

70. Nehra D, Howell P, Pye JK, Beynon J. Assessment of combined bile acid and pH profiles using an automated sampling device in gastro-oesophageal reflux disease. Br J Surg 1998;85:134-7.

71. Gillen P, Keeling P, Byrne PJ, Healy M, O'Moore RR, Hennessy TP. Importance of duodenogastric reflux in the pathogenesis of Barrett's oesophagus. Br J Surg 1988;75:540-3.

72. Smythe A, O'Leary D, Johnson AG. Duodenogastric reflux after gastric surgery and in gastric ulcer disease: continuous measurement with a sodium ion selective electrode. Gut 1993;34:1047-50.

73. Marshall REK, Anggiansah A, Owen WA, Manifold DK, Owen WJ. Effect of omeprazole 20mg twice daily on duodenogastric and gastro-oesophageal bile reflux in Barrett's oesophagus. Gut 1998;43:603-6.

74. Baldini F, Falciai R, Scheggi AM, Bechi P. A new fibreoptic sensor for bile reflux. In: Proceedings Optical Fibres and Sensors 1988, New Orleans, Louisiana, 1988. Norwood, Massachusetts: Artech, 1988:353-6.

75. Bechi P, Falciai R, Baldini F, Cosi F, Pucciani F, Boscherini S. A new fibreoptic sensor for ambulatory enterogastric reflux detection. Fiberoptic, Medical and Flourescent Sensors and Applications 1992;1648:130-5.

76. Bechi P, Pucciani F, Baldini F, Cosi F, Falciai R, Mazzanti R, Castagnoli A, Passeri A, Boscherini S. Long-term ambulatory enterogastric reflux monitoring. Validation of a new fiberoptic technique. Dig Dis Sci 1993;38:1297-306.

77. Vaezi MF, Lacamera RG, Richter JE. Validation studies of Bilitec 2000: an ambulatory duodenogastric reflux monitoring system. Am J Physiol 1994;267:G1050-7.

78. Ostrow JD. Bilitec to quantitate duodenogastric reflux: is it valid? Gastroenterology 1995;108:1332-4.

79. Kauer WKH, Burdiles P, Ireland AP, Clark GW, Peters JH, Bremner CG, DeMeester TR. Does duodenal juice reflux into the esophagus of patients with complicated GERD? Evaluation of a new fibreoptic sensor for bilirubin. Am J Surg 1995;169:98-104.

80. Sears RJ, Champion GL, Richter JE. Characteristics of distal partial gastrectomy patients with esophageal symptoms of duodenogastric reflux. Am J Gastroenterol 1995;90:211-5.

81. Marshall REK, Anggiansah A, Owen WA, Owen WJ. Bile in the oesophagus: how important is it in patients with an intact stomach? Br J Surg 1997;84:62.

82. Oberg S, Ritter MP, Crookes PF, Fein M, Mason RJ, Gadensytatter M, Bremner CG, Peters JH, DeMeester TR. Gastroesophageal reflux disease and

mucosal injury with emphasis on short-segment Barrett's esophagus and duodenogastroesophageal reflux. J Gastrointest Surg 1998;2:547-53.

83. Stipa F, Stein HJ, Feussner H, Kraemer SJ, Siewert JR. Assessment of non-acid esophageal reflux: comparison between long-term reflux aspiration test and fibre-optic bilirubin monitoring. Dis Esoph 1997;10:24-8.

84. Stein HJ, Kauer W, Feussner H, Siewert JR. Bile reflux in benign and malignant Barrett's esophagus: effect of medical acid suppression and Nissen fundoplication. J Gastrointest Surg 1998;2:333-41.

85. Manifold DK, Anggiansah A, Marshall REK, Owen WJ. Effect of omeprazole on antral duodenogastric reflux in Barrett's oesophagus. Gut 1999;44:A112.

86. Iftikhar SY, James PD, Steele RJ, Hardcastle JD, Atkinson M. Length of Barrett's oesophagus: an important factor in the development of dysplasia and adenocarcinoma. Gut 1992;33:1155-8.

87. Spechler SJ, Zeroogian JM, Antonioli DA, Wang HH, Goyal RK. Prevalence of metaplasia at the gastroesophageal junction. Lancet 1994;344:1533-6.

88. Blot WJ, Devesa SS, Kneller RW, Fraumeni JF, Jr. Rising incidence of adenocarcinoma of the esophagus and gastric cardia. JAMA 1991;265:1287-9.

89. Blot WJ, Devesa SS, Fraumeni JF. Continuuing climb in rates of esophageal adenocarcinoma: an update. JAMA 1993;270:1320.

90. Weston AP, Krmpotich P, Makdisi WF, Cherian R, Dixon A, McGregor DH, Banerjee SK. Short segment Barrett's esophagus: clinical and histological features, associated endoscopic findings, and association with gastric intestinal metaplasia. Am J Gastroenterol 1996;91:981-6.

91. Loughney T, Maydonovitch CL, Wong RK. Esophageal manometry and ambulatory 24-hour pH monitoring in patients with long and short segment Barrett's esophagus. Am J Gastroenterol 1998;93:916-9.

92. Oberg S, DeMeester TR, Peters JH, Hagen JA, Nigro JJ, DeMeester SR, Theisen J, Campos JMR, Crookes PF. The extent of Barrett's esophagus depends on the status of the lower esophageal sphincter and the degree of esophageal acid exposure. J Thorac Cardiovasc Surg 1999;117:572-80.

93. DeMeester SR, DeMeester TR. Columnar mucosa and intestinal metaplasia of the esophagus: 50 years of controversy. Ann Surg 2000;231:303-21.

94. Kauer WKH, Peters JH, DeMeester TR, Ireland AP, Bremner CG, Hagen JA. Mixed reflux of gastric and duodenal juice is more harmful to the esophagus than gastric juice alone. Ann Surg 1995;222:525-33.

95. Marshall REK, Anggiansah A, Owen WA, Owen WJ. The temporal relationship between oesophageal bile reflux and pH in gastro-oesophageal reflux disease. Eur J Gastroenterol Hepatol 1998;10:385-92.

96. D'Onofrio V, Bovero E, G.O.S.P.E., Iaquinto G. Characterisation of acid and alkaline reflux in patients with Barrett's esophagus. Dis Esoph 1997;10:16-22.

97. Nebel OT, Fornes MF, Castell DO. Symptomatic gastroesophageal reflux: incidence and precipitating factors. Am J Dig Dis 1976;21:953-6.

98. Sloan S, Rademaker AW, Kahrilas PJ. Determinants of gastroesophageal junction competence: hiatal hernia, lower esophageal sphincter or both. Ann Intern Med 1992;117:977-82.

99. Mittal RK. Pathophysiology of gastroesophageal reflux disease: motility factors. In Castell DO, Richter JE eds, The Esophagus, 3rd ed. Philadelphia: Lippincott, Williams and Wilkins, 1999:317-419.

100. Kahrilas PJ, Dodds WJ, Hogan WJ, Kern M, Arndorfer RC, Reece AC. Esophageal peristaltic dysfunction in peptic esophagitis. Gastroenterology 1986;91:897-904.

2.4 Endoscopic Classification of Gastro-esophageal Reflux Disease

Jan G. Hatlebakk and Arnold Berstad

1. INTRODUCTION

Endoscopy has gained a major role in the diagnostic workup and long-term follow-up of patients with gastro-esophageal reflux disease (GERD). In a quite unique way, it allows the physician to inspect the mucosa of the upper gastrointestinal tract, thereby enabling him to identify and classify the typical reflux-induced lesions. Furthermore, it lets him detect conditions that might predispose the patient to gastro-esophageal reflux or might be an alternative explanation for the symptoms. Only through endoscopic examination biopsies can be taken to further study mucosa pathology. The finding of reflux esophagitis in a patient with typical reflux-induced symptoms is for most purposes an adequate basis for making the diagnosis of GERD. Well-informed patients are aware of the importance of their physician having actually seen and evaluated the diseased mucosa for premalignant changes and other abnormalities. The disease spectrum of GERD is immense and includes at one extreme patients with purely symptomatic disease, with no endoscopically visible abnormalities, but at the other extreme patients with severe endoscopic changes, with a potential for developing complications. The potential of endoscopy to discriminate between mild and severe disease is based on the relative stability of the course of the disease. In the majority of patients, endoscopy shows its maximum severity at the time of the first endoscopic examination. Less than 20% develop more severe reflux esophagitis with time[1]. After 5 years of symptomatic disease, the condition is usually very stable. The role of endoscopy in GERD also seems to vary between countries. The reason for this may be historic and is linked to workup and management in dyspeptic patients in general. In most patients with dyspeptic symptoms, symptom evaluation alone is quite insufficient for making a firm diagnosis. Therefore, even patients with typical symptoms of gastro-esophageal reflux are examined with endoscopy to rule out other disease, such as peptic ulcer disease and cancer. In patients with heartburn as the predominant gastrointestinal symptom, other pathology is found only infrequently and presumably less frequently as peptic ulcer disease and gastric cancer are becoming less prevalent. In a recent study of 573 patients with heartburn as main symptom, only 20 patients (3%) had peptic ulcers and no patient had cancer. This speaks against routinely doing upper endoscopy in patients strongly suspected of having GERD, due to limited diagnostic gain and some discomfort for the patient. Nevertheless, endoscopy should be performed routinely in patients above the age of 40-50 and in patients with weight loss or dysphagia, as the possibility of cancer is clearly higher[2]. Therefore, endoscopy should still be the basis for diagnosis in most GERD patients. The increase in the incidence of Barrett's esophagus and esophageal and proximal gastric adenocarcinoma should lead to more frequent use of early endoscopy, possibly a "once in a lifetime" endoscopy that may detect metaplasia at an early stage and constitute a basis for the long-term management of the individual patient. As will be discussed later, it can be difficult to detect metaplasia in an area of extensive reflux esophagitis. In this setting, the option for taking biopsies is unique for endoscopy, which although of disputed importance in uncomplicated GERD, is very important once a stricture or possible metaplasia is encountered.

2. HISTORY

Ulcerations or erosions of the distal esophagus were first described in the medical literature at the turn of the century[3]. They were usually found in post mortem studies, were sometimes associated with duodenal ulcers, and in some reports it was speculated that they might represent a local infection. Histologically was found a lesion penetrating into the submucosa. The first series of esophageal ulcerations diagnosed in vivo by rigid esophagoscopy was published in 1929 by Chevalier Jackson[4]. With the increasing use of endoscopy, peptic ulcer disease, gastritis and carcinoma of the upper gastrointestinal tract were described and correlations of these lesions with histologic findings in biopsies were made at an early

H.W. Tilanus and S.E.A. Attwood (eds.), Barrett's Esophagus, 121–135.
© 2001 *Kluwer Academic Publishers. Printed in the Netherlands.*

stage. The suggestion was first made by Winkelstein in 1935 that the most common type of esophagitis could be causally associated with reflux of gastric contents to the distal esophagus, and he called it "peptic esophagitis"[5]. The condition was first called reflux esophagitis by Allison in 1946[6] and the condition was more frequently described in the literature[7-9] and diagnosed by rigid endoscopy over the next decades. What we today consider the typical endoscopic appearance of reflux esophagitis was not described until later, with the increasing use of endoscopy, and particularly with the advent of flexible fibrescopes. Until around 1970 side-viewing fibreoptic endoscopes limited the frequency of diagnosing reflux esophagitis. Over the next few decades, endoscopy came to supplant radiologic methods in the diagnosis of GERD. There are important advantages of endoscopy over x-ray methods in some, but not all diagnostic areas. Endoscopy is superior when evaluating mucosal changes, as shown in a study which included 40 patients with symptomatic gastroesophageal reflux. Reflux esophagitis seen at endoscopy was graded according to Behar[10]. Only 20 patients had some sort of radiographic abnormalities, usually thickened folds or ulcerations, whereas the finding of a ring or a hiatal hernia was considered not diagnostic[11]. In patients with no esophagitis at endoscopy only 14 % had abnormal radiograms, in those with grade 2 esophagitis (friability or exudation) 17 %, grade 3 (erosion or ulceration) 50 %, grade 4 (severe stricture or ulceration) 100 %. The observation of barium reflux to the esophagus was nonspecific for GERD. The so-called reticular pattern of the esophageal mucosa was found to correlate with esophageal pathology, but was not specific for metaplasia[12]. On the other hand, motility abnormalities can not be readily evaluated with endoscopy. The presence and configuration of a hiatal hernia can often be more easily evaluated with x-ray.

An important role for both endoscopy and radiology in gastro-esophageal reflux disease is to exclude predisposing conditions or other disease, as symptoms of GERD are far from specific.

3. WHY CLASSIFY REFLUX ESOPHAGITIS?

An experienced endoscopist employing careful technique should seldom overlook well-defined reflux esophagitis, a finding with obvious diagnostic and therapeutic implications in most patients. Very often this finding is recorded very briefly as "esophagitis" or "inflammatory changes", with no attempt to describe the finding further or indicate the severity and extent of the lesions. The role of endoscopy in the diagnosis of GERD is partly dependent on the endoscopist's need to and ability to classify the severity of mucosal damage. The finding of minimal lesions or more severe reflux esophagitis may have widely different implications for the therapy and care for the patient. In case of only minimal lesions being present, this may provide an explanation for the patient's symptoms and suggest a choice of symptomatic therapy, as felt needed. In case of more severe reflux esophagitis, the patient will inevitably need more intensive medical therapy or surgery, and will need follow-up to verify healing of the lesions. Not all gastroenterologists are experienced with or even do endoscopies, but will need simple and precise information, preferably as a numerical value, to indicate the severity of disease. More than any other easily accessible parameter, grade of esophagitis will provide this information. The severity of reflux esophagitis has prognostic importance for healing and relapse in each single patient, even with potent antisecretory medication[13-16]. Grade 1 reflux esophagitis (Savary-Miller or Berstad) heals more rapidly than grade 2 or 3 esophagitis. Relapse of reflux symptoms or esophagitis, however, seems relatively independent of severity of endoscopic changes[17,18]. The importance of obtaining complete healing of reflux esophagitis is disputed. Most authorities agree that complete healing of mild to moderate esophagitis is not always a necessity. On the other hand, metaplasia has been shown to develop from up to 22% of patients with severe erosive or ulcerative esophagitis[19], and it is possible that even shorter periods of relapse, for instance if the patient runs out of medication, may result in extension of the area of metaplastic mucosa. Healing of esophagitis may also prevent a gradual bloodloss and development of iron deficiency anaemia in patients with reflux esophagitis. The information on severity and extent of reflux esophagitis should to some extent decide the choice of long-term medication and therapeutic strategy. The concept of the "once in a lifetime endoscopy" is based on the fact that in most patients the severity of reflux esophagitis is relatively stable and does not aggravate much with time[1,20]. In fact, most patients with peptic strictures will already have this complication at the time of their first endoscopy and only infrequently does a stricture develop during follow-up for reflux esophagitis[21]. An early endoscopic examination is often useful in the management of GERD patients, although a later endoscopy, after >5 years of reflux symptoms, primarily to look for Barrett's esophagus is probably an even better indication[22]. Precise information on previously observed severity of reflux esophagitis is important for the clinician when doing control endoscopies looking for improvement or resolution of the lesions. It may not always be a requirement (or at all possible) to achieve complete healing, but significant improvement is likely to prevent complications developing over time. This improvement should be quantified in terms of grades of esophagitis. It can be quite difficult to discriminate metaplastic epithelium in an area of severe esophagitis, but this diagnosis is easier when the patient has been under acid suppressive therapy for 6-12 weeks and inflammatory lesions have more or less resolved. A precise classification of endoscopic findings is also important when following the effect of therapy in individual patients over longer periods of time (years). Significant deterioration may suggest the need for more intensive therapy and repeat endoscopies. The need for precise classification of reflux esophagitis is never more obvious than in clinical studies in which either selected subgroups or a wider population of GERD patients are treated according to a protocol and results are compared between different drugs or other treatment modalities. Traditionally, inclusion of patients has been based on endoscopic criteria, and although this may not be an ideal and complete way to judge the severity of disease, at least it represents a quite specific inclusion criterion. To avoid enrolling patients with dubious GERD and to avoid imbalance between study arms, the study should be stratified with regard to grade of esophagitis. Furthermore, precise data on classification and distribution of patients will enable us to make comparisons between studies and do meta-analyses. Last, but not least: grading of reflux esophagitis by a well accepted classification system ensures that the endoscopist is systematic and reflected on what lesions to accept as evidence for the presence of reflux esophagitis, resorting to additional investigations with manometry and 24-hour pH-metry (only) when in doubt. It will also make it easier to discriminate between reflux-induced and infectious lesions of the

esophagus. It is important to establish a clear-cut diagnosis, and to avoid that dubious changes are interpreted as esophagitis. The endoscopist will avoid overdiagnosis of GERD and expensive and futile overtreatment of patients.

4. WHAT IS REFLUX ESOPHAGITIS AND WHAT IS NOT

In severe cases of reflux esophagitis, there is usually little doubt about the nature of the changes in the distal esophagus. In less severe cases, the endoscopic image should be studied very closely to assess the presence of the typical changes associated with abnormal gastro-esophageal reflux. Certain minor changes in color or texture of the mucosa must be accepted as nonspecific or part of the normal spectrum. There has been considerable controversy regarding which endoscopically visible changes should be considered as part of the spectrum of reflux esophagitis. In particular, there has been disagreement about what minimal lesions that should be accepted as specific for reflux esophagitis. Edema is described as loss of the fine vascular pattern just proximal to the z-line and sometimes blurring it, but this has been shown to be a relatively nonspecific finding[23]. Alternatively, edema has been defined as increased thickness of the folds in the distal esophagus, reducing the distance between them and sometimes resulting in a cobblestone pattern. In our experience, this is an infrequent finding and its significance is doubtful. Diffuse redness of the mucosa, not confined to the folds and not well demarcated, was associated with abnormal gastro-esophageal reflux in only 55% of the patients in one series[24]. In the era of video endoscopy, one might expect diffuse redness to be an even less reproducible finding. Well demarcated red streaks, spots or spears (Figure 1) confined to the ridge of the folds in the distal esophagus are of greater significance, however. More severe lesions of this kind will still be centered on the folds and penetrate into the valleys in-between (Figure 2) or even bridge the valleys.

Such broader lesions will usually be covered with a layer of inflammatory exudate including fibrin. Erosions will then be whitish in color, either thin and translucent or more dense, a thicker layer not easily removed by rinsing gently with water. These "erosive" lesions are probably the most specific findings in patients with reflux esophagitis but similar lesions can still be found in some cases of viral or fungal infections of the esophagus. Ulcerations and strictures will deform the lumen (Figure 3).

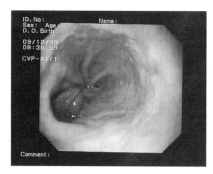

Figure 1. Mild reflux esophagitis, seen as a tiny spear of redness extending proximally from the ora serreta at 2 o'clock. With less air insufflated, the lesion would be seen to be located on the crest of a fold. This would be classified as Berstad grade 1 or Los Angeles grade A.

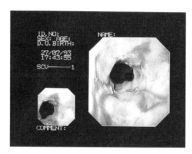

Figure 2. Moderate reflux esophagitis, with lesions wider than the folds and covered with a fibrinous exudate. This would be classified as Savary – Miller grade 2 or Los Angeles grade B.

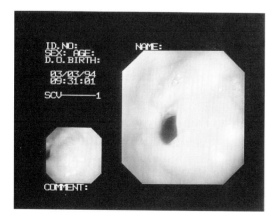

Figure 3. Severe reflux esophagitis, an ulceration within a peptic stricture. This would be graded as Savary – Miller grade 4 (Savary – Miller 1967, see table 1 and 2) or Berstad grade 3. It would not be classified by the Los Angeles classification, since these changes represent complications of reflux esophagitis.

In a recent study, 64 untreated patients with classical reflux symptoms and some extent of endoscopic changes in the distal esophagus, had several easily available observations and measures made[25]. These were subsequently correlated with the severity of acid gastro-esophageal reflux as determined by 24-hour pH-metry within a few days of the endoscopic examination. The tested variables were the following: axial extent of changes (measured in cm), width of the lesions (wider than the fold or not), presence of whitish exudate in the lesions, metaplastic spots or tongues, and presence and length of a hiatal hernia (measured in cm). Multiple linear regression analysis showed that only the width of the lesions ($p<0.01$) and presence of whitish exudate in the lesions ($p<0.001$) correlated significantly with percent total time esophageal pH <4.0. Certainly, correlation with severity of gastro-esophageal reflux may not be the only criterion for selecting features to base a classification of reflux esophagitis upon. In particular, features that can be shown to have prognostic importance should also be considered. Interobserver variation is another important and somewhat neglected aspect of endoscopy. It is important to select a classification system with features that can be reliably recognized and communicated between observers. In general, interobserver agreement has been found to be disappointingly low for overall grading of esophagitis, but particularly so for grade 1 and when inexperienced endoscopists were involved. In a study which included 150 dyspeptic patients, reflux esophagitis was diagnosed in 22.7, 32.7 and 35.3% of patients, respectively, by three endoscopists, and kappa values were estimated at between 0.34 and 0.47 (poor) for grade 1, but 0.68-0.79 (good) for grades 2-4[26]. Gustavsson and coworkers made video recordings from the distal esophagus in 28 patients with GERD before and after therapy with ranitidine and these were graded for reflux esophagitis by three experienced endoscopists. Video tapes were reexamined blindly by the same endoscopists to assess their ability to grade esophagitis reproducibly over time. Kappa-values between 0.44 and 0.74 were found for *inter*observer variation, but significantly better, between 0.63 and 0.91, for *intra*observer variation[27].

Interobserver variation was also investigated by the group working on the Los Angeles classification, asking expert as well as trainee endoscopists to grade esophagitis from still photographs and video images[28]. The observations were compared by kappa statistics, which showed excellent agreement between endoscopists (kappa values 0.7-0.9) with regard to the presence of severe esophagitis with complications (stricture, ulcer, metaplasia). The presence of mucosal breaks was also reliably recorded (kappa values 0.81-0.84), but the length and presence of exudate in lesions was problematic (kappa values around 0.4). Minor lesions such as increased vascularity, friability and localized erythema were recorded with a relatively high degree of agreement by experienced endoscopists (kappa values around 0.8), but not by endoscopists in training (kappa values 0.2-0.4). The main problems emerging from these studies were related to discriminating intermediate severities of reflux esophagitis (grades B and C, see Table 10).

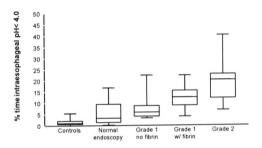

Figure 4. Esophageal acid exposure in patients with varying severity of endoscopic reflux esophagitis. Grades 1 and 2 according to the Berstad classification. Grade 1: Red streaks or spots along the ridge of the folds in the distal esophagus, covered or not with fibrinous exudate. Grade 2: Broader lesions, each involving the entire width of a fold or coalescing into fields of erythema, covered or not with fibrinous exudate. See Table 9.

Certain classifications of reflux esophagitis have included more sophisticated estimations of the extent of tissue damage. Percentage of the mucosal area in the distal esophagus affected by inflammation is used in the Hetzel[18] and Tytgat classifications but is clearly difficult to estimate with any precision[29]. The axial extent of lesions is in our experience also an unreliable measure to make, and is partly for that reason an unimportant variable to use (see above). The length of the *individual* lesions are used in the Tytgat and the Los Angeles classifications, the width of lesions in the Berstad and Los Angeles classification systems and the number of folds involved in the most recent Savary - Miller classification. Presence or absence of fibrinous exudate in the lesions, probably an important observation as discussed above, is included in the Ottenjann classification based on Savary – Miller and tentatively in the Berstad classification. Further details are commented on in the discussion on each single classification system. Different

classifications have emphasized different elements of the endoscopic appearance of reflux esophagitis, and may all be justifiable to some extent, but are likely to be associated with varying intra- and interobserver error, a problem which has not been adequately investigated. American classifications have usually accepted erythema, color unevenness, indistinct z-line and friability as criteria for grade 1 esophagitis, whereas European systems have not[30]. Inclusion of minor lesions of doubtful significance may increase interobserver variation[26] and will compromise the reliability of the diagnosis[31].

5. METAPLASIA IN GERD

Metaplastic changes were first described as the finding of columnar epithelium at the margin of ulcerations located in the anatomical tubular esophagus. While the diagnosis of metaplasia ultimately depends on histologic examination of bioptic material, the condition should be suspected at endoscopy, as often subtle changes in the color and texture of the mucosa. The successful recognition of metaplasia depends on routinely identifying the ora serrata or z-line, the transition from distal columnar epithelium to proximal squamous epithelium. If this transition seems to take place within the tubular esophagus, metaplasia should be suspected and a few biopsies will reliably assess the presence of intestinal type of metaplastic mucosa. The ora serrata can sometimes be found just beneath the upper esophageal sphincter, in a location in which it can easily be overlooked if it is not searched for systematically. The ora serrata can be asymmetric and one or more tongues or spots of metaplasia can be found to extend for several centimeters proximally, into the distal esophagus (see Figure 5).

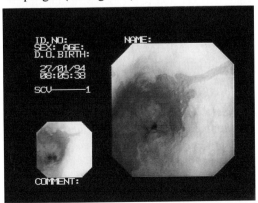

Figure 5. Circumferential metaplasia in the mid part of the esophagus, complicated with a stricture. In biopsies high-grade dysplasia was found, but no adenocarcinoma.

These spots in the distal esophagus should be held apart from an inlet patch, a remnant of embryonic columnar epithelium sometimes found in the proximal esophagus. Previously, three types of Barrett's esophagus were described and little attempt was made to discriminate between them. Today emphasis is placed on the intestinal type as precursor for dysplastic changes and adenocarcinoma of the esophagus and the cardia region of the stomach, whereas the cardia and gastric fundic type are of less clinical significance. For practical purposes, the three types of metaplastic epithelium can be found intermingled in the same patient[32]. Furthermore, areas without and with dysplastic changes can be found close together in the same operative preparation. The present definition of Barrett's esophagus depends on the identification of the intestinal type of metaplasia. In Barrett's esophagus, with metaplasia occurring either circumferentially or as short-segment metaplasia, the color of the mucosa is salmon-red to pink, rather than the faint whitish color of the esophageal epithelium (see Figure 6).

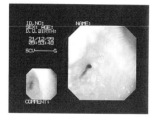

Figure 6. Circumferential metaplasia with islands of whitish squamous epithelium, having appeared within the metaplastic mucosa after long term therapy with acid-suppressive medication.

The color seems independent of the severity of inflammation found in the lamina propria, beneath the epithelial lining. The transition zone between the two types of epithelium is usually quite sharp, but in case of severe reflux esophagitis, always located in the transition zone if present, it can be blurred and it is then quite difficult to discriminate metaplasia from esophagitis. The metaplastic mucosa is homogenous in color and texture and the finding of a nodule or frank tumor is alarming, and biopsies must be taken, directed at this lesion in particular. Very often, particularly during or after successful acid suppressive or surgical therapy, islands of squamous epithelium can be seen to appear within previously homogenous metaplastic epithelium (see Figure 7).

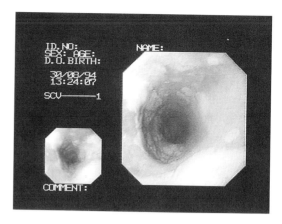

Figure 7. Circumferential metaplasia with islands of whitish squamous epithelium, having appeared within the metaplastic mucosa after long-term therapy with acid-suppressive medication.

Metaplastic mucosa is usually intact, with no adherent exudate except in presence of an ulceration, in which case the lumen is often deformed, commonly as a crater. Ulcerations are usually located either on the borderline between columnar and squamous epithelium (marginal or "Wolf - Marshak - Som ulcer") or less commonly anywhere in the distal tubular esophagus ("Barrett's ulcer")[33]. Both types of ulcers are usually localized posteriorly. Strictures in Barrett's esophagus are not uncommon, and are usually to be found in the transition zone between squamous and columnar epithelium. A peptic stricture must be discriminated from an adenocarcinoma by taking multiple biopsies.

6. ROUTINE ENDOSCOPY IN THE GERD PATIENT

The technique required for evaluating the endoscopic appearance in patients with suspected GERD is demanding. Esophageal lesions should be actively looked for in all patients. All too often, findings suggestive of reflux esophagitis are overlooked due to the patient vomiting, some bleeding occurring at the cardia, a need to cut short the examination, or insufficient technique. It is equally important to look for alternative causes for reflux symptoms such as heartburn, including a peptic ulcer or cancer, or other lesions causing an outflow obstruction from the stomach.

It is always advisable to inspect the entire esophagus when inserting the endoscope, and identify the ora serrata or z-line. Any minimal lesions of reflux esophagitis are usually located close to the z-line and it may be necessary to rinse gently with water to remove mucus or foam covering this area. One should spend a moment to actively decide whether there are lesions present that are compatible with reflux esophagitis. This may be the only time when this can be done reliably. Lesions due to vomiting may conceal the ora serrata and mask any esophagitis present, or on the contrary make it look more severe.

The endoscope should always be retroflexed in the gastric body, to inspect the cardia region for the presence of an ulcer or a tumor. It is also usually possible to see an open hiatus esophagi and a hiatal hernia from below. Often, the z-line can be seen within the dome of the hernia and even observe reflux esophagitis. With some care, a retroflexed scope can be withdrawn to inside the hernia. Occasionally, reflux esophagitis, such as short red spears or streaks can be seen only in this view. In our opinion, it is of some importance to detect a sliding hiatal hernia. Although the prevalence increases with age even in asymptomatic individuals, large hernias are usually associated with abnormal gastro-esophageal reflux[34]. The finding of a hiatal hernia is important and should prime the endoscopist to look particularly closely for even minor lesions of reflux esophagitis. The authors believe that a certain number of accurate measures should be made in every patient suspected of esophageal disease. These measurements should be made when retracting the endoscope after partly emptying the stomach of air, and should be given as distance from the lower incisors. The first measure is the level of the hiatus esophagi of the diaphragm, the observation of which might be facilitated by asking the patient to "sniff" briefly. Next, on further retraction of the scope, comes the level of the cardia, usually easily seen as the point where the wall collapses around the instrument. The interval between these points is the axial length of a hiatal hernia. If the cardia is difficult to observe clearly, as is often the case and particularly so in patients with Barrett's esophagus, the proximal end of the gastric folds within the hiatal hernia should be accepted as the proximal end of the hernia. The distal and proximal extent of all lesions within the body of the stomach, including esophagitis and metaplasia, should be recorded. In our experience, one to three photographic images of the distal esophagus should be made in all patients suspected of having GERD, particularly so in an untreated patient. It is extremely useful to keep these photographs in the patient's records for future reference. This may be particularly important in certain cases, such as patients enrolled in clinical studies, patients being considered for anti-reflux surgery etc. A photographic record may obviate the need to discontinue medication to verify the diagnosis and severity of disease at a future date and improves communication between gastroenterologist and surgeon.

7. THE IDEAL CLASSIFICATION OF REFLUX ESOPHAGITIS

When Monnier and coworkers presented the latest modification of the Savary and Miller classification in 1989, they had reviewed the literature for published and well described classification systems for reflux esophagitis and had reached the impressive number of thirty-four[35]. If nothing else, this is proof that no single system is perfect and fulfills all needs of gastroenterologists, surgeons, otorhinolaryngeologists and others working in the field of esophagology. More precisely, there are different traditions in different fields of medicine and in different parts of the world. North American classifications have relied on other ("softer") criteria than European classifications, usually less reliable variables, such as edema and diffuse redness of the mucosa. Endoscopists will feel different needs according to their field of interest. Most classifications of reflux esophagitis are empiric and are not validated with regard to histology, 24-hour pH-metry or prognostic importance of the findings. A classification system primarily intended for everyday clinical use should be simple, with few grades, and easy to remember, so that the endoscopist only rarely needs to look up the precise description in the literature. The less experienced endoscopists should be able to grasp the classification and utilize it with confidence. It should be clinically and prognostically meaningful. Such a classification can be felt to be crude, lumping together a wide spectrum of endoscopic changes within each grade. These classifications have most often also included as the most severe grade what is actually complications of GERD, such as peptic strictures, ulcers and metaplasia. In a classification primarily intended for research purposes, other motivations may take precedence. In order to establish even limited improvement in severity of reflux esophagitis, a more detailed classification is needed. Precise measurements of width and axial length of lesions in centimeters or even millimeters can be acceptable in this case, although this may sometimes require the use of a measuring rod. Some groups have included more endoscopic variables than simply reflux esophagitis, such as the MUSE system, which also includes metaplasia, ulcerations and peptic strictures. The Tytgat New System was defined to reconcile the many existing classification systems, primarily for research purposes, in order to make meta-analyses of treatment results from many published clinical studies, employing a variety of systems. The simplification of classification into a system that can be used for both routine clinical work and research seems important, since research results may seem less relevant if not directly applicable to everyday medicine, without a translation. Recent attempts at achieving such a consensus are therefore extremely welcome and important. The classifications that include complications of reflux esophagitis, such as ulcerations, metaplastic changes and peptic strictures should be avoided. The presence of such elements must be described but it may seem superfluous to grade them in this context and it is theoretically and practically difficult to grade them together with esophagitis. It is not uncommon to find metaplasia or a stricture with no endoscopic signs of esophagitis, particularly so during therapy. A classification system for reflux esophagitis should not just signal the existence of complications, particularly so since some complications are almost irreversible with conventional therapy, and the classification will not reflect considerable improvement in the condition. The great majority of patients with GERD have no complications, but the endoscopic appearance of reflux esophagitis varies considerably. It is important in any classification system that there is more than just one grade of uncomplicated reflux esophagitis. The description of reflux esophagitis should not rely on histologic examination, since this will delay important decisions regarding the management and therapy of a patient. Furthermore, classification systems should not rely on histologic terms or assumptions about an underlying histopathological process. Endoscopic appearance of reflux esophagitis should not be described in histological terms, as the relationship can be quite variable. On the other hand it is essential not to include observations of doubtful importance (see above!).

8. EARLY DESCRIPTIONS AND CLASSIFICATIONS

The best early descriptions of reflux esophagitis came from investigators who worked with rigid esophagoscopes. These early descriptions focused mainly on ulcerations, but also on diffuse redness and edema of the mucosa, most often to be considered as normal findings in recent years. More severe lesions were considered similar to peptic ulcers[4]. Associated findings such as hiatal hernia and metaplastic mucosa were not well defined at endoscopy until the fifties.

Early reports failed to recognize the role of the "erosion" or more correctly the "mucosal break" as the minimal lesion to recognize and base a classification upon. In the early years of endoscopy, it was focused primarily on identifying ulcers or peptic strictures and any less significant aberrations were described as "esophagitis" with no further qualification. An example of an early classification is that of Behar, which subdivides esophagitis into three grades: Grade 1: friability or exudation; grade 2: erosion or ulceration; grade 3: severe ulceration or stricture [10].

9. THE SAVARY – MILLER CLASSIFICATION

M. Savary and G. Miller, working in the field of otorhinolaryngeology in Switzerland, first published their newly developed classification in 1967. It was later included in an endoscopic atlas[33] showing a wide range of images recorded primarily during rigid esophagoscopy. The original four-graded classification is shown here in Table 1, with its French text, whereas the most commonly used English translation, taken from the somewhat revised English edition of the atlas, is shown in Table 2. Compared with other classifications or descriptions in use at the time, it represented a significant improvement. The basis for the new classification was the "erosion", a lesion usually covered with a whitish layer[36, 37]. In later publications, Savary and coworkers have objected to the inclusion of "discrete erythematous lesions, without further qualification" as grade 1 esophagitis in modifications of their classification[37]. Such has been the almost universal recognition and acceptance of the Savary - Miller classification that unless the opposite is explicitly stated, it is often assumed that whenever grade of esophagitis is stated, it is assumed that it is judged by this classification.

TABLE 1. The 1967 Savary and Miller classification system for reflux esophagitis, as originally published in French[36].

Stade I	Macules congestives ou exsudats pseudomembraneux isolés coiffant la crête des plis muqueux dans la région sus-vestibulaire postérieur
Stade II	Confluence des lésions qui prennent un caractère nettement érosif
Stade III	Extension circonférentielle des lésions avec infiltration pariétale
Stade IV	Réalisation des complications (sténose, ulcère de jonction, raccourcissement oesophagien fixé)

TABLE 2. The 1967 Savary - Miller classification system for reflux esophagitis, as translated into English in "The Esophagus"[33].

Stage I	One or more supravestibular, non-confluent mucosal lesions with erythema or exudate or superficial erosions.
Stage II	The erosive and exudative mucosal lesions confluent without covering the entire circumference of the esophagus
Stage III	The erosive and exudative lesions cover the whole esophageal mucous membrane circumferentially and lead to inflammatory infiltration of the wall without stricture
Stage IV	Appearance of chronic mucosal lesions (ulcer, fibrosis of the wall, stricture, short esophagus, scarring with columnar epithelium)

TABLE 3. The latest version of the Savary - Miller classification system for reflux esophagitis, as published in English in 1989[35].

Grade I	Single, erosive or exudative lesion, oval or linear, taking only one longitudinal fold.
Grade II	Noncircular multiple erosions or exudative lesions taking more than one longitudinal fold, with or without confluence.
Grade III	Circular erosive or exudative lesion.
Grade IV	Chronic lesions: ulcer(s), stricture(s), or short esophagus, isolated or associated with lesions of grades I, II or III.
Grade V	Islands, fingerlike forms or circumferential distribution of Barrett's epithelium isolated or associated with lesions of grades I through IV.

The basic lesion of the Savary - Miller classification is the "touche peptique" [36], usually a fibrin covered lesion. This ensured a high specificity, but lowered the sensitivity of recognizing the fundamental grade 1 lesion. This important point may seem to have been less emphasized in the English translation and later modifications.

Savary and coworkers have continued to defend and develop the Savary - Miller classification. It continues to have some obvious shortcomings, including the inclusion of complications within the classification. It is also a weakness that it is resorted to histopathological terms (erosions, fibrosis, exudative lesions...) when describing what is essentially a macroscopic observation.

Due to the multitude of modifications and translations of the Savary - Miller classifications, one often encounters confusion about what is actually meant by a certain grade of esophagitis by Savary - Miller, especially so after the introduction of the most recent

revision, shown in Table 3[38]. It is therefore always advisable to include the precise description and a reference for it in protocols, articles and research reports (i.e. as a table). The most recent version still includes complications (Grades IV and V).

9. MAJOR MODIFICATIONS OF THE SAVARY- MILLER CLASSIFIACTION

Over the next decades, several versions and adaptations of the Savary - Miller classification appeared in print. Colin-Jones and coworkers revised it according to their notion that minor reflux-induced lesions were not necessarily covered with a fibrinous exudate. They describe grade 1 as "discrete erythematous lesions immediately proximal to the mucosal junction"[39]. Others have added more disputable endoscopic changes, including erythema, edema and friability, as grade 1 esophagitis, which would seem to compromise the specificity of the classification[26].

TABLE 4. The Savary - Miller classification system for reflux esophagitis, as revised by Ottenjahn and coworkers[40].

Grade Ia	Red spots without fibrinous coat
Grade Ib	Red spots with fibrinous coat
Grade IIa	Red stripes without fibrinous coat
Grade IIb	Red stripes with fibrinous coat
Grade III	Confluent lesions
Grade VI	Complications (e.g., stenoses, Barrett's ulcers)

TABLE 5. The Savary - Miller classification system for reflux esophagitis, as revised for use in clinical studies[13].

Grade 0	Normal esophageal mucosa; no abnormalities noted
Grade I	Erythema or diffusely red mucosa; edema causing accentuated folds
Grade II	Isolated round or linear erosions extending from the gastro-esophageal junction upwards in relation to the folds
Grade III	Confluent erosions extending around the entire circumference or superficial ulceration, but without stenosis
Grade VI	Complicated: erosions as described above plus deep ulceration, stricture, or columnar epithelium lined esophagus

TABLE 6. The Savary - Miller classification system for reflux esophagitis, as revised by Gustavsson et al. for use in clinical studies[27].

Grade I	Erythema, edema.
Grade II	Scattered erosions.
Grade III	Confluent erosions longitudinally.
Grade IV	Confluent erosions circumferentially.
Grade V	Deep ulcerations or stricture

Ottenjahn decided to discriminate between lesions that were red and those that were covered by a white fibrinous coat, as shown in Table 4[40]. Other more extensive modifications to the Savary - Miller classification have been made for use in clinical studies, but these are often primarily aimed at excluding patients with complications, and sometimes also excluding patients with disputable endoscopic changes. Unfortunately, details about severity and extent of reflux esophagitis are often lost . This is particularly the case with the classification used in several clinical studies with omeprazole (Table 5). Gustavson and coworkers also elaborated the Savary - Miller classification for use in clinical studies and studies on interobserver variation in endoscopy of GERD patients, as briefly referred to above[27]. An important point in this classification is the very concise description of each grade, see Table 6.

10. TYTGAT NEW SYSTEM

This classification (Table 7) was created primarily for performing a meta-analysis of medical treatment results in patients with reflux esophagitis [41] and it was therefore necessary to reclassify the severity of esophagitis into a single grading system[30]. Grade 1 in this classification corresponds to diffuse erythema and other "minor lesions", and is less than would be accepted as definite reflux esophagitis by current thinking. The authors attempt to reconcile older and current concepts of reflux esophagitis and state that in grade 1 esophagitis, there is no "break in the mucosa". In the meta-analyses mentioned, grade 1 has been excluded.

From grade 2 on, it is superficially based on the first versions of the Savary - Miller classification and what is more important, it is largely compatible with most published European classifications. It was probably never intended as a classification for routine clinical use and has not been employed in any prospective clinical study.

TABLE 7. The Tytgat New System, a classification system for reflux esophagitis intended primarily for meta-analysis of published clinical studies[41].

Grade I	Mild, patchy, or rather diffuse erythema at the level of the squamocolumnar junction, minor friability, and loss of the shininess of the squamous mucosa, but there is no break in the mucosa.
Grade II	One or more discrete superficial erosions seen as red dots or streaks with or without adherent whitish exudate. These superficial erosions involve less than 10 percent of the mucosal surface or less than the distal 5 cm of the squamous segment of the esophagus above the gastro-esophageal junction.
Grade III	Confluent but non-circumferential lesions seen as defects, which merge either longitudinally or laterally. Less than 50 percent of the overall mucosal surface of the distal 5cm of the esophagus is involved.
Grade IV	Circumferential erosions or exudative lesions at the level of the squamocolumnar junction, regardless of the extent along the distal esophagus.
Grade V	Deep ulceration anywhere along the esophagus or various degrees of stricturing.

TABLE 8. The Hetzel classification of reflux esophagitis[18].

Grade 0	No mucosal abnormalities
Grade I	No macroscopic erosions but erythema, hyperemia, or mucosal friability
Grade II	Superficial erosions involving <10 % of the mucosal surface of the last 5 cm of esophageal squamous mucosa
Grade III	Superficial erosions or ulceration involving 10-50 % of the mucosal surface of the last 5 cm of esophageal squamous mucosa
Grade IV	Deep peptic ulceration anywhere in the esophagus or confluent erosion of >50% of the mucosal surface of the last 5 cm of esophageal squamous mucosa.

11. THE HETZEL CLASSIFICATION

A more widely used classification of reflux esophagitis is that of Hetzel and coworkers, as shown in Table 8[18]. In its description of uncomplicated esophagitis, it goes into more details than the Savary – Miller classifications, and introduces an estimate of the total mucosal area involved in the distal 5cm of the tubular esophagus. It is difficult to tell how well this works in practice, but a recent study showed a very low interobserver agreement (mean kappa values of 0-0.15) when considering the percentage of the distal esophageal mucosal area affected by esophagitis[29]. Complications of esophagitis are not included.

12. THE BERSTAD CLASSIFICATION

Berstad developed this classification as a result of experience with a variety of classifications in clinical therapeutic studies, after observing a surprisingly low interobserver agreement between investigators. From the outset it was developed as a simple classification for combined research and routine clinical use. It was first published in 1986[42] and is shown in Table 9. It is currently used mainly in Scandinavia[43] and has been employed in a number of clinical studies[2, 15, 44, 45].

The "minimal lesion" of the classification is the red spot or streak, which may not be an "erosion" in histological terms. The red lesion is always located on the crest of a fold and is often somewhat diffusely delineated compared with a metaplastic spot. In its center it may be covered with a fibrinous layer, varying from a milky white translucent layer to a thicker, snow white layer, always adherent and not possible to rinse away. The red lesion may be a streak, often thread-thin, a spot or just a spear originating at the z-line. It is most often found within 2cm of the z-line, and sometimes there are fibrin-covered lesions distally and just red spots more proximally. Grade 2 is defined as a lesion wider than the crest of a fold, an assessment that is fairly easy to make. Axial lengths have on the contrary been judged as too difficult to estimate precisely, and have partly for that reason not been included as a criterion for the classification When validating this classification by histology and 24-hour intraesophageal pH-metry it became apparent that absence or presence of fibrinous exudate in the lesions was of particular significance[25]. Sixty-four patients with typical symptoms of gastro-esophageal reflux and reflux esophagitis by this classification were divided into three groups: Grade 1 without (N=25) or with (N=23) fibrinous exudate or Grade 2 (N=16) reflux esophagitis.

TABLE 9. The Berstad classification system for reflux esophagitis[15]

Grade I	Red streaks or spots along the ridge of the folds in the distal esophagus, covered or not by fibrinous exudate
Grade II	Broader lesions, each involving the entire width of a fold or coalescing into fields of erythema, covered or not by fibrinous exudate
Grade III	Stricture or endoscopically visible ulcer in the distal esophagus

TABLE 10. The Los Angeles classification system for reflux esophagitis, most recent version[29].

Grade A	One (or more) mucosal break(s) no longer than 5mm, that does not extend between the tops of two mucosal folds.
Grade B	One (or more) mucosal break(s) more than 5mm, that does not extend between the tops of two mucosal folds.
Grade C	One (or more) mucosal break(s) that is continuous between the tops of two or more mucosal folds but which involves less than 75% of the circumference.
Grade D	One (or more) mucosal break(s) which involves at least 75% of the esophageal circumference.

Median percent total time esophageal pH<4.0 was 5.9, 12.5 and 20.25, respectively, significantly different between groups (Figure 4). Acid clearance time (mean duration of episodes) and supine acid exposure were also significantly different between all three groups, whereas daytime acid exposure was not. The fibrinous layer has been thought to signify a deeper lesion, exposing the deeper epithelial layers and lamina propria. Different emphasis is therefore placed on Grade 1 without fibrin or with a fibrinous layer, which is often very thin, milky white and translucent. Biopsies from the streaks show in general more inflammatory changes than biopsies taken in-between the streaks. Some infiltration of inflammatory cells is always present in Grade 2 lesions, but seldom in grade 1 lesions without fibrinous exudate (unpublished data). Healing of reflux esophagitis generally goes through several stages, initially by the disappearance of the fibrinous layer and later by narrowing and disappearance of the red fields or stripes. This process would be classified as Grade 2 with fibrin changing to Grade 2 without fibrinous exudate and then grade 1 and 0. Grade 1 with fibrin changes to Grade 1 without and then "grade 0", signifying full healing. The Berstad grading system has been used in several clinical studies and has been found to have prognostic importance, in that patients with grade 1 heal more rapidly on standard therapy with omeprazole 20mg or lansoprazople 30mg daily[15]. On the other hand, grade of esophagitis did not predict time until relapse of reflux esophagitis or reflux symptoms during maintenance therapy with lansoprazole 15 or 30mg daily[46].

12. THE LOS ANGELES CLASSIFICATION

An international expert group has worked systematically to develop and document a new classification of the endoscopic findings in patients with gastro-esophageal reflux disease. It was realized from the outset that a simple revision of an existing system would be insufficient, for several reasons. Unclear descriptions, adaptations and misuse of existing systems and inappropriate terminology made this impossible. The development process has gone through several stages employing amongst other things the studies on interobserver variation that have been referred to previously[28]. The exact description of each grade has changed somewhat since it was initially proposed during the World Congress of Gastroenterology in Los Angeles in 1994. Its most recent and presumably final version is shown in Table 10. The studies on interobserver agreement have mainly been used to identify the "hardest" variables suitable for inclusion in the classification[29]. Compared to previous classifications, the Los Angeles classification represents a further attempt to subdivide the classification of uncomplicated reflux esophagitis into four grades, based on both axial length and width of the lesions. Inherent in this more complicated classification is the problem with interobserver agreement and the possibly limited prognostic importance of finding each grade. One could argue that it has become too detailed for routine clinical use, but the LA classification has been favorably received by clinical

TABLE 11. The MUSE classification system for reflux esophagitis[37].

Metaplasia	M_0	Absent.
	M_1	Isolated islands.
	M_2	Non-circular.
	M_3	Circumferential.
Ulcer	U_0	Absent.
	U_1	Junctional ulcer. "Wolf or Savary ulcer".
	U_2	Barrett's ulcer.
	U_3	Double or multiple ulcers
Stricture	S_0	Absent.
	S_1	Stricture with diameter <9mm.
	S_2	Stricture with diameter >9mm.
	S_3	Stricture with short esophagus.
Erosions	E_0	Absent.
	E_1	Erosion involving one fold.
	E_2	Erosion(s) involving two or more folds.
	E_3	Circumferential lesions.

researchers. Studies on interobserver variability have shown that the main problem has been to discriminate between short (Grade A) and long (Grade B) axial extension of the lesions. There has also the problem of identifying circumferential esophagitis reliably, since the entire z-line may not always be clearly visible at endoscopy [29].

Therefore, an Estimate of the percentage of the circumference involved (more or less than 75%) has been used instead. Studies employing intraesophageal 24-hour pH-metry have also been performed and recently published, showing a significant trend towards increasing acid exposure with increasing grade of esophagitis. Mean percent esophageal pH < 4.0 in 159 patients with GERD was for 9.3 for Grade 1, 13.7 for Grade B, 11.7 for Grade C and 19.1 for Grade D, respectively, whereas mean percent time pH < 4.0 in those with no endoscopic evidence of esophagitis was 6.7 % [29]. The Los Angeles classification has been used in a few clinical studies, one of which showed some prognostic impact of grade of reflux esophagitis on healing rates[47].

13. MUSE

The MUSE system was presented by David Armstrong and coworkers and is a comprehensive system to describe the complete spectrum of esophageal mucosal lesions of GERD[37]. It therefore includes not only reflux esophagitis, but also signals the existence of and severity of its complications, as shown in Table 11. The acronym MUSE is made from the individual components Metaplasia– Ulcer– Stricture– Esophagitis.

The grading could in a hypothetical case be given as $M_0U_1S_1E_3$ in a patient with severe, circumferential reflux esophagitis with a single distal ulceration and some narrowing of the luminal diameter. The reflux esophagitis component is adapted from the most recent version of the Savary - Miller classification (grades I-III). It is an attempt to focus on the wider spectrum of esophageal tissue damage in GERD and is primarily intended for clinical research, as the data are well suitable for computerized analysis.

In one study, employing the MUSE system was found to increase the information value of the endoscopic examination, as compared with the widely used earlier Savary - Miller classification[48]. In 22/33 cases analyzed, there were additional endoscopic findings in addition to reflux esophagitis. In this study, metaplasia was judged to be present in 18, ulcer in 2, but stricture in none before therapy. As discussed above, metaplasia was commonly over-diagnosed in the untreated patient and biopsies and/or a control endoscopy after therapy is required.

It must be recognized that the main value of this classification is that the requirement for routinely assessing the presence or absence of common complications is likely to increase the sensitivity and precision of endoscopy in GERD patients.

14. CONCLUSION

Endoscopy is likely to become even more important in the future diagnosis, therapy and follow-up of patients with GERD, and in particular – Barrett's esophagus. Although not a complete source of information on the severity and prognosis of GERD, particularly not so in the patient with atypical symptoms such as chest pain of uncertain origin or airways symptoms, endoscopy is a highly relevant source of information to base management of the patient upon. In this chapter, we have reviewed past and current concepts of classifying gastro-esophageal reflux disease according to endoscopic criteria. The clinician should be familiar with at least one contemporary classification of reflux esophagitis, the one in active use in his institution or region, to facilitate communication between endoscopist, gastroenterologist and surgeon. This should preferably be either the latest revision of the Savary and Miller classification, the Berstad or Los Angeles classification. The same classification should be used for both research and clinical work. In the era of international multicenter clinical trials, there is an obvious need for agreement on a limited number of well validated classifications. Hopefully, within a reasonable period of time, it will be agreed upon routine use of one classification system, at least for research purposes.

It is of increasing importance to recognize and biopsy Barrett's esophagus in an era when structured follow-up and surgical, medical and endoscopic therapy of this premalignant condition can be offered. If endoscopy (with adequate taking of biopsies) can be used to identify patient groups at risk for developing metaplasia, this will facilitate follow-up of patients.

REFERENCES

1. Ollyo J-B, Monnier P, Fontolliet C, Savary M. The natural history, prevalence and incidence of reflux oesophagitis. Gullet 1993;3(Suppl.1):3-10.
2. Hatlebakk JG, Hyggen A, Madsen PH, Walle PO, Schultz T, Mowinckel P, Bernklev T, Berstad A on behalf of The Norwegian Heartburn Study Group. Heartburn treatment in primary care: randomized, double blind study for 8 weeks. BMJ 1999;319:550-3.
3. Tileston W. Peptic ulcer of the oesophagus. Amer J Med Sci 1906;132:240-65.
4. Jackson C. Peptic ulcer of the esophagus. JAMA 1929;92:369-70.
5. Winkelstein A. Peptic esophagitis: A new clinical entity. JAMA 1935;104:906-11.
6. Allison PR. Peptic ulcer of the esophagus. J Thoracic Surg 1946;15:308.
7. Wolf BS, Marshak RH, Som HL, Winkelstein A. Peptic esophagitis, peptic ulcer of the esophagus and marginal esopagogastric ulceration. Gastroenterology 1955;29:744-66.
8. Jackson C, ed. Bronchoesophagology. Philadelphia: Saunders, 1950.
9. Barrett NR. Chronic peptic ulcer of the oesophagus and "oesophagitis". Br J Surg 1950;38:175-82.
10. Behar J, Brand DL, Brown FC, Castell DO, Cohen S, Crossley RJ, Pope CE 2nd, Winans CS. Cimetidine in the treatment of sSymptomatic gastroesophageal reflux: a double blind controlled trial. Gastroenterology 1978;74:441-8.
11. Ott DJ, Gelfand DW, Wu WC. Reflux esophagitis: Radiologic and endoscopic correlation. Radiology 1979;103:583-8.
12. Vincent ME, Robbins AH, Spechler SJ, Schwartz R, Doos WG, Schimmel EM. The reticular pattern as a radiographic sign of the Barrett esophagus: an assessment. Radiology 1984;153:333-5.
13. Sandmark S, Carlsson R, Fausa O, Lundell L. Omeprazole or ranitidine in the treatment of reflux esophagitis. Results of a double-blind, randomized, Scandinavian multicenter study. Scand J Gastroenterol 1988;23:625-32.
14. Koelz HR, Birchler R, Bretholz A, Bron B, Capitaine Y, Delmore G, Fehr HF, Fumagalli I, Gehrig J, Govers JJ, Halter F, Hammer B, Kayarseh L, Kobler E, Miller G, Münst G, Pelloni S, Realini S, Schmid P, Voiroi M, Blum AL. Healing and relapse of reflux esophagitis during treatment with ranitidine. Gastroenterology 1986;91:1198-205.
15. Hatlebakk JG, Berstad A, Carling L, Svedberg L-E, Unge P, Ekström P, Halvorsen L, Stallemo A, Hovdenak N, Trondstad R, Kittang E, Lange OJ. Lansoprazole versus omeprazole in short-term treatment of reflux oesophagitis. Scand J Gastroenterol 1993;28:224-8.
16. Dent J, Yeomans ND, Mackinnon M, Reed W, Narielvava FM, Hetzel DJ, Solcia E, Shearman DJC. Omeprazole vs. ranitidine for prevention of relapse in reflux oesophagitis. A controlled double blind trial of their efficacy and safety. Gut 1994;35:590-8.
17. Hatlebakk JG, Johnsson F, Vilien M, Carling L, Wetterhus S, Thögersen T. The effect of cisapride in maintaining symptomatic remission in patients with gastro-oesophageal reflux disease. Scand J Gastroenterol 1997;33:1100-6.
18. Hetzel DJ, Dent J, Reed WD, Narielvala FM, Mackinnon M, McCarthy JH, Mitchell B, Beveridge BR, Laurence BH, Gibson GG, Grant AK, Shearman DJC, Whitehead R, Buckle PJ. Healing and relapse of severe peptic esophagitis after treatment with omeprazole. Gastroenterology 1988;95:903-12.
19. Brossard E, Monnier P, Ollyo J-B, Fontolliet C, Lévy F, Krayenbühl M, Savary M. Serious complications - stenosis, ulcer and Barrett's epithelium - develop in 21.6% of adults with erosive reflux esophagitis. Gastroenterology 1991;100:A36.
20. Kuster E, Ros E, Toledo-Pimentel V, Pujol A, Bordas JM, Grande L, Pera C. Predictive factors of the long term outcome in gastro-oesophageal reflux disease: six year follow-up of 107 patients. Gut 1994;35:8-14.
21. Ben Rejeb M, Bouché O, Zeitoun P. Study of 47 consecutive patients with peptic esophageal stricture

compared with 3880 cases of reflux esophagitis. Dig Dis Sci 1992;37:733-6.

22. DeVault KR, Castell DO, and The Practice Parameters Committee of the American College of Gastroenterology. Updated guidelines for the diagnosis and treatment of gastroesopgafeal reflux disease. Am J Gastroenterol 1999;94:1434-42.

23. Johnson LF, DeMeester TR, Haggitt RC. Endoscopic signs of gastroesophageal reflux objectively evaluated. Gastrointest Endosc 1976;22:151-5.

24. Johnsson F, Joelsson B, Gudmundsson K, Greiff L. Symptoms and endoscopic findings in the diagnosis of gastroesophageal reflux disease. Scand J Gastroenterol 1987;22:714-8.

25. Hatlebakk JG, Berstad A. Endoscopic grading of reflux oesophagitis: What observations correlate with gastro-oesophageal reflux? Scand J Gastroenterol 1997;32:760-5.

26. Bytzer P, Havelund T, Møller Hansen J. Interobserver variation in the endoscopic diagnosis of reflux esophagitis. Scand J Gastroenterol 1993;28:119-25.

27. Gustavsson S, Bergström R, Erwall C, Krog M, Lindholm CE, Nyrén O. Reflux esophagitis: Assessment of therapy effects and observer variation by video documentation of endoscopy findings. Scand J Gastroenterol 1987;22:585-91.

28. Armstrong D, Bennett JR, Blum AL, Dent J, de Dombal FT, Galmiche J-P, Lundell L, Marguiles M, Richter JE, Spechler SJ, Tytgat GNJ, Wallin L. The endoscopic assessment of esophagitis: A progress report on observer agreement. Gastroenterology 1996;111:85-92.

29. Lundell LR, Dent J, Bennett JR, Blum AL, Armstrong D, Galmiche JP, Johnsson F, Hongo M, Richter JE, Spechler SJ, Tytgat GNJ, Wallin L. Endoscopic assessment of oesophagitis: clinical and functional correlates and further validation of the Los Angeles classification. Gut 1999;45:172-80.

30. Tytgat GNJ. Endoscopy of the esophagus. In: Cotton PB, Tytgat GNJ, Williams CB, eds. Annual of Gastrointestinal endoscopy. London: Current Science, 1990:15-26.

31. Richter JE. Severe reflux esophagitis. Gastrointest Endosc Clin North Am 1994;4:677-98.

32. Monnier P, Savary M. Contribution of endoscopy to gastro-oesophageal reflux disease. In: Sandberg N, Walan A, eds. Function and disease of the oesophagus. Stockholm: Smith Kline and French AB, 1984:26-44.

33. Savary M, Miller G. L'oesophage. Manuel et atlas d'endoscopie. Soleure, Suisse: Verlag Gassmann AG, 1977.

34. Petersen H. The clinical significance of hiatus hernia. Scand J Gastroenterol 1995;211:19-20.

35. Ollyo JB, Lang F, Fontolliet C, Monnier P. Savary-Miller's new endoscopic grading of reflux oesophagitis: A simple, reproducible, logical, complete and useful classification. Gastroenterology 1990;98:A100.

36. Savary M. Endoscopie - Maladie peptique oesophagienne et gastrites herniaires. Médecine et Hygiène 1968;831:789-91.

37. Armstrong D, Monnier P, Nicolet M, Blum AL, Savary M. Endoscopic assessment of oesophagitis. Gullet 1991;1:63-7.

38. Ollyo JB, Gontollier C, Brossard E, Lang F. La nouvelle classification de Savary des oesophagites de reflux. Acta Endoscopica 1992;22:307.

39. Colin-Jones DG. Histamine-2-receptor antagonists in gastro-oesophageal reflux. Gut 1989;30:1305-8.

40. Ottenjahn R, Siewert JR, Heilmann K. Treatment of reflux esophagitis: results of a multicentre study. In: Siewert JR, Hölscher AH, eds. Diseases of the esophagus. Berlin: Springer-Verlag, 1988:1123-9.

41. de Boer WA, Tytgat GNJ. Review article: drug therapy for reflux oesophagitis. Aliment Pharmacol Ther 1994;8:147-57.

42. Berstad A, Weberg R, Frøyshov Larsen I, Hoel B, Hauer-Jensen M. Relationship of hiatus hernia to reflux oesophagitis. A prospective study of coincidence, using endoscopy. Scand J Gastroenterol 1986;21:55-8.

43. Lööf L, Götell P, Elfberg P. The incidence of reflux oesophagitis. A study of endoscopy reports from a defined catchment area in Sweden. Scand J Gastroenterol 1993;28:113-8.

44. Hatlebakk JG, Berstad A. Lansoprazole 15 and 30 mg daily in maintaining healing and symptom relief in patients with reflux oesophagitis. Aliment Pharmacol Ther 1997;11:365-72.

45. Wilhelmsen I, Hatlebakk JG, Olafsson S. On demand therapy of reflux oesophagitis - A study of symptoms, patient satisfaction and quality of life. Aliment Pharmacol Ther 1998;13:1035-40.

46. Hatlebakk JG, Berstad A. Prognostic factors for relapse of reflux oesophagitis and symptoms during 12 months of therapy with lansoprazole. Aliment Pharmacol Ther 1997;11:1093-100.

47. Carlsson R, Dent J, Watts R, Riley S, Sheikh R, Hatlebakk J, Haug K, de Groot G, van Oudevorst A, Dalväg A, Junghard O, Wiklund I, and The International GORD Study Group. Gastro-oesophageal reflux disease in primary care - an international study of different treatment strategies with omeprazole. Eur J Gastroenterol Hepatol 1998;10:119-24.

48. Armstrong D, Blum AL, Terrey J-P. A comparison of two methods for the endoscopic assessment of reflux oesophagitis. Gastroenterology 1993;104:A35.

2.5 OPTIMAL SURGICAL THERAPY FOR ANTI REFLUX DISEASE

Glyn G. Jamieson and David I. Watson

1. INTRODUCTION

The aim of anti reflux surgery is to restore, as closely as possible, a normally functioning hiatal/lower esophageal sphincter complex. This implies the unimpeded passage of swallowed material, while at the same time preventing liquid and solid gastric contents from refluxing into the esophagus, but allowing gas to be vented (belched) if the stomach becomes distended. This chapter documents the procedures which have been used to try and achieve these aims. In reality, anti reflux surgery is very effective at preventing solid and liquid reflux, and usually does not impede the passage of food through the esophagus. However, it is less successful in allowing patients to decompress their stomach through belching.

2. SELECTION OF PATIENTS FOR ANTIREFLUX SURGERY

Patients selected for surgery fall into three general groups:
1. Patients who have failed to respond (or have responded only partially) to medical therapy)
2. Patients whose symptoms are fully controlled by medications, but who do not wish to continue lifelong medication
3. Patients who present with a complication of gastro-esophageal reflux disease.

Failure of medical treatment can be defined as continuing symptoms of reflux while on an adequate dose of acid suppression. In most countries this means at least a standard dose of a proton pump inhibitor for a minimum period of three months. In some countries such as Australia and Belgium, where government imposed prescribing restrictions limit the availability of proton pump inhibitors to less than the full range of reflux patients, some patients will be selected for surgery who have only been treated with H2 receptor antagonists. Cost has become a significant issue in some countries, and in Australia despite prescribing restrictions, medication for reflux consumes more than 10% of national expenditure on prescription drugs. Proton pump inhibitors are more effective for the control of the symptom of heartburn than volume regurgitation, and it

is the latter symptom which is often the dominant problem in patients who have failed on medical therapy. In this group of patients, the response to surgery is usually more predictable if the patient has had a good response to acid suppression in the past, or at least has had some symptom relief from medication. If patients have had no response to proton pump inhibitors, then great caution is necessary. The patients' symptoms may be due to something other than reflux, despite concurrent objective evidence of reflux (which can be asymptomatic). Such patients will not benefit from anti reflux surgery, at least in a symptomatic sense.

The second group of patients are those who have had an excellent response to therapy (usually cure of heartburn) but who do not wish to be dependent on drugs to be symptom free. These patients are often relatively young and so face a lifetime of taking acid suppressant therapy. This also raises cost implications, as discussed above. Although costs vary from country to country, there is no doubt that decades of anti reflux medication is more costly than an anti reflux operation.

The third group of patients are those who present with a complication of gastro-esophageal reflux. Some patients present with difficulty in swallowing due to stricture formation.

The treatment of peptic esophageal strictures has been greatly altered since proton pump inhibitors became available, and this is one area where the role of surgery seems to have lessened.[1] In the past, surgery was the only effective treatment for strictures. If a stricture was densely fibrotic and undilatable, this usually meant resection of the esophagus. Fortunately it is now unusual to see patients with such advanced strictures. If a patient is young and fit, then many would see optimal treatment as antireflux surgery and dilatation. However, many patients who develop strictures are elderly or infirm and the use of proton pump inhibitors with dilatation is usually very effective in this group. When gastro-esophageal regurgitation spills over into the respiratory tree, this can cause chronic respiratory illness, such as recurrent pneumonia or asthma. This is a firm indication for anti reflux surgery, as proton pump inhibitors' predominant action is to block acid

H.W. Tilanus and S.E.A. Attwood (eds.), Barrett's Esophagus, 137–147.

secretion, and the volume of reflux is not greatly altered. Such problems as halitosis, chronic cough, chronic laryngitis, chronic pharyngitis, chronic sinusitis and loss of enamel on teeth are sometimes attributed to gastro esophageal reflux. Whilst there is little doubt that on occasions such problems do arise in refluxing patients, these problems in isolation are not reliable indications for surgery. As acid is usually the damaging agent, anti reflux surgery is probably not advisable unless proton pump inhibition unequivocally reverses the problem. At present it remains an open question whether Barrett's esophagus alone is an indication for antireflux surgery. There is little argument that patients with Barrett's esophagus who have reflux symptoms should be selected for surgery, largely as outlined previously, on the basis of their symptoms and their response to medications, not simply because they have a columnar lined esophagus[2]. There is some experimental evidence to suggest that continuing reflux may be deleterious in regard to malignant change in esophageal mucosa [3] and one prospective randomized trial has suggested that antireflux surgery gives superior results to drug therapy in this patient group[4]. However, proton pump inhibitors were only introduced into the medical arm of that trial in its later years. There is emerging evidence that abolition of symptoms with proton pump inhibition does not equate to "normalizing" the pH profile in a patient's esophagus[5]. Since anti reflux surgery usually does abolish reflux, this may become a further reason to recommend surgery in patients with Barrett's esophagus. There is no evidence to support the contention that either surgical or medical treatment of reflux in patients with Barrett's esophagus consistently leads to regression of the columnar lining[6] although in the future it is possible that a combination of medical or surgical therapy with ablation of the columnar lining might offer a better long term outcome for this group of patients.

3. PREOPERATIVE INVESTIGATIONS

Apart from the assessment of each patient's general suitability for surgery by determining comorbidities, some specific investigations should be performed before undertaking anti reflux surgery.

3.1 ENDOSCOPY

Endoscopy is a prerequisite. It enables esophagitis to be documented (confirming reflux disease), strictures to be dilated,

esophageal tumors to be excluded, and other gastro-esophageal pathology to be documented and treated. The position of the squamocolumnar junction and the presence and size of any hiatus hernia is also assessed.

3.2 MANOMETRY

Manometry is used to exclude primary motility disorders such as achalasia. It is also able to document the adequacy of esophageal peristalsis[7]. The presence of weak peristaltic amplitudes or poor propagation of peristalsis is not a contraindication to antireflux surgery. Although many surgeons recommend a tailored approach to patient selection by choosing a partial fundoplication in patients with poor peristalsis[8,9] there is no strong evidence to support this approach[10,11]. Evidence from one randomized trial[12] and two uncontrolled case series[10,11] has shown good results following the Nissen procedure in patients with very poor peristalsis. Nevertheless, common sense suggests that a partial fundoplication procedure is likely to be safer in patients with a true adynamic esophagus. Manometry also assists in the precise placement of a pH probe if pH monitoring is required.

3.3 ESOPHAGEAL Ph MONITORING

While many surgeons advocate the routine assessment of patients with 24-hour ambulatory pH monitoring before antireflux surgery, we use a selective approach. This test is not sufficiently accurate to be regarded as the "gold standard" for the investigation of reflux, and if an abnormal pH profile is used to select patients for surgery, up to 20% of patients who have reflux esophagitis and typical reflux symptoms will be excluded unnecessarily from antireflux surgery. Hence, we apply this investigation in patients with endoscopy negative reflux disease, and in patients with atypical symptoms[7]. The test's ability to clarify whether symptoms are associated with reflux events is useful for the assessment of these patients. The role of bile reflux (Bilitec) monitoring has yet to be defined in gastro-esophageal reflux disease, although in the future the measurement of bile reflux may be helpful in patients who fail to respond to acid suppression.

4. OPERATIONS AVAILABLE

To the non-surgeon, it might seem that there is a bewildering array of operations available for the treatment of reflux. In fact, the fundoplication introduced by Rudolf Nissen in 1956, or some variant of it, is overwhelmingly the most popular antireflux operation in the world today. Total fundoplications, such as the Nissen, or partial fundoplications, whether anterior or posterior, probably all work in a similar fashion[13,14] and that fashion may be as much mechanical as physiological, as it has been demonstrated that these procedures are effective, not only when placed in the chest in vivo[15] but also on the bench top, i.e. ex vivo [13]. The principles of fundoplication are to mobilize the lower esophagus and to wrap the fundus of the stomach, either partially or totally, around the esophagus. When the esophageal hiatus is enlarged, it is narrowed by sutures to prevent para-esophageal herniation postoperatively, and also to prevent the wrap being pulled up into the chest (although the fundoplication will work in the chest, other complications such as gastric ulceration and gastric obstruction sometimes occur in this situation). Complications of reflux such as fibrotic stricturing with shortened esophagus, are seen much less frequently today than in the past. In this circumstance, in order to provide a long enough esophagus to reach the abdomen, an esophageal lengthening (Collis) procedure is often undertaken. The upper lesser curvature of the stomach is used to produce the new esophagus and the stomach is then wrapped around this.

4.1 MECHANISMS OF ANTIREFLUX OPERATIONS

Exactly how various procedures work is often debated, and the range of possible mechanisms put forward is an indication of the lack of consensus on the mode of action of an antireflux operation. Some of the proposed mechanisms include;

1) The creation of a floppy valve which maintains close apposition between the abdominal esophagus and the gastric fundus. As intra-gastric pressure rises the intra-abdominal esophagus is compressed by the adjacent fundus.
2) Exaggeration of the flap valve at the angle of His.
3) Increase in the basal pressure generated by the lower esophageal sphincter.
4) Reduction in the triggering of transient lower esophageal sphincter relaxations.
5) Reduction in the capacity of the gastric fundus, thereby speeding proximal and total gastric emptying.
6) Prevention of effacement of the lower esophagus (which effectively weakens the lower sphincter).

Since the procedures seem to work, even ex vivo [13] it seems likely that the first two mechanisms account for the efficacy of the majority of anti reflux procedures. The increase in lower esophageal sphincter pressure following surgery does not seem important, since it has been demonstrated repeatedly that there is no correlation between efficacy and sphincter pressure, and in some partial fundoplication procedures there is very little increase in pressure, yet reflux is well controlled [16,17]. The trend towards increasingly looser and shorter total fundoplications or greater use of partial fundoplication procedures suggests that there is no such thing as a fundoplication which is "too loose".

5. TECHNIQUES OF ANTIREFLUX SURGERY

A range of different antireflux operations are currently performed and all have their advocates. No one procedure currently yields perfect results i.e. 100% cure of reflux and no side effects. Despite this, published reports can be found which support every known procedure, and it is probably better to consider results from randomized trials when assessing the merits of these procedural variants (see below), rather than relying on uncontrolled outcomes reported by advocates of a single procedure. It should also be recognized that the experience of the operating surgeon is of great importance for achieving a good post-operative outcome[18]. Variability can be reduced, but not eliminated, by detailed technical descriptions and effective surgical training. The arrival of laparoscopic antireflux surgery has also changed the way in which the vast majority of antireflux surgery is now performed. Over the last decade this approach has become standard for primary antireflux surgery, making operation more acceptable to patients and their physicians.

5.1 NISSEN FUNDOPLICATION (Figure 1)

This is probably the most commonly performed antireflux operation worldwide. Nissen originally described a procedure which entailed mobilization of the esophagus from the diaphragmatic hiatus, reduction of any hiatus hernia into the abdominal cavity, preservation of the vagus nerves, and mobilization of the posterior gastric fundus around behind the esophagus, without dividing the short gastric vessels, and suturing of the posterior fundus to the anterior wall of the fundus using non-absorbable sutures, thereby achieving a complete wrap of stomach around the intra-abdominal esophagus[19].

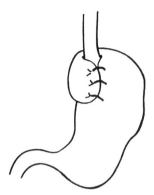

Figure 1.

The original fundoplication was 5 cm in length and an esophageal bougie was not used to calibrate the wrap. Because this procedure was associated with an incidence of persistent post-operative dysphagia, gas bloat syndrome and an inability to belch, the procedure has been progressively modified in an attempt to improve long-term outcomes. Most surgeons now agree that calibration of the wrap with a large (52 Fr or bigger) intra-esophageal bougie, and shortening the fundoplication to 1 to 2 cm in length achieves a better outcome [20,21]. Furthermore, whilst the need for routine hiatal repair was uncertain in the era of open surgery, most surgeons routinely include this step during laparoscopic antireflux surgery. Omission of this step is associated with a high incidence of post-operative hiatal herniation[22]. The hepatic branch of the vagus nerve is usually preserved during this procedure. Until the advent of laparoscopic surgery, the issue of division vs non-division of the short gastric vessels was rarely discussed. However, following anecdotal reports of increased problems with post-operative dysphagia following laparoscopic Nissen fundoplication without division of the short gastric vessels [23,24], this aspect of surgical technique has become a much-debated topic. Routine division of the short gastric vessels during fundoplication, to achieve full fundal mobilization and thereby ensure a loose fundoplication, is thought by some to be an essential step during laparoscopic (and open) Nissen fundoplication[20,21]. This opinion has gained credibility from the publication of studies which have compared experience with division of the short gastric vessels with historical experience with a Nissen fundoplication performed without dividing

these vessels [23,25]. However, other uncontrolled studies of Nissen fundoplication either with or without division of the short gastric vessels confuse the issue further, as good results have been reported whether these vessels were divided or not[26,27]. Three randomized trials have been reported which investigate this aspect of technique. Luostarinen et al reported the outcome of a small trial of division versus no division of the short gastric vessels during open total fundoplication. Fifty patients were entered into this trial, and the most recent report described outcomes following a median 3-year follow-up period [28]. Both procedures effectively corrected endoscopic esophagitis. However, there was a trend towards a higher incidence of disruption of the fundoplication (5 versus 2), and reflux symptoms (6 versus 1) in patients whose short gastric vessels were divided, and furthermore 9 out of 26 patients who underwent vessel division developed a post-operative sliding hiatus hernia, compared to only 1 out of 24 patients whose vessels were kept intact. The likelihood of long term dysphagia, or gas-related symptoms was not influenced by mobilizing the gastric fundus in this trial. In 1997, we reported a randomized trial which enrolled 102 patients undergoing a laparoscopic Nissen fundoplication, to have a procedure either with or without division of the short gastric blood vessels[29]. No difference in overall outcome was demonstrated at short term follow-up of 6 months, with the exception of increased operating time if the vessels were divided. In particular, this trial failed to show that dividing the short gastric vessels during laparoscopic Nissen fundoplication reduced the incidence or severity of dysphagia following surgery, nor was there any significant difference in lower esophageal sphincter pressure, esophageal emptying time, or barium meal X-ray appearances. Longer-term follow-up, however, is needed to assess the durability of each operative variant. A further trial, with similar numbers to the above has been reported only in abstract form. It found that there were more early re-operations required because of severe dysphagia in the group of patients in whom short gastrics were not divided[30]. Nevertheless, the evidence from these trials does not establish the proposition that the short gastric vessels need to be divided routinely during either laparoscopic or open Nissen fundoplication.

5.2 POSTERIOR PARTIAL FUNDOPLICATION (Figure 2)

A variety of fundoplication operations have been described in which the fundus is wrapped

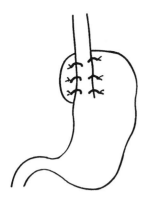

Figure 2.

partially round the back of the esophagus, with the aim of reduction of the possible side effects of total fundoplication due to overcompetence of the cardia i.e. dysphagia, and gas related problems. Toupet described a posterior partial fundoplication in which the fundus is passed behind the esophagus and sutured to the left lateral and right lateral walls of the esophagus, as well as to the right diaphragmatic pillar, creating a 270° posterior fundoplication[31]. A very similar procedure was described by Lind[32]. This entails a 300° posterior fundoplication, which is constructed by suturing the fundus to the esophagus at the left and right lateral positions, and additionally anteriorly on the left, leaving a 60° arc of esophageal wall uncovered anteriorly. The hiatus is repaired if necessary. Have such procedures achieved better results than the Nissen? Thor and Silander[33] reported a small trial in 1989, with follow-up extending to five years. They randomized 31 patients, to undergo either a Nissen or a Toupet fundoplication. The Nissen wrap was 4 cm in length, and it was calibrated over a 40 Fr bougie, the esophageal hiatus was not repaired, the hepatic branch of the vagus nerve was divided routinely, and the short gastric vessels were not divided. A good or excellent outcome was achieved in 8/12 of the Nissen group and 18/19 of the Toupet group. However, because of the small number of patients enrolled, this difference was not significant. Three of the patients who underwent Nissen fundoplication underwent further surgery for dysphagia. In each instance this was for the development of a 'slipped Nissen'. No re-operations were required in the Toupet group. The incidence of re-operation for the 'slipped Nissen' phenomenon, however, is far in excess of the low rates reported in other more recent studies[20,34,35].

Walker et al reported the results of a randomized trial in 1992[34]. This study compared a Nissen fundoplication (3 cm long, with selective division of the short gastric

vessels, and calibrated over a 40 Fr bougie), with a 300° posterior partial fundoplication (Lind). As only 26 patients were enrolled in each group, lack of statistical power is a weakness of this study, as with the preceding study. New dysphagia was seen equally in both groups at early (6 weeks) and late follow-up, and the incidence of gas bloat problems was also identical. Lundell et al have reported in several publications the outcome of a trial into which 137 patients were entered, of Nissen fundoplication without dividing the short gastric vessels versus a Toupet partial fundoplication. Early outcomes at 6 months follow-up were similar[36]. Interestingly at 5 years follow-up[35] there was a trend towards more dysphagia following partial than Nissen, although in all instances the symptom was reported to be mild. On the other hand, flatulence was commoner after Nissen fundoplication at 2 and 3 years but not at other earlier or later time intervals. Long-term relaps rate was similar for the two procedures at 3 years (6% following Toupet, 5% after Nissen). Reoperation was more common following Nissen fundoplication, with one patient in the Toupet group undergoing further surgery for severe gas bloat symptoms, and five of the Nissen group undergoing reoperation for post-operative para-esophageal herniation. Hiatal repair was performed infrequently in this trial, and in only one of the five patients who developed a postoperative hernia. A further recent reanalysis of the data from this trial sought to answer the question of whether a tailored approach to antireflux surgery should be applied[12]. There were no demonstrable disadvantages for either procedure in those patients who had manometrically abnormal peristalsis before surgery. Following the introduction of laparoscopic techniques, Laws et al[37] recently reported a small trial in which 39 patients were randomized to undergo either a laparoscopic Nissen or Toupet fundoplication. Again, no significant short-term outcome differences were demonstrated between the two procedures. If one combines all the data of the Nissen versus posterior fundoplication trials together, the available evidence appears to support the view that the only differences in outcome between the total fundoplication and the posterior fundoplication, is in the wind related problems. Certainly, the hypothesis that dysphagia is less of a problem following a posterior partial fundoplication has not been substantiated by these trials. Although this pooled data is essentially short term follow-up (because most trials have not reported longer term outcomes), the longer term data of

Lundell et al suggest these results may be representative of the longer term also [35].

5.3 ANTERIOR PARTIAL FUNDOPLICATION (Figure 3)

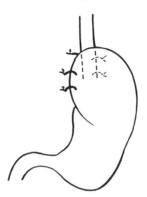

Figure 3.

Several anterior fundoplication procedures have been described, and all purport to reduce the incidence of dysphagia and other side effects. The Belsey Mark IV procedure entails a 240° anterior partial fundoplication which is usually performed through a left thoracotomy approach [38]. The distal esophagus is mobilized, sutured to the gastric fundus, and sutured to the diaphragm. Any hiatus hernia is repaired, and the anterior two-thirds of the abdominal esophagus is covered by the fundoplication. This procedure has been common in cardiothoracic surgical practice in the past, although the open thoracic access is associated with significant morbidity, and for this reason it has fallen from favor since the arrival of laparoscopic antireflux surgery. A minimally invasive thoracoscopic approach has been recently described, although clinical outcomes remain unreported [39] and anecdotal reports suggest the procedure is difficult to perform, and it has not been taken up. The Dor procedure is an anterior hemifundoplication which involves suturing of the fundus to the left and right sides of the esophagus [40]. The Dor procedure is commonly used in combination with an abdominal cardiomyotomy for achalasia as it is unlikely to cause dysphagia, and it may reduce the risk of gastro-esophageal reflux following cardiomyotomy. A 120° anterior fundoplication has also been described [17]. This entails reduction of any hiatus hernia, posterior hiatal repair, suture of the posterior esophagus to the hiatal pillars posteriorly, suture of the fundus to the diaphragm to accentuate the angle of His, and creation of an anterior partial fundoplication by suturing the fundus to the esophagus on the right antero-lateral aspect. Satisfactory medium term reflux control

following open surgery has been reported for this procedure, and a low incidence of gas related problems. However, published laparoscopic experience is limited [41] and its application has been limited to a few centers only. In 1999 we reported the first prospective randomized trial to compare a Nissen fundoplication with an anterior partial fundoplication technique [16]. Both procedures were performed laparoscopically. This study enrolled 107 patients to undergo either a Nissen or anterior partial fundoplication. The partial fundoplication variant entailed a 180° fundoplication which was anchored to the right hiatal pillar and the esophageal wall. Whilst, no overall outcome differences between the two procedures were demonstrated at 1 and 3 months follow-up, at 6 months patients who underwent an anterior fundoplication were less likely to experience dysphagia for solid food, were less likely to be troubled by excessive passage of flatus, were more likely to be able to belch normally, and the overall outcome was better. These differences have continued to be evident 2 years following surgery, and control of reflux has been similar following partial fundoplication (unpublished data). Despite this data, this trial has not resolved which procedure will be the most appropriate in the long term.

5.4 HILL PROCEDURE

Hill described a procedure which is often regarded as a gastropexy rather than a fundoplication [42]. However, it also plicates the cardia, and when examined endoscopically the intragastric appearances are similar to a fundoplication. The procedure entails suturing the anterior and posterior phreno-esophageal bundles to the pre-aortic fascia and the median arcuate ligament. Whilst excellent results have been reported by Hill [42,43] it has not been applied widely because most surgeons have difficulty understanding the anatomical principles, and in particular the so-called phreno-esophageal bundles are not clear structures. Hill also emphasizes the need for intra-operative manometry. This is not widely available, limiting the dissemination of his technique. Furthermore, this operation, like the Belsey, has been a casualty of the laparoscopic era and it now appears to be disappearing into the pages of history.

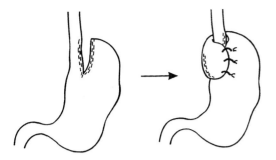

Figure 4.

5.5. COLLIS PROCEDURE (Figure 4)

The Collis procedure is useful for patients whose esophagogastric junction cannot be reduced below the diaphragm [44]. However, this situation has become uncommon in recent years, possibly due to the reduced incidence of stricture formation which has accompanied the introduction of effective medical therapy for reflux. The Collis procedure entails the construction of a tube of gastric lesser curve to construct an abdominal length of esophagus, around which a fundoplication is then fashioned. It is often constructed by using a circular end to end stapler to create a transgastric window, and a linear cutting stapler is used from this hole up to the angle of His to construct the neo-esophagus. Laparoscopic and thoracoscopic techniques for this procedure have been described, although long term outcomes are not available[45,46]. A disadvantage of this procedure is that the gastric tube does not have peristaltic activity, and furthermore it can secrete acid. This leads to a relatively poor overall success rate for this procedure, although this may be due to the end stage nature of the reflux disease which led to the choice of the procedure in the first place.

5.6. ANATOMICAL REPAIR

Earlier in the twentieth century it was believed that gastro-esophageal reflux was associated with an anatomical derangement at the esophageal hiatus of the diaphragm due to the development of a hiatus hernia, and this provided the basis for the first surgical treatment for reflux. This was popularized by Allison in the UK and Harrington in the USA, both of whom advocated "anatomical" repair of hiatus hernia. Using an open transthoracic approach, this procedure involved the reduction of the hiatus hernia, narrowing of the hiatal ring and accentuation of the angle of His. This successfully corrected pathological reflux, and early follow-up reported excellent results in around 90% of cases. At twenty year follow-up, however, this figure had dropped to 66% in Allison's hands[47] and partly as a result

of this the operation fell into disfavor, despite the fact that excellent long term outcomes had been reported by some other surgeons. However, one thing which these early operations demonstrated was that restoration of normal hiatal anatomy, without a fundoplication, resulted in control of gastro esophageal reflux symptoms in the short term, without the side effects typically associated with total fundoplication.

6.   LAPAROSCOPIC ANTIREFLUX SURGERY

Laparoscopic fundoplication was first reported in 1991 [48,49] and it has rapidly established itself as the procedure of choice for reflux disease[50,51] with the vast majority of antireflux procedures now being performed this way. The results of several large prospectively followed series have been published, with short and medium term (up to 3 years) outcomes available[52-54]. Overall results from these studies suggest that laparoscopic antireflux surgery is effective, and that it results in an overall reduction in the short-term morbidity associated with surgery for reflux. However, several complications unique to the laparoscopic approach have been described[55]. Long-term results remain unknown, although it is probably reasonable to extrapolate outcomes from open surgery if the same principles have been adhered to. In terms of curing reflux, the laparoscopic Nissen procedure has been successful, with only a 2% incidence of recurrence of reflux at 2 to 3 years follow-up. It is likely that this procedure will be as durable as open fundoplication, where a 70-80% success rate can be expected up to 25 years follow-up[56,57]. It has been suggested that dysphagia could be more common following laparoscopic fundoplication, although this impression may be erroneous due to the more intense nature of the prospective follow-up applied in many centers. Furthermore, in our experience, the rate of dysphagia has actually been lowered by fundoplication, with a reduction in incidence from approximately 30% before surgery to less than 10% at 12 months following surgery[29,58] and for the majority of these patients dysphagia has not been troublesome in the long term. The overall satisfaction rate of laparoscopic antireflux surgery has been quite high, with about 90% of patients stating that, given the opportunity, they would have the operation again. However, up to 10% of patients are dissatisfied. Some of this dissatisfaction is because of a complication of the original surgery. In our experience this has usually been either the development of a para-esophageal hernia (which accounts for about half of all reoperations), or because of continuing troublesome dysphagia (with either the wrap or the hiatus being too tight). Some patients are dissatisfied, however, even though their reflux has been cured and they have not had any complications[59]. This is usually because they do not like the flatulence which can follow the procedure. It is also important to recognize that there is a learning curve associated with this form of surgery, and we have demonstrated that the first 20 patients in an individual surgeon's experience are associated with a high complication rate, and as experience increases the reoperation rates fall to below 5% and probably to below 2%[18]. There are no specific contraindications to the laparoscopic approach, and the repair of giant hiatal hernias, and reoperative antireflux surgery are both feasible (although technically more demanding). There are some differences between the management of patients during and after laparoscopic and open fundoplication procedures. Laparoscopic surgery may increase the risk of thromboembolic complications and therefore prophylaxis for deep vein thrombosis is mandatory. Other differences are primarily due to the accelerated recovery following laparoscopic surgery. Our practice is to avoid the use of a nasogastric tube, commence oral intake within 24 hours of surgery, and to arrange a Barium meal X-ray within 2 days of surgery to check the post-operative anatomy at a time when problems are easily corrected. On several occasions we have detected an asymptomatic para esophageal hernia which has been easily corrected within a few days of surgery.

Non-randomized comparisons between open and laparoscopic fundoplication have generally shown that laparoscopic surgery requires more operating time than the equivalent open surgical procedure[60,61] that the incidence of post-operative complications is reduced, the length of post-operative hospital stay is shortened by 3 to 7 days, patients return to full physical function between 6 to 27 days quicker, and overall hospital costs are reduced following laparoscopic antireflux surgery. The efficacy of reflux control appears to be similar between the two approaches. Six randomized controlled trials have been reported which compare a laparoscopic Nissen fundoplication with its open surgical equivalent[62-67]. However, all describe early results, and two of the studies have been reported as published abstracts only. Nevertheless, the results of these trials, with one exception, confirm advantages for the laparoscopic approach, albeit less dramatic than the advantages expected from the results of non-randomized studies.

The one exception is the most recent trial[67] and it was a multicenter trial in 103 patients randomized to open or laparoscopic fundoplication. It was found that seven patients in the laparoscopic group had troublesome dysphagia compared to only one in the open group at 3 months follow-up. Longer follow-up was not reported. The reasons for their finding being different from the other five studies and the non-randomized studies, may relate to a type I statistical error. Furthermore, with longer follow-up, this difference could even disappear. Their study does, however, underline the importance of many studies being required to establish true outcomes.

7. OPTIMAL ANTI REFLUX – A TAILORED APPROACH

At various times, groups expert in anti reflux surgery have advocated a tailored approach, most often on the basis of preoperative abnormalities of esophageal motility. Even though the approaches advocated have seemed reasonable, there has been little scientific evidence produced to substantiate such approaches. As randomized studies of variations in technique become available, it may well prove possible to use a scientifically based tailored approach to anti reflux surgery. One such approach which is used by the senior author, is outlined below. While we have used what scientific evidence is available to us at present, we should emphasize that much of what follows is based on reasoned opinion rather than on scientifically proven facts. We should emphasize also, that as far as possible we place patients in randomized trials, since without such trials we will never know if approaches such as outlined below, are correct or not.

7.1 TOTAL FUNDOPLICATION

This remains the gold standard against which other procedures are compared. Therefore, this is used whenever there is evidence of severe reflux disease or complicated reflux disease; e.g, patients with strictures, Barrett's esophagus or erosive esophagitis, in spite of proton pump inhibitors. In all of these situations it is important to totally eliminate reflux. A total fundoplication is used in younger patients (<40 y) on the grounds that it is the operation with the longest track record of durability. We use a total fundoplication in any patient who has retained some degree of peristaltic activity regardless of the amplitude or consistency of contractions. We also tend to use a total fundoplication in patients having re-operative surgery if it has proven necessary to take down the previous operation, which is usually the case.

7.2 ANTERIOR FUNDOPLICATION

We use this in patients who have had an esophagomyotomy for achalasia. The fundoplication is stitched to the edges of the cut muscle in order to hold the lower esophagus widely open. We prefer the anterior to the posterior fundoplication as the former maintains a straighter lower esophageal axis. Both a total and a posterior fundoplication act as a buttress behind the esophagus, pushing the abdominal segment forwards.

This is a potential source of dysphagia in patients with an adynamic esophageal body, which is the situation in patients with achalasia.

7.3 ANATOMICAL REPAIR /90° ANTERIOR FUNDOPLICATION

This repair is associated with the least dysphagia and wind related problems. Therefore, we use it in any patient who thinks that such problems would greatly spoil an otherwise good outcome from operation, and in any patient whom we judge will be greatly troubled by dysphagia or wind related problems. We also use it routinely in patients with a totally aperistaltic esophagus on preoperative motility testing. This repair is also used routinely in older patients (>70 y) since long term durability is not the same issue as in young patients. Our practice has varied in patients following repair of an intra thoracic stomach. Increasingly, we have used this procedure rather than total fundoplication for the following reasons. First, preoperative motility is not always obtained in such patients. Second, many of these patients do not have a reflux problem, and in such patients it seems severe to impose on them the early dysphagia and later wind related problems of a total fundoplication. Third, it eliminates the need to pass a bougie after repair of the large hiatal defect. Since this bougie is passed "blind" through the thoracic cavity, we have had the experience of it being passed through the esophagus in the chest above the repair. (The esophagus of course had been extensively mobilized in the chest).

This repair is also used routinely in patients with endoscopy negative reflux – either negative per primum or rendered endoscopy negative by proton pump inhibition.

7.4 COLLIS-NISSEN OPERATION

When a patient has a shortened esophagus as a result of fibrous stricturing, it is appropriate to lengthen the esophagus using a Collis gastroplasty – followed by a fundoplication around the neo-esophagus. All of the operations described above we undertake laparoscopically, except this operation, which we undertake as an open procedure. This is because we have used the procedure much less than some surgeons, who believe that the problem of short esophagus is more prevalent than we do. We have undertaken the procedure in considerably less than 1% of our patients. Some surgeons require there to be at least 4-5 cm of esophagus below the diaphragm so that the fundoplication sits comfortably below the diaphragm. Provided we can construct the fundoplication below the diaphragm, we accept this as adequate. We accept that ultimately this may lead to a higher recurrence rate of herniation of the fundoplication, but to date this has not been a problem in our series, and furthermore, the Collis procedure is associated with its own inherent risk of morbidity, which should be balanced against the risk of post-operative herniation if this procedure is omitted.

8. SUMMARY

At a time when medical therapy for gastro esophageal reflux disease is often very effective, many clinicians thought that surgery for the condition would disappear in much the same way that elective surgery for peptic ulcer disease disappeared. In some ways, paradoxically, quite the opposite has occurred in many countries. This has been due in part to the development of laparoscopic anti reflux surgery, to the fact that medical treatment only deals with one aspect of reflux (the acid), to the fact that the good effects of drug therapy seem to diminish with time in some patients, to the high cost to the patient or to society, of continued drug therapy, and to the reluctance of some patients to be dependent on drugs over a lifetime. The recent demonstration that chronic reflux is associated with a greatly increased risk of developing adenocarcinoma of the esophagus will no doubt add to the reasons for patients choosing cure of their problem by anti reflux surgery. It therefore behooves us, as surgeons, to fine tune our operations to the point that nearly all patients will be glad they made the decision for surgery.

REFERENCES

1. Bischof G, Feil W, Riegler M, Wenzl E, Schiessel R. Peptic esophageal stricture: is surgery still necessary? Wei Klin Wochenschr 1996;08:267-71.
2. Farrell TM, Smith CD, Metreveli RE, Johnson AB, Galloway KD, Hunter JG. Fundoplication provides effective and durable symptom relief in patients with Barrett's esophagus. Am J Surg 1999;178:18-21.
3. Attwood SE, Smyrk TC, DeMeester TR, Mirvish SS, Stein HJ, Hinder RA. Duodenesophageal reflux and the development of esophageal adenocarcinoma in rats. Surgery 1992;11:503-10.
4. Ortiz EA, Martinez de Haro LF, Parrilla P, Morales G, Molina J, Bermejo J, Liron R, Aguilar J. Conservative treatment versus antireflux surgery in Barrett's esophagus: long-term results of a prospective study. Br J Surg 1996;83:274-8.
5. Ortiz A, De Maro LT, Parrilla P, Molina J, Bermejo J, Munitiz V. 24-h pH monitoring is necessary to assess acid reflux suppression in patients with Barrett's esophagus undergoing treatment with proton pump inhibitors. Br J Surg 1999; 86:1472-4.
6. Sagar PM, Ackroyd R, Hosie KB, Patterson JE, Stoddard CJ, Kingsnorth AN. Regression and progression of Barrett's esophagus after antireflux surgery. Br J Surg 1995;82:806-10.
7. Waring JP, Hunter JG, Oddsdottir M, Wo J, Katz E. The preoperative evaluation of patients considered for laparoscopic antireflux surgery. Am J Gastroenterol 1995;90:35-8.
8. Kauer WKH, Peters JH, DeMeester TR, Heimbucher J, Ireland AP, Bremner CG. A tailored approach to antireflux surgery. J Thorac Cardiovasc Surg 1995;110:141-7.
9. Little AG. Gastro-esophageal reflux and esophageal motility diseases; Who should perform antireflux surgery? Ann Chir Gynaecol 1995;84:103-5.
10. Beckingham IJ, Cariem AK, Bornman PC, Callanan MD, Louw JA. Esophageal dysmotility is not associated with poor outcome after laparoscopic Nissen fundoplication. Br J Surg 1998;85:1290-3.
11. Baigrie RJ, Watson DI, Myers JC, Jamieson GG. The outcome of laparoscopic Nissen fundoplication in patients with disordered pre-operative peristalsis. Gut 1997;40:381-5.
12. Rydberg L, Ruth M, Abrahamsson H, Lundell L. Tailoring antireflux surgery: A randomized clinical trial. World J Surg 1999;23:612-8.
13. Watson DI, Mathew G, Pike GK, Jamieson GG. Comparison of anterior, posterior and total fundoplication using a viscera model. Dis Esoph 1997;10:110-4.
14. Watson DI, Mathew G, Pike GK, Baigrie RJ, Jamieson GG. Efficacy of anterior, posterior and total fundoplication in an experimental model. Br J Surg 1998;85:1006-9.
15. Collard JM, De Koninck XJ, Otte JB, Fiasse RH, Kestens PJ. Intrathoracic Nissen fundoplication: long-term clinical and pH-monitoring evaluation. Ann Thorac Surg 1991;51:34-8.
16. Watson DI, Jamieson GG, Pike GK, Davies N, Richardson M, Devitt PG. A prospective randomised double blind trial between laparoscopic Nissen fundoplication and anterior partial fundoplication. Br J Surg 1999;86:123-30.
17. Watson A, Jenkinson LR, Ball CS, Norris TL. A more physiological alternative to total fundoplication for the surgical correction of resistant gastro-esophageal reflux. Br J Surg 1991;78:1088-94.
18. Watson DI, Baigrie RJ, Jamieson GG. A learning curve for laparoscopic fundoplication. Definable, avoidable, or a waste of time? Ann Surg 1996;224: 198-203.
19. Nissen R. Eine einfache operation zur beeinflussung der refluxoesophagitis. Schweiz Med Wochenschr 1956;86:590-2.
20. DeMeester TR, Bonavina L, Albertucci M. Nissen fundoplication for gastresophageal reflux disease. Evaluation of primary repair in 100 consecutive patients. Ann Surg 1986;204:9-20.
21. DeMeester TR, Stein HJ. Minimizing the side effects of antireflux surgery. World J Surg 1992;16:335-6.
22. Watson DI, Jamieson GG, Devitt PG, Mitchell PC, Game PA. Paraesophageal hiatus hernia: an important complication of laparoscopic Nissen fundoplication. Br J Surg 1995;82:521-3.
23. Hunter JG, Swanstrom L, Waring JP. Dysphagia after laparoscopic antireflux surgery. The impact of operative technique. Ann Surg 1996;224:51-7.
24. Dallemagne B, Weerts JM, Jehaes C, Markiewicz S. Causes of failures of laparoscopic antireflux operations. Surg Endosc 1996;10:305-310.
25. Donahue PE, Bombeck CT. The modified Nissen fundoplication - reflux prevention without gas bloat. Chir gastroent 1977;11:15-27.
26. Rossetti M, Hell K. Fundoplication for the treatment of gastroesophageal reflux in hiatal hernia. World J Surg 1977;1:439-444.
27. DeMeester TR, Bonavina L, Albertucci M. Nissen fundoplication for gastresophageal reflux disease. Evaluation of primary repair in 100 consecutive patients. Ann Surg 1986;204:9-20.
28. Luostarinen ME, Isolauri JO. Randomized trial to study the effect of fundic mobilization on long-term results of Nissen fundoplication. Br J Surg 1999;86: 614-8.
29. Watson DI, Pike GK, Baigrie RJ, Mathew M, Devitt PG, Britten-Jones R, Jamieson GG. Prospective double blind randomised trial of laparoscopic Nissen fundoplication with division and without division of short gastric vessels. Ann Surg 1997;226:642-52.
30. Dalenback J, Lonroth H, Blomqvist A, Lundell L. Improved functional outcome after laparoscopic fundoplication by complete gastric fundus mobilization. Gastroenterology 1998;114: 1384.
31. Toupet A. Technique d'oesophago-gastroplastie avec phrenogastropexie appliquee dans la cure radicale des hernies hiatales et comme complement de l'operation d'heller dans les cardiospasmes. Med Acad Chir 1963;89: 394.
32. Lind JF, Burns CM, MacDougal JT. 'Physiological' repair for hiatus hernia - manometric study. Arch Surg 1965;91:233-7.
33. Thor KBA, Silander T. A long-term randomized prospective trial of the Nissen procedure versus a modified Toupet technique. Ann Surg 1989;210:719-24.
34. Walker SJ, Holt S, Sanderson CJ, Stoddard CJ. Comparison of Nissen total and Lind partial transabdominal fundoplication in the treatment of gastro-esophageal reflux. Br J Surg 1992;79:410-4.
35. Lundell L, Abrahamsson H, Ruth M, Rydberg L, Lonroth H, Olbe L. Long-term results of a prospective randomized comparison of total fundic wrap (Nissen-Rossetti) or semifundoplication (Toupet) for gastro-esophageal reflux. Br J Surg 1996;83:830-5.
36. Lundell L, Abrahamsson H, Ruth M, Sandberg N, Olbe LC. Lower esophageal sphincter characteristics and esophageal acid exposure following partial or 360° fundoplication: Results of a prospective, randomized clinical study. World J Surg 1991; 5:115-21.
37. Laws HL, Clements RH, Swillies CM. A randomized, prospective comparison of the Nissen

versus the Toupet fundoplication for gastresophageal reflux disease. Ann Surg 1997;225:647-54.

38. Belsey R. Mark IV repair of hiatal hernia by the transthoracic approach. World J Surg 1977;1:475-81.

39. Nguyen NT, Schauer PR, Hutson W, Landreneau R, Weigel T, Ferson PF, Keenan RJ, Luketich JD. Preliminary results of thoracoscopic Belsey Mark IV antireflux procedure. Surg Lapar Endosc 1998;8:185-8.

40. Dor J, Himbert P, Paoli JM, Miorclerc M, Aubert J. Treatment of reflux by the so-called modified Heller-Nissen technic. Presse Med 1967;75:2563-9.

41. Watson A, Spychal RT, Brown MG, Peck N, Callender N. Laparoscopic 'physiological' antireflux procedure: preliminary results of a prospective symptomatic and objective study. Br J Surg 1995;82:651-6.

42. Hill LD. An effective operation for hiatal hernia: an eight year appraisal. Ann Surg 1967;166:681-92.

43. Aye RW, Hill LD, Kraemer SJM, Snopkowski P. Early results with the laparoscopic Hill repair. Am J Surg 1994;167:542-6.

44. Jobe BA, Horvath KD, Swanstrom LL. Postoperative function following laparoscopic Collis gastroplasty for shortened esophagus. Arch Surg 1998;133:867-74.

45. Swanstrom LL, Marcus DR, Galloway GQ. Laparoscopic Collis gastroplasty is the treatment of choice for the shortened esophagus. Am J Surg 1996;171:477-81.

46. Falk GL, Harrison RI. Laparoscopic cut Collis gastroplasty: a novel technique. Dis Esoph 1998;11:260-2.

47. Allison PR. Hiatus hernia: a 20-year retrospective survey. Ann Surg 1973;178:273-6.

48. Geagea T. Laparoscopic Nissen's fundoplication: preliminary report on ten cases. Surg Endosc 1991;5:170-3.

49. Dallemagne B, Weerts JM, Jehaes C, Markiewicz S, Lombard R. Laparoscopic Nissen fundoplication: Preliminary report. Surg Lapar Endosc 1991;1:138-43.

50. Jamieson GG, Watson DI, Britten-Jones R, Mitchell PC, Anvari M. Laparoscopic Nissen fundoplication. Ann Surg 1994;220:137-45.

51. Hinder RA, Filipi CJ, Wetscher G, Neary P, DeMeester TR, Perdikis G. Laparoscopic Nissen fundoplication is an effective treatment for gastresophageal reflux disease. Ann Surg 1994;220:472-83.

52. Gotley DC, Smithers BM, Rhodes M, Menzies B, Branicki FJ, Nathanson L. Laparoscopic Nissen fundoplication - 200 consecutive cases. Gut 1996;38:487-91.

53. Trus TL, Laycock WS, Branum G, Waring JP, Mauren S, Hunter JG. Intermediate follow-up of laparoscopic antireflux surgery. Am J Surg 1996;171:32-5.

54. Anvari M, Allen C. Laparoscopic Nissen fundoplication. Two-year comprehensive follow-up of a technique of minimal paraesophageal dissection. Ann Surg 1998;227:25-32.

55. Watson DI, Jamieson GG. Antireflux surgery in the laparoscopic era (Review). Br J Surg 1998;85:1173-84.

56. Rossetti M, Hell K. Fundoplication for the treatment of gastresophageal reflux in hiatal hernia. World J Surg 1977;1:439-44.

57. Luostarinen M, Isolauri J, Laitinen J, Koskinen M, Keyrilainen O, Markkula H, Lehtinen E, Uusitalo A. Fate of Nissen fundoplication after 20 years. A clinical, endoscopical, and functional analysis. Gut 1993;34: 1015-20.

58. Watson DI, Jamieson GG, Pike GK, Game PA, Devitt PG. Laparoscopic vs anterior fundoplication; a randomised double blind controlled trial. Aust NZ J Surg 1999;69: (Suppl):A57 (Abstract).

59. Watson DI, Chan ASL, Myers JC, Jamieson GG. Illness behaviour influences the outcome of laparoscopic antireflux surgery. J Am Coll Surg 1997;184:44-8.

60. Rattner DW, Brooks DC. Patient satisfaction following laparoscopic and open antireflux surgery. Arch Surg 1995;130:289-94.

61. Peters JH, Heimbucher J, Kauer WKH, Incarbone R, Bremner CG, DeMeester TR. Clinical and physiological comparison of laparoscopic and open Nissen fundoplication. J Am Coll Surg 1995;180:385-93.

62. Laine S, Rantala A, Gullichsen R, Ovaska J. Laparoscopic vs conventional Nissen fundoplication. A prospective randomized study. Surg Endosc 1997;11:441-4.

63. Watson DI, Gourlay R, Globe J, Reed MWR, Johnson AG, Stoddard CJ. Prospective randomised trial of laparoscopic versus open Nissen fundoplication. Gut 1994;35:(supplement 2):S15.(Abstract)

64. Franzen T, Anderberg B, Tibbling L, Johansson KE. A report from a randomized study of open and laparoscopic 360° fundoplication. Surg Endosc 1996;10:582.(Abstract).

65. Heikkinen T-J, Haukipuro K, Koivukangas P, Sorasto A, Autio R, Sodervik H, Makela H, Hulkko A. Comparison of costs between laparoscopic and open Nissen fundoplication: a prospective randomized study with a 3-month followup. J Am Coll Surg 1999;188:368-76.

66. Perttila J, Salo M, Ovaska J, Gronroos J, Lavonius M, Katila A, Lahteenmaki A, Pulkki K. Immune response after laparoscopic and conventional Nissen fundoplication. Eur J Surg 1999;165:21-8.

67. Bais JE, Bartelsman JFWM, Bonjer HJ, Cuesta MA, Go PMNYH, Klinkenberg-Kohl EC, van Lanschot JJB, Nadorp JHSM, Smout AJPM, van der Graaf Y, Gooszen HG. Laparoscopic or conventional Nissen fundoplication for gastro esophageal reflux disease: randomised clinical trial. The Lancet 2000;355:170-4.

2.6 SURGICAL TREATMENT OF DUODENO-GASTRO ESOPHAGEAL REFLUX

Attila Csendes, Patricio Burdiles and Owen Korn

Classically, pathologic acid reflux into the esophagus has been considered as a consequence of an excessive and prolonged contact of esophageal mucosa to acid and pepsin refluxed from the stomach[1]. However since several years, reflux esophagitis in absence of acid reflux after total gastrectomy or in patients with achlorhydria has been described, suggesting the injurious effect of bilio-pancreatic components[2,3]. The term "alkaline esophagitis" was introduced and widely used to describe this condition, in which duodenal content produces a severe injury to the esophageal mucosa. It has also been called "bile reflux". However both term are incorrect. On one hand, duodenal contents contain more than just bile and on the other hand, alkaline reflux suggests an alteration caused by an alkaline agent (ph greater than 7), which is very rare in clinical practice and a pH > 7 does not correlate with reflux of duodenal contents. It has been shown that the addition of bile salts to gastric refluxed material in experimental models can potentiate the deleterious effect of acid and pepsin to the esophageal mucosa, even keeping a pH below 4[1,4]. In humans, the presence of bile salts has been described together with acid in the refluxed material into the esophagus, confirming the hypothesis that acid reflux can be a mixture of gastric and duodenal content, keeping the pH less than 4[5,6]. Therefore the term "duodeno-gastro-esophageal reflux" has been proposed (DGER), and this chapter will deal mainly with its surgical treatment and alternatives. It has been clearly shown by experimental studies that entero or duodenoesophageal reflux can induce:

a) Severe epithelial damage with ulcers
b) Intestinal metaplasia and strictures
c) Dysplasia and adenocarcinoma of the distal esophagus[7,8].

In an effort to determine the presence of duodenal reflux into the esophagus, continuous ambulatory esophageal 24-hrs pH studies, were performed and excessive exposition to pH above 7 was demonstrated in patients with severe esophagitis and Barrett's esophagus, suggesting that this high pH was due to duodeno-esophageal reflux[9-11]. At present is has been demonstrated that in more than 95% of the time, a pH above 7 in the esophagus is due to retained food, inadequate calibration of antimonium electrode, dental sepsis and/or retention of saliva with deficient esophageal peristalsis[12] and therefore it was not a precise measure of duodeno-esophageal reflux. Therefore, Bechi developed a new method in 1992, consisting in a portable spectro-photometer which uses bilirubine as a direct and physiological index of duodeno-gastro-esophageal reflux, easily recognized by its characteristic optic absorption curve at 454 nm[13]. This new method allowed to assess in an easy and physiological way the presence of duodeno-esophageal reflux, which was very significant in patients with Barrett's esophagus, compared to patients with reflux esophagitis or to controls[14]. With these new studies the group of DeMeester proposed 5 postulates in patients with BE, including the following pathophysiological findings:[9,15].

a) An incompetent lower esophageal sphincter.
b) Impaired esophageal peristalsis.
c) Pathologic acid reflux.
d) Acid hypersecretion in some cases.
e) Excessive duodeno-esophageal reflux.

We have added recently a sixth constant finding, which is the presence of a pathologic dilated cardia or esophagogastric junction[16,17]. Patients with BE have a wide spectrum of presentation. The modern diagnosis of BE is based on the presence of intestinal metaplasia at the distal esophagus and esophago-gastric junction, provided it is in continuity with gastric mucosa[18,19]. The extent of this specialized columnar epithelium with intestinal metaplasia at the distal esophagus can be different[20,21]. We have recently evaluated 228 patients with short or long segment of BE all of them having intestinal metaplasia at the distal esophagus. The main findings are shown in table 1.

It can clearly be seen that there is a severe structural alteration of the lower esophageal sphincter, with pathological acid reflux and a severe duodeno-gastro-esophageal reflux. When considering patients with Barrett's esophagus to surgical treatment, we have noticed two main points:

a) The majority of surgeons include in 1 group all reflux esophagitis patients submitted

H.W. Tilanus and S.E.A. Attwood (eds.), Barrett's Esophagus, 149–158.

TABLE 1. Clinical, endoscopic and functional results in patients with intestinal metaplasia at the distal esophagus

	Short segment BE (n=117)	Long segment BE (n=111)	
Age	52.6 ± 13	52.8 ± 12	p>0.4
Males (%)	52	55	
Endoscopy (%)			
Hiatal hernia	30	70.2	P<0.001
Erosive esophagitis	87.2	98.2	p>0.4
Low grade dysphagia	11.1	21.6	P<0.01
Manometry			
LESP (mmHg)	8.3 ± 4	6 ± 4	p>0.18
Total length (mm)	30 ± 10	31 ± 12	p>0.10
Abdominal length (mm)	5.5 ± 6	5.5 ± 6	p>0.8
% incompetent LES	85	91	p.0.7
24-hrs pH-study			
% of time with pH<4	18 ± 16	28.8 ± 20	P<0.0001
Bilitec study			
% of time with bilirubin			
Absorbance>0.2 in 24hrs	15.8 ± 12	20.3 ± 20	p>0.45

to surgery, without separating the results in patients with or without BE. From 1990 up to now, we have reviewed more than 200 papers dealing with surgery for reflux esophagitis, either open or by laparoscopic route and only 9 of them mention the BE group as a separate group from non-BE patients[22-30].

b)   In the majority of the surgical reports the late follow up is missing. Even more there are some papers with just 3 or 6 months of follow up. The importance of separating patients with BE from non BE cases is based on the hypothesis that if the final results are included in only 1 group, the eventual "bad" results of patients with BE are "buffered" with the eventual "good" results in non BE patients. For example, if 100 cases are operated on and followed up, the careful preoperative analysis of them can reveal that 80 patients had only reflux esophagitis and 20 patients had BE. The 80 non BE cases have at 8 to 10 years 90% of good results, which means that 72 are well and 8 had failure of the antireflux procedure. From the 20 BE cases, 50% of them will have good results, which means that 10 are well and 10 are with recurrence. Therefore, the final results of 100 cases as a group will be 82% of good results and 18% of bad results, while among the BE the bad results were 50%.
The results of 9 surgical groups in the management of patients with BE by classic or laparoscopic antireflux surgery are shown in Table 2. The majority of the reports have very few patients with a short follow up. In 7 of

them appearance of adenocarcinoma or dysplastic changes are reported. Very few mention objective measurements such as 24-h pH monitoring. We have performed two prospective studies in patients with BE submitted to classic open antireflux surgery. The first study regards a late follow up of 152 patients with long segment BE submitted to classsic antireflux surgery, followed for more than 8 years[30]. The main final results are seen in table 3. The final late results were not satisfactory with appearance of dysplasia or adenocarcinoma at a mean time of 8 years after surgery. The second study regarded a prospective randomized controlled trial[31] comparing Nissen fundoplication with Hill posterior gastropexy with calibration of the cardia in 164 patients (table 4). Among them 125 were no BE cases and 39 had non complicated BE. The late results demonstrated that both procedures had very similar results, but significant differences were seen among patients with non BE compared to patients with BE. Therefore our group, based on these bad late results of classic antireflux surgery in patients with BE and knowing that the presence of duodenal reflux is an important key factor in the pathogenesis of BE (even previous to the Bilitec era), proposed to perform two different operations in patients with BE with intestinal metaplasia, based mainly on the principle of bile diversion". Medical treatment with proton pump inhibitors can decrease, but not abolish DGER.

TABLE 2. Results of antireflux surgery in patients with Barrett's esophagus.

Authors	N° cases	Mean Follow up (years)	%Good Results	% time pH less than 4	Appear. Dysplasia N° Cases	Appear. Adenoca N° Cases
DeMeester (1990)	35	3	77	n.d.	0	0
Williamson (1990)	37	5	81	38	4	3
Mc Entee (1991)	21	1.8	90	n.d.	2	0
Attwood (1992)	19	3	79	n.d.	0	1
Sagar (1995)	46	-	-	n.d.	0	1
Ortiz (1996)	30	5	90	17	1	1
Mc Donald (1996)	113	6.5	82	n.d.	0	3
Csendes (1998)	152	8	40	50	15	4
Patti (1999)	38	2	93	n.d.	0	0

n.d. : not done

TABLE 3. Final results of 152 patients with long segment BE treated by classic open antireflux surgery.

Preoperative length of history:	110 months
Cases with peptic ulcer or stricture	78 patients
Length Barrett's esophagus:	64 mm
Mean follow up:	108 months (96% of follow)
Operative mortality:	0.7%
Visick I-II	40%
Visick III-IV	60%
Appearance dysplasia	15 patients (10%)
Appearance adenocarcinoma	4 patients (2.8%)

TABLE 4. Final results of a prospective randomized study comparing Nissen Fundoplication and Hill posterior gastropexy with cardial calibration (n = 162)

- Operative mortality: 0
- Follow up: 92 months
      (95% follow up)
- Fundoplication (Visick I-II)
      a) Non BE   83%
      b) BE   24%
- Posterior gastropexy with cardial calibration (Visick I-II)
      a) Non BE   81%
      b) BE   22%

Three different studies using Bilitec have shown that DGER is decreased in the majority of BE cases, but the amount of DGER is still much higher than in controls[32,34]. If medical treatment stops, DGER may return to the pre-treatment values. Similar findings can be observed after classic antireflux surgery when the patients are evaluated late after surgery. Nissen fundoplication can reduce the episodes of acid and duodenal reflux into the distal esophagus, but never abolishes them[30,32]. As a consequence, many years after surgery, the lower esophageal sphincter can loose its competence and DGER can increase again, resulting in the development of dysplasia and adenocarcinoma[30]. Therefore, in patients with BE, in whom an important DGER has been documented, we proposed not only to perform an antireflux procedure, but also to modify or improve some of the other pathological findings in patients with BE by performing:

a)   Improvement of an incompetent lower esophageal sphincter by antireflux surgery (either fundoplication or calibration of the cardia)

b)   A highly selective vagotomy or selective vagotomy with antrectomy in order to decrease the acid secretion.

c)   A Roux-en-Y loop of 60 cm long to eliminate duodenal reflux.

For this, two different types of surgery were performed:

1)   Duodenal switch procedure plus highly selective vagotomy and antireflux surgery[35] (Figure 1).

2)   Selective or truncal vagotomy, partial distal gastrectomy, antireflux surgery and Roux-en-Y anastomosis with a 50 cm long limb[36] (Figure 2).

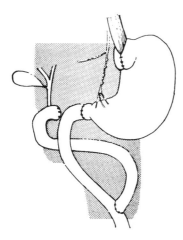

Figure 1. Duodenal switch procedure plus highly selective vagotomy and antireflux surgery

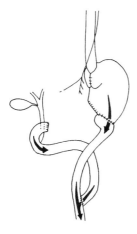

Figure 2. Selective or truncal vagotomy, partial distal gastrectomy, antireflux surgery and Roux-Y anastomosis with a 50 cm long limb.

The duodenal switch procedure consist of 4 surgical steps.

a) Highly selective vagotomy, in order to decrease acid secretion and to avoid anastomotic ulcers at the duodeno-jejunal anastomosis.

b)   Antireflux surgery, either a 360° total fundoplication or "calibration" of the cardia (a tight fundoplication) plus posterior gastropexy.

c)   Duodenal switch by performing a duodeno jejunal anastomosis with a 60 cm long Roux-en-Y jejunal limb.

d)   Closure of the crurae of the diaphragm and anterior fundophrenopexy.

The acid supression and bile diversion operation consists of 5 main surgical steps:

a)   Selective or truncal vagotomy, in order to decrease the gastric acid secretion.

b)   Antireflux surgery, either 360° total fundoplication or "calibration" of the cardia plus posterior gastropexy.

c)   Distal partial gastrectomy, in order to abolish gastrin release and therefore to decrease significantly gastric acid secretion and to avoid acid reflux.

d)   Gastrojejunostomy with a 60 cm long Roux-en-Y jejunal limb.

e)   Closure of the crurae of the diaphragm and anterior fundophrenopexy.

Selective vagotomy is performed in the same way as HSV, with division of both nerves of Latarjet. Completion of this vagotomy is similar to HSV, exposing at least 5 cm of the distal esophagus. Always 2 to 3 short vessels are divided in order to mobilize the gastric fundus for a proper antireflux surgery without tension. Partial distal gastrectomy is performed by using mechanical staplers with preservation of the gastroepiploic vessels of the greater curvature. Careful attention is given in order to avoid a dependent sump, by including sufficient greater curvature[37]. The duodenum is divided and closed 1 to 2 cm distal to the pylorus by using a stapler. The end-to-side gastrojejunostomy is performed with a 60 cm long Roux-en-Y limb[30]. The main clinical results are shown in table 5.

The duodenal switch procedure had no mortality, while vagotomy and partial gastrectomy showed a mortality rate of 1.0%. At the late follow up there were significantly better results in Visick score after vagotomy and partial gastrectomy compared to duodenal switch procedure. This difference can be explained by the results shown in table 6, were acid and duodenal reflux studies are evaluated before and after surgery.

It can be seen that duodenal reflux is completely eliminated after both procedures by the 60 cm long Roux-en-Y jejunal limb. However, there is much more acid reflux persisting after duodenal switch procedure than after vagotomy and partial gastrectomy, because this latter procedure can supress completely gastric acid secretion. A very important beneficial effect of duodenal diversion was the regression of low grade

TABLE 5. Clinical results of bile diversion operation.

	Duodenal Switch Procedure(n=75)	Truncal Vagotomy/Partial gastrectomy Roux-Y anastomosis (n=195)
Operative mortality	0	2 (1%)
Postoperative morbidity	12	4.1
Follow up (%)	95	92
Months follow up	55	94
Visick I and II	75	96
Visick III and IV	25	4
Appearance of dysplasia	0	0
Appearance of adenocarcinoma	0	0

TABLE 6. Acid and duodenal reflux before and after surgery

	Duodenal switch procedure		Truncal vagotomy/Partial gastrectomy Roux-Y anastomosis	
	Preop.	Postop.	Preop.	Postop.
24 hrs pH-studies				
% in time with pH less				
Than 4 in 24 hrs.	24.8 ± 1.9	4.8 ± 5.7	23.8 ± 15	1.8 ± 1.1
Bilitec studies				
% of time with bilirubin				
With absorbance rate				
>0.2 in 24 hrs.	23.5 ± 17	0.7 ± 0.7	20.8 ± 22	1.15 ± 1.3

dysplasia in more than 50% of the cases after both procedures and no progression or appearance of dysplasia was seen in any patients, confirming the importance of duodenal reflux in the development of this pre neoplastic histological changes in patients with intestinal metaplasia at the distal esophagus. Gastric emptying of solids evaluated 6 months after both operation is shown in table 7.

No significant differences were seen between both procedures and control subjects. The results of acid secretion can be seen in table 8. Vagotomy plus partial gastrectomy produced a significant and permanent decrease of acid secretion, while patients with classic antireflux surgery or patients with duodenal switch and showed a decreased but persisting acid secretion[39-53]. Knowing that the main pathogenic alterations in patients with Barrett´s esophagus are the presence of an incompetent lower esophageal sphincter together with acid and duodenal pathologic reflux into the esophagus, we propose to treat these patients in an other way, not only by improving sphincter competence, but also by abolishing acid secretion and eliminating completely and definitively duodenal reflux. In this way a possible recurrence of reflux and late complications as dysplasia or adenocarcinoma are avoided. As a consequence, vagotomy and partial gastrectomy with a Roux-en-Y

anastomosis was performed in 195 patients with BE. The careful close follow up of these cases has shown that in 54 cases followed more than 60 months, with a mean follow up of 103 months, reflux esophagitis and its complications have been controlled completely in 85% while 15% have some reflux symptoms or esophagitis easily controlled by medical treatment. This late recurrence of reflux is mainly due to pathologic acid reflux in some patients, because duodenal reflux is completely abolished by this surgical technique. A recent paper published by Salminen et al has reached to the same conclusion after performing pH studies in patients submitted to vagotomy, partial gastrectomy and Roux-en-Y anastomosis, but without antireflux surgery[54]. Healing of severe esophagitis was observed in spite of the persistance of abnormal acid reflux and this finding leaded the authors to conclude that reflux of duodenal content can play a major role in the development of severeesophagitis. This operation has been employed by many authors as a solution after second or third failure of a classic antireflux surgery[55-73] or in some selected patients with esophageal stricture[58-60,63,64,73-75]. However as a primary operation for complicated Barrett´s esophagus has been employed only by Fékéte[50,51] and by Spencer[59,64]. The first experimental data concerning this operation

TABLE 7. Gastric emptying of solids in controls and in patients submitted to bile diversion operation

	Controls n=30	Duodenal Switch n=39	Partial gastrectomy/Truncal vagotomy n=28	
T ½ (minutes)	84 ± 26	74 ± 22	104 ± 70	n.s
% retention				
- 60 minutes	61 ± 112	50 ± 21	62 ± 26	
- 90 minuten	41 ± 17	38 ± 18	50 ± 30	n.s.
- 120 minuten	30 ± 15	22 ± 19	41 ± 30	

TABLE 8. Gastric acid secretion before and after antireflux procedures

	Classic Antireflux Surgery n = 18	Duodenal Switch Procedure n = 22	Truncal Vagotomy Partial Gastrectomy n = 23
BAO Preop Postop % reduction	1.9 ± 1.2 0.7 ± 0.4 63	2.8 ± 1.0 1.2 ± 0.7 58	4.7 ± 2.3 0.2 ± 0.1 96
PAO Preop Postop % reduction	24.9 ± 18.0 12.5 ± 4.5 48	23.5 ± 7.8 11.7 ± 5.0 50	22.8 ± 7.8 2.9 ± 1.6 87

came from the Mayo Clinic in 1956[76], when localized resection of the cardia was performed in dogs (abolition of LES) and a bilateral vagotomy and antrectomy were added to eliminate cephalic and gastric phase of acid secretion. However, a gastroduodenostomy anastomosis was performed and later, recurrent strictures or regurgitation and failures were documented. The first clinical approach was performed by Wells and Johnston in 1955[55] who reported excellent results in 12 patients with GERD by performing this operation. Later Holt and Large in 1961[56], treated 11 patients with esophageal strictures with this procedure. They were examined 8 to 17 years later and the primary good results persisted[57]. Payne et al in 1970[58] employed the principle described by Ellis, but performed a Roux-en-Y anastomosis instead of a gastroduodenostomy in 15 patients, with 73% of good results, but no postoperative endoscopies were performed. Later, other authors have also employed this operation, mainly in failed antireflux surgery or severe esophageal strictures as described previously. The largest experience is that reported by Fékéte[66,67] who performed this operation in 83 patients, 42 of them with Barrett's esophagus with 80% of excellent results. Washer et al[64] performed a prospective randomized trial comparing Nissen fundoplication versus antrectomy and Roux-en-Y anastomosis in patients with primary severe esophagitis demonstrating good results in 65% after Nissen fundoplication versus 95% after Roux-en-Y anastomosis (p < 0.01). In our patients, we have demonstrated that this procedure can be performed safely with minimal postoperative morbidity and excellent late results in 94% of the cases. In the early stage of our experience we had two deaths, but since many years and more than 130 cases operated no mortality has occurred. Postoperative morbidity is minimal. However, some surgical details are important. We always try to perform a truncal or selective bilateral vagotomy. The incidence of a recurrent anastomotic ulcer is extremely low (2 cases among 195), because it has been shown that gastric denervation with bilateral vagotomy is very complete[77,78]. The area of resected stomach must be standard. It is important to perform an antiperistaltic gastrojejunal anastomosis as suggested by Ferguson et al[37] avoiding gastric stasis. Besides, partial distal gastrectomy should include sufficient greater curvature, so that the dependent sump is avoided[37]. This means that it is necessary to. perform at least a hemigastrectomy. Larger resections[79] produce dumping, loss of weight, anemia and diarrhea. The length of the jejunal limb must be 50-60 cm[38]. If the Roux limb is less than 50 cm long, enteric reflux into the gastric stump can occur[80,81]. Gastric stasis was not a real serious clinical problem. We had

TABLE 9. Comparison of results of different surgical procedures in patients with Barrett's esophagus (n=429)

Type operation	n	Operative Mortality	Late results (%) Visick I-II	Visick III-IV	Appearance Dysplasia	Adenoca
Classic antireflux surgery	152	1 (0.7%)	39	61	15	4
Duodenal Switch	75	0	70	30	0	0
TV + PG Roux-en-Y	195	2 (1%)	97	3	0	0
Esophagectomy	7	1 (14%)	100	0	-	-

only 1 patient who had a stricture of the anastomosis after surgery, but was managed medically. Gastric emptying of solids were in normal range, although 25% of the cases had a slower emptying, but without clinical impact. We have not seen the so-called Roux syndrome in any patient, as described by other authors[38,80,81]. After surgery, a significant improvement in sphincter pressure occurred, with a good recovery of sphincter function. Peptic ulcer of the esophagus healed in almost all cases between 3 to 6 months after surgery and no recurrence has been seen. The stricture which was present in 54 cases resolved completely in 51 (94%), leaving only a slight scar and a small decrease of the internal diameter of the squamous columnar junction. Late complications due to the gastric resection were seldom seen: severe dumping was an infrequent finding, diarrhea was episodic and mild during the first 6 months after surgery. The loss of weight which is routinely seen, has been secondary to a lesser food intake due in part to the antireflux surgery, in part to loss of accomodation and receptive relaxation due to vagotomy[82] and in part to a less reservoir secondary to gastrectomy. However in the great majority this loss of weight was very well tolerated because usually the patients were overweighed. In few cases (8 patients) severe diarrhea and loss of weight was a real problem for more than 1 year. One of the most important aspect in our study was the 24-hr pH measurements before and after surgery, as well as the Bilitec studies. Only 1 previous study reported pH studies after surgery, but without referral to duodenal reflux studies. We have demonstrated that acid reflux into the esophagus drops dramatically after surgery to subnormal levels, indicating an almost complete gastric acid suppression, which is permanent on time. In the same way, duodenal reflux into the esophagus is completely abolished by this surgical procedure. We believe that the elimination of the reflux into

the esophagus containing a mixture of acid and duodenal content will completely eliminate the appearance of dysplasia and adenocarcinoma in BE[7,30,83,88]. Up to now the late control has confirmed that in no patient these histological changes have occurred. Even if the antireflux procedure looses and fails, because no acid and no duodenal reflux exists within the esophagus[30]. We advice to perform in these patients also an antireflux surgery, in order to avoid persisting reflux and regurgitation as reported by Salminen et al[54]. The surgical management of complex problems related to GERD, specially after failed procedures, has been controversial as evidenced by the wide variety of techniques that have been advocated under such circumstances. Redo surgery employing the classic antireflux procedures, with variation as Nissen-Collis, Belsey-Collis, Thal-Nissen techniques, partial esophageal resection with esophagogastrostomy, interposition of short intestinal segment or total esophagectomy have been employed[89-92].

However, these operations do not have satisfactory results, because they are based on anatomical principles and not on the solution of the pathogenic factors that cause reflux. In table 9 we present the summary of our final results in the surgical management of 429 patients with Barrett's esophagus[36]. The best results have been obtained with vagotomy, partial gastrectomy and Roux-en-Y anastomosis. In summary, this operation is based in the fact that: a) patients with BE show several abnormalities in the foregut which include incompetent LES, impairment in the esophageal clearance, severe gastroesophageal acid reflux and frequent duodeno esophageal reflux, b) late results of classic antireflux procedure in BE are poor with a high recurrence rate due to a progressive loosening of the wrap[30] and c) the esophageal damage produced by the injurious component of the refluxate. We have observed that simple correction of the valve is insufficient because it does not abolishes but only diminishes the GE reflux. In patients with BE and therefore with impaired esophageal clearance even few reflux episodes can maintain or induce more damage. With the "suppression diversion" antireflux procedure the quality of the corrected valve is secondary and the main goal is to avoid the

reflux of injurious components of the refluxate instead of avoiding the refluxate itself which is almost always impossible. Our late results support this hypothesis and we propose this surgical procedure as an alternative treatment in patients with complicated BE.

REFERENCES

1. Harmon JW, Johnson LF, Maydonivitch CL. Effects of acid and bile salts on the rabbit esophageal mucosa. Dig Dis Sci 198;26:65-72.
2. Helsingen H. Oesophagitis following total gastrectomy. A follow up study on 9 patients 5 years or more after operation. Acta Chir Scand 1959;118:190-201.
3. Palmer DE. Subacute erosive ("peptic") esophagitis associated with achlorhydria. N Engl J Med 1960;262:927-9.
4. Lillemoe KD, Johnson LE, Harmon JW. Alkaline esophagitis: a comparison of the ability of components of gastroduodenal contents to injure rabbit mucosa. Gastroenterology 1983;85:621-8.
5. Gotley DC, Morgan AP, Cooper MJ. Bile acid concentrations in the refluxate of patients with reflux oesophagitis. Br J Surg 1988;75:587-90.
6. Gotley DC, Morgan AP, Ball D, Owens RW, Cooper MJ. Composition of gastroesophageal refluxate. Gut 1991;32:1093-9.
7. Attwood SEA, Smyrk TC, DeMeester TR, Mirvisch SS, Stein HJ, Hinder RA. Duodenoesophageal reflux and the development of adenocarcinoma in rats. Surgery 1992;111:503-10.
8. Fein M, Peters JH, Chandrasoma P, Ireland AP, Öberg S, Ritter Mp, Bremner CG, Hagen JA DeMeester TR. Duodenoesophageal reflux induces esophageal adenocarcinoma without exogenous carcinogen. J Gastroint Surg 1998;2:260-8.
9. Pellegrini CA, DeMeester TR, Wernly JA, Johnson LF, Skinner DB. Alkaline gastroesophageal reflux. Am J Surg. 1978;75:177-84.
10. Stein HJ, Haeft S, DeMeester T. Functional foregut abnormalities in Barrett's esophagus. J Thorac Cardiovasc Surg 1993;105:107-11.
11. Stein HJ, DeMeester TR, Hinder RA. Outpatient physiological testing and surgical management of foregut motor disorders. Curr Probl Surg 1992;24:418-555.
12. Devault KR, Georgeson S, Castell DO. Salivary stimulation mimics esophageal exposure to refluxed duodenal content. Am J Gastroenterol 1993; 88:1040-3.
13. Bechi P, Paucciani F, Baldini F, Cosi F, Falciai R, Mazzanti R, Castagnli R, Pesseri A. Long-term ambulatory enterogastric reflux monitoring. Validation of a new fiberoptic technique. Dig Dis Sci 1993;38:11297-1306.
14. Kauer WKH, Burdiles P, Ireland AP, Clark GNB. Does duodenal juice reflux into the esophagus of patients with complicated GERD? Evaluation of a fiberoptic sensor for bilirubin. Am J Surg 1995;169:98-104.
15. Öberg S, Clark GWB, DeMeester TR. Barrett's esophagus: update of pathophysiology and management. Hepato-gastroenterol 1998;45:1348-56.
16. Csendes A, Miranda M, Espinoza M, Velasco N, Henríquez A. Perimeter and location of the muscular esophagogastric junction or cardia in control subjects and in patients with reflux esophagitis or achalasia. Scand J Gastroent 1981;16:951-6.
17. Korn O, Csendes A, Burdiles P, Braghetto I, Stein HJ. Dilatation of the cardia and competence of the lower esophageal shincter. J Gastrointest Surg 2000, accepted for publication.
18. Spechler SJ, Goyal RK. The columnar lined esophagus, intestinal metaplasia and Norman Barrett. Gastroenterology. 1996;110:614-21.
19. Giuli R. The Barrett committed meeting on the International Society for Diseases of the Esophagus. Dis Esoph 1996;9:157-8.
20. Csendes A, Smok G, Sagastume H, Rojas J. Estudio prospecitvo endoscópico y biópsico de la prevalencia de metaplasia intestinal en la unión gastroesofágica en controles y en pacientes con reflujo gastroesofágico. Rev Méd Chile 1998;126:155-61.
21. Csendes A, Burdiles P, Smok G, Rojas J, Flores N, Domic S, Quiroz J, Henríquez A. Hallazgos clínicos, endoscópicos y magnitud del reflujo de contenido gástrico y duodenal en pacientes con metaplasia intestinal cardial y esófago de Barrett corto, comparados con controles. Rev Méd Chile 1999;127:1321-8.
22. De Meester TR, Atwood SEA, Smyrk TC, Therkildsen DH, Hinder RA. Surgical therapy in Barrett's esophagus. Ann Surg 1990;212:528-42.
23. Williamsom WA, Ellis FH Jr, Gibb SP, Shahian DM, Aretz HT. Effect of antireflux operation on Barrett's mucosa. Ann Thorac Surg 1990;49:537-42.
24. Mc Entee, Stuart RC, Byrne PJ, Nolan N, Hennessy TPJ. An evaluation of surgical and medical treatment of Barrett's esophagus. Gullet 1991;1:169-72.
25. Atwood SEA, Barlow AP, Norris TL, Watson A. Barrett's esophagus: effect of antireflux surgery on symptom control and development of complications. Br J Surg 1992;79:1050-4.
26. Sagar PM,Ackroid R, Hosie KB, Patterson JE, Stoddard CS, Kingnorth AN. Regression and progression of Barrett's esophagus after antireflux surgery. Br J Surg 1995;82:806-10.
27. Ortiz A, Martinez de Haro LF, Parrilla P, Morales G, Molina J. Conservative treatment versus antireflux surgery in Barrett's esophagus: long-term results of a prospective study. Br J Surg 1996;83:274-8.
28. Mc Donald ML, Trastek VF, Allen MS, Deschamps C, Pairolero PC. Barrett's esophagus: does an antireflux procedure reduce the need for endoscopic surveillance? J Thorac Cardiovasc Surg 1996;111:1135-40.
29. Patti MG, Arcerito M, Feo CV, Worth S, De Pinto M, Gibbs VC, Gantert D, Ferrell LF, Way LW. Barrett's esophagus a surgical disease. J Gastroint Surg 1999;3:397-4.
30. Csendes A, Braghetto I, Burdiles P, Puente J, Korn O, Díaz JC, Maluenda F. Long term results of classic antireflux surgery in 152 patients with Barrett's esophagus: clinical, radiologic, endoscopic, manometric and acid reflux test before and late after operation. Surgery 1998;123:645-57.
31. Csendes A, Burdiles P, Korn O, Braghetto I, Huerta C, Rojas J. Late results of a randomized clinical trial comparing total fundoplication versus calibration of the cardia with posterior gastropexy. Br J Surg 2000,87(3);289-97.
32. Stein HJ, Kauer WKH, Feussner H, Siewert R. Bile reflux in benign and malignant Barrett's esophagus: effect of medical acid suppression and Nissen fundoplication. J Gastrointest Surg 1998;2:333-41.

33. Vaezi MF, Lacamera RG, Richter JE. Validation studies of Bilitec 2000: an ambulatory duodenogastric reflux monitoring system. Am J Physiol 1994;267: G1050-7.

34. Marshall REK, Anggiansah A, Manifold DK, Owen WA, Owen WJ. Effect of omeprazol 20 mg twice daily on duodeno-gastric and gastro-esophageal bile reflux in Barrett's esophagus. Gut 1998;43:603-6.

35. Csendes A, Braghetto I, Burdiles P, Díaz JC, Maluenda F, Korn O. A new physiological approach for the surgical treatment of patients with Barrett's esophagus. Ann Surg 1997; 226:123-33.

36. Csendes A, Braghetto I, Burdiles P, Korn O, Maluenda F, Diaz JC, Rojas J, Puente J, Constant - Neto M. Results of surgical treatment in 362 patients with Barrett's esophagus. Rev Chil Cir 1998;50:175-85.

37. Ferguson GH, Rose M, Maclennani I, Taylor TV, Torrance HB. Vomiting after Roux-en-Y biliary diversion. Relationship to surgical technique. Br J Surg 1990;77:548-50.

38. Shirmer BD. Gastric atony and the Roux syndrome. Gastroent Clin N Am 1994;23: 327-43.

39. Loustarninen M. Nissen fundoplication for reflux esophagitis. Ann Surg 1993;217: 329-37.

40. Rossetti ME, Liebermann - Meffert D, Brauner RB. The "Rossetti" modification of the Nissen fundoplication: technique and results. Dis Esoph 1996;9:251-7.

41. DeMeester TR. The "De Meester" modification: technique and results. Dis Esoph 1996; 9: 258-62.

42. Siewert JR, Stein HJ. Technical details, long-term outcome and causes of failure. Dis Esoph 1996; 9: 278-84.

43. Csendes A, Braghetto I, Korn O, Cortes C. Late subjective and objective evaluation of antireflux surgery in patients with reflux esophagitis. Analysis of 215 patients. Surgery 1989;105:374-82.

44. Larrain A, Csendes A, Pope C. Surgical correction of refux. An effective therapy for esophageal strictures. Gastroenterology 1975;69:578-83.

45. Ellis FH Jr, Garabedion M, Gibb S. Fundoplication for gastroesophageal reflux. Arch Surg 1973;107:186-92.

46. Skinner DB. Benign esophageal strictures. Adv Surg 1976;10:177-81.

47. Russell C, Hill L. Gastroesophageal reflux. Curr Probl Surg 1983;20:209-77.

48. Hermreck A, Coates N. Results of the Hill antireflux operation. Am J Surg 1980;140: 764-8.

49. Watson A. A clinical and pathophysiological study of a simple effective operation for the correction of gastro esophageal reflux. Br J Surg 1984;71:991-3.

50. Watson A. Lower esophageal sphincter characteristics after a simplified procedure for the correction of gastro esophageal reflux. Br J Surg 1985;72:1628-32.

51. DeMeester T, Johnson L. Evaluation of the Nissen anti reflux procedure by esophageal manometry and twenty four hour pH monitoring. Am J Surg 1975;129:94-100.

52. De Meester TR, Bonavina L, Albertucci M. Nissen fundoplication for gatroesophageal reflux disease. Ann Surg 1986;204: 9-20.

53. Johansson J, Johnsson F, Joelsson B, Flores Ch, Walther B. Outcome 5 years after 360° fundoplication for gastroesphageal reflux disease. Br J Surg 1993;80:46-9.

54. Salminen F, Salo F, Tuominen F, Rämö F, Färkkilä M, Mattila S. pH-metric analysis after successful antireflux surgery: comparison of 24-hour profiles in patients undergoing floppy fundoplication or Roux-en-Y duodenal diversion. J Gastrointest Surg 1997;1 494-8.

55. Wells C, Johnston JM. Hiatus hernia: surgical relief of reflux esophagitis. Lancet 1955;1:937-40.

56. Holt CJ, Large AM. Surgical management of reflux esophagitis. Ann Surg 1961;153: 555-62.

57. Weaver AW, Large AM, Walt AJ. Surgical management of severe reflux esophagitis. Eight to seventeen year follow-up study. Am J Surg 1970;119:15-20.

58. Payne WS. Surgical treatment of reflux esophagitis and stricture associated with permanent incompetence of the cardia. Mayo Clin Proc 1970;45:553-62.

59. Royston CM, Dowling BL, Spencer J. Antrectomy with Roux-en-Y anastomosis in the treatment of peptic esophagitis and stricture. Br J Surg 1975;62:605-7.

60. Payne WS. Surgical management of reflux induced esophageal stenosis: results in 101 patients. Br J Surg 1984;71:971-3.

61. Matikainen M. Antrectomy, Roux-en-Y anastomosis reconstruction and vagotomy for recurrent reflux esophagitis. Acta Chir Scand 1984;150:643-5.

62. De Miguel J. Tratamiento de ciertas estenosis pepticas del esófago mediante vagotomía, gastrectomía parcial y anastomosis gastrojejunal en Y de Roux. Rev Esp Enf Apar Dig 1985;67:511-16.

63. Rossetti M, Heitz P, Van Aaburg R. Die distal Y gastrecktomie bei komplexem und rezidereflux. Helo Anir Acta 1990;56:935-8.

64. Washer GF, Gear MWL, DowlingBL, Billison EW, Royston CMS, Spencer J. Randomized prospective trial of Roux en Y duodenal diversion versus fundoplication for severe reflux esophagitis. Br J Surg 1984;71:181-4.

65. Salo JA, Ala-Kulju KV, Heinniken SO, Kinilaalkso EO. Treatment of severe peptic esophageal stricture with Roux-en-Y partial gastrectomy, vagotomy and endoscopic dilation. J Thorac Cardiovasc Surg 1991;101:649-53.

66. Perniceni TM, Meusnier H, Gayet B, Fékéte F. Traitment de esophagitis peptiques compliquées. Presse Med 1959;18:819-22.

67. Feketé F, Paeron D. What is the place of antrectomy with Roux-en-Y in the treatment of reflux disease? World J Surg 1992;16:349-55.

68. Salo JA, Lempinen M, Kivilaakso E. Partial gastrectomy with Roux-en-Y reconstruction in the treatment of persistent or recurrent esophagitis after Nissen fundoplication. Br J Surg 1985;72:623-5.

69. Herrington JL, Mody B. Total duodenal diversion for treatment of reflux esophagitis was controlled by repeated antireflux procedure. Ann Surg 1976;183:636-44.

70. Dieger NA, Jamieson GG, Brithen-Jones R, Teu S. Reoperation after failed antireflux surgery. Brit J Surg 1994;81:1159-61.

71. Ellis FH Jr, Gibb SP. Esophageal reconstruction for complex benign esophageal disease. J Thorac Cardiovasc Surg 1990;99:192-9.

72. Gotley DC, Ball DE, Owen RW, Williamson RCN, Cooper MJ. Evaluation and surgical correction of esophagitis after partial gastrectomy. Surgery 1992;111:29-36.

73. Ellis FH Jr, Gibb SP. Vagotomy, antrectomy and Roux-en-Y diversion for complex reoperative gastroesophageal reflux disease. Ann Surg 1994;220:536-43.

74. Herseling EJ, Slooff MJM, Bleichrodt RP, Jansen N, Edens EJ. Gastrectomy and Roux-Y duodenal diversion as treatment for severe reflux esophagitis. In Diseases of the Esophagus, Edited by JR Siewert and AH Holscher. Ed. Springer-Verlag 1987, pp:1248-10.

75. Burmeister R, Garcia C, Apablaza S, Benavides C, Maluenda S, Covacevic S, Riquelme R. Complicated

gastroesophageal reflux. Rev Chil Cir 1997;49:477-82.

76. Ellis FH Jr. Experimental aspects of surgical treatment of reflux esophagitis and esophageal stricture. Ann Surg 1956;143:465-70.

77. Csendes A. Late results of elective surgical treatment in patients with duodenal ulcer. Cuad Chil Cir 1990;34:96-116.

78. Csendes A. Braghetto I, Burdiles P, Díaz JC, Maluenda F, Korn O. Morbidity of elective surgery in duodenal ulcers (1978-1993). Gold standard for laparoscopic surgery. Rev Chil Cir 1995;47:209-16.

79. Csendes A, Amdrup E, Parada M. A peroperative technique for determining the extent of gastrectomy. Surg.Gynec Obstet 1979;149:81-4.

80. Van-der-Migle HCJ, Beekheus H, Blecchrodt RP, Kleibenker JH. Transit disorder of the gastric renmant and Roux limb after Roux-en-Y gastrojejunostomy: relation to symptomatology and vagotomy. Br J Surg 1993;80:60-4.

81. Mathias JR, Fernández A, Sninsky CA, Clench MH, Dayis RM. Nausea, vomiting and abdominal pain after Roux-en-Y anastomosis: motility of the jejunal lumb. Gastroenterology 1985;88:101-7.

82. Kelly M, Kennedy T. Motility changes in stomach after proximal gastric vagotomy. Br J Surg 1975;62:215-20.

83. Attwood SEA, DeMeester TR, Bremmer CG, Barlow AP, Hinder RA. Alkaline gastroesophageal reflux: implications in the development of complications in Barrett's columnar - lined lower esophagus. Surgery 1989;106:764-70.

84. Attwood SEA. Alkaline gastroesophageal reflux and esophageal carcinoma: experimental evidence and clinical implications. Dis Esoph 1994;7:87-91.

85. Smith RRC, Hamilton Sr, Boctwolt JK, Rogus EL. The spectrum of carcinoma arising in Barrett's esophagus: a clinicopathological study of 26 patients. Am J Surg Pathol 1984;119:563-72.

86. Cameron AJ, Ott BJ, Payne WS. The incidence of adenocarcinoma in columnar lined (Barrett's) esophagus. New Eng J Med 1985;313:857-9.

87. Haggrilt RC, Tryzelaar J, Ellis FX, Colcher M. Adenocarcinoma complicating columnar lined (Barrett's) esophagus. Am J Clin Pathol 1978;70:1-5.

88. Brand DL, Ylisaker JT, Gelfard M, Pope CE. Regression of columnar esophageal (Barrett's) epithelium after anti-reflux surgery. New Engl J Med 1980;302:844-8.

89. Stirling MC, Orringer MB. The combined Collis-Nissen operation for esophageal reflux strictures. Ann Thorac Surg 1988;45:148-53.

90. Pearson GF, Cooper JD, Patterson GA, Ramirez J, Todd TR. Gastroplasty and fundoplication for complex reflux problems. Ann Surg 1987;206 473-81.

91. Waters PF, Pearson GF, Todd TR, Patterson GA, Goldberg M. Esophagectomy for complex benign esophageal disease.Thorac Cardiovasc Surg 1988;95:378-88.

92. Ellis FH Jr, Gibb SP. Esophageal reconstruction for complex benign esophageal disease. J Thorac Cardiovasc Surg 1990;99:192-9.

3.1 HISTOPATHOLOGY OF BARRETT'S ESOPHAGUS

Herman van Dekken

1. INTRODUCTION

The first accurate description of the presence of columnar lined mucosa in the distal esophagus was reported by Barrett in 1950[1]. He described gastric mucosa extending into the esophagus for varying distances, in some patients as far as the aortic arch. This condition, later termed Barrett's esophagus, needs to be distinguished from congenital islands of ectopic gastric mucosa. These are found in approximately 10% of individuals undergoing upper endoscopy[2], and are mostly found in the cervical esophagus[3]. Esophageal adenocarcinomas evidently associated with Barrett's esophagus were reported shortly after Barrett's original observations in the early fifties[4] (Fig. 1).

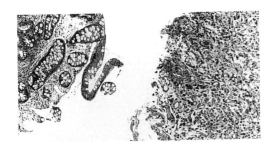

Figure 1 . Barrett's esophagus and Barrett's adeno-carcinoma (endoscopic biopsy). Metaplastic Barrett's mucosa is seen on the left, poorly differentiated adenocarcinoma with signet ring tumor cells is depicted on the right. H&E, 5X objective

Initially three types of Barrett's esophagus were discerned, i.e. gastric-fundic type epithelium with parietal and chief cells, junctional type epithelium with cardiac mucous glands, and specialized columnar epithelium with intestinal type goblet cells[5]. The intestinal type was always the most proximal, the gastric-fundic type the most distal epithelium, with the junction type being interposed. It suggests sampling errors due to variation and appearance of the squamocolumnar junction (Z-line), which does not necessarily coincides with the gastro-esophageal junction. Indeed, in the last decades it became clear that only the specialized type mucosa with goblet cells (intestinal metaplasia) carries an increased risk of developing adenocarcinoma[6-9]. Therefore only

the intestinal type should be classified as Barrett's esophagus, a condition with premalignant implications (Fig. 2).Barrett's esophagus is the single most important risk factor in the development of adenocarcinoma of the esophagus, which increases at an alarming rate[10,11]. There is predominance amongst white people, with a male to female ratio of, approximately, 3:1. The prevalence of this condition further increases with age[12]. Smoking and alcohol have only a weak relation with development of adenocarcinoma[13,14]. The length of the affected segment however is important[14,15]. In the past only a small percentage of patients with Barrett's esophagus was identified, and most patients with adenocarcinoma in Barrett's esophagus were not detected at an early stage[16]. Due to more sophisticated surveillance strategies more patients with Barrett's esophagus are detected at early stages[17]. Endoscopic biopsies then allow a definitive diagnosis of Barrett's esophagus and also assessment of histological (premalignant) changes.

2. DEFINITION OF BARRETT'S ESOPHAGUS.

In Barrett's esophagus the squamous cell epithelium has undergone metaplastic change to columnar epithelium, presumably as a result of long standing gastro-esophageal reflux[18]. At present, cancer risk in Barrett's esophagus is considered to be restricted to patients with intestinal metaplasia, i.e., the presence of goblet cells in the epithelial lining[6-9]. The transformed mucosa may have a foveolar, sometimes villous pattern with irregular spaced pits, crypts and glands. Often non-specific inflammation is found, occasionally ulcerating[19,20]. The metaplastic epithelium mainly consists of two cell types, i.e. columnar cells and goblet cells. Further, few neuroendocrine and Paneth cells might be discerned. The goblet cells contain acid mucin, and they stain well with Alcian Blue at low pH. The columnar cells resemble gastric mucous cells and intestinal epithelial cells, although a brush border is not present usually[21]. They contain a mixture of sialomucins and sulphomucins (at neutral pH), and in general do not exhibit staining with Alcian Blue[22] (Fig. 3). Barrett's epithelium needs to be distinguished

H.W. Tilanus and S.E.A. Attwood (eds.), Barrett's Esophagus, 159–166.

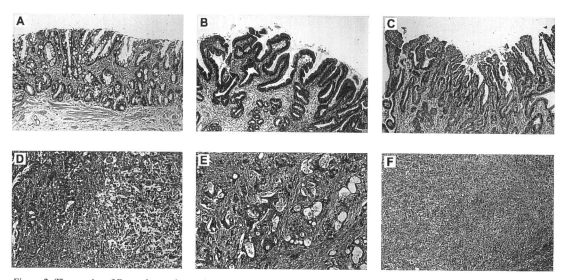

Figure 2. Three pairs of Barrett's esophagus (A-C) with adjacent adenocarcinoma (D-F) in resection specimens, illustrating the metaplasia-dysplasia-carcinoma sequence. A] Metaplastic, non-dysplastic, mucosa, adjacent to poorly differentiated adenocarcinoma (D). B] Low grade dysplasia can be seen together with moderately differentiated adenocarcinoma (E). C] High grade dysplastic Barrett's epithelium and a predominantly undifferentiated carcinoma (F). H&E, 5X objective

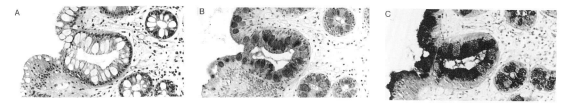

Figure 3. Mucin histochemistry of Barrett's metaplasia (A-C). A] H&E of metaplastic, non-dysplastic, intestinal type epithelium. B] Alcian Blue (at low pH) reveals acid mucin in goblet cells. C] Periodic acid-Schiff reaction (PAS; neutral pH) displays the mucin content of columnar cells, as well as (some) goblet cells. 20X objective.

from ectopic gastric mucosa, which is not considered a premalignant lesion[2,3]. These islands of congenital tissue are mostly found in the proximal esophagus, and therefore in general will not cause diagnostic difficulties. They usually consists of patches of (ciliated) columnar cells without goblet cells being present, and appear as embryonic gastric mucosa. A further distinction should be made with normal intramucosal mucous glands, which aid lubrication and are mainly confined to the lower part of the esophagus. The discrimination between Barrett's esophagus and gastric cardia with intestinal metaplasia is difficult, if not impossible. However, intestinal type metaplasia in the gastric cardia frequently occurs in a focal fashion within the setting of carditis, and the focal appearance might help to discriminate (Fig. 4).

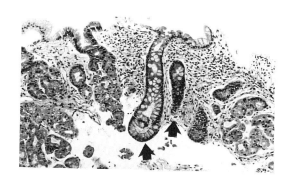

Figure 4. Focal intestinal metaplasia at the gastro-esophageal junction. A few metaplastic glands can be discerned (arrows) in a biopsy of gastric mucosa. H&E, 10X objective

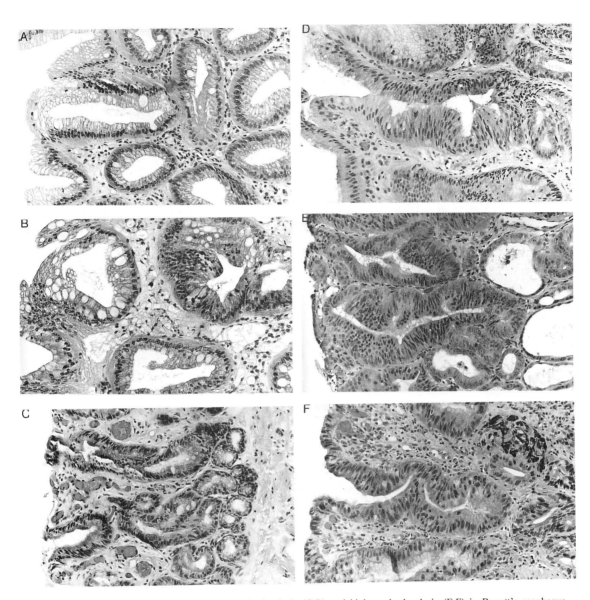

Figure 5. Examples of metaplasia (A,B), low grade dysplasia (C,D) and high grade dysplasia (E,F) in Barrett's esophagus without adenocarcinoma (endoscopic biopsies). A,B] Two examples of intestinal metaplasia without dysplasia: There are numerous goblet cells, the nuclei are basically located in the cells without stratification, and there is no cytonuclear atypia. C,D] Low grade dysplasia: The number of goblet cells is markedly reduced, the nuclei are still basically located, but there is little stratification at several locations, and mild atypia is present. E,F] High grade dysplasia: Goblet cells are generally absent, nuclei are also located at the luminal margin, there is profound stratification with atypia, and mitoses are present in the upper parts of the crypts. H&E, 20X objective

4. DYSPLASIA IN BARRETT'S ESOPHAGUS

Histopathologically, the development of an adenocarcinoma appears to be preceded by epithelial dysplasia (Fig. 5). Often, surrounding an adenocarcinoma in Barrett's esophagus, dysplastic changes can be found. Furthermore, longitudinal follow-up studies have documented the gradually increasing severity of dysplasia eventually resulting in adenocarcinoma. These observations suggest that dysplastic changes might be taken as early indicators of incipient malignancy. This is important because on the one hand patients with

Barrett's esophagus have a 30-40 fold increased risk for esophageal adenocarcinoma, but on the other hand only a low percentage of Barrett's esophagus patients eventually develop cancer. Low grade dysplasia is rather indolent and not a reliable hallmark for malignancy[23].However, there is no doubt that severe dysplasia in Barrett's mucosa is an indication for surgery, since it runs a high risk of developing into adenocarcinoma[24-26]. Often, when such a lesion is resected, focally infiltrative cancer is identified in the specimen. The grading of dysplasia, however, is rather subjective and lacks in interobserver agreement. Dysplasia is defined as neoplastic proliferation within epithelial glands without affecting the basement membrane. In rare cases this might have the appearance of an adenomatous formation[27] (Fig. 6). Dysplasia in Barrett's esophagus is classified as low or high grade in a fashion comparable to dysplasia in inflammatory bowel disease[28]. This implies that the grade of dysplasia should be determined by the features of the most dysplastic region, either surface or base (Fig. 7).

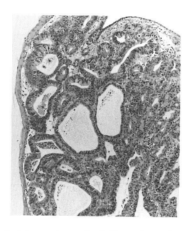

Figure 6. Adenomatous polyp in Barrett's esophagus. High grade dysplastic polyp, partially covered with squamous epithelium. H&E, 10X objective

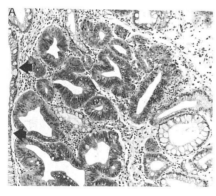

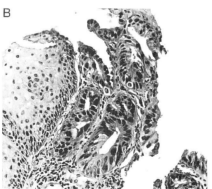

Figure 7. Dysplasia below surface epithelium in Barrett's esophagus (A,B). A] High grade dysplastic glands are present below non-dysplastic surface epithelium (arrows). B] Focal high grade dysplasia below squamous cell epithelium. H&E, 10X (A) and 20X (B) objective, respectively

The criteria for the grading of dysplasia in Barrett's esophagus are cited from Haggitt et al.[6].

- Low grade dysplasia.
The crypt architecture tends to be preserved and distortion, if present, is mild; the nuclei may be stratified, particularly near the base of the crypts, but the stratification does not reach the apical surfaces of the cells; nuclei are enlarged, crowded, and hyperchromatic; mitotic figures may be present in the upper portion of the crypt; and goblet and columnar cell mucus is usually diminished or absent, but goblet cells in which the mucus droplet does not communicate with the surface may be observed. The abnormalities extend to the mucosal surface.

- High grade dysplasia.
Distortion of crypt architecture usually is present and may be marked; it is composed of branching and lateral budding of crypts, a villiform configuration of the mucosal surface, or intraglandular bridging of epithelium to form a cribriform pattern of 'back-to-back' glands; nuclear abnormalities are present as in low grade dysplasia, but stratification reaches the crypt luminal surface, there may be a loss of nuclear polarity, i.e. not perpendicular to the basement membrane, and the nuclei often vary markedly in size, shape, and staining characteristics. Goblet and columnar cell mucus is usually absent. The abnormalities extend to the mucosal surface. In addition, it might be difficult to reliably exclude (micro)invasion within the lamina propria in cases of high grade dysplasia. In fact, beginning microinvasion, defined by an irregular epithelial stromal interface, is considered an integral part of high grade dysplasia in Barrett's esophagus[29] (Fig. 8). Another phenomenon that needs attention is the discrimination of reactive changes from true dysplasia. Especially when ulceration is present one should be cautious in the interpretation of cellular atypia. In these cases it is best to wait for repeat biopsies after adequate anti-reflux therapy. Reactive changes may lead to mild nuclear and cellular atypia, which might be classified as low grade dysplasia. Reactive cytonuclear changes are usually mainly present in the deeper parts of the glands, and do not involve the mucosal surface. This feature can be used to discriminate reactive atypia from true dysplasia. However, in case of doubt the classification 'indefinite for dysplasia' should be applied.

A

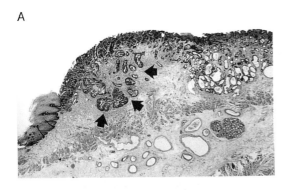

B

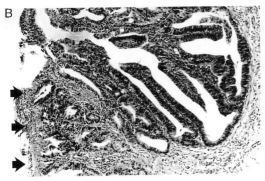

Figure 8. Intramucosal adenocarcinoma in Barrett's esophagus (A,B). A] A well-defined focus of intramucosal adenocarcinoma in high grade dysplastic Barrett's mucosa (pT1; arrows). B] A large atypical gland with a cribriform-like growth pattern amid high grade dysplasia (arrows), suspicious for invasive carcinoma. There is currently no consensus to correctly classify these lesions. Microinvasion is "accepted" within the concept of high grade dysplasia in Barrett's epithelium. However, the large atypical gland could be designated (focal) adenocarcinoma based on growth pattern and cytonuclear atypia. H&E, 1.25 (A) and X (B) objective, respectively

4.   SHORT-SEGMENT   BARRETT'S ESOPHAGUS

Intestinal metaplasia at the gastro-esophageal junction has gained great interest recently, since it might be involved in the rapid increase of adenocarcinomas in this region over the past 20 years[30,31]. The significance of short-segment Barrett's esophagus (intestinal metaplasia limited to the distal 3 cm of the tubular esophagus), which is increasingly being found both endoscopically and histologically, remains controversial. In most cases it seems associated with reflux disease. At present, the risk of developing dysplasia and adenocarcinoma due to short-segment Barrett's esophagus is considered to be low[32-34]. In an endoscopic study by Weston et al.[32] short-segment Barrett's was suspected in 15-20% of cases, and roughly half of these patients had symptoms of reflux disease. Histopathology confirmed the short-segment Barrett esophagus in half of these cases. Another report also mentioned the high prevalence of

intestinal metaplasia in biopsies, when an endoscopic diagnosis of short-segment Barrett's was made[33]. Thus, short-segment Barrett's esophagus is a frequent finding in patients undergoing upper endoscopy, and, importantly, it has also been related to dysplasia[32,34]. The prevalence of dysplasia appeared two times higher in long-segment Barrett's esophagus, than in short segments of Barrett's esophagus[34]. Therefore, agreement exists that patients with short-segment Barrett's esophagus require surveillance, until long-term follow-up studies have clarified its cancer risk.

5. INTESTINAL METAPLASIA AT THE GASTROESOPHAGEAL JUNCTION

Analyses of cancer incidence data in the United States and Western Europe have revealed steadily rising rates of adenocarcinomas of both esophagus and gastric cardia[30,31]. Esophageal and gastric cardia adenocarcinomas have in common that they arise around the gastro-esophageal junction[35]. Esophageal adenocarcinoma is strongly correlated with Barrett's esophagus. Cameron et al.[36] found a 100% correlation between esophageal adenocarcinoma and the presence of Barrett's esophagus. The same authors reported that in patients with a junction adenocarcinoma, which was defined as a tumor centered less than 2 cm from the junction, Barrett's esophagus was present in about half of cases. They concluded that adenocarcinomas of the gastro-esophageal junction are associated with short and long segments of Barrett's esophagus. Intestinal metaplasia at the gastro-esophageal junction was also observed by others[17,37]. All of this might explain the rising frequency of adenocarcinomas at this location. Whether this is related to intestinal metaplasia of the gastric cardia, or to the presence of Barrett's esophagus, or both, is not clear[36,38] (Fig. 9). Intestinal metaplasia of the gastro-esophageal junction is found in approx. 10-40% of patients without long segments of Barrett's mucosa[17,39,40]. Spechler et al.[17] reported that 15-20% of adults undergoing elective upper endoscopy had segments of intestinal metaplasia at the gastro-esophageal junction, which were not recognized by endoscopy. Trudgill et al.[39] also concluded that intestinal metaplasia at the junction is a common finding. In general, it is found in the setting of gastritis or related to gastro-esophageal reflux disease. Histologically, it may be difficult to discern a short-segment Barrett's esophagus from (focal) intestinal metaplasia of the gastric cardia. Recently, it was reported that cytokeratin staining could discriminate between esophageal and gastric cardia metaplasia[41] (Fig. 10). In contrast to Barrett's metaplasia, intestinal metaplasia in the gastric cardia is presently not considered to carry a risk of developing adenocarcinoma. Several studies have suggested that it is strongly related to Helicobacter pylori infection and signs of gastritis elsewhere in the stomach[42-44]. It is clear that distinction between the two sites is essential for patient management.

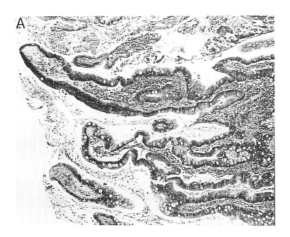
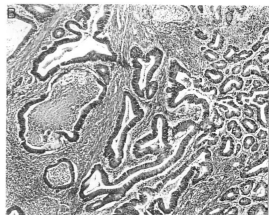

Figure 9. Gastric cardia intestinal metaplasia and dysplasia (A), adjacent to adenocarcinoma (B). H&E, 5X objective

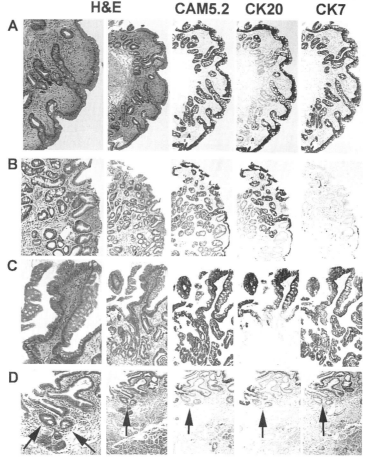

Figure 10. Keratin immunohistochemistry of intestinal metaplasia at the gastro-esophageal junction. H&E, cytokeratin 7 (CK7), cytokeratin 20 (CK20), and a pan-keratin control (CAM5.2) stained sections of:
A] Long-segment Barrett control.
B] Gastric antrum control.
C] Short-segment Barrett's esophagus.
D] gastric cardia intestinal metaplasia (focal; arrows).
Note staining of the superficial part of the epithelium by cytokeratin 20 in all specimens, whereas cytokeratin 7 shows immunoreactivity with the entire epithelium in Barrett's metaplasia, but is negative in gastric intestinal metaplasia.

REFERENCES

1. Barrett NR. Chronic peptic ulcer of the oesophagus and oesophagitis. Br J Surg 1950;38:175-82.
2. Borhan-Manesh F:Farnum JB. Incidence of heterotopic gastric mucosa in the upper oesophagus. Gut 1991;32:968-72.
3. Van Asche C:Rahm A Jr:Goldner F:Crumbaker D. Columnar mucosa in the proximal esophagus. Gastrointest Endosc 1988;34:324-6.
4. Morson BC:Belcher JR. Adenocarcinoma of the oesophagus and ectopic gastric mucosa. Br J Cancer 1952;6:127-30.
5. Paull A:Trier JS:Dalton MD:Camp RC:Loeb P:Goyal RK. The histologic spectrum of Barrett's esophagus. N Engl J Med 1976;295:476-80.
6. Haggitt RC. Barrett's esophagus:dysplasia and adenocarcinoma. Hum Pathol 1994;25:982-93.
7. Thompson JJ:Zinsser KR:Enterline HT. Barrett's metaplasia and adenocarcinoma of the esophagus and gastroesophageal junction. Hum Pathol 1983;14:42-61.
8. Hamilton SR:Smith RRL. The relationship between columnar epithelial dysplasia and invasive adenocarcinoma arising in Barrett's esophagus. Am J Clin Pathol 1987;87:301-12.
9. Reid BJ:Blount PL:Rubin CE:Levine DS:Haggitt RC:Rabinovitch PS. Flow-cytometric and histological progression to malignancy in Barrett's esophagus: Prospective endoscopic surveillance of a cohort. Gastroenterology 1992;102:1212-9.
10. Haggitt RC. Adenocarcinoma in Barrett's esophagus: A new epidemic. Hum Pathol 1992;23:475-6.
11. Blot WJ. Esophageal cancer trends and risk factors. Sem Oncology 1994;21:403-10.
12. Cameron AJ:Lomboy CT. Barrett's esophagus: Age:prevalence and extent of columnar epithelium. Gastroenterology 1992;103:1241-5.
13. Gray JR:Coldman AJ:MacDonald WC. Cigarette and alcohol use in patients with adenocarcinoma of the gastric cardia or lower esophagus. Cancer 1992;69:2227-31.
14. Menke-Pluymers MBE:Hop WCJ:Dees J:van Blankenstein M:Tilanus HW. Risk factors for the development of an adenocarcinoma in columnar lined (Barrett) esophagus. Cancer 1993;15:1155-8.
15. Iftikhar SY:James PD:Steele RJ:Hardcastle JD:Atkinson M. Length of Barrett's esophagus: An important factor in the development of dysplasia and adenocarcinoma. Gut 1992;33:1155-8.
16. Menke-Pluymers MBE:Schoute NW:Mulder AH:Hop WCJ:van Blankenstein M:Tilanus HW. Outcome of surgical treatment of adenocarcinoma in Barrett's esophagus. Gut 1992;33:1454-8.
17. Spechler SJ:Zeroogian JM:Antonioli JA:Wang HH:Goyal RK. Prevalence of metaplasia at the gastro-esophageal junction. Lancet 1994;344:1533-6.
18. Spechler SJ:Goyal RK. Barrett's esophagus. New Engl J Med 1986;315:362-71.
19. Petras RE:Sivak MV:Rice TW. Barrett's esophagus. A review of the pathologist' role in diagnosis and management. Pathol Annu 1991;26:1-32.
20. Reid BJ. Barrett's esophagus and esophageal adenocarcinoma. Gastroenterol Clin North Am 1991;20:817-34.
21. Levine DS:Rubin CE:Reid BJ:Haggitt RC. Specialized metaplastic columnar epithelium in Barrett's esophagus: A comparative transmission electron microscopy study. Lab Invest 1989;60:418-32.
22. Jass JR. Mucin histochemistry of the columnar epithelium of the oesophagus: A retrospective study. J Clin Pathol 1981;34:866-70.
23. Burke AP:Sobin LH:Shekitka KM:Helwig EB. Dysplasia of the stomach and Barrett esophagus: A follow-up study. Mod Pathol 1991;4:336-41.
24. Hameeteman W:Tytgat GNJ:Houthoff HJ:van den Tweel JG. Barrett's esophagus: Development of dysplasia and adenocarcinoma. Gastroenterology 1989;96:1249-56.
25. Miros M:Kerlin P:Walker N. Only patients with dysplasia progress to adenocarcinoma in Barrett's esophagus. Gut 1991;32:1441-6.
26. Levine DS:Haggitt RC:Blount PL Rabinovitch PS:Rusch VW:Reid BJ. An endoscopic biopsy protocol can differentiate high-grade dysplasia from early adenocarcinoma in Barrett's esophagus. Gastroenterology 1993;105:40-50.
27. Lee RG. Adenomas arising in Barrett's esophagus. Am J Clin Pathol 1986;85:629-32.
28. Riddell RH:Goldman H:Ransohoff DF:Appelman HD:Fenoglio CM:Haggitt RC:Ahren C:Correa P:Hamilton SR:Morson BC:Sommers SC:Yardley JH. Dysplasia in inflammatory bowel disease: Standardized classification with provisional clinical applications. Hum Pathol 1983;14:931-66.
29. Cameron AJ:Carpenter HA. Barrett's esophagus:high-grade dysplasia:and early adenocarcinoma: A pathological study. Am J Gastroenterol 1997;92:586-91.
30. Blot WJ:Devesa SS:Kneller RW:Fraumeni JF. Rising incidence of adenocarcinoma of the esophagus and gastric cardia. JAMA 1991;265:1287-9.
31. Powell J:McConkey CC. The rising trend in esophageal adenocarcinoma and gastric cardia. Eur J Cancer Prev 1992;1:265-9.
32. Weston AP:Krmpotich P:Makdisi WF:Cherian R:Dixon A:McGregor DH:Banerjee SK. Short segment Barrett's esophagus: Clinical and histological features:associated endoscopic findings:and association with gastric intestinal metaplasia. Am J Gastroenterol 1996;91:981-6.
33. Pereira AD:Suspiro A:Chaves P:Saraiva A:Gloria L:de Almeida JC:Leitao CN:Soares J:Mira FC. Short segments of Barrett's epithelium and intestinal metaplasia in normal appearing oesophagogastric junctions: The same or two different entities? Gut 1998;42:659-62.
34. Hirota WK:Loughney TM:Lazas DJ:Maydonovitch CL:Rholl V:Wong RK. Specialized intestinal metaplasia:dysplasia:and cancer of the esophagus and esophagogastric junction: Prevalence and clinical data. Gastroenterology 1999;116:277-85.
35. Wijnhoven BPL:Siersema PD:Hop WCJ:van Dekken H:Tilanus HW. Adenocarcinomas of the distal esophagus and gastric cardia are of the clinical entity. Br J Surg 1999;86:529-35.
36. Cameron AJ:Lomboy CT:Pera M:Carpenter HA. Adenocarcinoma of the esophagogastric junction and Barrett's esophagus. Gastroenterology 1995;109:1541-6.
37. Morales TG:Sampliner RE:Bhattacharyya A. Intestinal metaplasia of the gastric cardia. Am J Gastroenterol 1997;92:414-8.
38. Clark GWB:Smyrk TC:Burdiles P:Hoeft SF:Peters JH:Kiyabu M:Hinder RA:Bremner CG:DeMeester TR. Is Barrett's metaplasia the source of adenocarcinomas of the cardia? Arch Surg 1994;129:609-14.
39. Trudgill NJ:Suvarna SK:Kapur KC:Riley SA. Intestinal metaplasia at the squamocolumnar junction in patients attending for diagnostic gastroscopy. Gut 1997;41:585-9.
40. Nandurkar S:Talley NJ:Martin CJ:Ng TH:Adams S. Short segment Barrett's esophagus: Prevalence:diagnosis and associations. Gut 1997;40:710-5.

41. Ormsby AH:Goldblum JR:Rice TW:Richter JE:Falk GW:Vaezi MF:Gramlich TL. Cytokeratin subsets can reliably distinguish Barrett's esophagus from intestinal metaplasia of the stomach. Hum Pathol 1999;30:288-94.
42. El-Serag HB:Sonnenberg A:Jamal MM:Kunkel D:Crooks L:Feddersen RM. Characteristics of intestinal metaplasia in the gastric cardia. Am J Gastroenterol 1999;94:622-7.
43. Goldblum JR:Vicari JJ:Falk GW:Rice TW:Peek RM:Easly K:Richter JE. Inflammation and intestinal metaplasia of the gastric cardia: The role of gastroesophageal reflux and H. pylori infection. Gastroenterology 1998;114:633-9.
44. Chen YY:Antonioli DA:Spechler SJ:Zeroogian JM:Goyal RK:Wang HH. Gastroesophageal reflux disease versus Helicobacter pylori infection as the cause of gastric carditis. Mod Pathol 1998;11:950-6.

3.2 THE METAPLASIA-DYSPLASIA-CARCINOMA SEQUENCE OF BARRETT'S ESOPHAGUS

Anthony C Woodman, Janusz A Z Jankowski and Neil A Shepherd

1. INTRODUCTION

Characterization of the clinical and molecular pathology of the metaplasia-dysplasia-carcinoma sequence of Barrett's esophagus (columnar-lined esophagus, CLO) has only recently begun to resolve the complexities of the disease first described and debated nearly 50 years ago[1]. As with many of the clinical and histopathological features of the disease, the molecular pathology of CLO does not readily or necessarily comply with the known molecular events that occur in other common epithelial neoplasms. Yet failure to unravel the complexities of the pathogenesis of CLO and the molecular pathology of the neoplastic sequence of CLO is potentially devastating: the dramatic increase in the incidence of esophageal adenocarcinoma in Western communities continues at an almost epidemic manner, greater than any other common epithelial malignancy[2,3]. Advances in the understanding of the pathological and molecular mechanisms involved in the metaplasia-dysplasia-adenocarcinoma sequence will surely result in the development of markers of early stages of carcinogenesis and this, in combination with surveillance, has the potential to allow identification of patients at high risk of neoplastic change. This will in turn allow earlier intervention, either by molecular therapy, or perhaps more likely in the near future, early application of ablative or surgical methods of treatment. In this chapter, the pathogenesis and the clinical and molecular pathology of the metaplasia-dysplasia-adenocarcinoma sequence of CLO will be discussed, concentrating on the advances made in our understanding of the molecular changes that underpin the sequence. The following chapter (3.3) also reviews the genetic alterations, but is mainly focussed on Barrett's carcinoma rather than Barrett's metaplasia and dysplasia.

2. PATHOGENESIS AND ETIOLOGY OF METAPLASIA - ANIMAL AND CLINICAL STUDIES

The establishment of reliable and robust animal models of Barrett's esophagus has dramatically advanced the understanding of the pathology of the metaplastic changes that occur in Barrett's esophagus. Studies have demonstrated that esophageal mucosal regeneration occurs with glandular rather than squamous mucosa in the presence of chronic gastro-esophageal reflux, especially acid reflux into the esophagus[4,5]. Recognizing that Barrett's patients have decreased lower esophageal sphincter pressures, the increased frequency and duration of esophageal acid exposure coupled with delayed esophageal acid clearance were postulated as being the main causative events[6-9]. Although esophageal mucosa is relatively resistant to acid reflux alone, unless it occurs at pH1-1.3, acid and pepsin in gastric refluxate cause severe esophagitis in animal and human models. More recently, studies of duodeno-gastro-esophageal reflux into the esophagus have suggested a greater role for such refluxate, and especially bile, in the pathogenesis of CLO.

Several animal and patient-based studies have demonstrated that mixed reflux of acid and bile salts is significantly more destructive than acid reflux alone, suggesting a possible synergistic interaction existing between bile (especially taurine conjugates) and acid[8,9]. Ambulatory clinical studies using the Bilitec fibre-optic system have demonstrated a graded increase in both acid *and* duodenogastroesophageal reflux from controls to patients with esophagitis, and significantly CLO patients exhibited the highest values[6]. Furthermore, conjugated bile acids have been implicated as the component of duodenal fluid which cause mucosal injury. This is of particular significance since the high pH environment created by proton pump inhibitors inactivates these bile acids, whilst bile reflux in non-acidic circumstances, for example in partial gastrectomy patients, does not cause mucosal injury. In the animal model of Barrett's esophagus used by Gillen and colleagues (Fig. 1),[5] repair of mucosal defects was by columnar epithelium in the presence of mixed acid and bile reflux mimicking Barrett's metaplasia, whilst regenerative healing of squamous epithelium only occurred in the presence of bile reflux without acid.

H.W. Tilanus and S.E.A. Attwood (eds.), Barrett's Esophagus, 167–180.
© 2001 *Kluwer Academic Publishers. Printed in the Netherlands.*

2.1 EPITHELIAL REPAIR PROCESSES IN THE METAPLASIA OF CLO

Our understanding of repair mechanisms have been developed and refined in recent years. Early reports suggested that the repair of damaged esophageal mucosa by metaplastic glandular epithelium represented ingrowth of cardiac glandular epithelium in continuity with the injured esophageal mucosa[10,11]. However the elegant animal experiments of Hennessy's group,[5,12] in which a barrier of normal squamous mucosa was left between the gastric cardia and the area of esophageal mucosal damage (Fig. 1), have demonstrated re-epithelialisation of these defects by columnar epithelium. Furthermore, in the canine model,[5] esophageal gland ducts were seen in continuity with the surface columnar epithelium, suggesting that these were the cells of origin of Barrett's mucosa. Recent evidence from a variety of animal models and in human CLO patients support this concept of a multipotential stem cell in the native glandular structures of the esophagus (Fig. 2)[13,14]. Wright[15] has suggested that CLO is a form of ductular migration, similar to gastric metaplasia of the duodenum and the so-called "ulcer-associated cell lineage", arising from the esophageal gland ducts (Fig. 3). He proposes that there is evidence for CLO being such a glandular epithelial repair mechanism in that it actively secretes peptides that promote epithelial repair[15]. Against this is the evidence, promoted by some, that metaplasia occurs from pluripotential stem cells within the squamous mucosa of the esophagus[16].

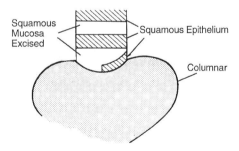

Figure 1. A diagram of the animal experiments of Gillen and colleagues. On induction of acid reflux, the squamous bar across the lower esophagus ensured that any developing glandular epithelium in the denuded squamous area above must be metaplastic and did not evolve from gastric mucosa below. Reproduced with permission of the British Journal of Surgery (Blackwell Science Publications) (from Gillen P, Keeling P, Byrne PJ, West AB, Hennessy TJP. Experimental columnar metaplasia in the canine esophagus. Br J Surg 1988;75:113-5.)

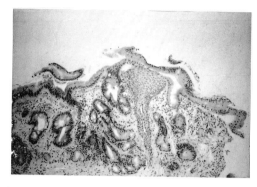

Figure 2. Evidence for multipotential stem cells within native esophageal structures comes partly from CLO patients treated with powerful acid suppressing drugs. Here a small squamous island, itself a metaplastic phenomenon within CLO, can be seen developing from an esophageal gland duct.

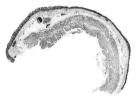

Figure 3. A wholemount section from an esophageal resection specimen. The close proximity of a small island of CLO metaplasia to an underlying esophageal submucosal gland suggests, at least, that the CLO may have arisen from such native esophageal structures.

2.2 ROLE OF HELICOBACTER PYLORI IN THE METAPLASIA OF CLO

There is much interest in the role of *Helicobacter pylori* (HP) in the pathogenesis of CLO and its progression to adenocarcinoma. There is an increasing body of evidence linking so-called ultra-short segment CLO (USSCLO; now better termed intestinal metaplasia {IM} of the cardia) with HP infection and intestinal metaplasia elsewhere in the stomach[17-19]. Conversely, there is increasing evidence of a reciprocal relationship between HP and traditional/classical CLO and short segment CLO.[20,21] It has been suggested that gastric infection, especially pangastric, with cag-A positive strains of HP may be protective against CLO[20]. It may be therefore that the dramatic changes in the prevalence of CLO and esophago-cardiac adenocarcinoma are related to alterations in the prevalence of gastric HP infection[20]. It has been proposed that a crucial determinant of the predominant pathology of the upper gastro-intestinal tract, in evolutionary and epidemiological terms, is the time of acquisition of HP infection[20]. Thus ameliorating socio-economic circumstances and the widespread use of antibiotics may account for a dramatic reduction in HP gastritis in childhood and early adulthood in Western communities over the past few decades. This, in turn, may help to explain the proximal movement in the prevalence of gastric cancer and the increase in GORD, CLO and esophageal adenocarcinoma. Perhaps the most important pathogenic factor here is that highly prevalent helicobacter infection (especially cag-A positive HP), often contracted at a young age, leads to pangastritis and a reduction in acid output from the stomach because of the destructive inflammation within the gastric fundus[20]. The reduction in acid in turn may reduce the propensity to acid-induced reflux esophagitis and thus reduce the incidence of CLO-type metaplasia. Indiscriminate eradication of HP may not be a sensible strategy (at least for esophageal disease) and there must be careful consideration of potential risks as well as benefits of HP eradication policies[20].

3. PATHOLOGY OF THE METAPLASIA-DYSPLASIA-CARCINOMA SEQUENCE OF CLO

It is now accepted that there is a well-defined neoplastic progression from metaplasia through dysplasia to adenocarcinoma in CLO and that the classification of neoplastic change in CLO should conform to that given in Table 1.

TABLE 1. The classification of neoplastic change in CLO

-	Negative for dysplasia
-	Indefinite for dysplasia
-	Low-grade dysplasia
-	High-grade dysplasia
-	Intramucosal adenocarcinoma
-	Invasive adenocarcinoma

Significantly, the risk of developing esophageal adenocarcinoma is estimated to be 30 to 125-fold greater in patients with intestinal metaplasia than in patients without. Thus intestinal metaplasia is now thought to be the most significant metaplastic change within CLO in terms of neoplastic risk. Correlation of the biopsy diagnosis of high-grade dysplasia (HGD) with the findings in subsequent esophagectomy

specimens has shown that HGD coexists with invasive adenocarcinoma in 38-64% of cases[3,22]. This emphasizes the importance of a pathological diagnosis of HGD in CLO (Fig. 4) Yet although the detection of pre-malignant change and in particular HGD remains the best predictor of adenocarcinoma, it is profoundly reliant on accurate pathology and the associated anomalies of subjective assessment.

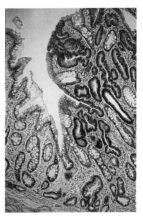

Figure 4. High-grade dysplasia in CLO. The cytological and architectural abnormalities (at right) contrast with the non-neoplastic mucosa at left.

3.1 LIMITATIONS OF CURRENT PATHOLOGICAL ASSESSMENT REGIMES.

It is usually not possible to distinguish dysplasia from non-dysplastic glandular mucosa using routine endoscopic techniques[23]. HGD and even adenocarcinoma can be detected in biopsies from macroscopically unremarkable Barrett's mucosa or can be associated with minimal visual abnormalities such as small erosions, plaques or polyps[24]. These problems are compounded by the vagaries of sampling, as foci of dysplasia may be missed if insufficient biopsies are taken or are poorly directed. Recommended biopsy protocols for patients being surveyed for dysplasia indicate four quadrant biopsies at 2cm levels within the CLO segment as well as multiple biopsies of any macroscopic abnormality such as nodules, erosions or plaques[24,25].

As well as the problems of the endoscopic recognition of dysplasia, there is also considerable inter-observer variation in the histological diagnosis of dysplasia, particularly for LGD[26]. As in other sites in the gastrointestinal tract, dysplasia is characterized by architectural and cytological abnormalities. In LGD there may be minimal architectural disturbance: the pathologist usually relies on

TABLE 2. Useful pathological criteria for the diagnosis of dysplasia in CLO[22]

Low grade
• Cytology approximates to that of mild or moderate adenomatous dysplasia
• Nuclei are enlarged, crowded, hyperchromatic and ovoid
• Mitotic activity may be substantial and atypical mitoses may be present
• Nuclear stratification is often present
• Architectural change, including villosity, may be present but in the appropriate cytological setting
• There is loss of the basal-luminal maturation/differentiation axis
High-grade
• Cytology approximates to that of severe adenomatous dysplasia
• Nuclei are enlarged, usually spheroidal, and have an open chromatin pattern with prominent nucleoli
• Mitotic activity may be substantial and atypical mitoses are usually present
• Nuclear stratification may be present but there is usually pronounced cellular disorganization
• Architectural change, including villosity, glandular budding and complex glandular structures, is usually present
• There is loss of the basal-luminal maturation/differentiation axis

cytological changes to make the diagnosis although villous architecture may be a feature (Table 2). In HGD there is more marked architectural abnormality including villous change and complex and/or cribriform glands. Nuclear stratification and cytological abnormality are usually present throughout the length of the glandular crypts. Intramucosal carcinoma is recognized by the presence of irregular groups of cells or single cells within the stroma eliciting a desmoplastic response. Whilst reasonable agreement can be achieved for the diagnosis of HGD, the main difficulty is in distinguishing LGD from reactive changes[26]. Indeed the intestinal-type glands often show marked nuclear 'activity' in contrast to the gastric-type mucosa and this has considerable propensity for the overdiagnosis of dysplasia [22]. Particularly given the patchwork nature of CLO, the juxtaposition of 'normal' gastric-type mucosa with hyperplastic intestinal-type mucosa can trap the unwary into an overdiagnosis of dysplasia[22]. However these hyperplastic changes are restricted to the deeper part of the gland, the proliferative zone, and normal maturation of the surface epithelial cells is seen. It is our belief that such surface maturation is the most important morphological differentiator between reactive pathology and dysplasia[22]. In contrast to regenerative epithelium, dysplasia, both LGD and HGD, shows loss of the basal–luminal maturation/differentiation axis with the cytological abnormalities extending to involve the surface epithelium. Perhaps the pathologist's single most problem in the identification of

dysplastic change in CLO is the lack of fully accepted and promulgated criteria: Table 2 gives our views on the morphological features that are most useful for the diagnosis of dysplasia in CLO.

The use of an "indefinite for dysplasia" category, analogous to that used in the grading of dysplasia in inflammatory bowel disease, is appropriate in those difficult borderline cases, often in the presence of active inflammation. Early re-endoscopy and multiple biopsies following treatment of the inflammation often resolve the issue. LGD is an indication for close endoscopic surveillance with multiple segmental and quadrantic biopsies. Clearly the early detection and diagnosis of pre-malignant change in CLO remain a priority if the number of cases of adenocarcinoma are to be dramatically reduced.

Yet routine pathology alone, for many of the reasons outlined, lacks the sensitivity to deliver. We believe it important to stress the problems of routine pathological diagnosis of neoplastic change in CLO because it is against this background that we should consider the potential benefits, not only in terms of our understanding of the pathogenesis and pathophysiology of the neoplastic sequence of CLO, but also in the management of individual patients, of our rapidly increasing knowledge of the molecular events that underpin the metaplasia-dysplasia-carcinoma sequence of CLO. As in much of clinical medicine today, the potential of molecular biology certainly as an adjunct to pathology is receiving significant attention. Elucidation of events at the molecular level will aid both the diagnosis and clinical management of CLO, for example by identifying markers useful in the identification progression risk, in addition to prognostic markers in patients who have already developed adenocarcinoma.

4. THE MOLECULAR PATHOLOGY OF THE METAPLASIA: DYSPLASIA: CARCINOMA SEQUENCE

A detailed understanding of the molecular mechanisms underlying the progression of CLO through the metaplasia-dysplasia-carcinoma sequence lags significantly behind the analogous colorectal adenoma-carcinoma sequence. Nevertheless a reasonable working model of the molecular events that underpin the progression of this neoplastic sequence in CLO now exists[14,27-30]. Figure 5 outlines the important pathogenic and molecular changes that putatively occur at different stages of the CLO neoplastic sequence.

Traditionally, the studies of the molecular pathology of the CLO neoplastic sequence have concentrated on five key areas[14].

- Abnormalities within the cell cycle and apoptotic regulatory pathways
- Oncogenic mutations and aberrant growth factor gene expression
- Alterations in cell adhesion
- Cytogenetic abnormalities and DNA instability
- Angiogenesis and proteolysis

Clearly, as in many organs and disease states, each of these aspects is critically important at different stages of the progression process. Yet it is equally important not to view each molecular event in isolation, but rather to take a global perspective. In reviewing the 'molecular timeline', we will focus upon current thinking related to:

- Chromosomal abnormalities and DNA instability
- Proliferation, immortality and cell death
- Disturbances in the cellular microenvironment

5. CHROMOSOMAL ABNORMALITIES AND DNA INSTABILITY

Investigations of gross abnormalities in chromosomal/genomic structures during the CLO neoplastic sequence have received much attention. Several studies have suggested that aneuploidy and alterations in DNA content *per se* can potentially be used as a marker to monitor the progression of CLO to adenocarcinoma[31-33]. These investigations have been supported by independent studies demonstrating that allelic losses (loss of heterozygosity; LOH), an early event in the neoplastic progression of CLO, presage the appearance of aneuploid populations[32,33]. The differential separation of cell populations according to their DNA content using flow cytometry, with subsequent molecular analysis for events such as LOH, comparative genomic hybridization (CGH), DNA mutations and aberrant gene expression has dramatically advanced the study of genetic abnormalities exhibited in cancer.

5.1 LOSS OF HETEROZYGOSITY (LOH)

Allelic loss on the short arm of chromosome 17 (17p) occurs in many tumors including colon, breast and bladder and has received considerable attention, not least because the p53 tumor suppressor gene is located here at 17p13.1 (vide infra)[32,36-45]. Apart from 17p, allelic losses have been described, in the CLO neoplastic progression, at an ever increasing number of loci including 9p, 5q, 13q, and 18q, and a picture of cytogenetic abnormalities in the neoplastic progression is emerging. A possible role for LOH in Barrett's esophagus was postulated when 17p and 5q allelic losses were identified in Barrett dysplasia and adenocarcinoma[34,46]. Subsequently LOH at 9p and 17p were described as early events in the Barrett's neoplastic progression[47-50].

Rather appropriately, Barrett and colleagues have recently proposed a model for LOH during the evolution of the cell lineage from CLO to esophageal adenocarcinoma[50]. The model proposes that allelic loss on 17p and 9p occur as early events, before the appearance of aneuploidy and cancer. The hypothesis advocated is "…..a progenitor clone undergoes expansion, with the development of genetic instability, enters a phase of clonal evolution that begins in pre-malignant cells, proceeds over a period of years and continues after the emergence of cancer"[50]. Allelic loss at 17p and 9p, as well as the related mutations (TP53 and CDKN2A), are proposed as early genetic abnormalities[51]. Subsequently during the neoplastic progression, bifurcation happens, and LOH at 5p, 13q and 18q occur in no obligate order. While Barrett *et al* did not show any

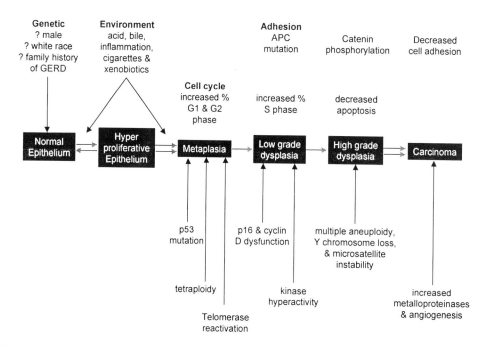

Figure 5. The pathogenic and molecular factors in the metaplasia-dysplasia-carcinoma sequence of CLO. This chapter has highlighted many of the molecular events depicted here although some, and particularly the stage at which they occur, remain somewhat speculative.

obligate order of appearance between 17p and 9p allelic loss,[50] it has been demonstrated that 9p LOH can be detected before 17p LOH[51]. Furthermore, 9p LOH in diploid populations is more common than LOH at 17p, suggesting that 9p LOH may occur in diploid cell populations, and thus before frank malignancy has developed. It is important to note that either abnormality can be detected in the absence of the other, raising the question as to whether these clones arise either independently of each other or from a common progenitor that had one or more abnormalities not being assessed in this study. If 17p and 9p LOH occur independently, patients with either one of the two abnormalities would have to be considered as potential subjects for the development of esophageal adenocarcinoma. A second hypothesis (17p and 9p LOH clone come from a common ancestor with genetic abnormalities not assessed yet) (Fig. 6) probably represents the common view of the progressive sequence.

Whilst the model shown in Figure 6 represents an excellent early attempt at refining and summarizing the important molecular changes in the CLO neoplastic sequence, it clearly remains a gross over-simplification of the complexities and interactions occurring during the progression. Indeed, LOH analysis of almost all 22

chromosomes has now been undertaken for esophageal adenocarcinoma. Frequent LOH has been located on chromosomes 3q, 4q, 5q, 6q, 9p, 9q, 11p, 12p, 12q, 13q, 17p, 17q and 18q[32,49] (for a summary of regions which show frequent LOH, see chapter 3.4, Table 2). Thus, whilst significant research is still required concerning LOH in CLO, it may well be the starting point for the cascade of events we know are involved in the progression to adenocarcinoma.

5.2 COMPARATIVE GENOMIC HYBRIDIZATION (CGH)

So far we have only considered LOH in isolation. Yet a recent study using comparative genomic hybridization highlights both chromosomal gain as well as loss[52]. In this study, the chromosomal alterations most often identified in Barrett's adenocarcinoma were: gains on 8q (80%), 20q (60%), 2p, 7p and 10q (47% each), 6p (37%), 15q (33%) and 17q (30%). Losses were observed predominantly on the Y-chromosome (76%) but also on chromosomes 4q (50%), 5q and 9p (43% each), 18q (40%), 7q (33%) and 14q (30%)[52]. High-level amplifications were observed on 8q23-qter, 8p12-pter, 7p11-p14, 7q21-31, 17q11-q23[52]. Recurrent chromosomal changes were also identified in metaplastic (gains on 8q, 6p, 10q,

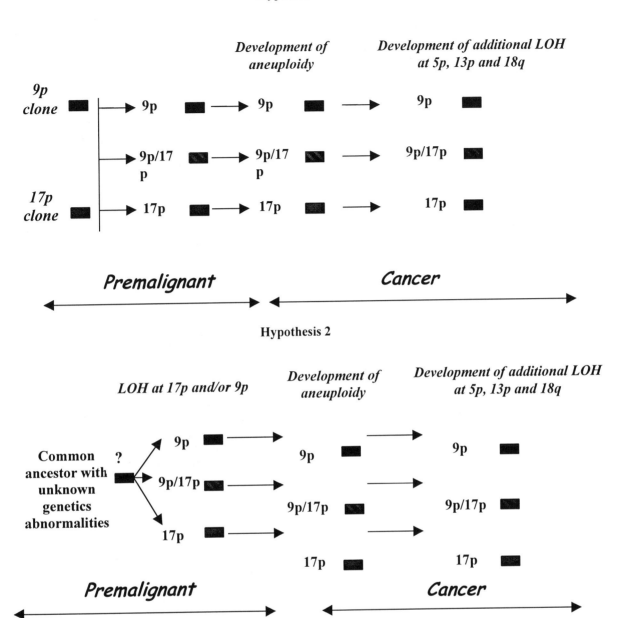

Figure 6. Two hypothesis of the influence of molecular events on the neoplastic progression of CLO

losses on 13q, Y, 9p) and dysplastic epithelium (gains on 8q, 20q, 2p, 10q, 15q, losses on Y, 5q, 9p, 13q, 18q)[52]. Novel amplified chromosomal regions on chromosomes 2p and 10q were also detected in both Barrett's adenocarcinoma and pre-malignant lesions[52]. An increase of the average number of detected chromosomal imbalances from CLO-type intestinal metaplasia (7.0 +/- 1.7), to LGD (10.8 +/- 2.2) and to HGD (13.4 +/- 1.1) were demonstrated. Furthermore invasive adenocarcinoma showed even higher levels (13.3 +/- 1.4), whilst metastatic disease

within lymph nodes showed the highest numbers (22 +/- 1.2). In the following chapter (3.4) Table 1 summarizes comparative genomic hybridization aberations of 3 other CGH-studies in esophageal adenocarcinomas and the candidate genes involved in the pathogenesis.

The conclusion of these complex studies is that, although the detection of common chromosomal alterations in pre-malignant lesions and adjacent carcinomas suggests a process of clonal expansion, the occurrence of several chromosomal changes in an apparently random order relative to one another is striking evidence that clonal evolution is much more complex than would be predicted by linear models[52]. This is probably a reflection of the existence of many divergent neoplastic subpopulations and highlights, once again, the complexities and divergence of the molecular changes in the CLO sequence. It also serves to accentuate one of the potential problems in using molecular analysis in the surveillance of Barrett's patients, in addition to the problems of sampling error[22].

6. ABNORMALITIES WITHIN THE CELL CYCLE AND APOPTOTIC REGULATORY PATHWAYS IN THE NEOPLASTIC SEQUENCE OF CLO

6.1 PROLIFERATION AND APOPTOSIS

The growth rate of any cell population is determined by the balance between proliferation and apoptosis[53]. Apoptosis, or programmed cell death, is one of the more important mechanisms of removing effete cells whilst those cells with DNA damage that cannot be repaired are usually eliminated by apoptosis[54]. Those that survive continue to proliferate, allowing propagation of genetic defects[54]. Changes are seen in the distribution of the proliferative zone of the crypt during the metaplasia-dysplasia-carcinoma sequence of CLO[55]. In dysplasia the proliferative zone expands from the proliferative zone to the luminal surface indicating disruption in the control of proliferation[56,57]. Conversely apoptosis is reduced in dysplasia and carcinoma, perhaps because of over-expression of bcl-2, resulting in a cell survival advantage in dysplasia and carcinoma[57,58]. Our studies have demonstrated the utility of the assessment of both proliferative activity and apoptosis in the differentiation of non-neoplastic mucosa and dysplasia, especially when analyzing the surface mucosa (Fig. 7 and 8)[57]. Perhaps semi-automation of such techniques offers some hope for the non-subjective demonstration of dysplasia in CLO[57,59].

6.2 CLONAL EXPANSION OF IMMORTAL POPULATIONS

The development of an immortal phenotype is clearly critical in carcinogenesis, and recent attention has implicated telomerase reactivation and aberrant chromosomal capping as important in this event[60-62]. Telomerase is a riboprotein responsible for the addition of telomeric repeat

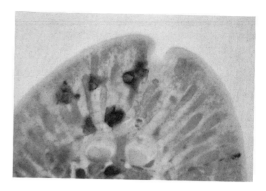

Figure 7. In our experience, apoptotic activity is most conveniently demonstrated by simple morphology. Here the villous surface of dysplastic CLO has been stained using CD45 immunohistochemistry and counterstained with haematoxylin. This allows apoptotic bodies (here sparse and represented by the small black dots (well seen centrally). The immunohistochemistry helps to differentiate apoptotic bodies from leukocytes (staining brown).

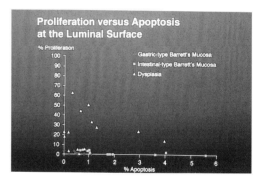

Figure 8. Proliferative activity compared with apoptotic activity at the luminal surface of CLO mucosa. Such a comparison allows a relatively good division between non-neoplastic CLO and dysplastic CLO, although there is inevitable overlap.

sequences (TTAGGG) to the ends of chromosomes, maintaining telomere length and hence the ability to replicate indefinitely. Recent studies, using a variety of methods to detect telomerase reactivation, have provided evidence that the development of an immortal phenotype is indeed an early event in Barrett's progression[63-65]. Our studies, using the telomeric repeat amplification protocol (TRAP), have demonstrated that 50% of cases demonstrating intestinal metaplasia also demonstrated telomerase activity[65]. This rose to 83% in cases of adenocarcinoma and is in accordance with the findings of others who have reported a marked increase in the levels of telomerase RNA during the transition from LGD to HGD to adenocarcinoma, using in situ hybridization to the telomerase RNA template (hTr)[63]. The study of telomerase during the neoplastic sequence of

CLO has also highlighted that a widespread cancer 'field' effect occurs: it has been recently reported that, in addition to the telomerase activity in metaplastic/dysplastic esophagus, telomerase reverse transcriptase activity was significant elevated in histologically normal squamous esophagus in patients with adenocarcinoma compared to normal tissue in patients with no esophageal malignancy[64]. In clinical practice, such a finding theoretically increases the chance of detecting early molecular changes in a minimal number of biopsies, whilst also supporting the practice of radical resection as opposed to local therapy, not only to remove all invasive tumor but also to remove potentially neoplastic tissue away from the tumor[64].

6.3 P53 AND TUMOR SUPPRESSOR GENES

Expression of the tumor suppressor gene p53, located on chromosome 17p, is of critical importance in the promotion of apoptosis in cells with mutant DNA. Whilst wild-type p53 exhibits a short half life and is present in low level, mutated p53 is over-expressed and detectable in many tumors,[38-44] including esophageal adenocarcinoma[32,36,37,45,46,66,67] (see chapter 3.4). In CLO progression, p53 is thought to be disrupted early in metaplasia-dysplasia-carcinoma sequence through gene loss, mutation or over-expression[27]. Studies of the expression of p53 in CLO and associated adenocarcinoma using immunohistochemistry (Fig. 9) have shown that p53 over-expression is relatively specific for HGD and adenocarcinoma but is of low sensitivity (around 50-60%)[36,37,45,66]. Others have suggested that p53 protein accumulation, as detected by immunohistochemistry, has a higher predictive value for malignant progression than the presence of low grade dysplasia and/or mucosa indefinite for dysplasia, demonstrated morphologically[67]. We would maintain that, of all markers currently available to the laboratory, p53 is probably the most useful in terms of substantiating a diagnosis of HGD (Fig. 9) and/or adenocarcinoma although low sensitivity remains a problem. However we would accept that all such markers should currently be regarded as experimental only, of use in research protocols, but as yet of unproven benefit in clinical practice[22].

The discovery of p53 homologues including p73 and p63 and that they can exist in multiple forms has greatly complicated the p53 field[68-70]. All members of the p53 family are transcription factors with very similar DNA binding domains

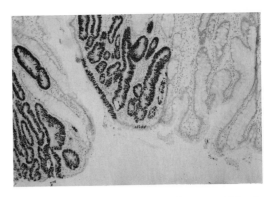

Figure 9. A dramatic demonstration of p53 specificity for high-grade dysplasia in CLO compared with the adjacent negative staining in non-neoplastic CLO mucosa.capable

of binding to p53 consensus sequences and transactivating downstream target genes[69-71]. However there is increasing evidence that there may be a differential ability to activate (or repress) p53-responsive elements[71,72]. Clinically this may be manifest by mutant p53 over-expression altering the properties of p63 and p73 in tumors. We have recently demonstrated an absolute concordance of over-expression of p63 and p53 in more advanced neoplasia, high-grade dysplasia and invasive adenocarcinoma, in CLO (Fig. 10) but have also shown that p63, unlike p53, may be expressed in non-neoplastic CLO mucosa, suggesting the possibility of a role in the control of the cell cycle in the metaplastic mucosa[45].

To understand the function of the p53 pathway and its critical role of carcinogenesis will require the detailed definition of all components of the p53 pathway in human cells and their complex interplay. Thus, while there is often a good correlation between p53 expression and the neoplastic phenotype, the relative failure of studies of p53 to equate with clinically useful parameters in neoplastic, and particularly frankly malignant, CLO may be due to the incomplete nature of our definition of the various components of the p53 pathway (including p63)[32,73].

6.4 ONCOGENES

Controversies surround the importance, in CLO neoplasia, of the oncogene c-erbB2, which produces a 185 kilodalton type 1 growth factor receptor with similarities to epithelial growth factor receptor (EGFR) and with tyrosine kinase activity. Over-expression of c-erbB2 appears to be a late event in the development of some adenocarcinomas arising from CLO,[74] and has been correlated with poor survival[53]. In another study, over-expression predicted a favorable response to chemotherapy[75]. The APC gene, which maps to chromosome 5q21, is a tumor suppressor gene involved in the control of growth and proliferation of epithelial cells, whose malfunction is central to the adenoma-carcinoma sequence of colorectal cancer. Studies have demonstrated loss of heterozygosity (LOH) for APC occurring in adenocarcinoma arising in CLO, in adjacent dysplastic columnar epithelium and also in adjacent non-dysplastic metaplastic epithelium[76,77].

However APC appears to have a more limited role in the development of esophageal adenocarcinoma compared to colorectal carcinogenesis.

As already described, a number of tumor suppressor gene loci have been demonstrated to show LOH in Barrett's cancers, the highest rates (all above 50%) being for VHL (chromosome 3p), CDKN2 (chromosome 9p), Rb (chromosome 13q) and DCC (chromosome 18q)[16,49, 51, 52]. For a more extensive review of oncogenes in Barrett's adenocarcinoma.

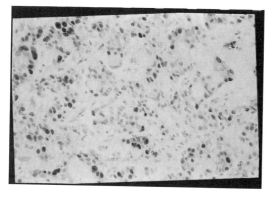

Figure 10. Immunohistochemistry of adenocarcinoma arising in CLO. There is absolute concordance of staining, representing protein over-expression, for p63 (Figure 10a) and p53 (Figure 10b) in these step sections.

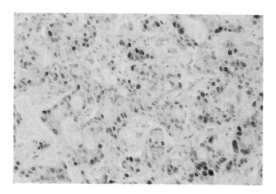

Figure 10b

6.5 COMPLEXITIES IN THE CELLULAR MICROENVIRONMENT

Metaplasia in CLO is postulated to arise as a consequence of clonal evolution of mucin-secreting epithelium from progenitor cells within the native squamous mucosa or alternatively from the adjacent native esophageal structures, the submucosal gland and/or its duct, primarily as a consequence of mucosal damage by gastro-esophageal reflux disease[29]. During the initiation phase of the CLO metaplasia, there is selection of clones of cells, which are better able to resist the injurious insults of duodenal or gastric reflux. Once GORD is corrected the metaplasia never regresses totally and only rarely reverses partially, suggesting that other factors in the environment are responsible for the maintenance/persistence of the metaplasia. At this stage of non-neoplastic metaplasia, there are no known common genetic alterations. However, the environmental mechanisms governing the early adaptive changes are now becoming clearer. It is apparent that, while the luminal microenvironment initiates the metaplasia, the mucosal microenvironment is important in remodelling and maintaining the metaplastic tissue. It is intriguing to note that both the inflammatory cell infiltrate and pattern of vascular development in inflamed esophageal epithelium have a cephalo-caudal distribution similar to that of distally located CLO. For example the degree of papillary elongation and the degree of inflammatory infiltrate are conventional histopathological indicators of the severity of esophagitis.

It is important to ask what molecules might be largely responsible for the bi-directional signalling between the metaplastic epithelial cells and the lamina propria. Cell adhesion abnormalities appear to be pivotal to the neoplastic progression of CLO. A variety of abnormalities of adhesion molecules have been described in CLO. These include CD44, traditionally a lymphocyte homing molecule. Expression of both standard form CD44 and splice variants containing CD44 v3 and v6 in esophageal adenocarcinoma are thought to convey a poor prognosis[78,79]. Furthermore abnormalities of the several members of the integrin family are also described[80, 81]. However it is alterations in E-cadherin expression and its interactions with other closely linked adhesion molecules which have received greatest attention in CLO.

6.6 E-CADHERIN EXPRESSION, NUCLEAR TRANSLOCATION AND THE ANGIO-GENESIS LINK

Loss of membranous E-cadherin expression occurs in metaplasia: in intestinal type Barrett's mucosa, 25% of cases show a reduction in immunoreactivity[82]. In dysplasia, expression of E-cadherin becomes further reduced and disorganised[83,84]. In functional terms, E-cadherin is closely linked to the proteins, alpha, beta and gamma catenin, which effectively provide intracytoplasmic communication with the membrane-bound E-cadherin. Catenin expression shows pronounced alterations in the progression of CLO through dysplasia to carcinoma[84]. Nuclear translocation of beta-catenin and gamma-catenin, in dysplasia and early carcinoma, may well be a critical step in neoplastic progression, the nuclear localization of these proteins having direct effects on transcription (Fig. 11)[84] Reduced E-cadherin expression in CLO tumors has been shown to correlate with shorter survival and expression of catenins may offer similar prognostic information[85]. In this regard phosphorylation of beta-catenin in both metaplastic cells and endothelial cells is one of the early events in the metaplasia-dysplasia-carcinoma sequence of CLO, and this is strongly associated with the degree of angiogenesis, tissue inflammation and the progression of metaplasia to dysplasia[86]. This molecule acts as an adhesion molecule when bound to E-cadherin. Beta-catenin can also function as a signalling molecule when it translocates in a complex to the nucleus, bound to Tcf, enabling transcription of genes of proliferation and migration[86].

Several mechanisms have been identified whereby beta-catenin can accumulate inside the cell. These are decreased breakdown as a consequence of APC or beta-catenin mutations such as those occurring in colorectal neoplasms[87] or increased tyrosine phosphorylation of beta-catenin as is common in CLO[86]. Increased transforming growth factor alpha stimulation of epidermal growth factor receptors is believed to be the major cause of tyrosine phosphorylation of beta-catenin in metaplastic cells. Although the data is preliminary, it is tempting to speculate that phosphorylated beta-catenin, in metaplastic cells, could increase COX-2 gene expression which in turn is known to stimulate angiogenesis by induction of VEGF. Thus not only could the nuclear localization of beta-catenin be important, in the neoplastic sequence of CLO (Fig. 11),

because it has the property to promote transcription, here it may also have a profound effect on stimulating the neoplastic phenotype through promotion of angiogenesis and also by instituting epithelio-stromal interactions critical for the progression of the malignancy.

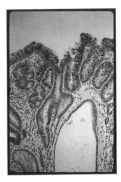

Figure 11.Nuclear translocation of beta-catenin demonstrated by immunohistochemistry in (a) high-grade dysplasia in CLO and (b) adenocarcinoma from the esophagus metastatic to a para-esophageal lymph node. The positive nuclei contrast with the adjacent negative staining in lymphocytes within the node.

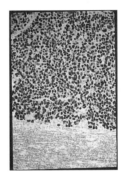

Figure 11b.

7. SUMMARY

As more information becomes available concerning the cytogenetic and molecular abnormalities encountered during the progression of CLO to adenocarcinoma, the more complex the picture becomes. Yet in turn the implications for the development of new diagnostic and therapeutic regimes are encouraging. In particular the coupling of minimally invasive methods of sampling such as balloon abrasion cytology[88,89] with molecular and cytogenetic tests may in turn offer the possibility of tailored cost-effective and appropriate diagnosis and therapeutic intervention earlier with a much greater chance of a successful outcome than is currently seen in routine practice. Application of these technologies to the clinical domain, can, with good fortune, continue to increase our knowledge of CLO at a greater rate than the incidence of Barrett's-related adenocarcinoma.

Hopefully it will eventually significantly impact on the considerably concerning prevalence of this disease in Western communities.

REFERENCES

1. Barrett NR. Chronic peptic ulcer of the esophagus and "oesophagitis". Br J Surg 1950;38:175-82

2. Blot W, Devesa SS, Fraumeni JF. Continuing climb in rates of esophageal adenocarcinoma:an update. JAMA 1993;270:1320.

3. Cameron AJ. Epidemiology of columnar-lined esophagus and adenocarcinoma. Gastroenterol Clin North Am 1997;26:487-93.

4. Bremner CG, Lynch VP, Ellis PH. Barrett's esophagus:congenital or acquired? An experimental study of esophageal mucosal regeneration in the dog. Surgery 1970;68:209-16.

5. Gillen P, Keeling P, Byrne PJ, West AB, Hennessy TPJ. Experimental columnar metaplasia in the canine esophagus. Br J Surg 1988;75:113-5.

6. Vaezi MF, Richter JE. Bile reflux in columnar lined esophagus. Gastroenterol Clin North Am 1997;26:565-82.

7. Vaezi MF, Richter JE. Synergism of acid and duodenogastresophageal reflux in complicated Barrett's esophagus. Surgery 1995;117:699-704.

8. Marshall REK, Anggiansah A, Owen WJ. Bile in the esophagus:clinical relevance and ambulatory detection. Br J Surg 1997;84:21-8.

9. Nehra D, Howell P, Pye JK, Beynon J. Assessment of combined bile acid and pH profiles using an automated sampling device in gastro-esophageal reflux disease. Br J Surg 1998;85:134-7.

10. Barrett NR. The lower esophagus lined by columnar epithelium. Surgery 1957;41:881-94.

11. Spechler SJ. The columnar-lined esophagus. History, terminology, and clinical issues. Gastroenterol Clin North Am 1997;26:455-66.

12. Li H, Walsh TN, O'Dowd G, Gillen P, Byrne PJ, Hennessy TPJ. Mechanisms of columnar metaplasia and squamous regeneration in experimental Barrett's esophagus. Surgery 1994;115:176-81.

13. Berenson MM, Johnson TD, Markowitz NR, Buchi KN, Samowitz WS. Restoration of squamous mucosa after ablation of Barrett's esophageal epithelium. Gastroenterology 1993;104:1686-91

14. Biddlestone LR, Barham CP, Wilkinson SP, Barr H, Shepherd NA. The histopathology of treated Barrett's esophagus:squamous re-epithelialisation following acid suppression, laser and photodynamic therapy. Am J Surg Pathol 1998;22:239-45.

15. Wright NA. Migrations of the ductular elements of gut-associated glands gives clues to the histogenesis of structures associated with responses to acid hypersecretory state:the origins of "gastric metaplasia" in the duodenum of the specialised mucosa of Barrett's esophagus and of pseudopyloric metaplasia. Yale J Biol Med 1996;6:147-53.

16. Jankowski JA, Wright NA, Meltzer SJ, Triadafilopoulos G, Geboes K, Casson AG, Kerr D, Young LS. Molecular evolution of the metaplasia-dysplasia-adenocarcinoma sequence in the esophagus. Am J Pathol 1999;154:975-84.

17. Morales TG, Sampliner RE, Bhattacharyya A. Intestinal metaplasia of the gastric cardia. Am J Gastroenterol 1997;92:414-8.

18. Goldblum JR, Vicari JJ, Falk GW, Rice TW, Peek RM, Easley K, Richter JE. Inflammation and intestinal metaplasia of the gastric cardia:the role of gastroesophageal reflux and H. Pylori infection. Gastroenterology 1998;114:633-9.

19. Hacklesberger A, Gunther T, Schultze V, Manes G, Dominguez-Munoz J-E, Roessner A, Marlfertheiner P. Intestinal metaplasia at the gastro-esophageal junction:Helicobacter pylori gastritis or gastro-esophageal reflux disease? Gut 1998;43:17-21.

20. Blaser MJ. Helicobacter pylori and gastric diseases. Br Med J 1998;316:1507-1510.

21. Henihan RDJ, Stuart RC, Nolan N, Gorey TF, Hennessy TPJ, O'Morain CA. Barrett's esophagus and the presence of Helicobacter pylori. Am J Gastroenterol 1998;93:542-46.

22. Shepherd NA. Dysplasia in Barrett's esophagus. Acta Endoscopica 2000;30:123-32.

23. Levine DS, Haggitt RC, Blount PL, Rabinovitch PS, Rusch VW, Reid BJ. An endoscopic biopsy protocol can differentiate high-grade dysplasia from early adenocarcinoma in Barrett's esophagus. Gastroenterology 1993;105:40-50.

24. Levine DS. Management of dysplasia in the columnar-lined esophagus. Gastroenterol Clin North Am 1997;26:613-34.

25. Riddell RH. The biopsy diagnosis of gastresophageal reflux disease, "carditis", and Barrett's esophagus, and sequelae of therapy. Am J Surg Pathol 1996;20:S31-S50.

26. Reid BJ, Haggitt RC, Rubin CE, Roth G, Surawicz CM, Van Belle G, Lewin K, Weinstein WM, Antonioli DA, Goldman H et al. Observer variation in the diagnosis of dysplasia in Barrett's esophagus. Hum Pathol 1988;19:166-78.

27. Reid B, Barrett M, Galipeau P, Sanchez C, Neshat K, Cowan D, Levine D. Barrett's esophagus:ordering the events that lead to cancer. Eur J Cancer Prev 1996;5:57-65.

28. Fitzgerald RC, Triadafilopoulos G. Recent developments in the molecular characterization of Barrett's esophagus. Dig Dis 1998;16:63-80.

29. Jankowski JA, Wright NA, Meltzer SJ, Triadafilopoulos G, Geboes K, Casson AG, Kerr D, Young LS. Molecular evolution of the metaplasia-dysplasia-adenocarcinoma sequence in the esophagus. Am J Pathol 1999;154:975-84.

30. Biddlestone LR, Bailey TA, Whittles CE, Shepherd NA. The clinical and molecular pathology of Barrett's esophagus. In Progress in Pathology, vol. 5 (eds Kirkham N, Lemoine NR), Greenwich Medical Media, London;in press.

31. Menke-Pluymers MB, Mulder AH, Hop WC, van Blankenstein M, Tilanus HW. Dysplasia and aneuploidy as markers of malignant degeneration in Barrett's esophagus. The Rotterdam Esophageal Tumor Study Group. Gut 1994;35:1348-51.

32. Gleeson CM, Sloan JM, McManus DT, Maxwell P, Arthur K, McGuigan JA, Ritchie AJ, Russell SE. Comparison of p53 and DNA content abnormalities in adenocarcinoma of the esophagus and gastric cardia. Br J Cancer 1998;77:277-86.

33. Rabinovitch PS, Reid BJ, Haggitt RC, Norwood TH, Rubin CE. Progression to cancer in Barrett's esophagus is associated with genomic instability. Lab Invest 1989;60:65-71.

34. Blount PL, Meltzer SJ, Yin J, Huang Y, Krasna MJ, Reid BJ. Clonal ordering of 17p and 5q allelic losses in Barrett dysplasia and adenocarcinoma. Proc Natl Acad Sci U S A. 1993;90:3221-5.

35. Blount PL, Galipeau PC, Sanchez CA, Neshat K, Levine DS, Yin J, Suzuki H, Abraham JM, Meltzer SJ, Reid BJ. 17p allelic losses in diploid cells of patients with Barrett's esophagus who develop aneuploidy. Cancer Res 1994;54:2292-5.

36. Flejou JF, Potet F, Muzeau F, Le Pelletier F, Fekete F, Henin D. Overexpression of p53 protein in Barrett's syndrome with malignant transformation. J Clin Pathol 1993;46:330-3.

37. Hardwick RH, Shepherd NA, Moorghen M, Newcomb PV, Alderson D. Adenocarcinoma arising in Barrett's esophagus:evidence for the participation of p53 dysfunction in the dysplasia/carcinoma sequence. Gut 1994;35:764-8.

38. Greenblatt MS, Bennett WP, Hollstein M, Harris CC. Mutations in the p53 tumor suppressor gene:clues to cancer aetiology and molecular pathogenesis. *Cancer Res* 1994 ;54 :4855-78.

39. Harris CC. p53 tumor suppressor gene:from basic research laboratory to the clinic - an abridged history. Carcinogenesis 1996;17:1187-98.

40. Hall PA, Meek D, Lane DP. p53:integrating the complexity. J Pathol 1996;180:1-5.

41. Levine AJ. p53, the cellular gatekeeper for growth and division. Cell 1997;88:323-31.

42. Vogelstein B, Kinzler KW. The genetic basis of human cancer. McGraw-Hill:New York, 1998.

43. Hahn WC, Counter CM, Lundberg AS, Beijersbergen RL, Brooks MW, Weinberg RA. Creation of human tumor cells with defined genetic elements. Nature 1999; 400:464-8.

44. Prives C, Hall PA. The p53 pathway. J Pathol 1999;187:112-26.

45. Hall PA, Woodman AC, Campbell SJ, Shepherd NA. The expression of the p53 homologue p63 and deltaNp63 in the neoplastic sequence of Barrett's esophagus:correlation with morphology and p53 protein. Gut 2000;in press.

46. Blount PL, Ramel S, Raskind WH, Haggitt RC, Sanchez CA, Dean PJ, Rabinovitch PS, Reid BJ. 17p allelic deletions and p53 protein overexpression in Barrett's adenocarcinoma. Cancer Res 1991;51:5482-6.

47. Galipeau PC, Cowan DS, Sanchez CA, Barrett MT, Emond MJ, Levine DS, Rabinovitch PS, Reid BJ. 17p (p53) allelic losses, 4N (G2/tetraploid) populations, and progression to aneuploidy in Barrett's esophagus. Proc Natl Acad Sci U S A 1996;93:7081-4.

48. Barrett MT, Sanchez CA, Galipeau PC, Neshat K, Emond M, Reid BJ. Allelic loss of 9p21 and mutation of the CDKN2/p16 gene develop as early lesions during neoplastic progression in Barrett's esophagus. Oncogene 1996;13:1867-73.

49. Dolan K, Garde J, Gosney J, Sissons M, Wright T, Kingsnorth AN, Walker SJ, Sutton R, Meltzer SJ, Field JK. Allelotype analysis of esophageal adenocarcinoma:loss of heterozygosity occurs at multiple sites. Br J Cancer 1998;78:950-7.

50. Barrett MT, Sanchez CA, Prevo LJ, Wong DJ, Galipeau PC, Paulson TG, Rabinovitch PS, Reid BJ. Evolution of neoplastic cell lineages in Barrett esophagus. Nat Genet 1999;22:106-9.

51. Galipeau PC, Prevo LJ, Sanchez CA, Longton GM, Reid BJ. Clonal expansion and loss of heterozygosity at chromosomes 9p and 17p in premalignant esophageal (Barrett's) tissue. J Natl Cancer Inst 1999;91:2087.

52. Walch AK, Zitzelsberger HF, Bink K, Hutzler P, Bruch J, Braselmann H, Aubele MM, Mueller J, Stein H, Siewert JR, Hofler H, Werner M. Molecular genetic changes in metastatic primary Barrett's adenocarcinoma and related lymph node metastases:comparison with nonmetastatic Barrett's adenocarcinoma. *Mod Pathol* 2000;13:814-24.

53. Jankowski J, Dover R. Cell proliferation, differentiation and cell death in epithelial cells of the esophagus;a critical review of biological markers and their applications to research and diagnosis. Gullet 1993;3:1-15.

54. Bellamy C, Malcomson R., Harrison D, Wyllie A. Cell death in health and disease:the biology and regulation of apoptosis. Sem Cancer Biol 1995;6:3-16.

55. Gillen P, McDermott M, Grehan D, Hourihane DO'B, Hennessy TPJ. Proliferating cell nuclear antigen in the assessment of Barrett's mucosa. Br J Surg 1994;81:1766-8.

56. Hong MK, Laskin WB, Herman BE, Johnston MH, Vargo JJ, Steinberg SM, Allegra CJ, Johnston PG. Expansion of the Ki-67 proliferative compartment correlates with degree of dysplasia in Barrett's esophagus. Cancer 1995;75:423-9.

57. Whittles CE, Biddlestone LR, Burton A, Barr H, Jankowski JAZ, Warner PJ, Shepherd NA. Apoptotic and proliferative activity in the neoplastic progression of Barrett's esophagus:a comparative study. J Pathol 1999;187:535-40.

58. Katada N, Hinder R, Smyrk T, Hirabayashi N, Perdikis G, Lund R, Woodward T, Klingler P. Apoptosis is inhibited early in the dysplasia-carcinoma sequence of Barrett esophagus. Arch Surg 1997;132:728-33.

59. Polkowski W, Baak J, van Lanschot J *et al*. Clinical decision making in Barrett's esophagus can be supported by computerized immunoquantitation and morphometry of features associated with proliferation and differentiation. J Pathol 1998;184:161-8.

60. Harley CB, Kim NW, Prowse KR, Weinrich SL, Hirsch KS, West MD, Bacchetti S, Hirte HW, Counter CM, Greider CW, et al. Telomerase, cell immortality, and cancer. Cold Spring Harb Symp Quant Biol. 1994;59:307-15.

61. Kim NW, Piatyszek MA, Prowse KR, Harley CB, West MD, Ho PL, Coviello GM, Wright WE, Weinrich SL, Shay JW. Specific association of human telomerase activity with immortal cells and cancer. Science 1994;266:2011-15.

62. Greider CW. Telomere length regulation. Ann Rev Biochem. 1996;65:337-65.

63. Morales CP, Lee EL, Shay JW. In situ hybridization for the detection of telomerase RNA in the progression from Barrett's esophagus to esophageal adenocarcinoma. Cancer 1998;83:652-9.

64. Lord RV, Salonga D, Daneberg KD, Peters JH, DeMeester TR, Park JM, Johansson J, Skinner KA, Chandrasoma P, DeMeester SR, Bremner CG, Tsai PI, Daneberg PV. Telomerase reverse transcriptase expression is increased early in the Barrett's metaplasia, dysplasia, adenocarcinoma sequence. J Gastrointest Surg 2000;4:135-42.

65. Cadd VA, Barr H, Shepherd NA, Warner PJ, Woodman AC. Development of an immortal phenotype in the metaplasia-dysplasia sequence of Barrett's esophagus. J Pathol 2000;in press.

66. Krishnadath KK, Tilanus HW, van Blankenstein M, Bosman FT, Mulder AH. Accumulation of p53 protein in normal, dysplastic, and neoplastic Barrett's esophagus. J Pathol 1995;175:175-80.

67. Younes M, Ertan A, Lechago LV et al. p53 protein accumulation is a specific marker of malignant potential in Barrett's metaplasia. Dig Dis Sci 1997;42:697-70.

68. Kaghad M, Bonnet H, Yang A, et al. Monoallelically expressed gene related to p53 at 1p36, a region frequently deleted in neuroblastoma and other human cancers. Cell 1997;90:809-19.

69. Yang A, Kaghad M, Wang Y, Gillett E, Fleming MD, Dotsch V, Andrews NC, Caput D, McKeon F. p63, a p53 homolog at 3q27-29, encodes multiple products with transactivating, death-inducing, and dominant-negative activities. Mol Cell 1998;2:305-16.

70. Hall PA, Campbell SJ, O'Neill M, Royston D, Nylander K, Carey FA, Kernohan NM. Characterisation of the expression of the p53 homologue, p63alpha and deltaNp63alpha in normal human tissues. Carcinogenesis;in press.

71. Zhu J, Jiang J, Zhou W, Chen X. The potential tumor suppressor p73 differentially regulates cellular p53 target genes. Cancer Res 1998;58:5061-5.

72. Nylander K, Bourdon JC, Bray S, Kay R, Hart I, Hall PA. Transcriptional activation of tyrosinase by p53 links UV irradiation to the protective tanning response. J Pathol;in press.

73. Flejou JF, Paraf F, Potet F, Muzeau F, Fekete F, Henin D. p53 protein expression in Barrett's adenocarcinoma:a frequent event with no prognostic significance. Histopathology 1994;24:487-9.

74. Hardwick RH, Shepherd NA, Moorghen M, Newcomb PV, Alderson D. c-erbB-2 overexpression in the dysplasia/carcinoma sequence of Barrett's esophagus. J Clin Pathol 1995;48:129-32.

75. Duhaylongsod FG, Gottfried MR, Ingehart JD, Vaughn AL, Wolfe WG. The significance of c-erb B-2 and p53 immunoreactivity in patients with adenocarcinoma of the esophagus. Ann Surg 1995;221:677-84.

76. Boynton RF, Blount PL, Yin J, Brown VL, Huang Y, Tong Y, McDaniel T, Newkirk C, Resau J, Raskind WH, Haggitt RC, Reid BJ, Meltzer SJ. Loss of heterozygosity involving the APC and MCC genetic loci occurs in the majority of human esophageal cancers. Proc Natl Acad Sci 1992;89:3385-7.

77. Zhuang Z, Vortmeyer AO, Mark EJ, Odze R, Emmert-Buck MR, Merino MJ, Moon H, Liotta LA, Duray PH. Barrett's esophagus:metaplastic cells with loss of heterozygosity at the APC gene locus are precursors to invasive adenocarcinoma. Cancer Res 1996;56:1961-64.

78. Castella E, Ariza A, Fernandez-Vasalo A, Roca X, Ojanguren I. Expression of CD44H and CD44v3 in normal esophagus, Barrett mucosa and esophageal carcinoma. J Clin Pathol 1996;49:489-92.

79. Lagorce-Pages C, Paraf F, Dubois S, Belghiti J, Flejou JF. Expression of CD44 in premalignant and malignant Barrett's esophagus. Histopathology 1998;32:7-14.

80. Bottger TC, Youssef V, Dutkowski P, Seifert J, Maschek H, Brenner W, Junginger T. Beta 1 integrin expression in adenocarcinoma of Barrett's esophagus. Hepatogastroenterology 1999;46:938-43.

81. Whittles C. PhD Thesis 'The Role of Apoptosis in the Progression of Barrett's Esophagus to Adenocarcinoma. Cranfield University:2000.

82. Jankowski JA, Newham PM, Kandemir O, Hirano S, Takeichi M, Pignatelli M. Differential expression of E-cadherin in normal, metaplastic and dysplastic esophageal mucosa:a putative biomarker. Int J Oncol 1994;4:441-8.

83. Bongiorno PF, Al-Kasspooles M, Lee SW, Rachwal WJ, Moore JH, Whyte RI, Oringer MB, Beer DG. E-cadherin expression in primary and metastatic thoracic neoplasms and in Barrett's esophagus. Br J Cancer 1995;71:166-72.

84. Bailey T, Biddlestone L, Shepherd N, Barr H, Warner P, Jankowski J. Altered cadherin and catenin complexes in the Barrett's esophagus-dysplasia-adenocarcinoma sequence:correlation with disease progression and dedifferentiation. Am J Pathol 1998;52:135-44.

85. Krishnadath KK, Tilanus HW, van Blankenstein M, Hop WCJ, Kremers ED, Dinjens WNM, Bosman FTJN. Reduced expression of the cadherin-catenin complex in esophageal adenocarcinoma correlates with poor prognosis. J Pathol 1997;182:331-8.

86. Jankowski J, Bruton R, Shepherd N, Sanders S. Catenin regulated transcription provides a global mechanism for cancer progression. Mol Pathol 1997;50:1-3.

87. Morin PJ, Sparks AB, Korinek V, Barker N, Clevers H, Vogelstein B, Kinzler KW. Activation of beta-catenin-Tcf signaling in colon cancer by mutations in beta-catenin or APC. Science 1997;275:1787-90.

88. Fennerty MB, DiTomasso J, Morales TG, Peterson D, Karmakar A, Fernandez T et al. Screening for Barrett's esophagus by balloon cytology. Am J Gastroenterol 1995;90:1230-2.

89. Falk GW, Chittajallu R, Goldblum JR, Biscotti CV, Geisinger KR, Petras RE et al. Surveillance of patients with Barrett's esophagus for dysplasia and cancer with balloon cytology. Gastroenterology 1997;112:1787-97.

3.3 GENETIC ALTERATIONS

B.P.L. Wijnhoven and W.N.M. Dinjens

1. INTRODUCTION

It is generally accepted that the transformation of a normal cell into a malignant tumor cell is caused by a multistep process of genetic and epigenetic alterations. These alterations render the cell independent of regulated proliferative and cell death pathways and deliver the cells with proliferative, invasive and metastasising capacities. As a consequence, a malignant tumor is generated composed of cells with an increased proliferative activity, a prolonged lifespan and with metastasising capacity. At least five to ten genetic alterations are necessary to generate the malignant phenotype and most tumors are characterised by genomic instability, facilitating the accumulation of mutations. The genomic instability occurs in two different forms; one characterised by microsatellite instability and the other by chromosomal instability[1]. The targets of the genomic instability are four classes of genes:

1. Proto-oncogenes. These are dominant genes with a regulated role in cell proliferation or inhibition of apoptosis. Upon activation of proto-oncogenes, by mutation, amplification, translocation, etc. these genes turn into oncogenes with unregulated, constitutive activity. This results in excessive stimulation of cell proliferation or inhibition of apoptosis.

2. Tumor suppressor genes. These recessive genes regulate cell growth by inhibition of proliferation or stimulation of apoptosis. By inactivation of both gene copies cell proliferation is activated or apoptosis is inhibited.

3. DNA mismatch repair genes. Inactivation of these recessive genes results in the accumulation of mutations and leads to the activation of proto-oncogenes and inactivation of tumor suppressor genes. Microsatellite instability is a hallmark of the inactivation of mismatch repair genes.[2]

4. Mitotic checkpoint genes. An inactivating mutation in one copy of these genes has a dominant effect on the phenotype (dominant-negative). Inactivation of mitotic checkpoint genes results in aneuploidy.[3]

1.1 PROTO-ONCOGENES

To date about 70 proto-oncogenes are known. They all act in signal transduction from extracellular stimuli to the nucleus or in regulation of gene expression. By this they confer roles in cell proliferation and apoptosis. In tumor cells these genes can be activated to become oncogenes by specific genetic alterations including gene mutation, amplification, translocation, insertion etc. The increased activity of oncogenes facilitates proliferation or prevents apoptosis and both contribute to the formation of a tumor.

Many oncogenes have been investigated in esophageal adenocarcinoma but only few show strong involvement in the majority of these tumors. Overexpression of the epidermal growth factor receptor (EGFR), its homologue c-erbB-2 and cyclin D1 has been found in a high percentage of esophageal adenocarcinomas. EGFR, cyclin D1 and bcl-2 alterations are found already in metaplastic and dysplastic conditions. Other oncogenes like the ras genes, c-myc and c-src appear to be involved in only a very minority of esophageal adenocarcinomas.

1.2 TUMOR SUPPRESSOR GENES

Tumor suppressor genes are normal cellular genes, which primarily are involved in cell proliferation, apoptosis, cell adhesion and gene expression regulation. These are recessive genes, which implies that both gene copies need to be inactivated to contribute to tumorigenesis. Functional inactivation of tumor suppressor genes can be caused by genetic as well as by epigenetic phenomena. Inactivation of both gene copies occurs by combinations of mutation, deletion of (part of) the gene or epigenetic silencing through promoter methylation. In the process of methylation, CG dinucleotides are methylated on cytosine residues and this renders the gene transcriptionally inactive. A number of tumor suppressor genes have been implicated in esophageal adenocarcinogenesis. P53 gene alterations, including mutation and loss, are the most common genetic lesions in human cancers. They occur at high frequency in esophageal high grade dysplasia and carcinoma. A second tumor suppressor gene involved in adenocarcinomas of the esophagus is p16 (CDKN2A, MTS1) located on chromosome 9p21. Loss of heterozygosity, homozygous deletions or somatic mutations in the p16 gene were detected at high frequency in both metaplasia, low and high grade dysplasia and adenocarcinomas. Furthermore, p16 gene silencing by promoter hypermethylation has been detected in esophageal adenocarcinomas.

1.3 MISMATCH REPAIR GENES

Genetic instability can be caused by impairment in DNA repair. Mismatch repair deficiency leads to a mutator phenotype resulting in the accumulation

H.W. Tilanus and S.E.A. Attwood (eds.), Barrett's Esophagus, 181–209.
© 2001 Kluwer Academic Publishers. Printed in the Netherlands.

of mutations. This deficiency is recognised in tumors by microsatellite instability (MSI) or the replication error (RER) phenotype. In tumors with underlying defects contractions or expansions of short repeat sequences (microsatellites) can be found.[2] To date six genes involved in mismatch repair are identified. The genes PMS1, PMS2, MLH1, MSH2, MSH6 and the recently discovered MBD4 (MED1) are all associated with microsatellite instability.[4,5] The mismatch repair deficiency leads to a genome wide accumulation of mutations, also in proto-oncogenes and tumor suppressor genes, and contributes as such in tumorigenesis. MSI has been found in only a minority of esophageal adenocarcinomas. Therefore, inactivation of mismatch repair genes is probably not an important mechanism in the genesis of these tumors.

1.4 MITOTIC CHECKPOINT GENES

A low percentage of Barrett's metaplasia and low grade dysplasia and the vast majority of esophageal high grade dysplasias and adenocarcinomas are characterised by chromosomal instability leading to an abnormal chromosome number (aneuploidy). Chromosome loss can result in inactivation of tumor suppressor genes whereas chromosome gain can play a role in proto-oncogene multiplication. The chromosomal instability is caused by mitotic checkpoint defects. To date eight human genes with a role in mitotic checkpoint control have been discovered.[3] Furthermore, the transforming viral T antigen has been shown recently to create chromosomal instability in human epithelial cells.[6] Involvement of this viral gene in human cancers remains to be established. Mutation analysis of the human mitotic checkpoint genes in aneuploid cancers revealed only few alterations. It is therefore anticipated that genes yet to be discovered are responsible for most of the checkpoint defects found in aneuploid cancers, including esophageal adenocarcinomas.

Genomic instability, at the nucleotide or at the chromosomal level, ultimately leads to the activation of proto-oncogenes and inactivation of tumor suppressor genes. It's believed that in human cells five to ten of these genes need to be altered in order to transform a normal cell into a malignant tumor cell. There are no proto-oncogenes or tumor suppressor genes that are activated or deleted in all cancers. Even comparable cancers from the same organ and cell type never share alterations in the same oncogenes and tumor suppressor genes completely. Although clear from a conceptual point of view, the relevant genetic alterations underlying comparable tumors, like esophageal adenocarcinomas, will show variation in the genes involved.

2. CELL PROLIFERATION AND APOPTOSIS (see also chapter 3.2)

2.1 CELL PROLIFERATION

Renewal of the gastro-intestinal epithelium fulfils the normal functions of maintaining the integrity of the mucosa, repairing mucosal injury, and replenishing the specialised cells of the epithelium. Alterations in epithelial proliferation, including an increase in the rate of proliferation and expansion of proliferating cells beyond the normal zone of proliferation, are closely linked to the predisposition for and development of GI cancer.

The fact that cell proliferation may be increased in Barrett's esophagus was first documented by autoradiographic studies using tritiated thymidine, which showed expansion of the proliferative compartment.[7,8] In order to assess the amount and distribution of cell proliferation in paraffin-embedded tissues, monoclonal antibodies have been developed to detect cell cycle modulators. Ki-67 is a nuclear antigen expressed in proliferating cells, (G1, S, G2 and M phases) but not in resting cells (G0 phase). Proliferating cell nuclear antigen (PCNA) is an indicator of cell cycle progression at the G1/S transition. Several studies used a monoclonal Ki-67 (MIB-1) and PCNA antibody to study the proliferative properties in Barrett's esophagus and adenocarcinomas. In general, an increased number of proliferating cells and an expansion of the proliferative compartment have been demonstrated in Barrett's esophagus and adenocarcinoma.[9-11] Effective intra-esophageal acid suppression decreased cell proliferation and favored differentiation in Barrett's epithelium, but had no effect on the grade of dysplasia.[12] PCNA immunostaining is mainly seen in the basal cells of the neck/foveolar epithelial compartment of the glands in Barrett's esophagus. However, in mucosa with high-grade dysplasia, the proliferative compartment extended upwards into the superficial layers of the glands.[13-15] The PCNA labelling index was highest in adenocarcinoma (25%) and in Barrett's intestinal type mucosa with high grade dysplasia (26%) compared with intestinal type mucosa with no significant dysplasia (20%) and Barrett's gastric type mucosa (12%).[14] Ki-67 staining pattern also correlated with the histologic findings in Barrett's esophagus: the number and localisation of Ki-67 positive nuclei was significantly different between non, low and high grade dysplastic Barrett's and adenocarcinoma.[13,16-19] Interestingly, the increased proliferative activity of intestinal metaplasia in the distal esophagus was similar to intestinal metaplasia at the gastroesophageal junction.[20] This supports an increased risk of carcinogenesis in patients with "short segments" of intestinal metaplasia at the GEJ.

Gillen *et al.* found a correlation between PCNA index in esophageal adenocarcinomas and grade of differentiation of the tumor, but there was no correlation between lymph node status and PCNA index.[11] Similarly, there was no correlation between the Ki-67 proliferation index and pathological features of the tumor or patient survival.[10,17]

2.2 OTHER PROLIFERATION MARKERS: POLYAMINES

Polyamines play an important role in cell proliferation and differentiation. Their overexpression correlates with malignant transformation. The enzyme ornithine decarboxylase (ODC) catalyses the rate-limiting step in the synthesis of polyamines and has a rapid turnover.[21] ODC is induced during cellular transformation by chemical carcinogens, viruses and oncogenes. Its expression is frequently enhanced in cancers and their precursors, as has been observed in Barrett's epithelium.[22] Furthermore, the enzyme activity is greater in patients with dysplastic Barrett's than in patients without dysplasia.[23] However, the concentration of the polyamines appears to stay constant. In adenocarcinomas increased levels of only the polyamine putrescine were found as compared to Barrett's epithelium and normal gastric epithelium, whereas the levels of spermidine, spermine and total polyamine values were lower in adenocarcinoma.[24] Moreover, the distinction between specialised and dysplastic columnar epithelium could not be made by measuring the polyamine content.[24] Nevertheless, because cell strains derived from metaplastic Barrett's tissue were growth inhibited by an inhibitor of ODC,[25] a possible role for these compounds in the treatment of (malignant progression of) Barrett's esophagus has been suggested.[26,27]

2.3 APOPTOSIS

Dividing normal cell populations maintain the balance between cell proliferation and cell loss. Apoptosis, or programmed cell death, is one of the mechanisms responsible for cell loss. The balance between cell proliferation and cell loss is important in maintaining a constant number of cells within a tissue. If there is increased proliferation, decreased apoptosis or both, uncontrolled growth occurs and this may result in tumor formation.[28] Furthermore, apoptosis provides a protective mechanism by removing senescent, DNA-damaged, or diseased cells that could either interfere with normal function or lead to neoplastic proliferation. Apoptosis itself can be

detected by use of immunohistochemical detection of DNA fragmentation as a marker of apoptosis.

2.3.1 Fas/APO-1
The Fas/APO-1 (CD95) gene encodes a transmembrane protein that is involved in apoptosis. Loss of its expression during carcinogenesis can result in the interruption of the apoptotic pathway.[29] Hughes *et al.* found that expression of Fas on the cell surface by oesophageal adenocarcinomas is reduced or absent whereas high levels of Fas mRNA were detected in these tumors.[30] Furthermore, they demonstrated in an oesophageal adenocarcinoma cancer cell line that wild-type Fas protein is retained in the cytoplasm. Apparently, retention of wild-type Fas protein within the cytoplasm may represent the mechanism by which malignant cells evade Fas-mediated apoptosis.[30]

2.3.2 Bcl-2
The bcl-2 proto-oncogene encodes a protein that blocks apoptosis.[31] Bcl-2 is normally expressed in regenerative crypt compartments of the gastrointestinal tract. Increased expression of bcl-2 oncogene is one mechanism by which apoptosis may be blocked in malignant cells and it is hypothesised that this results in a prolonged cellular life span, which renders the cells more susceptible to additional carcinogenic modifications.[13] In Barrett's epithelium, a negative correlation between apoptosis and bcl-2 expression was found confirming the inhibitory action of the protein on apoptosis.[13] However, bcl-2 expression is increased in reflux esophagitis, non dysplastic Barrett's and low grade dysplastic Barrett's epithelium (70-100% of patients), but low or virtually absent in high grade dysplasia (0-25% of patients) and carcinomas (0-40% of patients).[13,18,32,33] Apparently, inhibition of apoptosis by overexpression of bcl-2 protein occurs early in the dysplasia-carcinoma sequence of Barrett's esophagus. The resulting prolongation of cell survival may promote neoplastic progression and cells acquire other ways of avoiding apoptosis as malignancy appears.

A parallel increase in apoptotic rate and proliferation index with increasing histologic severity in intestinal metaplasia/dysplasia and carcinoma has also been noted and it was concluded that suppression of apoptosis does not seem to foster neoplastic growth in Barrett's esophagus and esophageal adenocarcinoma.[9] But others found few apoptotic cells in Barrett's high-grade dysplasia and adenocarcinoma.[32,34] It can be concluded that gradually increased and spatially distinguished cell proliferation is a well-established permanent alteration, whereas the role of apoptosis and bcl-2 seems less certain. Probably, the assessment of the ratio of proliferation to apoptosis may well be more important than the isolated assessment of either. Whittles *et al.* found an increase in the proliferation/apoptosis ratio with progression from metaplasia through dysplasia to adenocarcinoma and this may well be a useful and sensitive marker of neoplastic change in Barrett's esophagus.[10]

2.4 TELOMERASE

Telomeres play a role in chromosomal protection and replication. During normal somatic cell division, telomeres shorten. In contrast, immortalised and carcinoma cells show no loss of telomere length during cell division. Telomerase is a ribonucleoprotein complex that synthesises telomeric DNA located at the chromosomal ends, thereby maintaining telomere length. Telomerase activity has been demonstrated in carcinomas, but not in most normal human cells.[35] The increase in telomerase activity that accompanies most neoplastic and many preneoplastic conditions may permit the emergence of a population of immortalised cells, thereby facilitating the subsequent accumulation of genetic mutations.[36]

Telomerase activity was demonstrated in 87% of tissue extracts from esophageal squamous cell carcinomas, but remarkably, normal esophageal mucosa also showed telomerase activity.[37,38] By using in situ hybridization (ISH), Morales *et al.* detected telomerase RNA in Barrett's metaplasia (70%), in 90% of the low-grade dysplasias, and in 100% of the high-grade dysplasias and esophageal adenocarcinomas.[39] The increased expression of telomerase RNA was in the basal cells of the crypts and deep glands of Barrett's epithelium, similar to the zone of proliferative cells. Like in other renewal tissues, low levels of telomerase RNA were found in squamous epithelium of the esophagus, representing the population of stem cells located in the basal layer.[39] Interestingly, cardiac and fundic type Barrett's mucosa, which is not associated with an increased risk of adenocarcinoma, demonstrated telomerase RNA.[39] Therefore, telomerase is a potential marker for intestinal type differentiation of Barrett's epithelium.

3. DNA CONTENT AND CHROMOSOMAL ABNORMALITIES

3.1 DNA CONTENT/ANEUPLOIDY

Cells reproduce by duplicating their contents and then dividing in two. This mammalian cell division cycle is divided into several distinct phases (Fig. 1). Mitosis or M-phase is the actual process of nuclear division. Replication of the nuclear DNA usually occurs in the S-phase (S=synthesis) of the cell cycle. The interval between the completion of mitosis and the beginning of DNA synthesis is called the G1 phase (G=gap), and the interval between the end of DNA synthesis and the beginning of mitosis is called the G2-phase. G1, S, G2 and M are the traditional subdivisions of the standard cell cycle. The duration of the cell cycle varies depending on the tissue and cell type. Cells can exit the G1 phase and enter a quiescent phase, the G0 phase. Cells can also re-enter the cell cycle in the G1 phase from the G0 phase, a transition frequently regulated by growth factors and mitogenic stimuli. One can asses the relative position of the cell in the cell cycle by measuring the DNA content by flow cytometry (Fig. 2).

A normal cell has a chromosome number of 2N, for which the term *diploid* is applied. A cell with numerical aberrations is designated as *aneuploid*. When a suspension of single cells or nuclei is stained with a quantitative fluorescent DNA dye, the amount of fluorescence is directly proportional to the amount of DNA in each cell.

The cells can fall into three categories: those that have an unreplicated complement of DNA (2N) and therefore are in G1 phase, those that have a fully replicated complement of DNA and are in G2 or M phase (4N), and those that have an intermediate amount of DNA and are in S phase (2-4N).

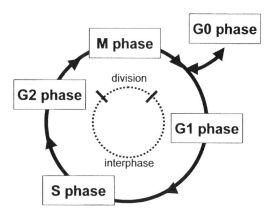

Figure 1. Schematic representation of the cell cycle. Mitosis (M phase) is the process of nuclear division. Replication of the DNA occurs in the S (synthesis) phase. The interval between M phase and S phase is called the G1 (gap) phase and the interval between the end of the S phase and beginning of mitosis the G2 phase. Cells can also exit the cell cycle and enter the G0 phase or quiescent state.

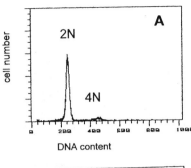

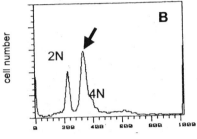

Figure 2.   DNA histograms of normal, non-tumorous cells (A) and tumor cells (B) as determined by flow cytometry. Note the aberrant peak (arrow) which refers to an increased aneuploid population of cells (figure kindly provided by C. Vissers, Erasmus University Rotterdam).

Evolution from a normal to a malignant cell may be associated with changes in total DNA content or ploidy. By using flow cytometry it is thus possible to provide objective information about the ploidy status of the tumor with reference to cells with a normal diploid amount of DNA. One of the advantages of flow cytometric analysis is that it can be done reliable on routine, paraffin-embedded mucosal biopsies. It has been shown that the evolution from normal esophagus to premalignant Barrett's metaplasia is frequently associated with abnormal DNA content, or aneuploidy and increased G2/M fraction (4N) of the metaplastic cells[40-42]. Moreover, abnormal DNA content shows a correlation with the histologic diagnosis of dysplasia and carcinoma[43,44]. Aneuploidy and increased tetraploidy were not found in esophagitis, but were detected in a low percentage of cases with intestinal type of metaplasia without dysplasia or indefinite for dysplasia, in a high percentage of cases with dysplasia and in all cases of adenocarcinoma[42]. Furthermore, flow cytometry detects a subset of patients whose biopsies are histologically indefinite or negative for dysplasia and carcinoma, but who have DNA content abnormalities similar to those otherwise seen only in dysplasia and carcinoma[42,45]. Therefore, this technique (in combination with histology) may be of use in screening patients with Barrett's esophagus for early signs of malignant change[46]. Indeed, prospective studies indicate that both aneuploidy and dysplasia may be prognostic factors for malignant transformation in Barrett's epithelium[41,46,47]. 70% of the patients with aneuploidy or increased G2/tetraploid fractions in biopsy specimens obtained during initial endoscopic evaluation developed high grade dysplasia or cancer.[41] Furthermore, none of the patients without flow cytometric abnormalities on initial evaluation showed progression to invasive carcinoma or high-grade dysplasia.[41] However, others report that histologic dysplasia and aneuploidy are often discordant.[48] Most discordance between several studies can be explained by methodological differences.

Some early Barrett's carcinomas appeared to be associated with a single aneuploid population of cells. Surrounding dysplastic epithelium often contained multiple, different overlapping aneuploid populations.[49] This suggests that neoplastic progression in Barrett's esophagus is associated with a process of genomic instability which leads to evolution of multiple aneuploid cell populations, with the ultimate development of a clone of cells capable of malignant invasion. It is suggested that chromosome instability, tetraploidization, and asymmetrical chromosome segregation during cell division are the result of deregulated cell cycle genes with multiple functions that normally exert active checks on the cell cycle processes including apoptosis and chromosome stability, e.g. p53 and k-ras genes.[50] This concept is supported by the finding that diploid cells with allelic loss of 17p (p53 gene locus) and p53 mutations of patients with Barrett's esophagus, develop increased 4N (G2/tetraploid) fractions and subsequently aneuploidy.[51,52] Furthermore, chromosomal instability is associated by defects in mitotic checkpoint genes.[3] As their precursor lesion, Barrett's adenocarcinomas often demonstrate aneuploidy. Several studies have consistently documented high levels of DNA aneuploidy, typically ranging from 50-100%.[45,53-59] Some studies report that tumors with abnormal nuclear DNA content are associated with increased lymph node metastases, advanced stage disease and/or poorer survival.[54,55,58,59] Moreover, DNA ploidy was shown to be an independent predictor of overall survival in patients with Barrett's adenocarcinoma after curative resection (R0)[55] and in lymph node-negative, R0-resected patients.[59] Others did not find a relationship between ploidy status and clinicopathological parameters.[53,57]

3.2 CHROMOSOMAL ABNORMALITIES

In Barrett's esophagus and Barrett's cancer chromosomal alterations have also been described based on karyotyping and in situ hybridisation (ISH) studies. Karyotyping and DNA ISH may also provide information on cell ploidy. The cytogenetic study of solid tumors by karyotyping is often unprofitable and strenuous and karyotypes are often complex and contain multiple numerical and structural rearrangements. In contrast, analysis of numerical chromosomal aberrations by non-isotopic ISH to isolated nuclei of solid tumors has proven to be efficient and successful. ISH on formalin-fixed paraffin embedded tissue sections created the possibility of chromosomal analysis in archival material. This has the great advantage of preserved morphology leaving different cell types distinguishable and enabling analysis of the tumorigenic cells only.

The most consistent numerical chromosomal abnormalities found in cytogenetic studies of dysplastic Barrett's mucosa and adenocarcinoma is loss of the Y-chromosome.[60-62] In esophageal adenocarcinoma Y-chromosome loss was found in 31 to 93% of the cases. In one study, the frequency of Y-chromosome loss in Barrett's mucosa increased along with grade of dysplasia and all cases of high-grade dysplasia showed Y-chromosome loss.[19] Although Barrett's esophagus and esophageal adenocarcinoma occur more commonly in men, no specific onco- or tumor suppressor genes have been assigned to the Y-chromosome. Perhaps, as genetic instability increases during malignant transformation of Barrett's esophagus, Y-chromosome loss randomly occurs. Other frequent numerical aberrations in esophageal adenocarcinomas are over representation of chromosomes 8, 14 and 20 and loss of chromosomes 4, 17, 18 and 21.[60,61,63,64] Karyotyping revealed frequent structural rearrangements in esophageal adenocarcinomas in the 1p, 3q, 11p-13, and 22p regions.[60,63] Furthermore, trisomies for chromosomes 5 and 7 and translocations involving chromosome 3 and 6 in Barrett's esophagus have been described.[62] Recently, common numeric chromosome abnormalities in 12 esophageal adenocarcinomas were identified using fluorescence ISH.[65] The most common numeric abnormalities detected were gains of chromosomes 6, 7, 11 and 12. In a subset of cases in which premalignant lesions were examined, aneusomy of these chromosomes was found to be an early change, frequently present in both Barrett's esophagus and dysplastic regions. It remains to be determined whether any of these abnormalities are predictive markers of progression to malignancy.

4. MICROSATELLITE INSTABILITY

A form of genetic instability that has recently been identified is microsatellite instability (MSI). Microsatellites are mostly highly polymorphic short, tandem repeat DNA sequences. They are abundantly and evenly distributed throughout the genome. MSI is caused by a failure of the DNA mismatch repair (MMR) system to repair errors that occur during the replication of DNA and is characterized by the accumulation of single

nucleotide mutations and alterations in length of simple, repetitive microsatellite sequences that occur throughout the genome. This widespread MSI is a characteristic feature of tumors from Hereditary Non-Polyposis Colorectal Cancer (HNPCC) kindreds.[66] The microsatellite instability detected in these tumors is a phenotypic manifestation of an underlying defect in DNA mismatch repair. Four genes involved in DNA MMR have been found to be mutated in the germ line of HNPCC families. The replication error (RER) phenotype is also associated with sporadic tumors including those of breast, stomach, bladder and lung.

Meltzer et al. reported microsatellite instability at one or more chromosomal loci of the 5 dinucleotide repeats tested in 2/28 (7%) patients with Barrett's metaplasia and 8/36 (22%) esophageal adenocarcinomas.[67] Among 25 flow cytometry sorted adenocarcinomas, instability occurred in 8 (32%). In 4 of these 8 positive cases, the diploid component of the tumor showed instability suggesting that the instability may develop as an early event in Barrett's associated neoplastic progression.[67] In a series of 69 esophageal adenocarcinomas, we found 7 MSI cases with 3 MSI markers tested.[68] However, there remains confusion as how to define the phenomenon of MSI, specifically, how many markers should be used, and how many must display instability before the tumor is defined as having MSI. Because of the absence of uniform criteria defining MSI, there has been considerable variability in the frequency of MSI reported within a given tumor type. According to more stringent definition of MSI, Gleeson et al. found that MSI is infrequent in Barrett's esophagus-associated adenocarcinomas and adenocarcinomas of the gastric cardia.[69,70] Alterations in microsatellite alleles were detected in all Barrett's adenocarcinomas, but only a single tumor (1/17=6%) exhibited ubiquitous somatic mutations throughout the genome (>45% of the loci tested) and a varying level of microsatellite alterations (ranging from 0.8 to 8.1% of loci tested) in the remaining (94%) tumors.[69] Gleeson et al. also detected a shared pattern of novel microsatellite alleles in premalignant and malignant Barrett's epithelium which is consistent with a process of clonal expansion underlying the histological progression of Barrett's epithelium. Several studies have confirmed the low prevalence of MSI, between 5-10%, in esophageal adenocarcinomas.[71-75] Interestingly, Wu et al. found a trend towards an improved survival for esophageal adenocarcinomas demonstrating MSI.[75] It is not yet known which mismatch repair genes are responsible for the microsatellite instability observed in Barrett's adenocarcinoma.

5. GENOME WIDE SCREENING FOR GENETIC ALTERATIONS

5.1 COMPARATIVE GENOMIC HYBRIDIZATION

In 1992 a new technique to screen the whole genome of cancer cells for genetic alterations was introduced: Comparative Genomic Hybridization (CGH).[76] This technique allows genome-wide screening for chromosomal imbalances without the need for metaphase cell preparations. In CGH, whole genomic tumor DNA and normal genomic control DNA are differentially labelled and cohybridized to normal metaphase chromosomes. After detection via different fluorochromes, the ratio of the fluorescence intensities generated by tumor and control probes allows one to identify over- and underrepresentations of chromosomes or chromosome segments in the tumor genome (Fig. 3).

Thus far, 4 studies have been published that applied this technique to a series of esophageal (Barrett and non-Barrett) adenocarcinomas, adenocarcinomas of the gastroesophageal junction and adenocarcinomas of the proximal stomach.[77-80] Multiple copy number imbalances at many locations in the genome were observed in all studies, suggesting genetic complexity. There were discrepancies between the studies in terms of chromosomal regions with gains and losses. However, there are also consistent areas of genetic gains and loss in these studies. Table 1 shows the most common regions of loss and gain and the candidate genes that may be involved in these cancers. Recently, Walch et al. published another CGH study in Barrett's metaplasia and adenocarcinoma (see chapter 3.2). Frequent gains are seen at 7p, 8q, 12q, 17q and 20q, and frequent loss at 4q, 5q, 9p and 18q. Most areas of loss and gain harbor known tumor suppressor genes or proto-oncogenes possibly involved in the tumorigenesis of esophageal adenocarcinomas. However, for example the amplicon 12q is not easily attributed to a candidate gene because this has not been described before as putative oncogenic site. The DNA copy gain of chromosome arm 20q is consistent with data from other carcinomas, including breast and colon cancer.[81] It is suggested that chromosome 20q harbors several proto-oncogenes whose activation contributes to tumorigenesis.[81]

So far, no studies on CGH analysis in Barrett's esophagus have been published. Preliminary data from our lab show that losses of chromosome 5q21-23 (APC, MCC), 9p21 (p16), 17p (p53) and 18q21 (DCC) are already present in low grade dysplastic Barrett's epithelium and that gains of chromosomes 7p12-15 (EGFR) and 17q21 (erBb-2) occur in the transition from low grade to high grade Barrett's dysplasia (Dr. H. van Dekken, personal communication).

5.2 ALLELOTYPING

Microsatellite allelotyping or loss of heterozygosity (LOH) analysis is also a useful technique to define areas of common deletion in esophageal adenocarcinomas. The LOH analysis uses polymorphic microsatellite repeats. These repeats are present on all chromosomes and multiple allelic forms (different sizes) are present. For example, the size of a repeat (=marker) on the long arm of chromosome 14 (14q) differs between the maternal and paternal chromosome. Frequent loss of one allele involving a chromosomal arm or locus suggests the presence, at or near that locus, of a tumor suppressor gene important in the tumor (Fig. 4). Therefore, LOH studies can lead to the identification of tumor suppressor genes that are inactivated in the metaplasia-dysplasia-carcinoma progression, and may therefore also be useful as biomarkers of future carcinogenesis in patients with Barrett's metaplasia and dysplasia undergoing endoscopic evaluation.

TABLE 1. Summary of CGH aberrations in esophageal adenocarcinomas and adenocarcinomas of the gastroesophageal junction. Where possible, the minimal region of overlapping loss or gain and the candidate genes are given.

chromosome number	Frequent gain (% of the tumors)				Frequent loss (% of the tumors)			
	van Dekken et al. n=28	**El-Rifai et al. n=8	Mosaluk et al. n=15	Candidate genes	van Dekken et al. n=28	**El-Rifai et al. n=8	Mosaluk et al. n=15	Candidate genes
1	1q (36)	1q (63)						
2		2q11-21.2 (63)						
3	3q (32)	3q21-qter (50)		CACY	3p14 (21)	3q21-qter (50)		FHIT, RCA1
4					4pq (54)	4q23-26 (75)	4p13-4q21(44)	
5	5p14 (32)				5q14-21 (36)	5q14-22 (75)	5q13-15 (53)	APC, MCC
6	6p12-21.1 (32)	6p11-21.3 (75)		MLV12 p :NRASL3, PIM-1 q: MYB				
7	7p12 (79)	7q21.2-22.1 (75)	7p11-15 (47)+ 7q21-22 (33)	EGFR, PGY1				
8	8q23-24.1	8q22.2-qter (63)	8q24 (53) + 8p23 (33)	MYC				
9	9q13.1		9q31-34 (27)		9p21 (29)	9p21-qter		p15/p16
12	12q21.1 (39)	12q13-14 (50)	12q21-24 (27)	FKHR		12q13-14 (50)		
13	13q (46)							
14				AKT2, IGF1R, BCL3	14q31-32.1 (46)			TSHR
15	15q25 (39)		15q26 (27)					
16					16q 23 (36)			
17	17q12-21 (29)	17q (75)	17q21 (47)	ERBB2	17p (27)			p53
18	18p (25)		18p11 (27)		18q21 (43)		18q (20)	DCC, DPC4, PI5
19	19q3l.1 (32)							
20	20p12 + 20q12-13 (86)	20q13 (100)	20q (47)	TGFβ p: PCNA q: MYBL2, PTPN1, PIPN1,AB1, AIB3				
21					21q21 (29)			
X	Xpq (32)							
Y					Y (64)		Y (71)	

Abbreviations used in the table are: MCC, mutated in colorectal cancer; APC, adenomatous polyposis coli; CDKN2A/B, cyclin dependent kinase 2A/2B; DCC, deleted in pancreatic carcinoma, locus 4; FHIT, fragile histidine triad gene; MLV12, MoMuLV integration site 2; NRASL3, v-ras neuroblastoma RAS-like oncogene 3; EGFR, epidermal growth factor receptor; MYC, v-myc myelocytomatosis oncogene; ERBB2, oncogene 2; TGFβ1, transforming growth factor β1; BCL3, B-cell CLL/lymphoma; AKT2, v-akt murine thymoma oncogene 2; PCNA, proliferating cell nuclear antigen; MYBL2, v-myb myelolastosis-like oncogene 2; PTPN1, protein tyrosine phosphatase nonreceptor type 1; TSHR, thyroid stimulating hormone receptor; IGF1R, insulin-like growth factor 1 receptor; PIM-1, proto-oncogene encoding a tyrosine kinase; PGY1, a multidrug resistance gene; FKHR, member of forkhead family of transcription factors, AIB1/3/4, steroid receptor coactivator genes; CACY, calcylin: calcium binding protein of S100 family; PI5, serine protease inhibitor; RCA1, regulator of cyclin A1.
* The study by Du Plessis et al. is not shown in this table since only 2 esophageal adenocarcinomas were studied.
** This study performed CGH analysis on xenografts of the gastroesophageal junction as well as proximal stomach.

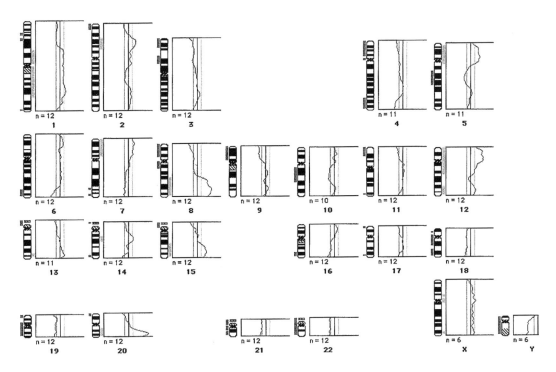

Figure 3.   Chromosomal ideograms showing DNA copy number changes detected by CGH in a male patient with an adenocarcinoma of the esophagus. Bars on the left and right side of the chromosomal ideograms indicate under- and overrepresentations of genetic material, respectively. Note the clear losses on 3p (FHIT), 5q (APC/MCC), 9p (p16), 18q (DCC/DPC4) and Y, as well as the gains on, 7p (EGFR), 8q (myc) and 20q (PCNA) (figure kindly provided by Dr. H. van Dekken, Erasmus University, Rotterdam).

Several groups have evaluated chromosomal regions for LOH in Barrett's esophagus-associated neoplasia and adenocarcinomas of the gastroesophageal junction. Four allelotyping studies have been performed on esophageal adenocarcinomas using a substantial number of polymorphic markers from (almost) every chromosomal arm.[73,74,82,83] In these studies, also the fractional allele loss (FAL) was calculated as the number of chromosomal arms displaying LOH divided by the number of informative chromosomal arms. It was suggested that FAL is an indicator of aneuploid DNA content and that the FAL reflects the quantity of genetic abnormality. In esophageal adenocarcinomas, the mean FAL was between 0.2 and 0.4, indicating that on average each tumor demonstrated LOH on 20-40% of its chromosomal arms.[73,74,82,83] This is significantly higher than the FAL in other carcinomas.[74] FAL was not related to grade of the tumor, survival or the level of ploidy, but a significant trend for FAL to increase with increasing depth of invasion was found.[73,74] Besides identification of regions that frequently show allelic loss, the background allelic loss can be estimated. The estimated background frequency of allelic loss, i.e. random loss of chromosomal regions due to genetic instability of

the tumor, was 0.23 in a study from Barrett et al. and 0.15 in a study from Dolan et al.[73,74] Table 2 summarises the regions of allelic loss in esophageal adenocarcinomas that occur with high frequency (>40% of the informative cases) and which presumably reflect true putative tumor suppressor gene loci.

In the following section we will discuss the chromosomal regions displaying frequent LOH and the (putative) tumor suppressor genes involved in the pathogenesis of Barrett's adenocarcinomas.

6. TUMOR SUPPRESSOR GENES

6.1 CHROMOSOME 3p: FHIT, VHL AND PPARγ

6.1.1 FHIT
Fragile sites are genomic regions that predispose for structural chromosome aberrations such as translocations or deletions, especially following exposure to toxins. The distribution of common fragile sites parallels the positions of neoplasia-associated chromosomal rearrangements, prompting the proposal that fragility disposes to

chromosomal rearrangements. Implicit in this hypothesis is that genes at fragile sites are altered by chromosome rearrangements and thus contribute to neoplastic growth.[103] Chromosome band 3p14.3 harbors the most inducible common fragile region. This region has been cloned and the Fragile Histidine Triad (FHIT) gene characterised. The FHIT gene is a promising candidate tumor suppressor gene, since aberrant transcripts have been found in a significant proportion of cancer-derived cell lines and primary tumors of the gastro-intestinal tract.[104,105] However, the role of FHIT as a tumor suppressor has been questioned: its apparent involvement might simply reflect its location within an unstable region of the genome.

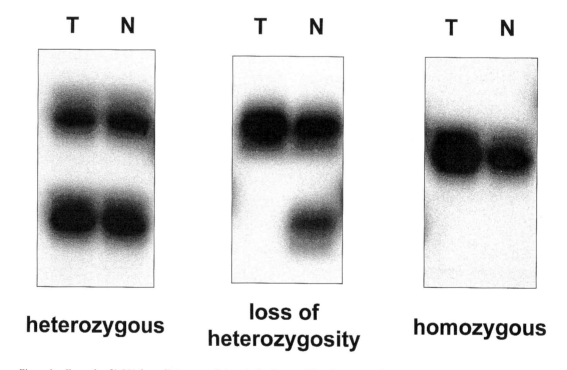

Figure 4.   Example of LOH (loss of heterozygosity) analysis of tumor (T) and corresponding normal (N) DNA derived from a single patient using polymorphic microsatellite repeats. The left panel shows a microsatellite marker for which the patient is heterozygous: there is a difference in size between both alleles. The panel in the middle shows a marker with LOH in the tumor when compared to corresponding normal DNA. The panel on the right shows a marker for which the patient is homozygous: no difference in size between the alleles.

In Barrett's esophagus and associated adenocarcinomas, alterations of the FHIT transcripts (FHIT mRNA lacking one or more exons or homo- or hemizygous deletions of the gene) were observed in 86 and 93%, respectively.[106] Another study found low rates of alterations in the FHIT open reading frame in primary esophageal cancers, although lack of expression of FHIT transcripts was common in esophageal cancer cell lines.[107] However, aberrant FHIT transcripts have also been detected in normal, non-cancerous tissues of the gastro-intestinal tract.[105] This suggests that the aberrant transcripts in the metaplastic and carcinomatous areas may have been induced by exposure to toxic agents (duodeno-gastroesophageal reflux) that affect the fragile site.[29,105]

6.1.2 VHL and PPAR

One study reported frequent (65%) loss of chromosome 3p encompassing 3p24-26. Among the candidate tumor suppressor genes on 3p, the Von Hippel Lindau (VHL) gene and the gene encoding the peroxidase proliferator activated receptor-gamma (PPARγ) are located within this region. The VHL gene is mutated in the germline of patients with VHL disease, which develop multiple benign and malignant tumors including pheochromocytomas, haemangiomas and pancreatic cysts.[108] PPARγ is a member of the nuclear receptor superfamily involved in fat cell differentiation and glucose homeostasis, but it also regulates differentiation and/or cell growth.[109] Loss of function mutations in this gene are found in colon cancer. We screened adenocarcinomas of the esophagus and gastroesophageal junction for genetic alterations in the VHL and PPARγ gene. However, we could not detect mutations in these genes (Lindstedt *et al.*, manuscript in preparation). Since we also detected a high percentage of LOH at the VHL locus, another putative tumor suppressor gene at 3p could be involved in the carcinogenesis of esophageal adenocarcinomas.

6.2 CHROMOSOME 5q: MCC AND APC

The MCC (mutated in colorectal carcinoma) gene is located on 5q.[110] LOH at the MCC locus has been reported in 63% of the cases with esophageal carcinoma.[87] So far, no reports have been published on MCC mutation analysis in esophageal adenocarcinomas. Observations from colorectal and gastric cancers suggests that, despite the high frequency of LOH of the MCC gene, mutation of the retained MCC allele is uncommon.[111,112]

TABLE 2. Summary of chromosomal regions which show frequent LOH (>40% of esophageal adenocarcinomas).

Chromosome Arm	No. of tumors with LOH/informative cases (%)	Minimal area of loss	Candidate genes	Mutations	References
3p	14/22 (64)	3p24-26	VHL, PPARγ	No	74
3q	11/17 (65)	3qter	unknown		83,84
4q	57/81 (70%)	4q21.1-22	unknown		82,83,85
		4q32-33	"		
		4q35	"		
5q	10/22 (45)	5q11.2-13.3	MSH3	?	74,83,86-88
	99/138 (72)	5q21-22	APC	rare	
			MCC	no	
			IRF-1	?	
5pq	4/9 (44)	5p12	unknown		89
	2/4 (50)	5q31.1	"		
6q	10/17 (56)	6qter	unknown		83
9p	81/131 (61)	9p21.1-22	p15	no	74,83,90-93
			p16	yes	
			IFNA	?	
9q	8/17 (47)	9qter	unknown		83
11p	8/15 (53)	11p15	p57KIP2, TSG101,WT2,	?	74
	14/23 (61)	11p15.5	H19	?	
12p	8/17 (47)	12pter	unknown		83
12q	11/17 (76)	12qter	unknown		83
13q	62/133 (47)		Rb	rare	73,74,94-97
16q	31/48 (65)	16q22	E-cadherin	none	98
17p	124/166 (75)	17p11.2-13.3	OVCA1/2, HIC1	?	73,82,83,94,96,99,100
			TP53	frequent	
17q	81/131 (63)	17q11.2-12	NF1, CSF3, erbB-2,	?	74,99,101,102
		17q21	ITB4,	?	
		17q24-25	BRCA1	?	
		17q25-ter	GH, TOC	?	
			unknown		
18q	40/68 (59)	18q22.1	DCC, DPC4	no	73,74,82
			Smad-2	?	

IFNA, interferon-alfa gene; NF1, neurofibromatosis gene; CSF3, colony stimulating factor 3; erbB-2, member of epidermal growth factor receptor family; ITB4, integrin-beta 4 ; MSH3, DNA mismatch repair gene; Rb, retinoblastoma; VHL, Von Hippel Lindau gene; PPARγ, peroxidase proliferator-activated receptor-γ; MCC, mutated in colorectal cancer; APC, adenomatous polyposis coli; IRF-1, interferon regulatory factor 1; TOC, tylosis esophageal cancer gene; DCC, deleted in colorectal carcinoma; DPC4, deleted in pancreatic carcinoma, locus 4; TP53, p53 tumor suppressor gene; BRCA1, breast cancer gene 1; WT2, Wilms's tumor suppressor gene; H19, gene involved in genomic imprinting; P57KIP2, a cyclin dependent kinase inhibitor; HIC1, zinc finger domain; OVCA1/2, ovarian cancer tumor suppressor genes 1 and 2; GH, growth hormone gene; Smad-2, signal transduction molecule involved in TGF-β signaling pathway. ?, no mutation analysis performed

This suggests that MCC does not function as a tumor suppressor gene in gastro-intestinal malignancies.

The APC gene is also a target of LOH on chromosome 5q21-22. LOH of the APC locus on 5q has been found in esophageal adenocarcinomas as well as in the surrounding high grade dysplastic Barrett's epithelium. Furthermore, the patterns of allelic loss of the APC gene were identical in all stages of neoplastic progression, suggesting the emergence of a clonal population of cells.[87] LOH has not been found in Barrett's metaplasia or low grade Barrett's dysplasia,[92] where alterations of the p53 tumor suppresor gene are already apparent. It is suggested that p53-LOH (17p)

precedes or is concurrent with APC allelic loss.[92,113] This is different from colon cancer, in which it is believed that 5q allelic loss precedes 17p allelic loss.[114] While APC mutations were found frequently in colorectal cancers, a very low rate of APC mutations in esophageal cancers was detected,[92,115,116] although in most studies not the whole coding sequence of the gene was screened for mutations. This raised the possibility that a gene distinct from APC may be the target of the frequent LOH on 5q. Ogasawara et al. (GE 1996) determined the smallest common deleted region in esophageal cancers.[115] They concluded that deletion of the APC locus may just be the result of large deletions on 5q and may not be important in esophageal carcinogenesis. The Interferon Regulatory Factor1 (IRF-1) gene or other gene(s) on 5q31.1 may be the true target of frequent deletions on 5q that may play an important role in the pathogenesis of the majority of esophageal carcinomas.[115]

6.3 CHROMOSOME 9p: P16

The progression of cells through the cell cycle is governed by genes encoding proteins transmitting positive (e.g. activated cyclins and cyclin-dependent kinases (CDKs)) and negative (e.g. inhibitors of CDK) signals. Three inhibitors of activated cyclin-CDK complexes controlling the G1 checkpoint of mammalian cells have recently been identified: p21, p27 and p16 (also known as p16INK4, CDKN2A or MTS1). The genes encoding these and other inhibitors of activated cyclin-CDK complexes are candidate tumor suppressor genes.

The p16 gene encodes a 16KDa protein. It forms complexes with CDK4 and CDK6, inhibiting their ability to phosphorylate the Rb protein (Fig. 5).

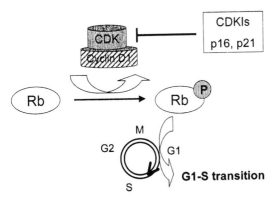

Figure 5.   Genes involved in cell cycle progression and inhibition. Cell cycle progression into S phase requires activation of cyclin dependent kinases (CDK) in association with cyclin D1. This active complex phosphorylates the retinoblastoma protein (Rb). Phosphorylated Rb is necessary in order to release its suppressant effect and enables the cell to enter the S phase. At the G1 checkpoint there are also negative regulatory signals controlling the cell cycle, namely inhibitors (CDKIs) of activated cyclin-CDK complexes (p16, p21).

Unphosphorylated Rb prevents the cell from entering the cell cycle (S phase). Thus inactivation of this gene may lead to uncontrolled cell growth. The p16 gene is located on chromosome 9p at 9p21, a locus at which frequent allelic loss occurs in esophageal adenocarcinomas.[90,92] Point mutations in exons 1 and 2 of the p16 gene are rare (ca. 5%) in esophageal adenocarcinomas, whereas p16 mutations were found more frequent

in squamous cell carcinomas.[91,107,117,118] Barrett et al. reported a higher prevalence (23%) of p16 gene mutations in adenocarcinomas with LOH of 9p21.[93] However, in that study only aneuploid cell populations were investigated, which are not representative for esophageal carcinomas in general and thus might explain the higher prevalence of p16 gene mutations. Therefore, the relatively low rate of p16 mutations observed coupled with the high frequency of LOH on chromosome 9 suggests that one or several tumor suppressor genes distinct from p16 may be the targets of allelic deletion. A potential candidate gene, p15 (MTS2/CDKN2B), a close homologue of p16 and located 20kb centromeric, is extremely rare altered in various types of human cancers, including esophageal adenocarcinomas.[93,117]

It is possible that p16 is inactivated by different mechanisms. Gonzalez et al. report homozygous deletions of the p16 gene in 3 of 12 (25%) esophageal adenocarcinomas.[92] However, these genetic changes were not present in patients with non-dysplastic Barrett's esophagus. p16 promoter hypermethylation may also be an alternative mechanism for p16 inactivation in esophageal adenocarcinomas. Indeed, data from two studies show that p16 promoter methylation (with or without p16 LOH) is a common mechanism of p16 inactivation during neoplastic progression in Barrett's esophagus, and is already present in non-dysplastic premalignant Barrett's epithelium.[119,120]

The possible prognostic significance of p16 LOH and/or p16 promoter methylation in malignant transformation of Barrett's metaplasia requires further elucidation by a prospective study design with a large number of patients. Recent data from the Fred Hutchinson Cancer Research Center in Seattle demonstrate that p16 inactivation may indeed be a useful biomarker to stratify patients' risk of progression to esophageal cancer.[121]

6.4   CHROMOSOME   13q: RETINO-BLASTOMA

The protein coded for by the normal retinoblastoma (Rb) gene is a critical regulatory molecule in the G1 phase of the cell cycle.[122] The protein is hypophosphorylated during most of G1 and becomes phosphorylated during late G1 and early S phase in order to release its suppressant effect and enable cells to progress through the cell cycle (Fig. 6). Mutations in Rb result in uncontrollable cell proliferation and predispose to numerous human tumors.

However, there has not been much evidence for its role in gastrointestinal tumors. LOH of 13q has been demonstrated in esophageal adenocarcinomas,[95] and this was associated with an unfavourable survival rate.[97] There are no reports on mutation analysis of the Rb gene in esophageal adenocarcinomas, but there are several reports on the expression of Rb protein during the progression of Barrett's metaplasia to adenocarcinoma. Loss of normal Rb staining was observed as the Barretts' metaplasia progressed to dysplasia and carcinoma, indicating accumulation of unstainable aberrant protein.[9,123] LOH of the Rb gene and gene product expression as detected by immunohistochemistry, however, were not significantly correlated. In contrast, there was a direct correlation between cyclin D1 (a cyclin-dependent kinase involved in cell cycle progression from the G1 to S phase) and Rb immunoreactivity.[97] The tumors that had cyclin D1 gene amplification and overexpression exhibited normal levels of Rb protein. By contrast, tumors with loss of expression of Rb did not show amplification of the cyclin D1 gene and expressed low levels of cyclin D1.[124] This is in keeping with the current knowledge on the interactions between cyclin D1 and Rb in cell cycle control.

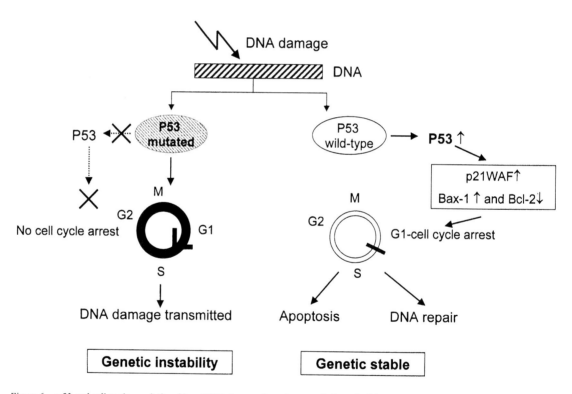

Figure 6.   p53 and cell cycle regulation. Upon DNA damage there is upregulation of wild-type p53 protein. This leads to increased transcription of p53 regulated genes (e.g. p21, bax-1,bcl-2) which inhibit the cell cycle. This facilitates DNA repair or the cell enters the apoptotic pathway. In this way p53 provides genomic stability. Mutations in the p53 gene render the p53 protein inactive and the damaged DNA is transmitted.

The inhibitory function of wild-type Rb protein in cell-cycle progression can be overcome by either loss of expression of the Rb gene or by increased expression of cyclin D1 (see also chapter on genes controlling the cell cycle).

6.5 CHROMOSOME 17p: P53

Mutations and deletions of the p53 gene are the most common genetic lesions in human cancers. The p53 protein functions in a homotetrameric complex as a transcription factor that induces expression of genes that facilitate cell cycle arrest, DNA repair and apoptosis. Upon DNA damage, upregulation of the wild type p53 protein leads to cell cycle arrest in the G1 phase. This inhibition of the cell cycle facilitates DNA repair or entering of the apoptotic pathway. In this way the p53 protein provides genomic stability: the DNA damage is repaired or the cell with damaged DNA undergoes apoptosis, so the DNA damage is not transmitted to the cell progeny (Fig. 6).

Mutations in the p53 gene, association with viral proteins or association with the cellular oncoprotein MDM2 render the p53 protein inactive, deprived from its normal function.[125] One mutant p53 protein in the tetrameric p53 complex abolishes the function of the entire complex. Furthermore, most mutant proteins have a much longer half-life than the wild type protein. This implicates that when a cell harbors one inactivating p53 mutation, the concentration of this protein will increase relative to the product of the wild type allele and the activity of the wild type protein will be inhibited by complexing with the mutant protein (dominant-negative). The prolonged half-life of the mutant p53 protein and the concomitant increased cellular p53 concentration makes visualisation by immunohistochemistry possible.

In a number of studies increasing p53 expression in the Barrett's metaplasia-dysplasia-carcinoma sequence has been reported, despite the rather low sensitivity of immunohistochemistry to detect p53 mutations[126] (see also chapter 3.2). For instance, mutant p53 proteins can escape detection by the antibodies depending on the type of mutation. On the contrary, high levels of p53 have been detected without evidence of p53 mutations. This is probably caused by cellular proteins that stabilise p53.[126] Most studies report a very low percentage of metaplasia cases with p53 protein

accumulation[16,127-132] although Kim et al. found 36% of metaplasia without dysplasia cases with p53 immunoreactivity.[133] p53 accumulation increases in low grade dysplasia to high grade dysplasia from less than 10 to more than 70% respectively.[129,130,132,134,135] From numerous immunohistochemical studies it is clear that in more than 50% of esophageal adenocarcinomas pronounced p53 overexpression is present.[128,130-132,135-138] An example of p53 immunostaining is shown in chapter 3.2, figure 9. With more sensitive molecular techniques to detect p53 alterations, such as single strand conformation polymorphism (SSCP) analysis, sequencing and LOH analysis, occasional cases of metaplasia and low grade dysplasia with p53 mutations have been found.[75,139,140] In high grade dysplastic Barrett's epithelium and invasive adenocarcinoma the prevalence of p53 mutations exceeds 40% and p53 locus LOH in these conditions is generally found in even higher percentages.[51,75,121,137,139-141]

In high grade dysplasia and in esophageal adenocarcinoma p53 mutations have been found even in diploid cell subpopulations from aneuploid tumors.[121,137] Furthermore, allelic loss of chromosome 17p often occurs before the loss of 5q during neoplastic progression.[113,132] These findings suggest that p53 mutation is an early event in esophageal adenocarcinogenesis. In conclusion, there is overwhelming evidence that p53 gene alterations are early and frequent events in esophageal adenocarcinomas and that this gene is associated with malignant transformation of Barrett's esophagus. Although prognostic significance of p53 alterations has been suggested, p53 abnormality alone is not sufficient to predict progression to cancer or disease outcome.[142-144]

6.6 CHROMOSOME 18q: DPC4 AND DCC

Allelotype analysis has shown that allelic loss of 18q was frequent in esophageal adenocarcinomas. However, mutational analysis of the deleted in pancreatic cancer (DPC4) gene did not reveal any mutations.[145] Therefore, DPC4 is unlikely to be the target gene on 18q21 and other candidates such as deleted in colorectal cancer (DCC) or as yet unidentified target genes can be involved.

7. PROTO-ONCOGENES

The proto-oncogenes encode a group of proteins that are normally involved either in signal transduction (from the plasma membrane to the nucleus) or the regulation of gene expression (Fig.

7). Mutated proto-oncogens are called oncogenes, because many mutations activate or increase the activity of the proteins, which results in excessive stimulation of cell proliferation.

7.1 GROWTH FACTORS AND THEIR RECEPTORS

7.1.1 EGF, TGF-α and EGFR
An important family of growth factors is the one that binds to the epidermal growth factor receptor (EGFR), including epidermal growth factor (EGF) and transforming growth factor-α (TGF-α). These growth factors act in an autocrine, paracrine and humoral way on growth and differentiation of the gastrointestinal tract.[146] EGF has a stimulatory effect on epithelial cell proliferation in the gastrointestinal tract and has been demonstrated in several gastrointestinal malignancies. EGF was found to be overexpressed in esophageal carcinomas. Although EGF is also expressed in Barrett's esophagitis, the expression of EGF does not discriminate between dysplastic and neoplastic epithelium.[147] Overexpression of its receptor EGFR in the esophagus did correlate with the degree of mucosal dysplasia and the occurrence of adenocarcinoma, suggesting that high expression levels may reflect increased malignant transformation potential in Barrett's mucosa.[17,147-149] Al-Kasspooles et al. found EGFR gene amplification in 30% of the esophageal adenocarcinomas and also in Barrett's metaplasia. However, there was no correlation between the level of EGFR expression by immunohistochemistry and the degree of EGFR gene amplification as determined by Southern blot analysis.[150] In addition to its correlation with the degree of dysplasia, the presence EGFR also correlates with the frequency of lymph node metastasis and poor survival.[17] Transforming growth factor-α (TGF-α) is structurally and functionally related to EGF and is expressed in many tissues including the gastrointestinal tract. TGF-α, as EGF, binds to the EGFR leading to activation of the intranuclear proto-oncogenes c-fos and c-myc, which are involved in the regulation of cell division and differentiation. TGF-α expression is increased in metaplastic, dysplastic and neoplastic tissue of the esophagus compared to normal mucosa.[147] The degree of abnormal expression becomes more marked as dysplasia increases and correlates with the proliferative index in Barrett's esophagus.[14,147,151] However, TGF-α expression in esophageal adenocarcinomas did not correlate with pathological or clinical follow-up data..[17] What emerges from all these data is that EGF/TGF-α and their receptor EGFR are important in the progression of normal esophageal squamous epithelium to metaplasia, dysplasia and finally carcinoma. It is possible that coexpression of

TGF-α, EGF and EGFR may be associated with autocrine growth regulation in normal gastrointestinal mucosa and neoplasia.[146]

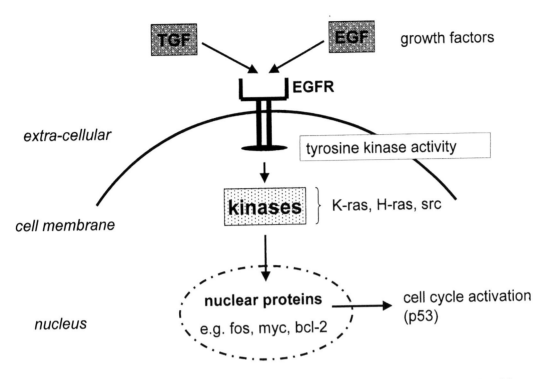

Figure 7.   Signal transduction from the cell membrane to the nucleus: the role of proto-oncogenes. Mutational activation of the genes encoding the growth factors and their receptors or the signal transduction pathway genes leads to constitutive activation of the cell cycle. (EGF, epidermal growth factor; TGF-α, transforming growth factor-α and their receptor EGFR).

7.1.2 c-erbB2

The c-erbB2 proto-oncogene (HER2/neu; chromosome 17q21) encodes a transmembrane glycoprotein with intrinsic tyrosine kinase activity that is homologous to, but distinct from the EGFR. Upon binding of specific ligands, the receptor is activated and promotes tumor cell proliferation. C-erbB2 protein overexpression and/or amplification of the c-erbB2 gene occur in approximately 10-70% of esophageal adenocarcinomas.[59,147,152-156] Overexpression of c-erbB2 was not demonstrated in dysplastic Barrett's epithelium suggesting that it is a late event in the dysplasia-carcinoma sequence.[153] But others detected strong membranous staining for c-erbB2 in 30% of high-grade dysplasia and in only 10% of adenocarcinomas.[133] c-erbB2 overexpression in adenocarcinomas correlated significantly with tumor invasion, lymph node involvement, distant metastasis and presence of residual tumor after resection.[59,156] Moreover, c-erbB2 overexpression was an (independent) prognostic factor for overall survival,[59,155] but others found no difference in survival between patients whose tumors overexpressed c-erbB2 and those that did not.[152] Recently, Friess et al. showed that 64% of the esophageal adenocarcinomas had overexpression of c-erbB3, another member of the EGFR family, but no correlation with clinico-pathological parameters was found.[157]

7.1.3 VEGF

The family of the vascular endothelial growth factor (VEGF) proteins includes potent and specific mitogens for vascular endothelial cells that function in the process of angiogenesis. VEGF is overexpressed in many tumors and promotes angiogenesis. Furthermore, VEGF is one of the molecules that are related to metastasis and prognosis in human cancers.[158] There have been several studies on VEGF expression in esophageal squamous cell carcinomas. VEGF expression was associated with tumor progression and poor prognosis.[159,160]

Kitadai et al. determined the angiogenic profile of human esophageal cancers.[161] Six esophageal cell lines, including one adenocarcinoma cell line, expressed VEGF mRNA and 60% of 119 resected tumors showed intense VEGF immunoreactivity and had significant more microvessels. VEGF expression correlated with tumor stage, venous and lymphatic invasion and there was a tendency for poorer survival of patients with VEGF-positive tumors.[161] No data are available on VEGF expression in the premalignant Barrett's epithelium, but expression is already observed in precursor lesions of colonic cancers (adenomas).[162] Further studies on VEGF expression in the neoplastic progression form Barrett's metaplasia to carcinoma are awaited.

7.1.4 FGF

The fibroblast growth factors (FGFs) are potent mitogens that possess angiogenic properties and the capability to regulate growth and differentiation of various cell types. They have been implicated in the development and progression of solid tumors, including carcinomas of the aerodigestive tract and gastro-intestinal tract. The expression of acidic and basic FGF (aFGF, bFGF) has also been studied in esophageal adenocarcinoma and Barrett's metaplasia. FGF is generally sequentially accumulated in the progression from metaplasia to neoplasia. Esophageal adenocarcinomas and high grade dysplastic Barrett's epithelium showed enhanced expression of aFGF mRNA and protein (immunohistochemistry) but not bFGF, when compared to low grade dysplasia and normal control epithelium.[163,164] This suggests that that aFGF may be a valuable prognostic marker.

The int-2 and hst-1 genes both encode growth factors of the fibroblast growth factor family (FGF). Both genes are located on chromosome 11q13. In esophageal squamous cell carcinomas, co-amplification of int-2 and hst-1 has been observed in 30-50% of primary tumors and appears to be related to higher probability of distant metastases and haematogenous recurrence after curative resection of esophageal carcinoma.[165,166] However, the correlation between 11q13 amplification and overexpression of hst-1 and/or int-2 is unclear.[167] No data on hst-1 and int-2 gene amplification are available for esophageal adenocarcinomas.

7.1.5 TGF-β

In contrast to TGF-α, TGF-β is a potent inhibitor of cell proliferation, an inducer of differentiation in epithelial cells of the intestine in vitro, and a suppressor of genomic instability.[168] There is some evidence that the TGF-β signaling pathway is involved in the initiation and progression of esophageal adenocarcinomas. First, TGF-β is expressed in non-dysplastic Barrett's epithelium, as well as esophageal adenocarcinomas.[169,170] Second, inactivating mutations occur in MADR2, an important component of the TGF-β signalling pathway in colon cancers.[171] The chromosomal localisation of the MADR2 gene is 18q21, which frequently shows LOH in esophageal adenocarcinomas. Finally, loss of expression of the functional receptor for TGF-β (TGF-β receptor type II) appears to be associated with Barrett's esophagus and esophageal adenocarcinomas.[170,172,173] However, the exact role of TGF-β and its receptor in Barrett's adenocarcinomas needs to be clarified.

7.2 RAS-FAMILY

The ras family of proto-oncogenes (H, K and N) encode specific proteins which appear to be essential components in normal cell division and differentiation. Ras proteins act as signal-transducing molecules in the cytoplasm. Mutational activation of K-ras promotes cell growth and may thereby contribute to initiation and/or progression of tumors.[174] Ras has not been shown to be mutated in most studies on Barrett's esophagus and esophageal adenocarcinomas.[175-177] On the other hand, increased H-ras expression in Barrett's carcinoma and amplification of the K-ras gene in esophageal adenocarcinomas has been reported.[178-180] Trautmann et al. reported, for the first time, point mutations in K-ras/codon 12 in biopsies from Barrett's esophagus and in esophageal adenocarcinomas, but these were rare.[181] Casson et al. found a K-ras mutation in an esophageal adenocarcinoma, but the frequency appears to be very low.[182] In conclusion, activation of the ras proto-oncogenes seems to be of little importance in Barrett's adenocarcinomas contrary to that observed in other carcinomas of the gastrointestinal tract (pancreatic and colon carcinomas).

7.3 C-MYC

The c-myc gene is located on chromosome 8q24. c-myc encodes a nuclear protein that is thought to regulate the transcription of other genes important for cell growth.[183] Activation of the c-myc gene occurs in a variety of human tumors and may contribute to tumor progression in both early and late stages by preventing the cell from entering the G0-resting phase. Amplification of c-myc has been observed in squamous cell carcinomas of the esophagus.[184,185] CGH and cytogenetic studies suggest that c-myc is the target gene of the high level 8q amplifications found in esophageal adenocarcinomas.[65,79,80] By using in situ hybridization, Abdelatif et al. found enhanced c-myc expression in dysplastic Barrett's epithelium and adenocarcinomas, but not in non-dysplastic Barrett's mucosa.[180] Lu et al. found amplification of of the c-myc oncogene in 1 out of 3 adenocarcinomas of the gastroesophageal junction.[184] On the contrary, Jankowski et al. could detect c-myc neither in esophageal adenocarcinomas nor in Barrett's epithelium.[178] It is possible that due to the short half life of c-myc it could not be detected with immunohistochemistry.[178] Presently, it is unclear whether amplification or mutation of c-myc play a significant role in the malignant progression of Barrett's esophagus, but it appears that it is of limited prognostic value in human esophageal carcinomas.[186]

7.4 SRC

The cellular oncogene c-src and its viral homologue v-src encode 60KDa, cytoplasmic, membrane-associated, protein-tyrosine kinases. A close correlation exists between elevated specific kinase activity and cell transformation. Src may deregulate cell-adhesion by anchorage-dependent growth control, thereby maintaining cells in the proliferative state.[187] Src activity is elevated in colon and breast carcinomas and neuroblastomas. In terms of preneoplastic tissues, colonic adenomas which show elevated src activity are at greatest risk for developing colon cancer.[188] Src activity is also elevated in dysplastic epithelia. The src activity was found to be 3 to 4 fold higher in Barrett's epithelium and 6 fold higher in esophageal adenocarcinomas than in control tissues.[189] Moreover, Jankowski et al. found that 20% of the esophageal adenocarcinomas and Barrett's esophagus expressed src.[178] These data suggest an important role for src in the malignant transformation of Barrett's esophagus and warrants further investigation.

7.5 PROSTAGLANDINS

Cyclo-oxygenase (COX) catalyses the rate-limiting step in prostaglandin (PG) synthesis. There are two different isoforms of COX, referred to as COX-1 and COX-2. COX-1 is constitutively expressed and involved for example in cytoprotection of the gastric mucosa. In contrast, COX-2 is normally absent in most tissues, but can be induced by pro-inflammatory or mitogenic stimuli. COX-2 is involved in a large number of processes fundamental for tumor development: apoptosis, cell adhesion, invasion and metastasis and angiogenesis.[190] The role of COX-2 in the development of colorectal cancer has received much attention. More than 80% of colorectal cancers have increased levels of COX-2. The use of COX-2 inhibitors such as aspirin, NSAIDs and selective COX-2 inhibitors is associated with a lower risk of colorectal cancer.[191]

Chronic esophagitis is associated with the excessive mucosal production of prostaglandin E2 (PGE2) and bile acids stimulate COX-2 expression in esophageal cells in vitro.[192,193] Two studies investigated the role of COX gene expression in esophageal adenocarcinomas in vivo. It was found that COX-2 is expressed (determined by immunohistochemistry and/or RT-PCR or western blotting) in 70-80% of the esophageal adenocarcinomas and also in corresponding Barrett's metaplasia.[194,195] This suggests that COX-2 overexpression is involved in the Barrett's associated neoplasia and that overexpression of this protein is an early event in the esophageal neoplastic transformation process. It was shown that selective inhibition of COX-2 in esophageal cancer cell lines induces apoptoic cell death and reduced proliferative activity.[195] Moreover, in an in vitro esophageal carcinoma model NSAIDs inhibited the synthesis of cyclo-oxygenase (COX) thereby reducing the synthesis of PGE2.[194] Among regular aspirin users, a 40-50% or even higher reduction in esophageal cancer risk was found.[196,197] These data indicate that the chemopreventive potential of NSAIDs in esophageal adenocarcinomas, by repressing the induction of COX-2 enzymes in esophagitis and Barrett's metaplasia, deserves further attention.

8. GENES INVOLVED IN CONTROLLING THE CELL CYCLE

The progression of cells through the cell cycle is governed by genes encoding proteins transmitting positive (e.g. activated cyclins and cyclin-dependent kinases (CDKs) and negative (e.g. inhibitors of CDK) signals. Cyclins form a family of proteins that complex with CDKs. Phosphorylation of the Rb protein by cyclin-CDKs is correlated with the transition across the G1 checkpoint (Fig. 5). Different cyclin-CDK complexes are required at various stages of the cell cycle.[198] CyclinD-CDK4-CDK6 acts in the G1 phase, cyclin E-CDK2 and cyclin A-CDK2 in G1 and S and cyclin A-cyclin BCDK-1 at G2-M transition. Cyclin-CDK activity is regulated by phosphorylation events and by CDK inhibitors (CDKI), which bind to the Cyclin-CDK complex and inhibit its activity and ability to phosphorylate the Rb protein. Unphosphorylated Rb prevents the cell from entering the cell cycle (S phase). Thus inactivation of the genes encoding CDKIs may lead to uncontrolled cell growth. There are two structurally related groups of CDKIs. One group forms the INK4 family that specifically inhibit cyclinD-CDK 4/6 complexes, such as p15, p16, p18 and p19.[199] P15 and p16 have been already discussed. The other group forms the Cip/Kip family and includes p21, p27 and p57 proteins, which seem to target preferentially cyclin-CDK complexes containing CDK2.

8.1 CYCLIN D1 (11q13)

Cyclin D1 is the key cyclin involved in progression from G1 to S. Cyclin D1 complexes with CDK4 and phosphorylates the Rb protein. Phosphorylation of Rb blocks the inhibitory function of the Rb protein and the cell progresses into S-phase. Cyclin D1 abnormalities, either gene amplification or overexpression lead to constitutive activation of the CDK-cyclin D1 pathway. Increased nuclear expression of cyclin D1 is observed in 22-64% of the esophageal adenocarcinomas, and is already present in Barrett's metaplasia.[97-200-202] The increased expression of cyclin D1 is especially frequent in the intestinal-type lesions and early stage tumors.[200,203] Amplification of the cyclin D1 gene was observed in 16-26% of the esophageal adenocarcinomas.[88,203] However, cyclin D1 immunoreactivity was not always associated with gene amplification.[97,204] Therefore, additional regulatory mechanism of protein expression probably exists. Finally, cyclin D1 was shown to be a prognostic marker in esophageal cancer.[202]

8.2 P27[Kip-1] (12p13)

The p27[Kip1] (p27) gene is located on chromosome 12p13. p27 is a cyclin-dependent kinase inhibitor. Overexpression of p27 induces a block during G1 in the cell cycle. In addition, high levels of p27[kip-1] have been found in G0/G1 quiescent cells. Levels of p27 decrease as the cell re-enter the cell cycle.[205] No structural alterations and only rare genetic mutations have been identified in the p27 gene in human tumors.[206] Abundance of p27 is regulated at the post-translational level by proteolytic degradation by the ubiquitin-proteasome pathway.[205] During the past two years a large number of studies reported decreased p27 expression in more aggressive tumors. Singh et al. found p27 protein expression and p27 mRNA to be increased in intensity and distributed throughout the glands of high-grade dysplastic Barrett's epithelium, indicating transcriptionally upregulation of p27.[207] In contrast, low p27 protein expression but elevated levels of p27 mRNA were found in 83% of esophageal adenocarcinomas, possibly due to post-transcriptional regulation of the gene. In addition to nuclear staining, cytoplasmic staining of p27 was noted in 48% and 26% of dysplasia and carcinomas, respectively.[207] Loss of nuclear and/or cytoplasmic staining for p27 correlated with higher histological grade, depth of invasion, presence of lymph node metastasis and shorter survival.[207] These findings suggest that the cell cycle inhibitor p27 may be overexpressed to counteract proliferative stimuli in Barrett's associated dysplasia. Loss of p27 or altered subcellular localisation as the process becomes invasive suggests an important role for this CDKI in preventing progression of Barrett's esophagus to adenocarcinoma.[169]

8.3 P21[WAF1/CIP1]

The G1-S phase of the cell cycle can also be down-regulated by inhibition of CDKs by p21[WAF1/CIP1] (p21). Nuclear expression of p21 is upregulated by the wild-type p53 tumor suppressor, but not mutated p53.[208] Absence of p53 staining and presence of p21 was proposed as an indication of wild-type p53 status.[209] P21 expression was elevated in Barrett's tissue classified as indefinite for dysplasia, low-grade dysplasia, high grade dysplasia and in Barrett's adenocarcinoma, but not in Barrett's epithelium negative for dysplasia.[210] Although p21 expression levels were similar for indefinite, dysplastic and adenocarcinoma stages, p53 scores for high grade dysplasia and adenocarcinoma were higher than those for low grade dysplasia.[210] No relationship between p21 and p53 staining in esophageal adenocarcinomas was found, indicating that there are also p53 independent pathways for the upregulation of p21.[127,210] The elevated nuclear p21 expression in Barrett's esophagus and adenocarcinoma does, most likely, not represent mutated protein.[211] P21 expression was significantly associated with prognosis: patients with p21 positive tumors showed a better prognosis than patients with p21 negative tumors.[202]

9. CELL-CELL ADHESION

It has long been known that cell-cell adhesion is generally reduced in human cancers. Reduced cell-cell adhesiveness removes contact inhibition of proliferation, thus allowing escape from growth control signals. Moreover, invasion and metastases, which are life-threatening properties of malignant tumors, are considered to be later, but critically important carcinogenic steps. Reduced cell-cell adhesiveness is considered to be indispensable for both early and late carcinogenic steps.

9.1 E-CADHERIN-CATENIN COMPLEX

In recent years, there has been an increasing interest in E-cadherin, which is the prime mediator of calcium-dependent cell-cell adhesion in normal epithelial cells. E-cadherin is bound via series of undercoat proteins, the catenins (alfa-, beta-, gamma- and p120-catenin), to the actin cytoskeleton (Fig. 8). This linkage between transmembranous cadherins and actin filaments of the cytoskeleton is necessary to form strong cell-cell adhesion. There is increasing evidence that modulation of this complex by different mechanisms is an important step in the initiation and progression of human cancers.[212]

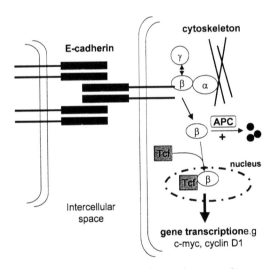

Figure 8. The E-cadherin-catenin complex connecting two adjacent epithelial cells. The extra-cellular domains of E-cadherin establish intercellular adhesion. The cytoplasmic tail of E-cadherin is linked to the actin cytoskeleton. The unbound cytoplasmic pool of beta-catenin is rapidly degraded by adenomatous polyposis coli (APC) gene product. Abnormalities in this degradation can lead to raised concentrations of unbound beta-catenin, which then binds to T-cell factor (Tcf) and translocates to the nucleus where it stimulates transcription of target genes.

In non-malignant epithelia, E-cadherin and the catenins show a membranous localisation at intercellular borders. In Barrett's adenocarcinomas, reduced membranous expression of E-cadherin as well as the catenins is observed in 60-80% of the tumors.[213-216] The expression of E-cadherin and alfa- and beta-

catenin correlated significantly with stage and grade of the carcinomas and with the occurrence of lymph node metastases. Reduced expression of E-cadherin and beta-catenin were significant prognosticators for survival, independent of stage of disease.[216] Moreover, abnormal or reduced expression has been shown to be associated with higher degrees of dysplasia in Barrett's esophagus.[214,217] This suggests that the E-cadherin-catenin complex may be useful as a marker for neoplastic progression from Barrett's metaplasia to adenocarcinoma and metastases. There have been several reports on somatic and germline E-cadherin gene mutations in poorly differentiated invasive tumors like lobular breast cancer and diffuse type gastric cancer.[218] E-cadherin mutations with loss of the remaining wild-type allele were also detected in the pre-invasive *in situ* component of these cancers.[218] However, no mutations could be detected in esophageal adenocarcinomas despite frequent LOH of the E-cadherin locus at 16q22.[98] Down-regulation of E-cadherin expression due to methylation of the E-cadherin promoter has been reported, but currently it is unknown whether this epigenetic phenomenon explains the reduced expression of E-cadherin found in esophageal adenocarcinomas. In some tumors the staining pattern of the E-cadherin-catenin complex is not always a reduction in membranous expression but shows redistribution from the cell membrane to the cytoplasm. Alterations in the phosphorylation status of E-cadherin and/or the catenins has been held responsible along with suppression of cell-cell adhesion.[218] Moreover, phosphorylation of beta-catenin may also promote angiogenesis, as discussed in chapter 3.2.

Besides establishing cell-cell adhesion, beta-catenin has been shown recently to function in cell signalling, has been elucidated over the past years.[220] Under normal conditions, beta-catenin is bound to the cytoplasmic tail of E-cadherin. Free beta-catenin in the cytoplasm is kept low by rapid degradation of unbound beta-catenin. In order to be degraded, beta-catenin is phosphorylated by a protein complex, of which the adenomatous polyposis coli (APC) protein is one of the members (Fig. 8). Inactivation of APC leads to an increase in cellular free beta-catenin that enters the nucleus of the cell, directly binds to transcription factors and activates gene expression. These target genes are involved in promoting cellular proliferation and migration, such as the c-myc oncogene and the cell cycle regulator cyclin D1. Besides inactivation of APC, mutations in phosphorylation sites of the beta-catenin gene can also lead to stabilisation of the protein. In esophageal adenocarcinomas, increased cytoplasmic and nuclear localisation of beta-catenin has been observed,[214] implicating involvement of APC inactivation or beta-catenin mutations with subsequent activation of the signal transduction pathway (see chapter 3.2, figure 11). However, inactivation of APC is rare and no mutations in beta-catenin could be detected.[68,116] This implicates that other proteins that function in this pathway should be involved.

9.2 SERINE PROTEASE SYSTEM

The serine protease system has been shown to play an important role in the invasive potential of a variety of tumors by breaking down the extracellular matrix. Urokinase plasminogen activator (uPA) is a serine protease. Consistent with its role in cancer spread, uPA has been shown to be a (independent) prognostic marker in a variety of malignancies: high levels of uPA predict poor outcome.[221] High levels of uPA were present in esophageal adenocarcinomas,[222,223] and a correlation with pT, pN and pM categories, tumor stage and lymphatic invasion was established.[224] Multivariate survival analysis showed that uPA was an independent prognostic factor for survival in adenocarcinoma of the esophagus.[224] Therefore, uPA antigen content could identify esophageal adenocarcinoma patients who will develop early tumor recurrences, thus providing a more accurate estimation of prognosis.

9.3 CD44 PROTEIN FAMILY

CD44 is a family of glycoproteins involved in cell-cell adhesion and cell-matrix interactions. As a result of alternative splicing of 10 exons (v1-10) more than 20 isoforms have been described. This cell surface protein is expressed as multiple isoforms in many normal and neoplastic tissues. Although the role of CD44 splice variants is not completely understood, the presence of certain splice variants was shown to correlate with metastatic behavior of several cancers, including gastrointestinal malignancies.[225] CD44-standard (CD44s) and its abnormal transcripts (CD44variant or CD44v) have been described in esophageal adenocarcinoma.[226-228] Increased CD44s expression was seen in 50-66% of the esophageal adenocarcinomas (Krishnadath, unpublished data).[226-228] Generally, no significant correlations were found between expression of CD44s and CD44v and grade or stage of the carcinomas. However, a significant correlation between CD44s, v6 and v10 expression and pT stage has been reported.[226-228] In Barrett's esophagus CD44s (but not CD44v6) expression increases along with dysplasia and the proliferation rate and increased CD44v6 was seen in an early stage of malignant transformation (Krishnadath, unpublished data).[228] On univariate analysis, cancers with increased CD44v6 expression or downregulation of CD44s had a poorer prognosis than those with reduced or no

expression (Krishnadath, unpublished data)[226,228] and expression of CD44v4 was an independent factor in prognosis.[226] Further studies on a larger patient cohort are required to validate the usefulness of CD44s and isoforms in clinical decision making.

9.4 CATHEPSIN B

The cysteine protease cathepsin B (CTSB) gene, which maps to 8p22, is a lysosomal enzyme that has been shown to be overexpressed or exhibit altered localisation in cancers.[229] Overexpression or altered localisation of CTSB is thought to result in degradation of basement membrane facilitating tumor invasion and metastasis. Altered expression of CTSB was found to be an independent predictor of poor prognosis in tumors of the lung, colon and breast. Hughes et al. found an amplicon at chromosome 8p22-23 resulting in CTSB gene amplification and overexpression.[230] Moreover, abundant extracellular expression of CTSB protein was found in 29 of 40 (73%) esophageal adenocarcinoma specimens by using immunohistochemical analysis.[230] These data support an important role for CTSB gene amplification and CTSB protein overexpression in esophageal adenocarcinomas and possibly other tumors as well. A possible association between CTSB gene amplification and protein expression and survival in esophageal adenocarcinomas has not been studied so far.

10. SUMMARY AND CONCLUSIONS

There is need for improved understanding of the molecular biology of Barrett's esophagus and adenocarcinoma. Despite ongoing efforts to characterise the molecular changes in Barrett's esophagus, its pathogenesis remains poorly understood. A wide variety of genetic events and mechanisms appear to play a role in the development and progression of Barrett's esophagus-associated neoplastic lesions. There have been attempts to correlate the pathophysiology with specific molecular alterations.[174,199,231-234] Table 3 summarises these molecular events. However, there is still no uniform molecular pathway of progression. In the next several years the subsequent genetic events critical for the initiation and progression of Barrett's adenocarcinoma will be further characterised and may clinically be useful as biomarkers for early cancer detection or prognostication. With the disturbing increase in incidence of Barrett's adenocarcinomas, further research into this area is vital.

TABLE 3. Summary of the genetic and epigenetic alterations and changes in protein expression that occurs in the progression from Barrett's esophagus to adenocarcinoma.

	Barrett's esophagus		*Adenocarcinoma*
	Metaplasia (without dysplasia)	*Dysplasia*	
Proliferation and apoptosis	↑ proliferation ↑ bcl-2 expression	↑ proliferative zone ↓ apoptosis ↑ ODC & polyamines expression ↑ telomerase expression	↑ proliferation & zone ↓ apoptosis ↑ ODC expression ↑ telomerase expression ↓ fas/APO-1 expression
Cell cycle and DNA content	↑ G1 & G2 phases aneuploidy (rare) ↑ cyclin D1	↑ S phase aneuploidy ↑ cyclin D1 ↑ p27 ↓ chromosoom Y	↑ G2/M aneuploidy ↑ cyclin D1 ↑ p27 ↓ chromosoom Y ↑ p21
Microsatellite instability	RER (rare)	RER (rare)	RER (rare)
Tumor suppressor genes	17p LOH & p53 expression p16 LOH (9p) & methylation	p53 mutations & LOH (17p) p16 LOH (9p) & methylation 5q LOH	p53 mutations & LOH (17p) p16 LOH & mutations & methylation 5q LOH see table 2 for other LOH regions
Oncogenes	↑ COX-2 ↑ src ↑ TGF-β	↑ COX-2 ↑ src ↑ TGF-β aFGF ↑ TGF-α	↑ COX-2 ↑ src ↑ TGF-β aFGF, bFGF ↑ TGF-α ↑ EGFR, EGF, TGF-α ↑ VEGF ↑ c-erbB2 expression
Cell-cell adhesion		catenin phosphorylation ↓ E-cadherin-catenin expression changes in CD44S+V expression	↓ E-cadherin-catenin expression changes in CD44S+V expression ↑ uPA ↑ cathepsin B

Abbreviations used in the table: RER, replication error phenotype; ODC, ornithine decarboxylase enzyme; LOH, loss of heterozygosity; COX-2, cyclo-oxygenase-2; EGFR epidermal growth factor receptor; VEGF, vascular endothelial growth factor; uPA, urokinase plasminogen activator; aFGF, acidic fibroblast growth factor; TGF-α/β, transforming growth factor α/β.

REFERENCES

1. Lengauer C, Kinzler KW,Vogelstein B. Genetic instabilities in human cancers. Nature, 1998; 396: 643-649.
2. Modrich P, Lahue R. Mismatch repair in replication fidelity, genetic recombination, and cancer biology. Annu Rev Biochem, 1996; 65: 101-133.
3. Cahill DP, Lengauer C, Yu J, et al. Mutations of mitotic checkpoint genes in human cancers. Nature, 1998; 392: 300-303.
4. Riccio A, Aaltonen LA, Godwin AK, et al. The DNA repair gene MBD4 (MED1) is mutated in human carcinomas with microsatellite instability [letter]. Nat Genet, 1999; 23: 266-268.
5. Lynch HT, de La Chapelle A. Genetic susceptibility to non-polyposis colorectal cancer. J Med Genet, 1999; 36: 801-818.
6. Hahn WC, Counter CM, Lundberg AS, Beijersbergen RL, Brooks MW, Weinberg RA. Creation of human tumour cells with defined genetic elements. Nature, 1999; 400: 464-468.
7. Herbst JJ, Berenson MM, McCloskey DW, Wiser WC. Cell proliferation in esophageal columnar epithelium (Barrett's esophagus). Gastroenterology,1978; 75: 683-687.
8. Pellish LJ, Hermos JA, Eastwood GL. Cell proliferation in three types of Barrett's epithelium. Gut, 1980; 21: 26-31.
9. Soslow RA, Remotti H, Baergen RN, Altorki NK. Suppression of apoptosis does not foster neoplastic growth in Barrett's esophagus. Mod Pathol, 1999; 12: 239-250.
10. Whittles CE, Biddlestone LR, Burton A, et al. Apoptotic and proliferative activity in the neoplastic progression of Barrett's oesophagus: a comparative study. J Pathol, 1999; 187: 535-540.
11. Gillen P, McDermott M, Grehan D, Hourihane DO, Hennessy TP. Proliferating cell nuclear antigen in the assessment of Barrett's mucosa. Br J Surg, 1994; 81: 1766-1768.
12. Ouatu-Lascar R, Fitzgerald RC, Triadafilopoulos G. Differentiation and proliferation in Barrett's esophagus and the effects of acid suppression. Gastroenterology, 1999; 117: 327-335.
13. Lauwers GY, Kandemir O, Kubilis PS, Scott GV. Cellular kinetics in Barrett's epithelium carcinogenic sequence: roles of apoptosis, bcl-2 protein, and cellular proliferation. Mod Pathol, 1997; 10: 1201-1208.
14. Jankowski J, McMenemin R, Yu C, Hopwood D, Wormsley KG. Proliferating cell nuclear antigen in oesophageal diseases;correlation with transforming growth factor alpha expression. Gut, 1992; 33: 587-591.
15. Hong MK, Laskin WB, Herman BE, et al. Expansion of the Ki-67 proliferative compartment correlates with degree of dysplasia in Barrett's esophagus. Cancer, 1995; 75: 423-429.
16. Polkowski W, van Lanschot JJ, Ten Kate FJ, et al. The value of p53 and Ki67 as markers for tumour progression in the Barrett's dysplasia-carcinoma sequence. Surg Oncol, 1995; 4: 163-171.
17. Yacoub L, Goldman H, Odze RD. Transforming growth factor-alpha, epidermal growth factor receptor, and MiB-1 expression in Barrett's-associated neoplasia: correlation with prognosis. Mod Pathol, 1997; 10: 105-112.
18. Rioux-Leclercq N, Turlin B, Sutherland F, et al. Analysis of Ki-67, p53 and Bcl-2 expression in the dysplasia-carcinoma sequence of Barrett's esophagus. Oncol Rep, 1999; 6: 877-882.
19. Krishnadath KK, Tilanus HW, van Blankenstein M, et al. Accumulation of genetic abnormalities during neoplastic progression in Barrett's esophagus. Cancer Res, 1995; 55: 1971-1976.
20. Gulizia JM, Wang H, Antonioli D et al. Proliferative characteristics of intestinalized mucosa in the distal esophagus and gastroesophageal junction (short-segment Barrett's esophagus): a case control study. Hum Pathol, 1999; 30: 412-418.
21. Rustgi AK. Biomarkers for malignancy in the columnar-lined esophagus. Gastroenterol Clin North Am, 1997; 26: 599-606.
22. Garewal HS, Sampliner R, Gerner E, Steinbronn K, Alberts D, Kendall D. Ornithine decarboxylase activity in Barrett's esophagus: a potential marker for dysplasia. Gastroenterology, 1988; 94: 819-821.
23. Garewal HS, Sampliner R, Alberts D, Steinbronn K. Increase in ornithine decarboxylase activity associated with development of dysplasia in Barrett's esophagus. Dig Dis Sci, 1989; 34: 312-314.
24. Gray MR, Wallace HM, Goulding H, Hoffman J, Kenyon WE, Kingsnorth AN. Mucosal polyamine metabolism in the columnar lined oesophagus. Gut, 1993; 34: 584-587.
25. Garewal HS, Gerner EW, Sampliner RE, Roe D. Ornithine decarboxylase and polyamine levels in columnar upper gastrointestinal mucosae in patients with Barrett's esophagus. Cancer Res, 1988; 48: 3288-3291.
26. Gerner EW, Garewal HS, Emerson SS, Sampliner RE. Gastrointestinal tissue polyamine contents of patients with Barrett's esophagus treated with alpha-difluoromethylornithine. Cancer Epidemiol Biomarkers Prev, 1994; 3: 325-330.
27. Garewal HS, Sampliner RE, Fennerty MB. Chemopreventive studies in Barrett's esophagus: a model premalignant lesion for esophageal adenocarcinoma. J Natl Cancer Inst Monogr, 1992; 51-54.
28. Sinicrope FA, Roddey G, McDonnell TJ, Shen Y, Cleary KR, Stephens LC. Increased apoptosis accompanies neoplastic development in the human colorectum. Clin Cancer Res, 1996; 2: 1999-2006.
29. Werner M, Mueller J, Walch A, Hofler H. The molecular pathology of Barrett's esophagus. Histol Histopathol, 1999; 14: 553-559.
30. Hughes SJ, Nambu Y, Soldes OS, et al. Fas/APO-1 (CD95) is not translocated to the cell membrane in esophageal adenocarcinoma. Cancer Res, 1997; 57: 5571-5578.
31. Reed JC. Bcl-2 and the regulation of programmed cell death. J Cell Biol, 1994; 124: 1-6.
32. Katada N, Hinder RA, Smyrk TC, et al. Apoptosis is inhibited early in the dysplasia-carcinoma sequence of Barrett esophagus. Arch Surg, 1997; 132: 728-733.
33. Goldblum JR, Rice TW. bcl-2 protein expression in the Barrett's metaplasia-dysplasia- carcinoma sequence. Mod Pathol, 1995; 8: 866-869.
34. Wetscher GJ, Schwelberger H, Unger A, et al. Reflux-induced apoptosis of the esophageal mucosa is inhibited in Barett's esophagus. Am J Surg, 1998; 176: 569-573.
35. Shay JW, Bacchetti S. A survey of telomerase activity in human cancer. Eur J Cancer, 1997; 33: 787-791.
36. Oshimura M, Barrett JC. Multiple pathways to cellular senescence: role of telomerase repressors. Eur J Cancer, 1997; 33: 710-715.
37. Bachor C, Bachor OA, Boukamp P. Telomerase is active in normal gastrointestinal mucosa and not up- regulated in precancerous lesions. J Cancer Res Clin Oncol, 1999; 125: 453-460.
38. Takubo K, Nakamura K, Izumiyama N, et al. Telomerase activity in esophageal carcinoma. J Surg Oncol, 1997; 66: 88-92.
39. Morales CP, Lee EL, Shay JW. In situ hybridization for the detection of telomerase RNA in the progression from Barrett's esophagus to esophageal adenocarcinoma. Cancer, 1998; 83: 652-659.
40. Levine DS, Reid BJ, Haggitt RC, Rubin CE, Rabinovitch PS. Correlation of ultrastructural aberrations with dysplasia and flow cytometric abnormalities in Barrett's epithelium. Gastroenterology, 1989; 96: 355-367.
41. Reid BJ, Blount PL, Rubin CE, Levine DS, Haggitt RC, Rabinovitch PS. Flow-cytometric and histological progression to malignancy in Barrett's esophagus:

prospective endoscopic surveillance of a cohort. Gastroenterology, 1992; 102: 1212-1219.

42. Reid BJ, Haggitt RC, Rubin CE, Rabinovitch PS. Barrett's esophagus. Correlation between flow cytometry and histology in detection of patients at risk for adenocarcinoma. Gastroenterology, 1987; 93: 1-11.

43. Gimenez A, Minguela A, Parrilla P, et al. Flow cytometric DNA analysis and p53 protein expression show a good correlation with histologic findings in patients with Barrett's esophagus. Cancer, 1998; 83: 641-651.

44. Montgomery EA, Hartmann DP, Carr NJ, Holterman DA, Sobin LH, Azumi N. Barrett esophagus with dysplasia. Flow cytometric DNA analysis of routine, paraffin-embedded mucosal biopsies. Am J Clin Pathol, 1996; 106: 298-304.

45. Haggitt RC, Reid BJ, Rabinovitch PS, Rubin CE. Barrett's esophagus. Correlation between mucin histochemistry, flow cytometry, and histologic diagnosis for predicting increased cancer risk. Am J Pathol, 1988; 131: 53-61.

46. Teodori L, Gohde W, Persiani M, et al. DNA/protein flow cytometry as a predictive marker of malignancy in dysplasia-free Barrett's esophagus: thirteen-year follow-up study on a cohort of patients. Cytometry, 1998; 34: 257-263.

47. James PD, Atkinson M. Value of DNA image cytometry in the prediction of malignant change in Barrett's oesophagus. Gut, 1989; 30: 899-905.

48. Fennerty MB, Sampliner RE, Way D, Riddell R, Steinbronn K, Garewal HS. Discordance between flow cytometric abnormalities and dysplasia in Barrett's esophagus. Gastroenterology, 1989; 97: 815-820.

49. Rabinovitch PS, Reid BJ, Haggitt RC, Norwood TH, Rubin CE. Progression to cancer in Barrett's esophagus is associated with genomic instability. Lab Invest, 1989; 60: 65-71.

50. Giaretti W. Aneuploidy mechanisms in human colorectal preneoplastic lesions and Barrett's esophagus. Is there a role for K-ras and p53 mutations? Anal Cell Pathol, 1997; 15: 99-117.

51. Blount PL, Galipeau PC, Sanchez CA, et al. 17p allelic losses in diploid cells of patients with Barrett's esophagus who develop aneuploidy. Cancer Res, 1994; 54: 2292-2295.

52. Galipeau PC, Cowan DS, Sanchez CA, et al. 17p (p53) allelic losses, 4N (G2/tetraploid) populations, and progression to aneuploidy in Barrett's esophagus. Proc Natl Acad Sci U S A, 1996; 93: 7081-7084.

53. Gleeson CM, Sloan JM, McManus DT, et al. Comparison of p53 and DNA content abnormalities in adenocarcinoma of the oesophagus and gastric cardia. Br J Cancer, 1998; 77: 277-286.

54. Finley RJ, Inculet RI. The results of esophagogastrectomy without thoracotomy for adenocarcinoma of the esophagogastric junction. Ann Surg, 1989; 210: 535-542; 542-543.

55. Bottger T, Dutkowski P, Kirkpatrick CJ, Junginger T. Prognostic Significance of Tumor Ploidy and Histomorphological Parameters in Adenocarcinoma of Barrett's Esophagus. Dig Surg, 1999; 16: 180-185.

56. McKinley MJ, Budman DR, Grueneberg D, Bronzo RL, Weissman GS, Kahn E. DNA content in Barrett's esophagus and esophageal malignancy. Am J Gastroenterol, 1987; 82: 1012-1015.

57. Sarbia M, Molsberger G, Willers R, et al. The prognostic significance of DNA ploidy in adenocarcinomas of the esophagogastric junction. J Cancer Res Clin Oncol, 1996; 122: 186-188.

58. Schneeberger AL, Finley RJ, Troster M, Lohmann R, Keeney M, Inculet RI. The prognostic significance of tumor ploidy and pathology in adenocarcinoma of the esophagogastric junction. Cancer, 1990; 65: 1206-1210.

59. Nakamura T, Nekarda H, Hoelscher AH, et al. Prognostic value of DNA ploidy and c-erbB-2 oncoprotein overexpression in adenocarcinoma of Barrett's esophagus [published erratum appears in Cancer, 1994; 73: 1785-1794.

60. Rodriguez E, Mathew S, Reuter V, Ilson DH, Bosl GJ, Chaganti RS. Cytogenetic analysis of 124 prospectively ascertained male germ cell tumors. Cancer Res, 1992; 52: 2285-2291.

61. Raskind WH, Norwood T, Levine DS, Haggitt RC, Rabinovitch PS, Reid BJ. Persistent clonal areas and clonal expansion in Barrett's esophagus. Cancer Res, 1992; 52: 2946-2950.

62. Garewal HS, Sampliner R, Liu Y, Trent JM. Chromosomal rearrangements in Barrett's esophagus. A premalignant lesion of esophageal adenocarcinoma. Cancer Genet Cytogenet, 1989; 42: 281-286.

63. Menke-Pluymers MB, van Drunen E, Vissers KJ, Mulder AH, Tilanus HW, Hagemeijer A. Cytogenetic analysis of Barrett's mucosa and adenocarcinoma of the distal esophagus and cardia. Cancer Genet Cytogenet, 1996; 90: 109-117.

64. Krishnadath KK, Tilanus HW, Alers JC, Mulder AH, van Dekken H. Detection of genetic changes in Barrett's adenocarcinoma and Barrett's esophagus by DNA in situ hybridization and immunohistochemistry. Cytometry, 1994; 15: 176-184.

65. Persons DL, Croughan WS, Borelli KA, Cherian R. Interphase cytogenetics of esophageal adenocarcinoma and precursor lesions. Cancer Genet Cytogenet, 1998; 106: 11-17.

66. Aaltonen LA, Peltomaki P, Mecklin JP, et al. Replication errors in benign and malignant tumors from hereditary nonpolyposis colorectal cancer patients. Cancer Res, 1994; 54: 1645-1648.

67. Meltzer SJ, Yin J, Manin B, et al. Microsatellite instability occurs frequently and in both diploid and aneuploid cell populations of Barrett's-associated esophageal adenocarcinomas. Cancer Res, 1994; 54: 3379-3382.

68. Wijnhoven BPL, Nollet F, de Both NJ, Tilanus HW, Dinjens WNM. Genetic alterations involving exon 3 of the beta-catenin gene do not play a role in adenocarcinomas of the oesophagus. Int J Cancer, 2000; 86: 533-537.

69. Gleeson CM, Sloan JM, McGuigan JA, Ritchie AJ, Weber JL, Russell SE. Ubiquitous somatic alterations at microsatellite alleles occur infrequently in Barrett's-associated esophageal adenocarcinoma. Cancer Res, 1996; 56: 259-263.

70. Gleeson CM, Sloan JM, McGuigan JA, Ritchie AJ, Weber JL, Russell SE. Widespread microsatellite instability occurs infrequently in adenocarcinoma of the gastric cardia. Oncogene, 1996; 12: 1653-1662.

71. Keller G, Rotter M, Vogelsang H, et al. Microsatellite instability in adenocarcinomas of the upper gastrointestinal tract. Relation to clinicopathological data and family history. Am J Pathol, 1995; 147: 593-600.

72. Muzeau F, Flejou JF, Belghiti J, Thomas G, Hamelin R. Infrequent microsatellite instability in oesophageal cancers. Br J Cancer, 1997; 75: 1336-1339.

73. Barrett MT, Galipeau PC, Sanchez CA, Emond MJ, Reid BJ. Determination of the frequency of loss of heterozygosity in esophageal adenocarcinoma by cell sorting, whole genome amplification and microsatellite polymorphisms. Oncogene, 1996; 12: 1873-1878.

74. Dolan K, Garde J, Gosney J, et al. Allelotype analysis of oesophageal adenocarcinoma: loss of heterozygosity occurs at multiple sites. Br J Cancer, 1998; 78: 950-957.

75. Wu TT, Watanabe T, Heitmiller R, Zahurak M, Forastiere AA, Hamilton SR. Genetic alterations in Barrett esophagus and adenocarcinomas of the esophagus and esophagogastric junction region. Am J Pathol, 1998; 153: 287-294.

76. Kallioniemi A, Kallioniemi OP, Sudar D, et al. Comparative genomic hybridization for molecular cytogenetic analysis of solid tumors. Science, 1992; 258: 818-821.

77. Du Plessis L, Dietzsch E, Van Gele M, et al. Mapping of novel regions of DNA gain and loss by comparative genomic hybridization in esophageal carcinoma in the Black and Colored populations of South Africa. Cancer Res, 1999; 59: 1877-1883.

78. El-Rifai W, Harper JC, Cummings OW, et al. Consistent genetic alterations in xenografts of proximal stomach and gastro-esophageal junction adenocarcinomas. Cancer Res, 1998; 58: 34-37.

79. Moskaluk CA, Hu J, Perlman EJ. Comparative genomic hybridization of esophageal and gastroesophageal adenocarcinomas shows consensus areas of DNA gain and loss. Genes Chromosomes Cancer, 1998; 22:305-311.

80. van Dekken H, Geelen E, Dinjens WN, et al. Comparative genomic hybridization of cancer of the gastroesophageal junction: deletion of 14Q31-32.1 discriminates between esophageal (Barrett's) and gastric cardia adenocarcinomas. Cancer Res, 1999; 59: 748-752.

81. Tanner MM, Tirkkonen M, Kallioniemi A, et al. Increased copy number at 20q13 in breast cancer: defining the critical region and exclusion of candidate genes. Cancer Res, 1994; 54: 4257-4260.

82. Hammoud ZT, Kaleem Z, Cooper JD, Sundaresan RS, Patterson GA, Goodfellow PJ. Allelotype analysis of esophageal adenocarcinomas: evidence for the involvement of sequences on the long arm of chromosome 4. Cancer Res, 1996; 56: 4499-4502.

83. Gleeson CM, Sloan JM, McGuigan JA, Ritchie AJ, Weber JL, Russell SE. Barrett's oesophagus: microsatellite analysis provides evidence to support the proposed metaplasia-dysplasia-carcinoma sequence. Genes Chromosomes Cancer, 1998; 21: 49-60.

84. Gleeson CM, Sloan JM, McGuigan JA, Ritchie AJ, Weber JL, Russell SE. Allelotype analysis of adenocarcinoma of the gastric cardia. Br J Cancer, 1997; 76: 1455-1465.

85. Rumpel CA, Powell SM, Moskaluk CA. Mapping of genetic deletions on the long arm of chromosome 4 in human esophageal adenocarcinomas. Am J Pathol, 1999; 154: 1329-1334.

86. Boynton RF, Blount PL, Yin J, et al. Loss of heterozygosity involving the APC and MCC genetic loci occurs in the majority of human esophageal cancers. Proc Natl Acad Sci U S A, 1992; 89: 3385-3388.

87. Zhuang Z, Vortmeyer AO, Mark EJ, et al. Barrett's esophagus: metaplastic cells with loss of heterozygosity at the APC gene locus are clonal precursors to invasive adenocarcinoma. Cancer Res, 1996; 56: 1961-1964.

88. Shimada Y, Imamura M, Shibagaki I, et al. Genetic alterations in patients with esophageal cancer with short- and long-term survival rates after curative esophagectomy. Ann Surg, 1997; 226: 162-168.

89. Peralta RC, Casson AG, Wang RN, Keshavjee S, Redston M, Bapat B. Distinct regions of frequent loss of heterozygosity of chromosome 5p and 5q in human esophageal cancer. Int J Cancer, 1998; 78: 600-605.

90. Tarmin L, Yin J, Zhou X, et al. Frequent loss of heterozygosity on chromosome 9 in adenocarcinoma and squamous cell carcinoma of the esophagus. Cancer Res, 1994; 54: 6094-6096.

91. Muzeau F, Flejou JF, Thomas G, Hamelin R. Loss of heterozygosity on chromosome 9 and p16 (MTS1, CDKN2) gene mutations in esophageal cancers. Int J Cancer, 1997; 72: 27-30.

92. Gonzalez MV, Artimez ML, Rodrigo L, et al. Mutation analysis of the p53, APC, and p16 genes in the Barrett's oesophagus, dysplasia, and adenocarcinoma. J Clin Pathol, 1997; 50: 212-217.

93. Barrett MT, Sanchez CA, Galipeau PC, Neshat K, Emond M, Reid BJ. Allelic loss of 9p21 and mutation of the CDKN2/p16 gene develop as early lesions during neoplastic progression in Barrett's esophagus. Oncogene, 1996; 13: 1867-1873.

94. Morgan RJ, Newcomb PV, Bailey M, Hardwick RH, Alderson D. Loss of heterozygosity at microsatellite marker sites for tumour suppressor genes in oesophageal adenocarcinoma. Eur J Surg Oncol, 1998; 24: 34-37.

95. Boynton RF, Huang Y, Blount PL, et al. Frequent loss of heterozygosity at the retinoblastoma locus in human esophageal cancers. Cancer Res, 1991; 51: 5766-5769.

96. Huang Y, Boynton RF, Blount PL, et al. Loss of heterozygosity involves multiple tumor suppressor genes in human esophageal cancers. Cancer Res, 1992; 52: 6525-6530.

97. Roncalli M, Bosari S, Marchetti A, et al. Cell cycle-related gene abnormalities and product expression in esophageal carcinoma. Lab Invest, 1998; 78: 1049-1057.

98. Wijnhoven BP, de Both NJ, van Dekken H, Tilanus HW, Dinjens WN. E-cadherin gene mutations are rare in adenocarcinomas of the oesophagus. Br J Cancer, 1999; 80: 1652-1657.

99. Dunn J, Garde J, Dolan K, et al. Multiple target sites of allelic imbalance on chromosome 17 in Barrett's oesophageal cancer. Oncogene, 1999; 18: 987-993.

100. Blount PL, Ramel S, Raskind WH, et al. 17p allelic deletions and p53 protein overexpression in Barrett's adenocarcinoma. Cancer Res, 1991; 51: 5482-5486.

101. Swift A, Risk JM, Kingsnorth AN, Wright TA, Myskow M, Field JK. Frequent loss of heterozygosity on chromosome 17 at 17q11.2-q12 in Barrett's adenocarcinoma. Br J Cancer, 1995; 71: 995-998.

102. Petty EM, Kalikin LM, Orringer MB, Beer DG. Distal chromosome 17q loss in Barrett's esophageal and gastric cardia adenocarcinomas: implications for tumorigenesis. Mol Carcinog, 1998; 22: 222-228.

103. Huebner K, Garrison PN, Barnes LD, Croce CM. The role of the FHIT/FRA3B locus in cancer. Annu Rev Genet, 1998; 32: 7-31.

104. Ohta M, Inoue H, Cotticelli MG, et al. The FHIT gene, spanning the chromosome 3p14.2 fragile site and renal carcinoma-associated t(3;8) breakpoint, is abnormal in digestive tract cancers. Cell, 1996; 84: 587-597.

105. Chen YJ, Chen PH, Lee MD, Chang JG. Aberrant FHIT transcripts in cancerous and corresponding non-cancerous lesions of the digestive tract. Int J Cancer, 1997; 72: 955-958.

106. Michael D, Beer DG, Wilke CW, Miller DE, Glover TW. Frequent deletions of FHIT and FRA3B in Barrett's metaplasia and esophageal adenocarcinomas. Oncogene, 1997; 15: 1653-1659.

107. Zou TT, Lei J, Shi YQ, et al. FHIT gene alterations in esophageal cancer and ulcerative colitis (UC). Oncogene, 1997; 15: 101-105.

108. Maher ER, Kaelin WG, Jr. von Hippel-Lindau disease. Medicine (Baltimore), 1997; 76: 381-391.

109. Vamecq J, Latruffe N. Medical significance of peroxisome proliferator-activated receptors. Lancet, 1999; 354: 141-148.

110. Kinzler KW, Nilbert MC, Vogelstein B, et al. Identification of a gene located at chromosome 5q21 that is mutated in colorectal cancers [see comments]. Science, 1991; 251: 1366-1370.

111. Sud R, Talbot IC, Delhanty JD. Infrequent alterations of the APC and MCC genes in gastric cancers from British patients. Br J Cancer, 1996; 74: 1104-1108.

112. Curtis LJ, Bubb VJ, Gledhill S, Morris RG, Bird CC, Wyllie AH. Loss of heterozygosity of MCC is not associated with mutation of the retained allele in sporadic colorectal cancer. Hum Mol Genet, 1994; 3: 443-446.

113. Blount PL, Meltzer SJ, Yin J, Huang Y, Krasna MJ, Reid BJ. Clonal ordering of 17p and 5q allelic losses in Barrett dysplasia and adenocarcinoma. Proc Natl Acad Sci U S A, 1993; 90: 3221-3225.

114. Vogelstein B, Fearon ER, Hamilton SR, et al. Genetic alterations during colorectal-tumor development. N Engl J Med, 1988; 319: 525-532.

115. Ogasawara S, Tamura G, Maesawa C, et al. Common deleted region on the long arm of chromosome 5 in esophageal carcinoma. Gastroenterology, 1996; 110: 52-57.

116. Powell SM, Papadopoulos N, Kinzler KW, Smolinski KN, Meltzer SJ. APC gene mutations in the mutation cluster region are rare in esophageal cancers. Gastroenterology, 1994; 107: 1759-1763.

117. Esteve A, Martel-Planche G, Sylla BS, Hollstein M, Hainaut P, Montesano R. Low frequency of p16/CDKN2 gene mutations in esophageal carcinomas. Int J Cancer, 1996; 66: 301-304.

118. Suzuki H, Zhou X, Yin J, et al. Intragenic mutations of CDKN2B and CDKN2A in primary human esophageal cancers. Hum Mol Genet, 1995; 4: 1883-1887.

119. Klump B, Hsieh CJ, Holzmann K, Gregor M, Porschen R. Hypermethylation of the CDKN2/p16 promoter during neoplastic progression in Barrett's esophagus. Gastroenterology, 1998; 115: 1381-1386.

120. Wong DJ, Barrett MT, Stoger R, Emond MJ, Reid BJ. p16INK4a promoter is hypermethylated at a high frequency in esophageal adenocarcinomas. Cancer Res, 1997; 57: 2619-2622.

121. Galipeau PC, Prevo LJ, Sanchez CA, Longton GM, Reid BJ. Clonal expansion and loss of heterozygosity at chromosomes 9p and 17p in premalignant esophageal (Barrett's) tissue. J Natl Cancer Inst, 1999; 91: 2087-2095.

122. Stiegler P, Kasten M, Giordano A. The RB family of cell cycle regulatory factors. J Cell Biochem Suppl, 1998; 30-31: 30-6.

123. Coppola D, Schreiber RH, Mora L, Dalton W, Karl RC. Significance of Fas and retinoblastoma protein expression during the progression of Barrett's metaplasia to adenocarcinoma. Ann Surg Oncol, 1999; 6: 298-304.

124. Jiang W, Zhang YJ, Kahn SM, et al. Altered expression of the cyclin D1 and retinoblastoma genes in human esophageal cancer. Proc Natl Acad Sci U S A, 1993; 90: 9026-9030.

125. Piette J, Neel H, Marechal V. Mdm2: keeping p53 under control. Oncogene, 1997; 15: 1001-1010.

126. Hall PA, Lane DP. p53 in tumour pathology: can we trust immunohistochemistry? J Pathol, 1994; 172: 1-4.

127. Moskaluk CA, Heitmiller R, Zahurak M, Schwab D, Sidransky D, Hamilton SR. p53 and p21(WAF1/CIP1/SDI1) gene products in Barrett esophagus and adenocarcinoma of the esophagus and esophagogastric junction. Hum Pathol, 1996; 27: 1211-1220.

128. Krishnadath KK, van Blankenstein M, Tilanus HW. Prognostic value of p53 in Barrett's oesophagus. Eur J Gastroenterol Hepatol, 1995; 7: 81-84.

129. Krishnadath KK, Tilanus HW, van Blankenstein M, Bosman FT, Mulder AH. Accumulation of p53 protein in normal, dysplastic, and neoplastic Barrett's oesophagus. J Pathol, 1995; 175: 175-180.

130. Rice TW, Goldblum JR, Falk GW, Tubbs RR, Kirby TJ, Casey G. p53 immunoreactivity in Barrett's metaplasia, dysplasia, and carcinoma. J Thorac Cardiovasc Surg, 1994; 108: 1132-1137.

131. Symmans PJ, Linehan JM, Brito MJ, Filipe MI. p53 expression in Barrett's oesophagus, dysplasia, and adenocarcinoma using antibody DO-7. J Pathol, 1994; 173: 221-226.

132. Ramel S, Reid BJ, Sanchez CA, et al. Evaluation of p53 protein expression in Barrett's esophagus by two-parameter flow cytometry. Gastroenterology, 1992; 102: 1220-1228.

133. Kim R, Clarke MR, Melhem MF, et al. Expression of p53, PCNA, and C-erbB-2 in Barrett's metaplasia and adenocarcinoma. Dig Dis Sci, 1997; 42: 2453-2462.

134. Jones DR, Davidson AG, Summers CL, Murray GF, Quinlan DC. Potential application of p53 as an intermediate biomarker in Barrett's esophagus. Ann Thorac Surg, 1994; 57: 598-603.

135. Younes M, Lebovitz RM, Lechago LV, Lechago J. p53 protein accumulation in Barrett's metaplasia, dysplasia, and carcinoma: a follow-up study. Gastroenterology, 1993; 105: 1637-1642.

136. Hamelin R, Flejou JF, Muzeau F, et al. TP53 gene mutations and p53 protein immunoreactivity in malignant and premalignant Barrett's esophagus. Gastroenterology, 1994; 107: 1012-1018.

137. Neshat K, Sanchez CA, Galipeau PC, et al. p53 mutations in Barrett's adenocarcinoma and high-grade dysplasia. Gastroenterology, 1994; 106: 1589-1595.

138. Flejou JF, Paraf F, Potet F, Muzeau F, Fekete F, Henin D. p53 protein expression in Barrett's adenocarcinoma: a frequent event with no prognostic significance. Histopathology, 1994; 24: 487-489.

139. Campomenosi P, Conio M, Bogliolo M, et al. p53 is frequently mutated in Barrett's metaplasia of the intestinal type. Cancer Epidemiol Biomarkers Prev, 1996; 5: 559-565.

140. Casson AG, Manolopoulos B, Troster M, et al. Clinical implications of p53 gene mutation in the progression of Barrett's epithelium to invasive esophageal cancer. Am J Surg, 1994; 167: 52-57.

141. Hardwick RH, Shepherd NA, Moorghen M, Newcomb PV, Alderson D. Adenocarcinoma arising in Barrett's oesophagus: evidence for the participation of p53 dysfunction in the dysplasia/carcinoma sequence. Gut, 1994; 35: 764-768.

142. Coggi G, Bosari S, Roncalli M, et al. p53 protein accumulation and p53 gene mutation in esophageal carcinoma. A molecular and immunohistochemical study with clinicopathologic correlations. Cancer, 1997; 79: 425-432.

143. Kimura H, Konishi K, Maeda K, et al. Flow cytometric analysis and immunohistochemical staining for the p53 protein and proliferating cell nuclear antigen in submucosal carcinoma of the esophagus. Hepatogastroenterology, 1999; 46: 285-289.

144. Kubba AK, Poole NA, Watson A. Role of p53 assessment in management of Barrett's esophagus. Dig Dis Sci, 1999; 44: 659-667.

145. Barrett MT, Schutte M, Kern SE, Reid BJ. Allelic loss and mutational analysis of the DPC4 gene in esophageal adenocarcinoma. Cancer Res, 1996; 56: 4351-4353.

146. Tahara E. Growth factors and oncogenes in human gastrointestinal carcinomas. J Cancer Res Clin Oncol, 1990; 116: 121-131.

147. Jankowski J, Hopwood D, Wormsley KG. Expression of epidermal growth factor, transforming growth factor alpha and their receptor in gastro-oesophageal diseases. Dig Dis, 1993; 11: 1-11.

148. Jankowski J, Coghill G, Tregaskis B, Hopwood D, Wormsley KG. Epidermal growth factor in the oesophagus. Gut, 1992; 33: 1448-1453.

149. Jankowski J, Murphy S, Coghill G, et al. Epidermal growth factor receptors in the oesophagus. Gut, 1992; 33: 439-443.

150. al-Kasspooles M, Moore JH, Orringer MB, Beer DG. Amplification and over-expression of the EGFR and erbB-2 genes in human esophageal adenocarcinomas. Int J Cancer, 1993; 54: 213-219.

151. Jankowski J, Hopwood D, Wormsley KG. Flow-cytometric analysis of growth-regulatory peptides and their receptors in Barrett's oesophagus and oesophageal adenocarcinoma. Scand J Gastroenterol ,1992; 27: 147-154.

152. Hardwick RH, Barham CP, Ozua P, et al. Immunohistochemical detection of p53 and c-erbB-2 in oesophageal carcinoma;no correlation with prognosis. Eur J Surg Oncol, 1997; 23: 30-35.

153. Hardwick RH, Shepherd NA, Moorghen M, Newcomb PV, Alderson D. c-erbB-2 overexpression in the dysplasia/carcinoma sequence of Barrett's oesophagus. J Clin Pathol, 1995; 48: 129-132.

154. Duhaylongsod FG, Gottfried MR, Iglehart JD, Vaughn AL, Wolfe WG. The significance of c-erb B-2 and p53 immunoreactivity in patients with adenocarcinoma of the esophagus. Ann Surg, 1995; 221.

155. Flejou JF, Paraf F, Muzeau F, et al. Expression of c-erbB-2 oncogene product in Barrett's adenocarcinoma: pathological and prognostic correlations. J Clin Pathol, 1994; 47: 23-26.

156. Polkowski W, van Sandick JW, Offerhaus GJ, et al. Prognostic value of Lauren classification and c-erbB-2 oncogene overexpression in adenocarcinoma of the esophagus and gastroesophageal junction. Ann Surg Oncol, 1999; 6: 290-297.

157. Friess H, Fukuda A, Tang WH, et al. Concomitant analysis of the epidermal growth factor receptor family in esophageal cancer: overexpression of epidermal growth factor receptor mRNA but not of c-erbB-2 and c-erbB-3. World J Surg, 1999; 23: 1010-1018.

158. Arii S, Mori A, Uchida S, Fujimoto K, Shimada Y, Imamura M. Implication of vascular endothelial growth factor in the development and metastasis of human cancers. Hum Cell, 1999; 12: 25-30.

159. Shimada Y, Imamura M, Watanabe G, et al. Prognostic factors of oesophageal squamous cell carcinoma from the perspective of molecular biology. Br J Cancer, 1999; 80: 1281-1288.

160. Inoue K, Ozeki Y, Suganuma T, Sugiura Y, Tanaka S. Vascular endothelial growth factor expression in primary esophageal squamous cell carcinoma. Association with angiogenesis and tumor progression. Cancer, 1997; 79: 206-213.

161. Kitadai Y, Haruma K, Tokutomi T, et al. Significance of vessel count and vascular endothelial growth factor in human esophageal carcinomas. Clin Cancer Res, 1998; 4: 2195-2200.

162. Wong MP, Cheung N, Yuen ST, Leung SY, Chung LP. Vascular endothelial growth factor is up-regulated in the early pre- malignant stage of colorectal tumour progression. Int J Cancer, 1999; 81: 845-850.

163. Soslow RA, Ying L, Altorki NK. Expression of acidic fibroblast growth factor in Barrett's esophagus and associated esophageal adenocarcinoma. J Thorac Cardiovasc Surg, 1997; 114: 838-843.

164. Soslow RA, Nabeya Y, Ying L, Blundell M, Altorki NK. Acidic fibroblast growth factor is progressively increased in the development of oesophageal glandular dysplasia and adenocarcinoma. Histopathology, 1999; 35: 31-37.

165. Itagawa Y, Ueda M, Ando N, Shinozawa Y, Shimizu N, Abe O. Significance of int-2/hst-1 coamplification as a prognostic factor in patients with esophageal squamous carcinoma. Cancer Res, 1991; 51: 1504-1508.

166. Chikuba K, Saito T, Uchino S, et al. High amplification of the hst-1 gene correlates with haematogenous recurrence after curative resection of oesophageal carcinoma. Br J Surg, 1995; 82: 364-367.

167. Kanda Y, Nishiyama Y, Shimada Y, et al. Analysis of gene amplification and overexpression in human esophageal- carcinoma cell lines. Int J Cancer, 1994; 58: 291-297.

168. Glick AB, Weinberg WC, Wu IH, Quan W, Yuspa SH. Transforming growth factor beta 1 suppresses genomic instability independent of a G1 arrest, p53, and Rb. Cancer Res, 1996; 56: 3645-3650.

169. Ellis FH, Jr., Loda M. Role of surveillance endoscopy, biopsy and biomarkers in early detection of Barrett's adenocarcinoma. Dis Esophagus, 1997; 10: 165-171.

170. Triadafilopoulo G, Kumble S. Transforming growth factor-b (TGFb) expression is enhanced in gastroesophageal reflux disease, Barrett's esophagus, and esophageal adenocarcinoma. Gastroenterology, 1996; 110: 1126.

171. Eppert K, Scherer SW, Ozcelik H, et al. MADR2 maps to 18q21 and encodes a TGFbeta-regulated MAD-related protein that is functionally mutated in colorectal carcinoma. Cell, 1996; 86: 543-552.

172. Souza RF, Garrigue-Antar L, Lei J, et al. Alterations of transforming growth factor-beta 1 receptor type II occur in ulcerative colitis-associated carcinomas, sporadic colorectal neoplasms, and esophageal carcinomas, but not in gastric neoplasms. Hum Cell, 1996; 9: 229-236.

173. Garrigue-Antar L, Souza RF, Vellucci VF, Meltzer SJ, Reiss M. Loss of transforming growth factor-beta type II receptor gene expression in primary human esophageal cancer. Lab Invest, 1996; 75: 263-272.

174. Polkowski W, van Lanschot JJ, Offerhaus GJ. Barrett esophagus and cancer: pathogenesis, carcinogenesis, and diagnostic dilemmas. Histol Histopathol, 1999; 14: 927-944.

175. Jiang W, Kahn SM, Guillem JG, Lu SH, Weinstein IB. Rapid detection of ras oncogenes in human tumors: applications to colon, esophageal, and gastric cancer. Oncogene, 1989; 4: 923-928.

176. Meltzer SJ, Zhou D, Weinstein WM. Tissue-specific expression of c-Ha-ras in premalignant gastrointestinal mucosae. Exp Mol Pathol, 1989; 51: 264-274.

177. Meltzer SJ, Mane SM, Wood PK, et al. Activation of c-Ki-ras in human gastrointestinal dysplasias determined by direct sequencing of polymerase chain reaction products. Cancer Res, 1990; 50: 3627-3630.

178. Jankowski J, Coghill G, Hopwood D, Wormsley KG. Oncogenes and onco-suppressor gene in adenocarcinoma of the oesophagus. Gut, 1992; 33: 1033-1038.

179. Sorsdahl K, Casson AG, Troster M, Van Meyel D, Inculet R, Chambers AF. p53 and ras gene expression in human esophageal cancer and Barrett's epithelium: a prospective study. Cancer Detect Prev, 1994; 18: 179-185.

180. Abdelatif OM, Chandler FW, Mills LR, McGuire BS, Pantazis CG, Barrett JM. Differential expression of c-myc and H-ras oncogenes in Barrett's epithelium. A study using colorimetric in situ hybridization. Arch Pathol Lab Med, 1991; 115: 880-885.

181. Trautmann B, Wittekind C, Strobel D, et al. K-ras point mutations are rare events in premalignant forms of Barrett's oesophagus. Eur J Gastroenterol Hepatol, 1996; 8: 799-804.

182. Casson AG, Wilson SM, McCart JA, et al. ras mutation and expression of the ras-regulated genes osteopontin and cathepsin L in human esophageal cancer. Int J Cancer, 1997; 72: 739-745.

183. Dang CV, Resar LM, Emison E, et al. Function of the c-Myc oncogenic transcription factor. Exp Cell Res, 1999; 253: 63-77.

184. Lu SH, Hsieh LL, Luo FC, Weinstein IB. Amplification of the EGF receptor and c-myc genes in human esophageal cancers. Int J Cancer, 1988; 42: 502-505.

185. Sarbia M, Loberg C, Wolter M, et al. Expression of Bcl-2 and amplification of c-myc are frequent in basaloid squamous cell carcinomas of the esophagus. Am J Pathol, 1999; 155: 1027-1032.

186. Miyazaki S, Sasno H, Shiga K, et al. Analysis of c-myc oncogene in human esophageal carcinoma: immunohistochemistry, in situ hybridization and northern and Southern blot studies. Anticancer Res, 1992; 12: 1747-1755.

187. Takekura N, Yasui W, Yoshida K, et al. pp60c-src protein kinase activity in human gastric carcinomas. Int J Cancer, 1990; 45: 847-851.

188. Cartwright CA, Kamps MP, Meisler AI, Pipas JM, Eckhart W. pp60c-src activation in human colon carcinoma. J Clin Invest, 1989; 83: 2025-2033.

189. Kumble S, Omary MB, Cartwright CA, Triadafilopoulos G. Src activation in malignant and premalignant epithelia of Barrett's esophagus. Gastroenterology, 1997; 112: 348-356.

190. Tsujii M, Kawano S, Tsuji S, Sawaoka H, Hori M, DuBois RN. Cyclooxygenase regulates angiogenesis induced by colon cancer cells. Cell, 1998; 93: 705-716.

191. Morgan G. Non-steroidal anti-inflammatory drugs and the chemoprevention of colorectal and oesophageal cancers. Gut, 1996; 38: 646-648.

192. Morgan GP, Williams JG. Inflammatory mediators in the oesophagus. Gut, 1994; 35: 297-298.

193. Zhang F, Subbaramaiah K, Altorki N, Dannenberg AJ. Dihydroxy bile acids activate the transcription of cyclooxygenase-2. J Biol Chem, 1998; 273: 2424-2428.

194. Zimmermann KC, Sarbia M, Weber AA, Borchard F, Gabbert HE, Schror K. Cyclooxygenase-2 expression in human esophageal carcinoma. Cancer Res, 1999; 59: 198-204.

195. Wilson KT, Fu S, Ramanujam KS, Meltzer SJ. Increased expression of inducible nitric oxide synthase and cyclooxygenase-2 in Barrett's esophagus and associated adenocarcinomas. Cancer Res, 1998; 58: 2929-2934.

196. Funkhouser EM, Sharp GB. Aspirin and reduced risk of esophageal carcinoma. Cancer, 1995; 76: 1116-1119.

197. Thun MJ, Namboodiri MM, Calle EE, Flanders WD, Heath CW, Jr. Aspirin use and risk of fatal cancer. Cancer Res, 1993; 53: 1322-1327.

198. Sherr CJ. Cancer cell cycles. Science, 1996; 274: 1672-1677.

199. Montesano R, Hollstein M, Hainaut P. Genetic alterations in esophageal cancer and their relevance to

etiology and pathogenesis: a review. Int J Cancer, 1996; 69: 225-235.

200. Arber N, Gammon MD, Hibshoosh H, et al. Overexpression of cyclin D1 occurs in both squamous carcinomas and adenocarcinomas of the esophagus and in adenocarcinomas of the stomach. Hum Pathol, 1999; 30: 1087-1092.

201. Arber N, Lightdale C, Rotterdam H, et al. Increased expression of the cyclin D1 gene in Barrett's esophagus. Cancer Epidemiol Biomarkers Prev, 1996; 5: 457-459.

202. Kuwahara M, Hirai T, Yoshida K, et al. p53, p21(Waf1/Cip1) and cyclin D1 protein expression and prognosis in esophageal cancer. Dis Esophagus, 1999; 12: 116-119.

203. Morgan RJ, Newcomb PV, Hardwick RH, Alderson D. Amplification of cyclin D1 and MDM-2 in oesophageal carcinoma. Eur J Surg Oncol, 1999; 25: 364-367.

204. Adelaide J, Monges G, Derderian C, Seitz JF, Birnbaum D. Oesophageal cancer and amplification of the human cyclin D gene CCND1/PRAD1. Br J Cancer, 1995; 71: 64-68.

205. Lloyd RV, Erickson LA, Jin L, et al. p27kip1: a multifunctional cyclin-dependent kinase inhibitor with prognostic significance in human cancers. Am J Pathol, 1999; 154: 313-323.

206. Ponce-Castaneda MV, Lee MH, Latres E, et al. p27Kip1: chromosomal mapping to 12p12-12p13.1 and absence of mutations in human tumors. Cancer Res, 1995; 55: 1211-1214.

207. Singh SP, Lipman J, Goldman H, et al. Loss or altered subcellular localization of p27 in Barrett's associated adenocarcinoma. Cancer Res, 1998; 58: 1730-1735.

208. el-Deiry WS, Tokino T, Velculescu VE, et al. WAF1, a potential mediator of p53 tumor suppression. Cell, 1993; 75: 817-825.

209. el-Deiry WS, Tokino T, Waldman T, et al. Topological control of p21WAF1/CIP1 expression in normal and neoplastic tissues. Cancer Res, 1995; 55: 2910-2919.

210. Hanas JS, Lerner MR, Lightfoot SA, et al. Expression of the cyclin-dependent kinase inhibitor p21(WAF1/CIP1) and p53 tumor suppressor in dysplastic progression and adenocarcinoma in Barrett esophagus. Cancer, 1999; 86: 756-763.

211. Shiohara M, el-Deiry WS, Wada M, et al. Absence of WAF1 mutations in a variety of human malignancies. Blood, 1994; 84: 3781-3784.

212. Perl AK, Wilgenbus P, Dahl U, Semb H, Christofori G. A causal role for E-cadherin in the transition from adenoma to carcinoma. Nature, 1998; 392: 190-193.

213. Jian WG, Darnton SJ, Jenner K, Billingham LJ, Matthews HR. Expression of E-cadherin in oesophageal carcinomas from the UK and China: disparities in prognostic significance. J Clin Pathol, 1997; 50: 640-644.

214. Bailey T, Biddlestone L, Shepherd N, Barr H, Warner P, Jankowski J. Altered cadherin and catenin complexes in the Barrett's esophagus- dysplasia-adenocarcinoma sequence: correlation with disease progression and dedifferentiation. Am J Pathol, 1998; 152: 135-144.

215. Jankowski JA, Newham PM, Kandemir O, Hirano S, Takeichi M, Pignatelli M. Differential expression of E-Cadherin in normal, metaplastic and dysplastic oesophageal mucosa: a putative biomarker. Int J Oncol, 1994: 441-448.

216. Krishnadath KK, Tilanus HW, van Blankenstein M, et al. Reduced expression of the cadherin-catenin complex in oesophageal adenocarcinoma correlates with poor prognosis. J Pathol, 1997; 182: 331-338.

217. Washington K, Chiappori A, Hamilton K, et al. Expression of beta-catenin, alpha-catenin, and E-cadherin in Barrett's esophagus and esophageal adenocarcinom. Mod Pathol, 1998; 11: 805-813.

218. Berx G, Becker KF, Hofler H, van Roy F. Mutations of the human E-cadherin (CDH1) gene. Hum Mutat, 1998; 12: 226-237.

219. Shiozaki H, Oka H, Inoue M, Tamura S, Monden M. E-cadherin mediated adhesion system in cancer cells. Cancer, 1996; 77: 1605-1613.

220. Pennisi E. How a growth control path takes a wrong turn to cancer. Science, 1998; 281: 1438-1439, 1441.

221. Duffy MJ, Maguire TM, McDermott EW, O'Higgins N. Urokinase plasminogen activator: a prognostic marker in multiple types of cancer. J Surg Oncol, 1999; 71: 130-135.

222. Sier CF, Verspaget HW, Griffioen G, Ganesh S, Vloedgraven HJ, Lamers CB. Plasminogen activators in normal tissue and carcinomas of the human oesophagus and stomach. Gut, 1993; 34: 80-85.

223. Hewin DF, Savage PB, Alderson D, Vipond MN. Plasminogen activators in oesophageal carcinoma. Br J Surg, 1996; 83: 1152-1155.

224. Nekarda H, Schlegel P, Schmitt M, et al. Strong prognostic impact of tumor-associated urokinase-type plasminogen activator in completely resected adenocarcinoma of the esophagus. Clin Cancer Res, 1998; 4: 1755-1763.

225. Mulder JW, Kruyt PM, Sewnath M, et al. Colorectal cancer prognosis and expression of exon-v6-containing CD44 proteins. Lancet, 1994; 344: 1470-1472.

226. Bottger TC, Youssef V, Dutkowski P, Maschek H, Brenner W, Junginger T. Expression of CD44 variant proteins in adenocarcinoma of Barrett's esophagus and its relation to prognosis. Cancer, 1998; 83: 1074-1080.

227. Castella E, Ariza A, Fernandez-Vasalo A, Roca X, Ojanguren I. Expression of CD44H and CD44v3 in normal oesophagus, Barrett mucosa and oesophageal carcinoma. J Clin Pathol, 1996; 49: 489-492.

228. Lagorce-Pages C, Paraf F, Dubois S, Belghiti J, Flejou JF. Expression of CD44 in premalignant and malignant Barrett's oesophagus. Histopathology, 1998; 32: 7-14.

229. Keppler D, Sameni M, Moin K, Mikkelsen T, Diglio CA, Sloane BF. Tumor progression and angiogenesis: cathepsin B & Co. Biochem Cell Biol, 1996; 74: 799-810.

230. Hughes SJ, Glover TW, Zhu XX, et al. A novel amplicon at 8p22-23 results in overexpression of cathepsin B in esophageal adenocarcinoma. Proc Natl Acad Sci U S A, 1998; 95: 12410-12415.

231. Jankowski JA, Wright NA, Meltzer SJ, et al. Molecular evolution of the metaplasia-dysplasia-adenocarcinoma sequence in the esophagus. Am J Pathol, 1999; 154: 965-973.

232. Fitzgerald RC, Triadafilopoulos G. Recent developments in the molecular characterization of Barrett's esophagus. Dig Dis, 1998; 16: 63-80.

233. Souza RF, Meltzer SJ. The molecular basis for carcinogenesis in metaplastic columnar-lined esophagus. Gastroenterol Clin North Am, 1997; 26: 583-597.

234. Barrett MT, Sanchez CA, Prevo LJ, et al. Evolution of neoplastic cell lineages in Barrett oesophagus. Nat Genet, 1999; 22: 106-109.

3.4   ENDOSCOPIC SURVEILLANCE

Richard E. Sampliner

1. THE RATIONALE FOR ENDOSCOPIC SURVEILLANCE OF BARRETT'S ESOPHAGUS

Barrett's esophagus is a recognized premalignant lesion for adenocarcinoma of the esophagus and gastric cardia. The rationale for endoscopic surveillance of patients with Barrett's esophagus is the early detection of high-grade dysplasia and adenocarcinoma of the esophagus in order to improve patient survival. It is well recognized that patients presenting with dysphagia and diagnosed with adenocarcinoma of the esophagus and Barrett's esophagus at the same time have a poor prognosis. The best data supporting endoscopic surveillance are three retrospective studies comparing outcome in surveyed and non-surveyed patients with Barrett's esophagus and adenocarcinoma of the esophagus. In the first reported series, 19 Barrett's patients undergoing surveillance diagnosed with cancer had a five year survival of 62% in contrast to 58 patients with prevalent adenocarcinoma in Barrett's esophagus with a five year survival of 20% [1]. This was subsequently confirmed in a series of 17 patients undergoing surveillance with a five year survival greater than 80% in contrast to a 20% five year survival in 35 patients not undergoing surveillance [2]. Four of the 17 surveyed patients had high-grade dysplasia and not cancer at the time of resection and if excluded from the analysis the improved survival was not statistically significant. In a 2-year follow-up of 16 patients undergoing surveillance the five year survival was 86% in contrast to a 43% survival in 54 patients not undergoing surveillance [3]. Will prospective data supporting these observations ever be available? This is unlikely in view of the large number of patients who would have to be followed over an extended time period. Such a study would have to be multicentered and very costly. Even using a high estimate of the annual incidence of cancer in Barrett's esophagus (1.3%), a randomized trial would require approximately five thousand patients followed 10 years [4].

2. THE NATURAL HISTORY OF DYSPLASIA

Unfortunately, our database on the natural history of dysplasia and the development of adenocarcinoma in Barrett's esophagus is limited. Prospective series come from five centers [5-10]. More than 150 patients have been followed from a baseline endoscopy with no dysplasia to cancer – 2% developed cancer over a follow-up of 3.6-10 years. Even fewer patients with low-grade dysplasia, 45, have been followed with 18% developing cancer over 1.5-4.3 years. In the majority of the patients low grade dysplasia does not progress or even persist. One hundred twenty seven patients with high-grade dysplasia have been followed from .2-9.5 years with 30% developing cancer. A recently reported series from the University of Washington highlights the problem of referral bias of patients with high-grade dysplasia versus having the opportunity to observe the entire natural history of dysplasia. If all patients with high-grade dysplasia are included, then 59% developed cancer over five years [11]. However, if only incidence cases are included, i.e. patients who were observed to develop high grade dysplasia, then a dramatically lower 30% went on to cancer. In other words, patients referred with high-grade dysplasia may well have a higher risk of cancer because they may be further along in their course of evolution to adenocarcinoma of the esophagus. The course of high-grade dysplasia is variable and not all patients progress to cancer.

In contrast to these endoscopic surveillance series, an observational study of patients with Barrett's esophagus suggests that few patients with Barrett's actually die from adenocarcinoma of the esophagus [12]. Although "only" 2.5% died of cancer, in fact this is a high death rate from esophageal cancer. Esophageal cancer represented 12.5% of the deaths from cancer, much higher than expected for the general population. Furthermore this large cohort of Barrett's patients with a mean follow up of 9 years had a mortality 50% in excess of an age and sex matched population for reasons not fully evident.

H.W. Tilanus and S.E.A. Attwood (eds.), Barrett's Esophagus, 211–216.
© 2001 *Kluwer Academic Publishers. Printed in the Netherlands.*

Surveillance Intervals

No Dysplasia	Low Grade Dysplasia	High Grade Dysplasia
2 endoscopies	Confirmed by repeat endoscopy	Confirm with repeat endoscopy and expert pathologist
↓	↓	↓
3 years	Annual until no dysplasia	Intervention

The wide range of the reported incidence of adenocarcinoma of the esophagus - 1 in 52 to 1 in 441 patient years of follow-up – adds to the controversy of the value of surveillance endoscopy [7,13]. The range is attributable to the variability of the number of Barrett's patients followed, the definition of Barrett's esophagus, i.e. the length and presence of intestinal metaplasia, the definition of an incidence case, i.e. the duration of follow up defined as a prevalence case, and the retrospective or prospective nature of the study. A recent analysis of the incidence of cancer highlights that those series with more patient-years of follow up report a lower incidence [14]. This is not surprising in view of a larger number of patients and/or a longer follow-up "diluting" the reported incidence of cancer. In 15 published studies the number of incidence cancers range from 1 to 6 with a total of only 52 (mean 3.5 per study). The size of the series range from 32 to 176 patients (mean 84 per study) [7-8,12-13,15-25].

3. SURVEILLANCE GUIDELINES

Most gastroenterologists see patients with Barrett's esophagus in their practice on a regular basis. Faced with the practical dilemma of how to manage the cancer risk, guidelines have been proposed for surveillance in patients with Barrett's esophagus. If a patient has no dysplasia on two endoscopies with systematic biopsies, then a 3-year interval for surveillance endoscopy and biopsy have been recommended [26]. If low grade dysplasia is found and a repeat endoscopy confirms that low grade dysplasia is the most severe grade present, then yearly endoscopy is probably adequate after confirmation of the grade of dysplasia with a repeat endoscopy. Because of the sampling problem, low-grade dysplasia may be found either adjacent to or overlying a frank carcinoma. Therefore, the finding of low-grade dysplasia is not necessarily reassuring. With the detection of high-grade dysplasia, the gastroenterologist is faced with the

dilemma of choosing between esophagectomy, continuing more intensive surveillance, or endoscopic ablative therapy. This dilemma results from the variability of the natural history of high-grade dysplasia ranging from apparent regression to a lower grade or no dysplasia to progression to cancer over a brief or prolonged (years) interval. Because this grade of dysplasia is a critical clinical decision point a repeat endoscopy should be performed to ensure that cancer is not already present. If high-grade dysplasia is detected at repeat biopsy, a pathologist expert in reading dysplasia in mucosal biopsies should confirm the diagnosis. The choice of a therapeutic intervention to eliminate high grade dysplasia is between esophagectomy, endoscopic mucosal ablation and endoscopic mucosal resection. The surgical data based on clinical esophagectomy series usually lacking an explicit endoscopic surveillance protocol demonstrate a 40% frequency of cancer in the resected specimen [27]. A series utilizing a rigorous research endoscopy protocol produces the capability of differentiating high-grade dysplasia from early adenocarcinoma in 9 patients subjected to esophagectomy [9]. In the usual clinical setting where such an endoscopy protocol is not followed, esophagectomy in a patient fit for surgery at an experienced center is reasonable. With the application of a research endoscopy protocol, ongoing surveillance is an option.

What are endoscopists doing in clinical practice? A survey in the United States prior to the publication of American College of Gastroenterology guidelines, revealed that 96% of gastroenterologists were performing surveillance endoscopy in patients with Barrett's esophagus [29]. On average these physicians saw 20 patients with Barrett's esophagus in their practice. Ninety-five percent of those responding performed surveillance endoscopy more often than every 3 years in patients who had no dysplasia on two sets of biopsies. Only 15% utilized jumbo biopsy forceps. Seventy three percent recommended esophagectomy for the finding of high-grade dysplasia. Interestingly, in spite of the widely perceived range of the lifetime cancer risk of a patient with Barrett's esophagus of 0.1-40% there was no relationship between the perceived cancer risk and the frequency of surveillance. A better understanding of the lifetime risk of cancer of an individual patient will help rationalize surveillance practice.

4. SURVEILLANCE COST

One of the barriers to surveillance in Barrett's esophagus is the cost. Assuming a cancer incidence of 0.4% per year, the cost for a five year surveillance interval is $98,000 per quality life year. For the dollars spent this represents a greater gain in life than heart transplantation or cervical cancer screening – two modalities currently practiced in the United States [30]. Such a decision analysis is sensitive to cancer incidence, surveillance intervals, and quality of life post esophagectomy. However, extending practitioner surveillance interval is a difficult process that will take years to accomplish.

Major advances could be made in reducing cost of surveillance with non-endoscopic detection of dysplasia. Non-endoscopic balloon cytology has been used to detect dysplasia. The sensitivity compared to biopsy was 80% for high-grade dysplasia or cancer but only 25% for low-grade dysplasia [31]. A more abrasive balloon may improve the yield. Additionally, the documentation that endoscopic mucosal ablation therapy is effective in decreasing the development of cancer would offer a less morbid and potentially less expensive approach than esophagectomy [32]. Not only would this change cost analyses, but it would also increase the number of patients with Barrett's eligible for surveillance. Patients who are not candidates for esophageal resection because of older age or comorbidity would be candidates for endoscopic ablation.

5. WHO TO SURVEY

Which patients with Barrett's esophagus should undergo surveillance? Although males more commonly have Barrett's esophagus than females, 90% of Barrett's patients with adenocarcinoma of the esophagus are male [33-35]. Additionally, Caucasians seem to have a unique predilection to the development of adenocarcinoma of the esophagus. As patients with Barrett's age both dysplasia and cancer are

more likely [36]. The highest yield of surveillance would therefore be older white males because of their greater risk of developing malignancy.

Candidates for Surveillance
Caucasian
Male
Age 50 and older
Dysplasia
p53 mutation

The decision to enroll an individual in a surveillance program is clearly difficult. Evidence based data demonstrating differential outcome in patient groups would clarify this decision process. As in any surveillance of a premalignant lesion, the issue of when to discontinue surveillance is important and has cost saving implications. Because an 80-year-old has a life expectancy of less than one decade, it would seem reasonable to discontinue surveillance in such an individual who has no evidence of dysplasia. Furthermore, in a younger patient who has major comorbidity, who would not tolerate esophageal resection or potentially repeated endoscopy for endoscopic therapy, surveillance should not be undertaken.

6. HOW TO SURVEY

How should surveillance be performed? Because inflammatory changes from reflux esophagitis can confound the reading of dysplasia, reflux symptoms should be controlled and erosive esophagitis healed for the performance of surveillance biopsies to avoid confounding the histologic interpretation. The number of biopsies necessary to rule out dysplasia is difficult to determine. The University of Washington recommends a rigorous surveillance protocol of four quadrant biopsies every 2cm. Once a patient has been found to have high-grade dysplasia, a 4-quadrant biopsy protocol every 1cm with a jumbo biopsy forceps is recommended. This represents an intensity of biopsy that is rarely followed in clinical practice. In a case report from this group, one patient had more than 60 biopsies per cm of metaplasia over less than 1 year. Only 15% of gastroenterologists use the recommended "jumbo" biopsy forceps which obtains biopsies with a larger sample volume [29]. In spite of using a jumbo biopsy forceps and following a 4-quadrant biopsy protocol every 2cm, the yield of cancer is not improved compared to a standard biopsy forceps [37]. Intense biopsy protocols require an additional person in the endoscopy suite handling and labeling biopsies as their sole function. It is a form of research endoscopy that requires more time than the standard upper endoscopy performed in a practice context. Until better methods are developed the number of biopsies obtained in patients will be a compromise between the ideal and the achievable. A more efficient biopsy technique retrieving multiple samples simultaneously is eagerly awaited. Once dysplasia is detected, the importance of separating different levels of biopsies becomes apparent. With separation the dysplastic area can be localized within 1-2cm and more intensely sampled on repeat endoscopy. The clinical endoscopist must be willing to spend the time to carefully sample the Barrett's esophagus over its entire length. Controversy exists as to the focality of dysplastic changes in Barrett's esophagus, estimates range from only one biopsy showing dysplasia in 69% of patients [38] to two thirds of patients having high grade dysplasia at more than one level of biopsies. Even if this controversy is clarified sampling will remain a problem with Barrett's esophagus. The problem of sampling is highlighted by a study which systematically mapped esophagectomy specimens form patients undergoing resection for high-grade dysplasia or early adenocarcinoma. The median surface area of Barrett's in this patient group was 32cm^2, low-grade dysplasia dysplasia 13cm^2, high grade dysplasia 1.3cm^2 and cancer 1.1cm^2 [39]. This is why optical techniques to demonstrate dysplasia represent a potential major breakthrough in our ability to survey Barrett's esophagus. Laser induced fluorescence can accurately detect high-grade dysplasia but has had a low specificity for nondysplastic Barrett's of 70% [40]. Light induced fluorescence endoscopy also detected high-grade dysplasia and early cancer [41]. Photodynamic diagnosis using 5-aminolevulenic acid as a photosensitizer can also demonstrate dysplasia [42]. These techniques remain to be validated. The

intensity and frequency of surveillance are driven by dysplasia. Although the interobserver agreement for the reading of high-grade dysplasia is good (86%), that for separating high grade dysplasia from intramucosal cancer and low grade dysplasia from other grades is only fair. Risk stratification could be further improved with the use of validated biomarkers. For example p53 mutation may help identify patients with low-grade dysplasia who will progress to cancer [43]. In a subgroup of Barrett's patients with high-grade dysplasia and cancer p53 mutation is widespread and apparently a field defect [44]. Such a biologic field defect which is easier to recognize than an isolated mutation would identify patients at greatest risk of cancer and simplify risk stratification. In one series of patients with Barrett's, patients with negative or low grade dysplasia and lacking aneuploidy or increased 4N fraction on flow cytometry had no cancer develop in 5 years [11]. Validation of this finding would enable at least a major reduction in the frequency of surveillance of such patients.

7. THE FUTURE

Reduction in the development of cancer in patients with Barrett's esophagus could be achieved with progress in a number of areas. A better understanding of the natural history of dysplasia would help better define surveillance intervals. Improved detection of dysplasia that would not be subject to sampling problems would facilitate surveillance. Risk stratification of individual patients would be enhanced with validation of demographic factors, optical detection of dysplasia and biologic markers. Then intensive surveillance could be focused on individuals with high risk based on age, gender, ethnicity, dysplasia and phenotypic or genotypic features. This progress would reduce cost and more importantly better serve patients with Barrett's esophagus.

REFERENCES

1. Streitz J, Andrews C, Ellis F. Endoscopic surveillance of Barrett's esophagus: does it help? J Thorac Cardiovasc Surg 1993;105:383-8.
2. Peters J, Clarck G, Ireland A, Chandrasoma P, Smyrk T, DeMeester T. Outcome of adenocarcinoma arising in Barrett's esophagus in endoscopically surveyed and nonsurveyed patients. J Thorac Cardiovasc Surg 1994;108:813-22.
3. vanSandick J, vanLanschot J, Kuiken B, Tytgat G, Offerhaus G. Impact of endoscopic biopsy surveillance of Barrett's oesophagus on pathological stage and clinical outcome of Barrett's carcinoma. Gut 1998;43:216-22.
4. Provenzale D, Kemp J, Arora S, et al. A guide for surveillance of patients with Barrett's esophagus. Am J Gastroenterol 1994;89:670-80.
5. Reid B, Weinstein W, Lewin K, et al. Endoscopic biopsy can detect high grade dysplasia or early adenocarcinoma in Barrett's esophagus without grossly recognizable neoplastic lesions. Gastroenterology 1988;94:81-90.

6. Robertson C, Mayberry J, Nicholson D, James P, Atkinson M. Value of endoscopic surveillance in the detection of neoplastic change in Barrett's oesophagus. Br J Surg 1988;75:760-3.

7. Hameetman W, Tytgat J, Houthoff H, VanDenTweek J. Barrett's esophagus: development of dysplasia and adenocarcinoma. Gastroenterology 1989;69:1249-56.

8. Miros M, Kerlin P, Walker N. Only patients with dysplasia progress to adenocarcinoma in Barrett's oesophagus. Gut 1991;32:1441-6.

9. Levine D, Haggitt R, Blount P, Rabinovitch P, Rusch V, Reid B. An endoscopic biopsy protocol can differentiate high grade dysplasia from early adenocarcinoma in Barrett's esophagus. Gastroenterology 1993;105:40-50.

10. Weston A, Badr A, Hassanein R. Prospective multivariate analysis of clinical, endoscopic, and histological factors predictive of the development of Barrett's multifocal high grade dysplasia or adenocarcinoma. Am J Gastroenterol 1999;94:3413-9.

11. Reid B, Levine D, Longton G, Blount P, Rabinovitch P. Predictors of progression to cancer in Barrett's esophagus: baseline histology and flow cytometry identify low and high risk patient subsets. Am J Gastroenterol 1999;94:2598(85).

12. VanDerBurgh A, Doos J, Hop W, VanBlankenstein M. Oesophageal cancer is an uncommon cause of death in patients with Barrett's oesophagus. Gut 1996;39:5-8.

13. Cameron A, Ott B, Payne W. The incidence of adenocarcinoma in columnar lined (Barrett's) esophagus. N Engl J Med 1985;313:857-9.

14. Shaheen N, Crosby M, Bozymski E. Is there publication bias in the reporting of cancer risk of Barrett's esophagus? Gastroenterology 1999;116:G0404.

15. Spechler S, Robbins A, Rubins H, et al. Adenocarcinoma and Barrett's esophagus: a overrated risk? Gastroenterology 1984;87:927-33.

16. Robertson C, Mayberry J, Nicholson D, James P, Atkinson M. Value of endoscopic surveillance in the detection of neoplastic change in Barrett's oesophagus. Br J Surg 1988;75:760-3.

17. Watson R, Porter K, Sloan J. Incidence of adenocarcinoma in Barrett's oesophagus and an evaluation of endoscopic surveillance. Eur J Gastroenterol 1991;3:159-62.

18. Ovaska J, Miettinen K, Kivilaakso E. Adenocarcinoma arising in Barrett's esophagus. Dig Dis Sci 1989;34:1336-9.

19. Bonelli L, GOSPE. Barrett's esophagus: results of a multicentric survey. Endoscopy 1993;25(suppl):652-4.

20. Iftikhar S, James P, Steele R, et al. Length of Barrett's oesophagus: an important factor in the development of dysplasia and adenocarcinoma. Gut 1992;33:1155-8.

21. Wright T, Gray M, Morris A, Gilmore I, Ellis A, Smart H, Myskow M, Nash J, Donnelly R, Kingsnorth A. Cost effectiveness of detecting Barrett's cancer. Gut 1996;39:574-9.

22. Drewitz D, Young M, Maples M, Ramirez F. The incidence of adenocarcinoma in Barrett's esophagus: a prospective study of 170 patients followed 4.8 years. Am J Gastroenterol 1997;92:212-5.

23. Katz D, Rothstein R, Schned A, Dunn J, SeaverK, Antonioli D. The development of dysplasia and adenocarcinoma during endoscopic surveillance of Barrett's esophagus. Am J Gastroenterol 1998;93:536-41.

24. O'Connor J, Falk G, Richter J. The incidence of adenocarcinoma and dysplasia in Barrett's esophagus. Am J Gastroenterol 1999;94:2037-42.

25. Williamson W, Ellis F, Gibb S, et al. Barrett's esophagus: prevalence and incidence of adenocarcinoma. Arch Intern Med 1991;151:2212-6.

26. Sampliner R, The Practice Parameters Committee of the American College of Gastroenterology. Practice guidelines on the diagnosis, surveillance, and therapy of Barrett's esophagus. Am J Gastroenterol 1998;93:1028-32.

27. Edwards M, Gable D, Lentsch A, Richardson J. The rationale for esophagectomy as the optimal therapy for Barrett's esophagus with high grade dysplasia. Ann Surg 1996;223:585-91.

28. Heitmiller R, Redmond M, Hamilton S. Barrett's esophagus with high grade dysplasia: an indication for prophylactic esophagectomy. Ann Surg 1996;224:66-71.

29. Gross G, Canto M, Hixson J, Powe N. Management of Barrett's esophagus: a national study of practice patterns and their cost implications. Am J Gastroenterol 1999;94:3440-7.

30. Provenzale D, Schmitt C, Wong J. Barrett's esophagus: a new look at surveillance based on emerging estimates of cancer risk. Am J Gastroenterol 1999;94:2043-53.

31. Falk G, Chittajallu R, Goldblum J, Biscotti C, Geisinger K, Petras R, et al. Surveillance of patients with Barrett's esophagus for dysplasia and cancer with balloon cytology. Gastroenterology 1997;112:1787-97.

32. Overholt B, Panjehpour M, Haydek J. Photodynamic therapy for Barrett's esophagus: follow up in 100 patients. Gastrointest Endosc 1999;49:1-7.

33. Streitz J, Ellis F, Gibb S, Balogh K, Watkins E. Adenocarcinoma in Barrett's esophagus. Ann Surg 1991;213:122-5.

34. Paraf F, Flejou J, Pignon J, Fekete F, Potet F. Surgical pathology of adenocarcinoma arising in Barrett's esophagus. Am J Surg Pathol 1995;19:183-91.

35. Hoff S, Sawyers J, Blanke C, Choy H, Stewart J. Prognosis of adenocarcinoma arising in Barrett's esophagus. Ann Thorac Surg 1998;65:176-81.

36. Gopal D, Faigel D, Magaret N, Fennerty M, Sampliner R, Garewal H, Falk G, Lieberman D. Risk factors for dysplasia in patients with Barrett's esophagus (BE): results from a multicenter consortium. Gastroenterology 1999;116:A175.

37. Falk G, Rice T, Goldblum J, Richter R. Jumbo biopsy forceps protocol still misses unsuspected cancer in Barrett's esophagus with high grade dysplasia. Gastrointest Endosc 1999;49:170-6.

38. Reid B, Blount P, Feng Z, Levine, D. Optimizing endoscopic biopsy detection of early cancers in Barrett's high grade dysplasia. Am J Gastroenterol 1999;94:2598(84).

39. Cameron A, Carpenter H. Barrett's esophagus, high grade dysplasia, and early adenocarcinoma: a pathological study. Am J Gastroenterol 1997;92:586.

40. Panjehpour M, Overholt B, Vo-Dihn T, Haggitt R, Edwards H, Buckley F. Endoscopic fluorescence detection of high grade dysplasia in Barrett's esophagus. Gastroenterology 1996;111:93-101.

41. Messmann H, Knuchel R, Baumler W, Holstege A, Scholmerich J. Endoscopic fluorescence detection of dysplasia in patients with Barrett's esophagus, ulcerative colitis, or adenomatous polyps after 5-aminolevulinic acid-induced protoporphyrin IX sensitization. Gastrointest Endosc 1999;49:97-101.

42. Haringsma J, Prawirodirdjo W, Tytgat G. Accuracy of fluorescence imaging of dysplasia in Barrett's esophagus. Gastroenterology 1999;116:G1832.

43. Younes M, Ertan A, Lechago L, Somoano J, Lechago J. p53 protein accumulation is a specific marker of

malignant potential in Barrett's metaplasia. Dig Dis Sci 1997;42:697-701.

44. Prevo L, Sanchez C, Galipeau P, Reid B. p53 mutant clones and field effects in Barrett's esophagus. Cancer Res 1999;59:4784-7.

3.5 SHORT SEGMENT BARRETT'S ESOPHAGUS AND INTESTINAL METAPLASIA AT THE GASTRO-ESOPHAGEAL JUNCTION

Shaun R. Preston and Geoffrey W. B. Clark

1. INTRODUCTION

Barrett's esophagus is a pathological entity in which the normal squamous mucosa of the lower esophagus is replaced by a metaplastic columnar mucosa. It is accepted to be a consequence of gastro-esophageal reflux disease (GERD) and is premalignant. It has been suggested that in health the normal distal esophagus may be lined by columnar mucosa for a distance of up to 2 cm,[1] placing the squamocolumnar junction within the lower esophagus. In clinical practice the landmarks which define the exact termination of the esophagus and the beginning of the stomach have proved difficult to measure with certainty, especially in patients with a hiatus hernia. Consequently, Barrett's esophagus, was previously only diagnosed when the columnar mucosa extended well into the esophagus, at least 3 cm proximal to the gastro-esophageal junction[2]. Other investigators have used different criteria ranging from 2 to 5cm[3,4]. However in the 1980s the accepted international standard for the diagnosis of Barrett's esophagus was a purely endoscopic diagnosis, made when the squamo-columnar junction (SCJ) was located more than 3cm above the proximal gastric folds.

Histological studies on the columnar lined esophagus demonstrate a variety of histological types: 1) gastric fundic epithelium, 2) junctional epithelium, or 3) a distinctive intestinal metaplastic epithelium termed specialized columnar epithelium[5]. Based upon histological examination of esophageal resection specimens specialized columnar epithelium (IM) is the mucosal type most strongly associated with both dysplastic change and adenocarcinoma formation[6]. Hence concern was raised about diagnosing Barrett's mucosa purely based upon endoscopy, especially in the light of reports of adenocarcinomas arising in shorter lengths of columnar lined esophagus (< 3 cm) harboring IM[7]. It was in this setting that a columnar lined esophagus measuring < 3 cm visible to the endoscopist with IM on biopsy became known as short segment Barrett's esophagus[7-11].

As interest in short segment Barrett's esophagus increased and physicians started to biopsy the "no go area" of the gastro-

esophageal junction the concept of "ultra short segment Barrett's" has emerged. The condition is diagnosed when biopsies from the gastro-esophageal junction reveal IM and the squamocolumnar junction is located at the site of the gastro-esophageal junction, in the absence of a columnar lining in the distal esophagus visible to the endoscopist[12,13]. In essence this is a histological diagnosis. This article reviews the current literature regarding short segment Barrett's esophagus and ultra short segment Barrett's in terms of etiology, premalignant potential and management. Terminology for the rest of the article is as follows:

1. long segment Barrett's esophagus (LSBE) refers to traditional Barrett's > 3 cm in length and containing specialized intestinal metaplasia on biopsy.

2. short segment Barrett's esophagus (SSBE) refers to a columnar lined esophagus, visible on endoscopy, measuring < 3 cm, with specialized intestinal metaplasia on biopsy.

3. intestinal metaplasia at the gastro-esophageal junction (CIM) refers to specialized intestinal metaplasia on biopsy obtained from the columnar lining juxtaposed to a normally positioned squamocolumnar junction. This terminology will encompass patients diagnosed as having ultra short segment Barrett's and those with intestinal metaplasia of the cardia.

2. LONG SEGMENT BARRETT'S ESOPHAGUS

The prevalence of Barrett's esophagus in patients undergoing endoscopy approaches 1% (0.97% of men and 0.49% of women)[14]. This prevalence increases with age and reaches a plateau in the seventh decade. The length of Barrett's esophagus does not increase with age, nor does it increase over time in those patients subjected to repeated endoscopic surveillance. The Italian multicenter GOSPE study[15] assessed the prevalence of Barrett's esophagus in 14,898 patients undergoing upper GI endoscopy. The incidence of Barrett's esophagus cited was 1.75%, however this figure refers to the number of patients with endoscopic appearances of Barrett's esophagus and/or grades 2, 3, and 4 (peptic stenosis)

H.W. Tilanus and S.E.A. Attwood (eds.), Barrett's Esophagus, 217–229.

esophagitis. When the definition was limited to those histologically diagnosed as Barrett's esophagus the prevalence fell to 0.75%. Cameron et al.[16] estimated the prevalence of Barrett's esophagus by two different methods and found that the prevalence of clinically diagnosed Barrett's esophagus was 21.6 /100,000, and that within the population as a whole, estimated from a series of 733 unselected autopsies was 21 fold higher at 376/100,000. This data suggests that many patients with Barrett's esophagus remain asymptomatic and are never diagnosed in the community at large.

Physiological studies show that 90% of patients have a mechanically defective lower esophageal sphincter and 93% have abnormal esophageal acid exposure on pH monitoring[17,18]. Further, patients with Barrett's esophagus have impaired esophageal body contractility characterized by reduced contraction amplitudes in the lower esophagus. In addition, most patients with Barrett's esophagus have frequent reflux of duodenal content, including bile, into their distal esophagus[19,20]. The premalignant potential of "Barrett's esophagus" is established, and it is accepted that patients with LSBE have a 30 to 40 fold increased risk of esophageal adenocarcinoma[21,22]. There is no convincing evidence that either medical treatment or surgical therapy causes regression of Barrett's esophagus. However the question to be addressed is whether or not therapy can prevent progression of Barrett's esophagus? McCallum et al.[23] showed that dysplasia developed in 19.7% of patients with LSBE treated medically during 4 years of follow up, compared to 3.4% of patients treated by anti-reflux surgery. Oritz et al.[24] reported similar results with 22% of patients with Barrett's esophagus developing dysplasia after a median of 4 years of medical treatment compared to 3% of patients treated by antireflux surgery. McDonald et al.[25] followed up 112 patients with Barrett's esophagus who had undergone antireflux surgery over a median of 6.5 years. Three developed adenocarcinoma, all within the first 3 years, suggesting that the malignant transformation may have already been initiated at the time of surgical therapy. None of the remaining 109 patients developed cancer during more than 12 years of follow up. Despite the evidence to suggest that surgical therapy may provide better protection against the risk of neoplastic progression for patients with LSBE there is a need for a properly conducted prospective randomized study to compare the outcome of current medical

therapy versus surgical therapy in Barrett's esophagus.

3. SHORT SEGMENT BARRETT'S ESOPHAGUS

3.1 DIAGNOSIS AND PREVALENCE

The prevalence of short segment Barrett's esophagus in patients undergoing diagnostic endoscopy has been cited at between 8 and 36 %[10,11]. In one study 156 patients undergoing diagnostic endoscopy had 2 biopsies taken from the columnar epithelium at the SCJ, to look for IM, and 1 biopsy from the squamous epithelium 2cm above this point, to look for esophagitis[13]. Fourteen patients had known LSBE and all had IM upon histological examination of the biopsies. Endoscopic examination of the remaining 142 patients, not known to have Barrett's esophagus, revealed 2 patients with LSBE. In 26 / 140 (18.6%) of patients without endoscopic evidence of LSBE biopsies showed specialized columnar epithelium. Two thirds of these patients had SSBE and one third had CIM. All 42 patients with IM, whether in LSBE or not, were caucasian despite 14% of the endoscopic population being non-caucasian. The male to female ratios were 1.7:1 in those patients with LSBE, 1.9:1 in those with 'short segment' Barrett's esophagus, and 0.8:1 in those without IM. This study may under represent the prevalence of SSBE as only two biopsies where taken from the SCJ.

Weston et al.[10] prospectively scrutinized the GEJ of 237 patients undergoing elective upper GI endoscopy and suspected SSBE in 18%. The criteria used to diagnose SSBE were the presence of any of the following endoscopic appearances:

1. An accentuated or serrated z-line in which short tongues of pink mucosa extending less than 2cm above the GEJ, with a minimum of 2 biopsies taken from each tongue;
2. 2. One or more small, patches of red to pink mucosa lying less than 2cm above the GEJ, with a minimum of one biopsy per patch;
3. Where the z-line was displaced cephalad to the GEJ, but by less than 2cm, by a continuous, circumferencial extension of pink mucosa, with 4 quadrant biopsies taken from the most proximal edge.

The biopsies were stained with H&E and those containing distended, barrel-shaped goblet cells, underwent confirmatory staining with Alcian blue at pH 2.5 to identify acid mucin.

IM was confirmed on biopsy in 19 of 40 patients (2 patients excluded because of previous Bilroth II surgery), a prevalence of 8%; none had dysplasia. Long segment Barrett's was identified in 45 patients (19%). The age of those with SSBE and LSBE was significantly older than for patients thought to have SSBE but in whom biopsies were non confirmatory.

The high prevalence of SSBE reported by Nandurkar et al.[11] differed from the above in the methodology and definitions used. Patients who were free of LSBE had two biopsies taken from the columnar epothelium at the squamocolumnar junction. The biopsies were stained with H&E and Alcian blue (pH 2.5), and SSBE was diagnosed in the presence of intensely staining Alcian blue positive goblet cells. One hundred and fifty eight patients were included in the analysis (66% women, mean age 50.8 years) and the prevalence of IM was 36% (95% CI 28.5-43.5), higher than the 18 and 24% reported from the USA[12,13]. This difference is purported to be due to the use of Alcian blue. The patients in Nandukar's study[11] were questioned regarding symptoms and logistic regression analysis performed to determine the independent risk factors for the presence of SSBE. They identified age (OR 1.3), histological esophagitis (OR 3.2) and inflammation at the gastro-esophageal junction (OR 5.9) as being statistically significant.

Byrne et al.[26] obtained 3 biopsies from the GEJ, 2 biopsies from 3 cm proximal to the GEJ (esophagus) and 2 biopsies from 3 cm distal to the GEJ (cardia), from 225 symptomatic patients attending for open-access endoscopy. All biopsies were stained using H&E and sections from GEJ and cardia were stained with PAS/Alcian blue (PAS/AB) and high-iron, diamine/Alcian blue (HID/AB). The sex ratio in this group was 53% male and the median age was 54.5 years. A new diagnosis of malignancy was made in 3.6% of patients, LSBE was identified in 8 patients (3.6%) and SSBE was identified in 15 patients (6.7%).

3.2 ETIOLOGY

SSBE is associated with gastro-esophageal reflux disease in a similar fashion to classical LSBE. Symptoms in patients with SSBE may be more prevalent (58-82%)[10,11] than observed with LSBE (60%). This has been explained by the fact that the SSBE group may lack the reduced sensivity characteristic of LSBE[27]. This however is not reported in all studies. Spechler et al.[13] showed that there was no difference in the percentage of patients with symptoms of GERD when comparing patients with LSBE, SSBE and those without evidence of a columnar lined esophagus. There was however a higher percentage of patients with histological and/or endoscopic esophagitis in the SSBE group compared to the LSBE group. The lack of correlation between SSBE and symptoms of GERD was also reported in the study of Nandurkar[11]. Byrne et al.[26] showed no correlation between the presence of IM and reflux disease, when assessed either by symptom questionnaire or endoscopic esophagitis. However the presence of IM was shown to correlate with the use of acid suppressant therapy. They noted that 91% of the patients with intestinal metaplasia were taking acid suppressant therapy, compared to 68.5% of subjects without intestinal metaplasia. This finding could reflect the severity or duration of symptoms in patients with IM, however it was also suggested by the authors that a direct link between SSBE and the use of acid suppressant therapy, possibly though alteration of the refluxate, might be plausible.

Detailed physiological studies have clarified the importance of reflux in SSBE. In a prospective evaluation of 241 consecutive patients undergoing upper GI endoscopy for reflux symptoms, the position of the GEJ, SCJ and diaphragmatic crura were recorded[9]. Biopsies were obtained from the distal squamous esophagus, and were present from columnar lined esophagus (4 quadrants at 2 cm intervals). In the absence of a visible columnar lined esophagus biopsies were taken 1 cm below the SCJ. Subjects underwent esophageal manometry (211, 88%) and 24 hour pH monitoring (204, 85%). This study demonstrated that 14% had SSBE and 15% had LSBE. It also documented that 81% of patients with LSBE had increased esophageal acid exposure (i.e. a composite DeMeester score >14.9) when compared with data collected from asymptomatic volunteers (Fig.1).

The duration of distal esophageal acid exposure to pH<4 was longer as one progressed from normal, to reflux without Barrett's, through SSBE and LSBE (Fig 2).

The cause of the increased acid exposure in the subjects with Barrett's esophagus was most commonly due to a mechanically defective lower esophageal sphincter (LES). Figure 3 shows the prevalence of a mechanically defective LES in each of the patient groups. Overall 62% of patients with SSBE had a defective LES. The prevalence of structurally abnormal LES components can be seen in Table 1.

TABLE 1. Prevalence of abnormal lower esophageal sphincter characteristics in each of the study groups (Clark et al 1997).

	Volunteers (n=50)	No Barrett's (n=146)	Barrett's <3 cm (n=32)	Barrett's ≥3 cm (n=33)
Resting pressure < 6 mmHg	0 (0%)[a]	36 (25%)	17 (43%)[b]	24 (73%)[b]
Overall length < 2 cm	0 (0%)[a]	26 (18%)	9 (28%)	13 (39%)[c]
Abdominal length< 1 cm	1 (2%)[a]	40 (27%)	10 (27%)	20 (61%)[d]

[a] $p < 0.05$ vs. each of the patient groups (Fishers exact).
[b] $p < 0.01$ vs. no Barrett's group (Chi square).
[c] $p < 0.05$ vs. no Barrett's group (Chi square).
[d] $p < 0.01$ vs. No Barrett's group & Barrett's <3 cm (Chi square)

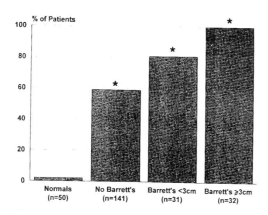

Figure 1. Prevalence of a positive composite score for increased esophageal acid exposure. *All patient groups were significantly different to normals, $p < 0.01$ and to each other $p < 0.05$. From Clark et al, J Gastrointest Surg 1997; 1, 113-122.

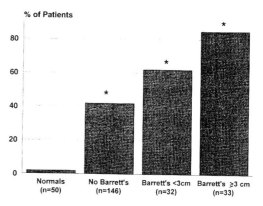

Figure 3. Prevalence of a mechanically defective lower esophageal sphincter. *All patient groups were significantly different to normals, $p < 0.01$ and to each other $p < 0.05$. From Clark et al, J Gastrointest Surg 1997; 1, 113-122.

Figures 4 and 5 show a progressive deterioration in the LES resting pressure, overall sphincter length and abdominal length as the groups progressed from no GERD to GERD to SSBE to LSBE. A reduction in the amplitude of distal esophageal contractions was also seen in patients with Barrett's esophagus compared with those who had GERD symptoms but no IM (Fig 6). This was noted throughout the lower 4/5 of the esophagus even in patients with SSBE. Significant differences also existed between the prevalence of hiatal hernia between the three groups, being present in 34% of those without IM, 55% of those with SSBE and 78% of those with LSBE. Loughney et al.[28] identified 28 patients with SSBE from a study of 203 consecutive patients undergoing endoscopy. Twenty two patients with SSBE underwent esophageal manometry and 24 hour pH monitoring. The results were compared to 18 LSBE patients and 15 symptomatic GERD

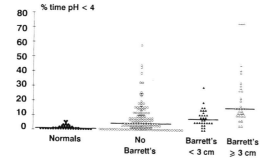

Figure 2. Scatter plot of the total percentage of time the esophageal pH was < 4 in each of the study groups. Horizontal line indicates the median. There was a significant difference between the groups ($\chi^2 = 82.6$, 3 df, $P < 0.01$, Kruskal-Wallis). All groups were significantly different from each other ($P < 0.01$, Mann-Whitney). . From Clark et al, J Gastrointest Surg 1997; 1, 113-122.

patients without Barrett's. The authors showed that both LSBE and SSBE patient groups were older than the non-Barrett's group. The resting LES pressure of the LSBE group was significantly lower than that of the SSBE group (5.2 mmHg compared with 12.3 mmHg). Both Barrett's groups had lower sphincter pressures than the non-Barrett's group (16.9mmHg). The SSBE group had a significantly lower mean total 24 hour pH score when measured at both the GOJ (65.4 compared with 174.3) and 5cm proximal to this point (40.5 compared with 112.3) compared to the LSBE group.

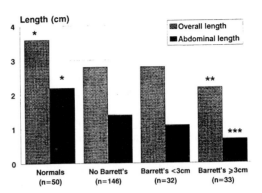

Figure 5. Overall length and abdominal length of the lower esophageal sphincter. The bars represent the median. *All groups were significantly different to normals, p,0.01 for both parameters. ** For overall length no Barrett's vs extended Barrett's, p,0.05. For abdominal length extended Barrett's vs no Barrett p ,0.01 & extended Barrett's versus short Barrett's p,0.05. From Clark et al, J Gastrointest Surg 1997;1:1130122.

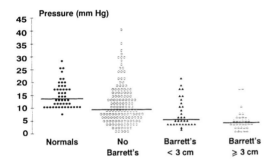

Figure 4. Scatter plot of the lower esophageal sphincter pressures in each of the study groups. Horizontal line indicates the median. There was a significant difference between the groups ($\chi^2 = 61.7$, 3 df, P<0.01, Kruskal-Wallis). All groups were significantly different from each other (P<0.05, Mann-Whitney). From Clark et al, J Gastrointest Surg 1997; 1, 113-122.

Both LSBE and SSBE groups had higher 24 pH scores than the non-Barrett's group indicating that the degree and length of acid exposure are important factors in the development of IM in the esophagus.

3.3. NATURAL HISTORY OF SHORT SEGMENT BARRETT'S ESOPHAGUS

The natural history of SSBE is unclear. It is not known whether SSBE remains static, regresses or progresses to LSBE. The evidence from LSBE is that there is no spontaneous regression[14,29]. Further Cameron et al.[14] showed that the length of LSBE was similar at all age groups studied suggesting that Barrett's esophagus develop over a short time period and once present remains static throughout life. If SSBE progresses to LSBE over time then one would expect the average age of those with SSBE to be less than those

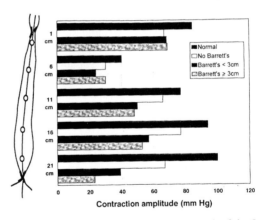

Figure 6. Median contraction amplitudes at each of the 5 levels of the esophagus for the different groups. There were significant differences between the groups at each of the lower 4 levels (Kruscal Wallis, 2 df, 6 cm X^2=18.1, 11 cm X^2=25.7, 16 cm X^2=39.1, 21 cm X^2=33.8). * Significantly different to normals (Mann Whitney, p<0.05). Additionally, extended Barrett's was significantly different to the short segment Barrett's group at the lower 3 levels (Mann Whitney, p<0.05). From Clark et al, J Gastrointest Surg 1997; 1, 113-122.

with LSBE. This is not the case. Loughney et al.[28] reported that the mean age of SSBE patients was 61.6 years, and 53.7 years in LSBE patients, while Clark et al.[9] showed similar ages for the two groups of Barrett's patients (SSBE 53 yrs, range 20 – 79, LSBE 51 yrs, range 35 – 80). The prevalence of IM at the normal gastro-esophageal junction appears to increase with age. Byrne et al.[26] reported no IM in patients under 30 years of age, IM in 15-

18% those 30-60 years of age, and in >30% in those 70-89 years of age.

3.4. SHORT SEGMENT BARRETT'S ESOPHAGUS AND RISK OF ADENOCARCINOMA

The above data is of concern when taken with the epidemiological studies from the US demonstrating a rapid increase in the incidence of esophageal adenocarcinoma during recent decades[30-32]. This rise predominantly affects caucasian males, the same population who has columnar lined esophagus irrespective of its length. Increases in the incidence of distal esophageal and junctional cancer have also been reported from the United Kingdom,[33] France and Switzerland,[34] Denmark[35] and Sweden[36]. The association between dysplasia and SSBE has been addressed in a small number of studies. Spechler et al.[13] detected low grade dysplasia in 1 of 26 patients (4%); Conio et al.[37] found low grade dysplasia in 3 of 32 patients (9%); and Weston et al.[10] did not find dysplasia in the 19 patients studied. Sharma et al.[38] detected dysplasia in 20/117 (11%), of which 85% were low grade and 15% high-grade dysplasia. Examination of the resected esophagus from those patients with junctional adenocarcinoma revealed high-grade dysplasia in 2 of the 4 patients found to have associated SSBE[7]. Clark et al.[39] examined the resection specimens of 13 patients with gastro-esophageal junction adenocarcinomas and SSBE. Dysplastic Barrett's epithelium was present in 10 patients (77%); most had high-grade changes. These limited data sets suggest that the incidence of dysplasia in SSBE is low, but high in those who progress to adenocarcinoma.

Clark and co-workers[9] reported 4 of 33 patients (12%) with SSBE had dysplasia (2 HGD, and 2 LGD) which was not different to the 19% (7/37) seen in those with LSBE (1 HGD, 6 LGD). In the same study the authors[9] evaluated 16 patients with small (<3 cm long) non-circumferencial adenocarcinomas associated with IM ('Barrett's adenocarcinomas') and the length of their Barrett's mucosa was recorded. The length of Barrett's was <3 cm in 4 of the 16 patients (25%), in all of whom evidence of HGD was present, suggesting that the metaplastic mucosa was the source of the adenocarcinoma. They concluded that SSBE is a premalignant condition. The median age of those with Barrett's adenocarcinoma (62.5 years) was significantly greater than those with SSBE (53 years) or LSBE (51 years).

Table 2 lists a number of case studies describing adenocarcinomas at the gastro-esophageal junction arising in association with SSBE[7,40-42]. Clark et al.[39] investigated the prevalence of specialized intestinal metaplasia in the resection specimens from 100 patients with adenocarcinoma of the distal esophagus and proximal stomach. They divided the tumors into three groups based upon where their epicenter lay: 'esophageal' if it lay in the esophagus; 'cardiac' if at the gastro-esophageal junction; and 'subcardiac' if in the stomach. They examined 48 esophageal tumors, 31 cardiac tumors, and 21 subcardiac tumors, and found IM, as identified upon H&E, in 79%, 42% and 5% of the specimens respectively, a statistically significant difference existing between all groups. The length of IM also differed significantly between the groups in that the mean length of IM measured at endoscopy was 7.4 ± 3.4 cm in the esophageal cancer group compared with 2.7 ± 1.8 cm in the cardiac cancer group. Only one patient with subcardiac cancer had IM limited to a 1cm segment that histologically was not dysplastic. The authors proposed that this might be an underestimate of the actual prevalence of adenocarcinoma arising from SSBE as a consequence of the metaplastic epithelium being 'cannibalized' by overgrowth of tumor. Analysis of the patient demographics demonstrated an increasing male preponderance with the more proximal cancers: male: female ratios being 2.5:1 for subcardiac; 5.2:1 for cardiac, and 15:1 for esophageal. Some clarity in the division of tumors originating around the gastro-esophageal junction has been afforded by the Siewert[43] classification. Tumors whose center lies within 5cm of the anatomical cardia are divided into three distinct entities:

Type I Adenocarcinoma of the distal esophagus which usually arises from an area of specialized intestinal metaplasia (i.e. Barrett's esophagus) and which may infiltrate the esophagogastric junction from above.

Type II True carcinoma of the cardia arising from the cardiac epithelium or short segments with intestinal metaplasia at the esophagogastric junction; this entity is also often referred to as 'junctional carcinoma'.

Type III Subcardial gastric carcinoma which infiltrates the esophago-gastric junction and distal esophagus from below.

Using this classification Siewert and Stein[44] studied 815 patients undergoing surgical resection between 1982 and 1997.

TABLE 2. Case reports of adenocarcinoma arising in short segment of Barrett's esophagus (M, male; NS, not stated; GERD, gastro-esophageal reflux disease).

Author	Patient Age(yrs)	Sex	Race	Resected Specimen	High Grade Dysplasia	Endoscopy	Reason
Schnell et al., 1992	66	M	White	T₁No	NS	2 x <2cm tongues No visible tumor	Asthma ?GERD
	62	M	White	T₁No	NS	2 x 1cm tongues No visible tumor	Long Hx reflux Chest pain
	66	M	White	T₁No	Yes	1 x 0.5cm tongue No visible tumor	Mild reflux Dyspepsia
	60	M	White	T₁No	Yes	1 x 1.5cm tongue No visible tumor	Known cirrhosis Exam of varices
Nishimaki et al., 1996	66	M	NS	T₁No	NS	Small tumor above Es-jej anastomosis (5mm tongue above es-jej anastomosis in resection specimen)	Reflux for 29yrs after total abdominal gastrectomy
Iqbal et al., 1997	47	M	White	T₁No	Yes	Short tongues No visible tumor	Reflux symptoms
Nandurkar et al., 1998	47	M	NS	T₁No	Yes	Erosive esophagitis 3mm nodule in <2cm tongue	Worsening reflux symptoms

They found a male preponderance of 8.2:1 for type I, 5.1:1 for type II, and 2.4:1 for type III; similar to those ratios demonstrated by Clark *et al.*[39] In addition, of the type I cancers 72% were associated with a hiatus hernia and 84% had a history of GERD, compared with 28 and 42% of type II, and 21 and 29% of type III cancers. The prevalence of IM also varied according to the tumor type: IM being present in the distal esophagus in 81% of type I tumors, 11% of type II tumors and 2% of type III tumors. The incidence of adenocarcinoma in patients with endoscopically diagnosed LSBE is around 1 per 100 patient years of follow up ranging from 1 in 52 to 1 in 441 patient years[30,45-49]. A similar figure for SSBE has not been published but the risk is thought to be lower. Since the number of patients with SSBE is greater than with LSBE it can be anticipated that adenocarcinomas of the gastro-esophageal junction will be encountered as frequently as those arising from the tubular esophagus. One prospective 'long-term' follow-up study of patients with SSBE has been published, with comparative data for LSBE[50]. Seventy four patients with SSBE (IM on biopsy confirmed with Alcian blue staining, <2 cm from the GEJ) and 78 with LSBE (mean length 6.9 ± 3.6 cm), newly diagnosed on elective upper GI endoscopy for the investigation of GERD were included. The groups were comparable for age and sex, however, the race ratio differed significantly between groups (white: black; SSBE = 8.25:1; LSBE = 38:1). The incidence of dysplasia at

diagnosis was 8.1% in the SSBE group (5 patients with LGD; 1 with HGD) and 19.2% in the LSBE group (11 with LGD; 4 with HGD). None of the patients with SSBE had adenocarcinoma at initial diagnosis while 12 (15.4%) of the LSBE patients had adenocarcinoma at their first endoscopy. Twenty-six patients with SSBE and 29 with LSBE were followed-up for more than one year. During follow-up 2 of 22 with SSBE but no index dysplasia, developed new LGD/indeterminate dysplasia. Within the LSBE group 6 of 15 patients went on to develop dysplasia (5LGD, 1HGD). The risk of developing *de novo* dysplasia was higher in the LSBE group when compared with the SSBE group. Of the 3 patients followed-up with index LGD and SSBE, all demonstrated resolution of dysplasia and remained clear 11, 19 and 31 months later.

3.5. SHOULD PATIENTS WITH SSBE UNDERGO BARRETT'S SURVEILLANCE?

It is accepted that the presence of IM in segments of SSBE increases the risk of the development of distal esophageal and possibly cardia adenocarcinoma. There is however inadequate data to quantify this risk as no prospective data exist. It is considered that the risk is lower than for LSBE. Maniatis & Brazer[51] propose that "cohorts with SSBE need to be followed prospectively to determine their risk for the development of esophageal adenocarcinoma" and that "until such data are available, Barrett's esophagus should be defined as the presence of specialized columnar epithelium of any length." Moreover if screening for dysplasia and cancer arising in Barrett's is to be undertaken, all patients with IM should be included, not just the minority with endoscopically visible LSBE. If patients with SSBE are indeed at significant risk of esophageal carcinoma routine biopsy of the columnar epithelium at the SCJ in all patients undergoing endoscopic examination irrespective of symptoms should be considered to identify these patients'. The Italian GOSPE study[37] Conio et al. evaluated 166 patients with short extensions (0.5-2.0cm) of metaplastic epithelium seen at endoscopy. Histological examination of biopsies demonstrated IM in 32 patients (19%). LGD was detected in 3 patients (prevalence 9.4%), each of whom had extension of Barrett's esophagus for only 1 cm in length. This group compares the prevalence of 9.4% with the 9.1% prevalence of dysplasia within a subset analysis of patients with LSBE from their previously published GOSPE multicenter study of Barrett's esophagus[15]. Consequently they recommend periodic endoscopic follow-up for all patients with a histological diagnosis of IM irrespective of the length of the metaplastic epithelium. Sharma et al.[52] performed a prospective evaluation of dysplasia in SSBE. They identified 59 patients with SSBE in whom the prevalence of dysplasia at initial endoscopy was 8.5%, (all LGD). Over an average 36.9 months follow-up 5/32 patients (15.6%) developed dysplasia, 3 LGD and 2 HGD. One patient was subsequently diagnosed with esophageal adenocarcinoma, 33 months after the initial diagnostic endoscopy, and 2 years after the diagnosis of HGD. It must be noted that the patient had 'a chronic nonhealing ulcer in his Barrett's mucosa'. In the discussion this group also recommended 'long-term endoscopic and histological surveillance of patients with SSBE'. Romero & Riddell[53] argue against surveillance of SSBE. They state that as a consequence of the high prevalence of SSBE and the low incidence of esophageal carcinoma, at 2-4 per 100,000 per year, even allowing for the increasing its incidence, any screening program for SSBE would be unlikely to be viable upon economic grounds. They also state that 'we do not as yet have evidence that endoscopic surveillance of LSBE has a significant impact upon the prolongation of life? Recommending surveillance endoscopy for a large percentage of the population without a clear idea of the expected outcome seems premature on the data provided'. This view and the same reasoning has also been

reported by Kapadia[54] and Ireland & DeMeester[55]. Further, Spechler[56] suggests that until the cancer risk is better defined, it is not recommended that endoscopists routinely obtain biopsy specimens from a healthy-appearing distal esophagus to look for specialized intestinal metaplasia.

4. INTESTINAL METAPLASIA AT THE GASTRO-ESOPHAGEAL JUNCTION AND GASTRIC CARDIA

4.1. PREVALENCE

Biopsies obtained from the columnar aspect of the squamocolumnar junction that appears normal at endoscopy may reveal specialized intestinal metaplasia[12,13]. Concurrent with the increase in incidence of esophageal adenocarcinoma has been the increase in incidence of gastric cardia cancer[57]. There are similarities between the two tumors and it has been proposed that cardia cancer may arise from foci of IM at a normally located Z-line[58]. Whether the location of this IM is termed gastro-esophageal junction or gastric cardia in origin is subjective but can be related to how far below the SCJ the biopsies are obtained. When the biopsy specimen contains both columnar and squamous elements this is clearly GEJ in origin. Most investigators would also include biopsies obtained at the level of the highest gastric folds as GEJ whereas biopsies obtained from > 1 cm below the normally located SCJ would be termed cardiac in origin. The descriptive difficulties are self evident and probably unnecessary. For the following discussion IM obtained from anywhere in this region will be termed CIM. Further many investigators use the terms SSBE and CIM interchangeably and may report mixed groups of patients composing both those with SSBE and CIM. Specialized intestinal metaplasia can be demonstrated in 37 to 48% of patients whose squamocolumnar junction is jagged, irregular or especially prominent at endoscopy[10,59] and also in up to 15% of patients with a normal Z-line displaying none of the above features. The use of Alcian blue (pH 2.5) staining increases the frequency of identifying specialized IM[11]. The data suggest that approximately 25% of the population attending for diagnostic endoscopy will have CIM particularly in caucasian populations. It is evident that the incidence and prevalence of CIM varies depending upon definitions used, and their stringency, to diagnose the condition. Byrne et al.[26] obtained 3 biopsies from the gastro-esophageal junction (GEJ), 2 biopsies from 3cm proximal to the GEJ (esophagus), and 2 biopsies from 3cm distal to the GEJ (cardia), from 194 patients with no visible columnar lining in the distal esophagus. They were stained using H&E and sections from GEJ and cardia were stained with PAS/Alcian blue (PAS/AB) and high-iron diamine/Alcian blue (HID/AB). IM was identified at the GEJ in 18.1% of patients, at the cardia in 4.6% and at both sites in 2.1% with H& E. When the same locations were stained with PAS/AB IM was reported in 58.7% at the GEJ, 34.0% at the cardia and 27.8% had IM at both sites. With HID/AB the reported rates of IM were 65.4%, 28.3%, and 24.2% respectively. The acid mucins expressed at the two sites differed with sulphomucins predominating at the GEJ (84.3%) compared to 58.2% at the cardia; sulphomucins being a characteristic of type III intestinal metaplasia, which carries the greatest cancer risk[60]. Sialomucins were present at high levels at both sites. The prevalence of IM at the GEJ and cardia reported in this study, using standard H&E staining, is similar to that of other studies[8,11,13]. The high frequency of IM seen using acid mucin staining far exceeds that of Nandurkar et al.[11] and may result from the inclusion of non-goblet cells containing acid mucins as 'more subtle forms of IM'. It has become recognized that metaplastic epithelium containing goblet cells recovered from the lower esophagus or GEJ is abnormal irrespective of exact location of origin[61]. When using H&E plus Alcian blue (pH 2.5) staining a group of cells are identified which are more common than genuine goblet cells. These cells look just like gastric columnar cells on H&E but stain with Alcian blue and are considered to represent a transitional type of metaplastic cell intermediate between gastric columnar cells and goblet cells. These cells are called transitional cells or 'columnar blues'[58]. The presence of these cells alone in a biopsy is not sufficient to make a diagnosis of Barrett's esophagus or of cardia intestinal metaplasia[10]. Weston and co-workers[62] recruited 183 patients who were attending for routine diagnostic or repeat surveillance endoscopy. For the 60 patients with LSBE (defined as the presence of specialized columnar epithelium extending ≥2 cm above the GEJ) 4 quadrant biopsies were taken every 2 cm from the columnar lined esophagus. Fifty nine patients with SSBE had ≥2 biopsies taken from each tongue of pink mucosa and ≥1 biopsy from each patch of pink mucosa, plus 4 biopsies from the GEJ. Those patients in whom the esophageal biopsy specimens showed either squamous or junctional epithelium and no specialized columnar epithelium served as controls (64 patients). Cardia (defined as the 2

cm segment distal to the GEJ) biopsies were obtained in all patients as well as gastric surveillance biopsies to determine the prevalence of non-cardia intestinal metaplasia. Biopsies were stained with H&E and sections containing distended barrel-shaped goblet cells, indicative of intestinal metaplasia were stained with Alcian blue. CIM was identified in 6 patients with SSBE (10%), 2 with classical LSBE (3%), and in none of the control group. Only one patient had dysplasia within CIM which was low grade. There was no difference in the prevalence of gastric IM between the three groups, with gastric IM being more prevalent than cardia IM. These findings suggest that the development of cardia IM occurs independently to the development of IM seen elsewhere in the stomach.

The prevalence and demographic details of patients with IM in the esophagus and GEJ was further investigated in a large US study[63]. Eight hundred and eighty three patients referred for gastroscopy consented to interview and to additional biopsies being taken at endoscopy, 56% were male and 68% caucasian. The presence of IM was determined by H&E staining of 2 biopsies taken from immediately distal to the SCJ, and from biopsies of all tongues of pink mucosa extending cephalad from the SCJ. Equivocal diagnoses were clarified by Alcian blue staining. IM was not identified in 738 (83%) of the patients who acted as the reference group. The prevalence of LSBE was 1.6%, that of SSBE 6.0%, and CIM 5.6%. There were significant differences in the sex and ethnic mix of the LSBE and SSBE groups, being predominantly male (88% and 70% (p<0.05)) and white (100% and 86% (p<0.05)). The population with CIM had the same sex and racial mix as the reference population but was older (median age 62yrs cf. 53yrs). The incidence of Helicobacter pylori infection was higher in the CIM group (21.3%) than the reference group (8.8%), SSBE (4.7%) or LSBE (2.5%) groups.

4.2. ETIOLOGY OF CIM

CIM is invariably associated with inflammation in the transitional zone epithelium[64] which has been termed carditis[65]. It was originally proposed that the identification of intestinal metaplasia at this site was a consequence of GERD[12,66]. Other investigators have reported that intestinal metaplasia at the gastro-esophageal junction is the consequence of Helicobacter pylori infection. Goldblum and co-workers[67] found that CIM was associated with intestinal metaplasia in other parts of the stomach, and with *H. pylori* carditis. The relationship of CIM with intestinal metaplasia elsewhere in the stomach and *Helicobacter pylori* gastritis was also demonstrated by Hacklesberger et al.[68] In their analysis of 23 patients with SSBE and 42 with CIM, they noted that patients with SSBE were younger than those with CIM, plus they were predominantly male, with higher reported GERD symptoms and erosive esophagitis. Those with SSBE had no correlation with the presence of gastric IM or *Helicobacter pylori* infection. However, we have shown that carditis is unrelated to *Helicobacter pylori* infection in over 60% of patients[64]. It has emerged that both views may be accurate and that intestinal metaplasia located at the gastro-esophageal junction may arise as a consequence of GERD or in relation to *Helicobacter pylori* infection. In patients with GERD the intestinal metaplasia and associated carditis is focal, whereas if the intestinal metaplasia is related to *Helicobacter pylori* there is usually a pangastritis[64]. Voutilainen et al.[69] characterized intestinal metaplasia at the gastro-esophageal junction into two types: type I; complete intestinal metaplasia consisting of columnar cells with absorptive capacity and neutral mucin content or type II/III; incomplete intestinal metaplasia consisting of columnar cells with secretory capacity containing acidic sialomucins or sulphomucins. Of 1058 dyspeptic subjects 22.6% had intestinal metaplasia at the gastro-esophageal junction. Thirteen percent had type I as the sole subtype, 6% had a mixture of complete and incomplete intestinal metaplasia and 3.6% had type II/III. Independent risk factors for type I intestinal metaplasia at the gastro-esophageal junction were age, antral predominant non-atrophic gastritis, antral predominant atrophic gastritis, and atrophic pangastritis. Type I intestinal metaplasia was also associated with *Helicobacter pylori* infection and carditis in univariate analysis. Independent risk factors for type II/III intestinal metaplasia at the gastro-esophageal junction were age, erosive esophagitis and carditis, but not *Helicobacter pylori* infection. Similar conclusions were drawn by Nandurkar et al.[11] who identified histological esophagitis and carditis as major risk factors for type II/III intestinal metaplasia at the gastro-esophageal junction but not *Helicobacter pylori* infection.

4.3. CIM AND RISK OF ADENOARCINOMA

Hirota et al.[63] reported the prevalence of dysplasia in patients with CIM was 2/47

(4.3%), compared to 4/50 (8.0%) in the SSBE group, and 2/13 in the LSBE group (2.5%). One patient in the CIM (2.1%) and SSBE groups (2.0%), plus two in the LSBE group (15.4%) had visible lesions, biopsies of which demonstrated adenocarcinoma. The prevalence of neoplasia was 0% for the reference group, 6.4% CIM, 10% SSBE, and 31% in LSBE. This data indicate that those with LSBE have the greatest risk of malignant transformation. In a recent prospective study[38] the incidence and prevalence of the development of dysplasia was assessed in 177 patients with SSBE and 76 patients with CIM. The prevalence of dysplasia at the initial endoscopy in the SSBE group was 11.3% (17/117 LGD and 3/117 HGD); and 1.3% in the CIM group (1/76 – LGD). Seventy-eight patients with SSBE and 34 with CIM were followed with annual endoscopy. Nine patients with SSBE developed dysplasia (7 LGD, 2 HGD) during follow up, compared with one in the CIM group (LGD), giving a dysplasia incidence of 4.6% per year for SSBE and 1.5% per year for CIM. Ten patients had both SSBE and CIM, of which 3 had LGD in their SSBE, but none had corresponding dysplasia in CIM. Comparative genomic hybridization (CGH) was used to address the question of whether distal esophageal, junctional and cardia cancers are one disease process or whether distinction can be made between the subtypes[70]. Eleven tumors localized to the distal esophagus with Barrett's metaplasia, 10 gastric cardia cancers and 7 tumors located at the gastro-esophageal junction without the presence of Barrett's mucosa were classed as GEJ tumors. The tumors were microdissected to enrich the tumor cell content and DNA extracted. CGH was performed upon the FITC-labelled tumor DNA and hybridized to normal male metaphases. It was demonstrated that loss of locus 14q31-32.1 occurred more frequently in Barrett's-related adenocarcinomas of the distal esophagus, than in cardia cancers. The junctional cancers however displayed an intermediate position suggesting that they were composed of a mixture of carcinomas occurring in undetected SSBE and true cardia cancers. This data suggests the presence of two tumor types with an area of overlap at the junction. There is no data to support surveillance of this group of patients and as the cancer risk appears to be low it is very unlikely to be worthwhile.

5. SUMMARY

Short segment Barrett's esophagus is a condition which is prevalent in caucasian males, is related to gastro-esophageal reflux and carries an increased risk for the development of adenocarcinoma. The risk appears to be lower than that associated with long segment Barrett's esophagus but higher than that associated with cardia intestinal metaplasia. The three disease states may represent the premalignant stage of Siewert I, II and III cancers. The increased risk correlates with the presence of type III intestinal metaplasia which is most prevalent in the esophagus. The understanding of SSBE has been made more complex by the identification of patients with IM immediately beneath a normal appearing SCJ and the inclusion of these patients into the SSBE group of some studies. This condition should be referred to as CIM and appears to carry a lower neoplastic risk than SSBE. CIM is a common finding

and is probably multifactoral in origin. In patients with reflux disease CIM is a focal lesion and often of the type II/III variety. In other patients CIM is part of a pangastritis, is usually of the type I variety and associated with gastric infection with *Helicobacter pylori*. The relationship between GERD, SSBE, LSBE and esophageal adenocarcinoma is established. However, much work remains to be done to clear the murky waters we call Barrett's esophagus. The importance of clarity of thought and careful study design has never been more important if we are to understand this condition which is implicated in the pathogenesis of adenocarcinoma of the esophagus and cardia, both of which are increasing in incidence throughout the Western world.

REFERENCES

1. Hayward J. The lower end of the esophagus. Thorax 1961;16:36-41.
2. SkinnerDB, Walther BC, Riddell RH et al. Barrett's esophagus:Comparison of benign and malignant cases. Ann Surg 1983;198:554-65.
3. McClave SA, Boyce HW Jr, Gottfried MR. Early diagnosis of columnar-lined oesophagus:a new endoscopic criterion. Gastrointest Endosc 1987;33:413-6.
4. Rothery GA, Patterson JE, Stoddard CJ, Day DW. Histological and histochemical changes in the columnar lined (Barrett's) oesophagus. Gut 1986;27:1062-8.
5. Paull A, Trier JS, Dalton MD, et al. The histological spectrum of Barrett's esophagus. N Engl J Med 1971;295:476-80.
6. Reid BJ, Haggitt RC, Rubin CE, Rabinovitch PS. Barrett's esophagus. Correlation between flow cytometry and histology in detection of patients at risk for adenocarcinoma. Gastroenterol 1987;93:1-11.
7. Schnell TG, Sontag SJ, Chejfec G. Adenocarcinomas arising in tongues or short segments of Barrett's esophagus. Dig Dis Sci 1992;37:137-43.
8. Johnston MH, Hammond AS, Laskin W, Jones DM. The prevalence and clinical characteristics of short segments of specialized intestinal metaplasia in the distal esophagus on routine endoscopy. Am J Gastroenterol 1996;91:1507-11.
9. Clark GWB, Ireland AP, Peters JH, Chandrasoma P, DeMeester TR, Bremner CG. Short-segment Barrett's esophagus:a prevalent complication of gastro-esophageal reflux disease with malignant potential. J Gastrointest Surg 1997;1:113-22.
10. Weston AP, Krmpotich P, Makdisi WF et al. Short segment Barrett's esophagus:clinical and histological features, associated endoscopic findings, and association with gastric intestinal metaplasia. Am J Gastroenterol 1996;91:981-6.
11. Nandurkar S, Talley NJ, Martin CJ, Ng THK, Adams S. Short segment Barrett's esophagus:prevalence, diagnosis and associations. Gut 1997;40:710-5.
12. Clark GWB, Ireland AP, Chandrasoma P, DeMeester TR, Peters JH, Bremner CG. Inflammation and metaplasia in the transitional epithelium of the gastro-esophageal junction:A new marker for gastro-

esophageal reflux disease. Gastroenterol 1994;106:A63.
13. Spechler SJ, Zeroogian JM, Antonioli DA, Wang HH, Goyal RK. Prevalence of metaplasia at the gastro-oesophageal junction. Lancet 1994;344:1533-6.
14. Cameron AJ, Lomboy CT. Barrett's esophagus:age, prevalence, and extent of columnar epithelium. Gastroenterol 1992;103:1241-5.
15. GOSPE (Gruppo Operativo per lo Studio delle Precancerosi dell'Esofago). Barrett's esophagus:epidemiological and clinical results of a multicentric survey. Int J Cancer 1991;48:364-8.
16. Cameron AJ, Zinsmeister AR, Ballard DJ, Carney JA. Prevalence of columnar-lined (Barrett's) esophagus. Comparison of population based clinical and autopsy findings. Gastroenterol 1990;99:918-22.
17. Iascone C, DeMeester TR, Little AG, Skinner DB. Barrett's esophagus. Functionalassessment, proposed pathogenesis and surgical therapy. Arch Surg 1983;118:543-9.
18. Attwood SEA, DeMeester TR, Bremner CG, Barlow AP, Hinder RA. Alkaline gastro-esophageal reflux: Implications in the development of complications in Barrett's columnar-lined lower esophagus. Surgery 1989;106:764-70.
19. Champion G. Richter JE. Vaezi MF. Singh S. Alexander R. Duodenogastro-esophageal reflux:relationship to pH and importance in Barrett's esophagus. Gastroenterol 1994;107:747-54.
20. Kauer WKH, Peters JH, DeMeester TR et al. Mixed reflux of gastric and duodenal juice is more harmful to the esophagus than gastric juice alone. The need for surgical therapy re-emphasized. Ann Surg 1995;222:525-33.
21. Iftikhar SY, James PD, Steele RJC, Hardcastle JD, Atkinson M. Length of Barrett's oesophagus:an important factor in the development of dysplasia and adenocarcinoma. Gut 1992;33:1155-8.
22. Reid BJ. Barrett's esophagus and esophageal adenocarcinoma. Gastroenterol Clin N Am 1991;20:817-34.
23. McCallum R.W., Polepalle S., Davenport K., Frierson H., Boyd S. Role of anti-reflux surgery against dysplasia in Barrett's esophagus. Gastroenterol 1991;100::A121.
24. Ortiz A, Martinez de Haro LF, Parrilla P et al. Conservative treatment versus antireflux surgery in Barrett's oesophagus:long-term results of a prospective study. Br J Surg 1996;83:274-8.

25. McDonald ML, Trastek VF, Allen MS, et al. Barretts's esophagus:does an antireflux procedure reduce the need for endoscopic surveillance? J Thorac & Cardiovasc Surg 1996;111:1135-8.

26. Byrne JP, Bhatnagar S, Hamid B, Armstrong GR, Attwood SEA. Comparative study of intestinal metaplasia and mucin staining at the cardia and esophagogastric junction in 225 symptomatic patients presenting for diagnostic open-access gastroscopy. Am J Gastroenterol 1999;94:98-103.

27. Winters C Jr, Spurling TJ, Chobanian SJ et al. Barrett's oesophagus. A prevalent, occult complication of gastro-esophageal reflux disease. Gastroenterology 1987;92:118-24.

28. Loughney T, Maydonovitch CL, Wong RKH. Esophageal manometry and ambulatory 24-hour pH monitoring in patients with short and long segment Barrett's esophagus. Am J Gastrenterol 1998;93:916-9.

29. Stein HJ, Siewert JR. Barrett's esophagus:pathogenesis, epidemiology, functional abnormalities, malignant degeneration, and surgical management. Dysphagia 1993;8:276.

30. Cameron AJ, Ott BJ, Payne WS. The incidence of adenocarcinoma in columnar-lined (Barrett's) esophagus. N Engl J Med 1985;313:857-9.

31. Blot WJ, Devesa SS, Kneller RW, et al. Rising incidence of adenocarcinoma of the esophagus and gastric cardia. JAMA 1991;265:1287-9.

32. Devesa SS, Blot WJ, Fraumeni JF. Changing patterns in the incidence of esophageal and gastric carcinoma in the United States. Cancer 1998;83:2049-3.

33. Powell J, McConkey CC. Increasing incidence of adenocarcinoma of the gastric cardia and adjacent sites. Br J Cancer 1990;62:440-3.

34. Tuyns AJ. Oesophageal cancer in France and Switzerland:recent time trends. Eur J Cancer Prev 1992;1:275-8.

35. Meller H. Incidence of cancer of the oesophagus, cardia and stomach in Denmark. Eur J Cancer Prev 1992;1:159-64.

36. Hansson L-E, Sparén P, Nyrén O. Increasing incidence of both major histological types of esophageal carcinomas amongst men in Sweden. Int J Cancer 1993;54:402-7.

37. Conio M, Aste H, Bonelli L. "Short" Barrett's esophagus:a condition not to be underestimated. Gastrointest Endosc 1994;40:111.

38. Sharma P, Weston AP, Morales T, Topalowski M, Mayo MS, Sampliner RE. Relative risk of dysplasia for patients with intestinal metaplasia in the distal oesophagus and in the gastric cardia. Gut 2000;46:9-13.

39. Clark GWB, Smyrk TC, Burdiles P et al. Is Barrett's metaplasia the source of adenocarcinoma of the cardia? Arch Surg 1994;129:609-14.

40. Iqbal M, Youngberg GA, Young MF, Thomas E. High grade dysplasia/esophageal adenocarcinoma in short segment Barrett's oesophagus. Southern Med J 1997;90:828-30.

41. Nandurkar S, Martin CJ, Talley NJ, Ma Wyatt J. Curable cancer in a short segment Barrett's oesophagus. Dis Esophagus 1998;11:284-7.

42. Nishimaki T, Watanabe K, Suzuki T, Hatakeyama K, Watanabe H. Early esophageal adenocarcinoma arising in a short segment of Barrett's mucosa after total gastrectomy. Am J Gastroenterol 1996;1856-7.

43. Siewert JR, Stein HJ. Classification of adenocarcinoma of the oesophagogastric junction. Br J Surg 1998;85:1457-9.

44. Siewert JR, Stein HJ. Adenocarcinoma of the gastro-esophageal junction. Classification, pathology and extent of resection. Dis Esoph 1996;9:173-82.

45. Robertson CS, Mayberry JF, Nicholson JF et al. Value of endoscopic surveillance in detection of neoplastic change in Barrett's oesphagus. Br J urg 1988;75:760-3.

46. Hameeteman W, Tytgat GNJ, Huthoff HJ, VanDerTweel JC. Barrett's esophagus:Development of dysplasia and adenocarcinoma. Gastroenterol 1989;96:1249-56.

47. Miros M, Kerlin P, Walker N. Only patients with dysplasia progress to adenocarcinoma in Barrett's oesophagus. Gut 1991;32:1441-6.

48. Levine DS, Haggitt RC, Blount PL et al. An endoscopic biopsy protocol can differentiate high grade dysplasia from early adenocarcinoma in Barrett's esophagus. Gastroenterol 1993;105:40-50.

49. Drewitz DJ, Sampliner RE, Garewal HS. The incidence of adenocarcinoma in Barrett's esophagus:A prospective study of 170 patients followed 4.8 years. Am J Gastroenterol 1997;92:212-5.

50. Weston AP, Krmpotich PT, Cherian R, Dixon A, Topalovski M. Prospective long-term endoscopic and histological follow-up of short segment Barrett's esophagus:comparison with the traditional long segment Barrett's esophagus. Am J Gastroenterol 1997(b);92:407-13.

51. Maniatis AG, Brazer SR. Is short segment Barrett's clinically significant?. Am J Gastroenterol 1995;90:1894-5.

52. Sharma P, Morales T, Bhattacharyya A, Garewal HS, Sampliner RE. Dysplasia in of short-segment Barrett's esophagus:a prospective 3-year follow-up. Am J Gastroenterol 1997;92:2012-6.

53. Romero Y, Riddell RH. Re:Sharma *et al.* Dysplasia and cancer risk of short-segment Barrett's esophagus. Am J Gastroenterol 1998;93:2639-40.

54. Kapadia CR. Short-segment Barrett's esophagus:prevalence, diagnosis, and associations. Gastroenterol 1998;114:409-10.

55. Ireland A, DeMeester TR. Short answer in short segment Barrett's oesophagus. Gut 1997;40:804.

56. Spechler SJ. The role of gastric carditis in metaplasia and neoplasia at the gastro-esophageal junction. Gastroenterol 1999;117:218-28.

57. Chow WH, Finkle WD, McLauglin JK, Frankl H, Zielk HK, Fraumeni JF Jr. The relation of gastro-esophageal reflux disease and its treatment to adenocarcinomas of the esophagus and gastric cardia. JAMA 1995;274:474-7.

58. Weinstein WM, Ippoliti AF. The diagnosis of Barrett's esophagus:goblets, goblets, goblets. Gastrointest Endosc 1996;44:91-5.

59. Cameron AJ, Kamath PS, Carpenter HC. Barrett's esophagus. The prevalence of short and long segments in reflux patients. Gastroenterol 1996;108:A65.

60. Filipe MI, Munoz N, Matko I et al.. Intestinal metaplasia types and the risk of gastric cancer:a cohort study in Slovinia. Int J Cancer 1994;57:324-9.

61. Donahue D. Navab F. Significance of short-segment Barrett's esophagus. Journal of Clinical Gastroenterol. 1997;25:480-4.

62. Weston AP, Krmpotich PT, Cherian R, Dixon A, Topalovski M. Prospective evaluation of intestinal metaplasia and dysplasia within the cardia of patients with Barrett's esophagus. Dig Dis Sci 1997(a);42:597-602.

63. Hirota WK, Loughney TM, Lazas DJ, Maydonovitch CL, Rholl V, Wong RKH. Specialized intestinal metaplasia, dysplasia, andcancer of the esophagus and esphagogastric junction:prevalence and clinical data. Gastroenterol 1999;116:277-85.

64. Bowrey DJ, Clark GWB, Williams GT. Patterns of gastritis in patients with gastro-esophageal reflux disease. Gut 1999;45:798-803.

65. Riddell RH. The biopsy diagnosis of gastro-esophageal reflux disesase, "carditis", and Barrett's esophagus, and sequelae of therapy. Am J Surg Pathol 1996;20:S31-50.

66. Oberg S, Peters JH, DeMeester TR et al. Inflammation and specialized intestinal metaplasia of cardiac mucosa is a manifestation of gastro-esophageal reflux disease. Ann Surg 1997;226:522-32.

67. Goldblum JR, Vicari JJ, Falk GW et al. Inflammation and intestinal metaplasia of the gastric cardia:the role of gastro-esophageal reflux and H. pylori infection. Gastroenterol 1998;114:633-9.

68. Hackelsberger A, Gunther T, Schultze V et al. Intestinal metaplasia at the gastro-oesophageal junction:Helicobacter pylori gastritis or gastro-oesopageal reflux disease? Gut 1998;43:17-21.

69. Voutilainen M, Fakkila M, Juhola M, Mecklin JP, Sipponen P. Complete and incomplete intestinal metaplasia at the oesophagogastric junction:prevalences and associations with endoscopic erosive oesophagits and gastritis. Gut 1999;45:644-8.

70. Van Dekken H, Geelen E, Dinjens WNM et al. Comparative genomic hybridization of cancer of the gastro-esophageal junction:deletion of 14Q31-32.1 discriminates between esophageal (Barrett's) and gastric cardia adenocarcinomas. Cancer Res 1999;59:748-7.

4.1 PREVENTION OF CANCER BY CONTROL OF REFLUX

Lars Lundell

1. INTRODUCTION

The average age of people presenting with esophageal adenocarcinoma is about 20 years older than that of patients with known or newly diagnosed Barrett's esophagus[1-3]. The long duration between development of Barrett's esophagus and its malignant degeneration is important to bear in mind since it suggests that there is a significant time interval during which therapeutic and/or preventive interventions may have the potential to be effective. The accessibility of the esophagus for inspection and biopsy and the observation that results of surgical treatment for esophageal adenocarcinoma are directly linked to the stage of the disease at the time of discovery, have led to the introduction of endoscopic surveillance for patients with Barrett's esophagus[4-8]. This approach has been supported by the reports that patients with esophageal adenocarcinoma detected within a surveillance program present at an early stage and have significantly better survival than those who present de novo[6-9]. Investigators have also found that the majority of patients with Barrett's adenocarcinoma do report a past history of chronic heartburn when specifically questioned. This point emphasizes the need to endoscope patients with chronic heartburn and take multiple biopsies from the distal esophagus even when the appearance may be relatively normal. In doing so, the physician can exclude or identify Barrett's esophagus prior to placing patients on long term therapy or offer antireflux surgery.

There are, however, a number of very important questions which have to be specifically addressed when discussing the different options available in cancer prevention. Firstly it has to be considered whether the respective therapies can prevent the occurrence of columnar metaplasia, secondly if the extent of columnar metaplasia can be reduced (regression), thirdly if the occurrence of intestinal metaplasia and dysplasia can be prevented and finally if regression of established dysplastic lesions is possible. If one or more of these prerequisites could be fulfilled, an important basis for prevention of adenocarcinoma of the esophagus has been created.

2. MARKERS OF CLINICAL SIGNIFICANCE?

Cancer develops in Barrett's esophagus by a multistep process in which specialised metaplastic epithelium progresses to high grade dysplasia and eventually to adenocarcinoma. Progression in Barrett's esophagus is associated with increased genomic instability and clonal evolution[10,11]. The process of clonal evolution is associated with the progressive accumulation of genetic abnormalities resulting in proliferative advantage and eventually development of cell clones with invasive capability forming an invasive carcinoma[12,13]. Several genetic errors are involved in this neoplastic progression including mutations of the P_{53} gene[14]. Barrett's esophagus is an excellent model to study the neoplastic progression and the genetic events preceding malignancy in vivo because the esophagus is an organ available for serial biopsies and Barrett's metaplasia is a well defined condition often diagnosed before malignancy appears. Furthermore, in a majority of cases with established adenocarcinoma of the esophagus there is a premalignant tissue surrounding the tumor making it possible to study genetic and other abnormalities during neoplastic progression[15,16]. The risk of malignant degeneration may be greater the longer the segment of Barrett's mucosa but even patients with short segments of intestinal metaplasia are at risk although at a considerable lower level [17,18]. The presence of dysplasia appears to predate the development of adenocarcinoma. The histological identification of dysplasia within Barrett's mucosa is at present the most reliable way of identifying patients who are already harboring adenocarcinoma or are at risk of developing one [19,25]. Dysplasia is defined as an equivocal neoplastic transformation, i.e. distinguishable from reactive and regenerative changes, but the ability to identify dysplasia may differ between pathologists. Investigators have searched for better indicators of malignancy with techniques such as flow cytometry to identify changes in the DNA ploidy and immunohistochemical techniques or polymerase chain reaction to look for specific chromosomal mutations. Most notably has been the use of P_{53} tumor suppression gene

231

H.W. Tilanus and S.E.A. Attwood (eds.), Barrett's Esophagus, 231–238.
© 2001 *Kluwer Academic Publishers. Printed in the Netherlands.*

abnormalities[26,27]. These techniques provide considerable insight into the neoplastic progression of Barrett's esophagus but at present do not provide a truly useful tool in the identification of patients who will develop adenocarcinoma. Although the extent of columnar metaplasia may be prognostically important there are difficulties in studying this specific parameter. Similarly, the loss of the "at risk" mucosa, i. e. intestinal metaplasia, in patients with Barrett's esophagus is also rare. In contrast the majority of patients with intestinal metaplasia of the cardia may be of significance for instance has it been reported that the cardia loose its intestinal metaplasia after fundoplication[28,29]. It has been suggested that the cardiac mucosa is dynamic and that it in contrast to intestinal metaplasia that extents several centimeters into the esophagus is much more readily reversed. The progression from columnar metaplasia to low and high grade dysplasia via intestinal metaplasia is characterized by an increase in the proliferation index and in inhibition of apoptosis. A sensitive quantitative measurement of this progression is reflected for instance by the expression levels of the genes involved. Inhibition of cox 2 receptor causes tumor regression in vitro and in animal models[30]. Furthermore, the use of cyclo-oxygenase inhibitors is associated with low incidence of GI-cancer. Recently it has been shown that cox 2 expression is stimulated by exposure of epithelial cells to bile acids and a marked change of cox 2 expression by the Barrett's epithelium has been measured after fundoplication[31]. The cytoskeleton protein villin has been selected as a marker of intestinal differentiation in Barrett's esophagus explants as well as in other cells. The villin expression in microvilli has been shown to be either absent or very low in esophageal adenocarcinoma. Proliferating cell nuclear antigen (PCNA) immunolocalisation is widely available and a simple technique and seems to be a valid indicator of cellular proliferation in Barrett's esophagus and has been correlated with other methods such as thymidin labeling [32-34]. A positive relationship has been demonstrated between PCNA staining and dysplasia and the reduction in the rate of cell proliferation in response to normalization of esophageal pH. Similar data would suggest that PCNA staining could serve as an adjunct in the assessment of patients with Barrett's esophagus and dysplasia.

3. REGRESSION OF COLUMNAR METAPLASIA AND/OR INTESTINAL METAPLASIA

A decrease in cancer risk might be anticipated if treatment could induce a regression of Barrett's epithelium with restitution of squamous epithelium. A number of case reports and non-randomized open label studies have indeed suggested that regression of Barrett's esophagus can be accomplished by anti reflux treatment. However, other studies could not confirm this[35-43]. One important aspect on the medical management of Barrett's esophagus is the recent observation that simple relief of reflux symptoms does not necessarily provide adequate evidence of control of esophageal acid exposure[44-47]. This is probably caused by the well-known decreased sensitivity of Barrett's epithelium to acid[48]. When one evaluates normal acid exposure while on therapy with a PPI, different "normal values" are obtained. This variability in what is considered normal may be of special significance based on the recent observations made in in vitro studies suggesting that even small acid pulses may induce proliferation and decreased differentiation in tissue culture from patients with Barrett's esophagus. It is therefore reasonable to assume that the long term goal of therapy should be to eliminate any acid exposure to this susceptible mucosa. Data have been presented to propose that this can be accomplished in most patients by giving a PPI for day acid control with bedtime H_2 receptor antagonist to control nocturnal acid [49]. This is also important when taking into account recent observations on the effect of improved control of esophageal acid exposure on histological markers of differentiation and proliferation (see above) within biopsy specimens from the epithelium of patients with Barrett's esophagus[33]. Barrett's cases in whom reflux was controlled by PPI doses from 15 – 60 mg daily demonstrated a significant decrease in proliferating cell nuclear antigen and a significant increase in villin expression, i. e. evidence of decreased proliferation and increased differentiation of respective tissue specimens. On the other hand, in patients in whom a "normalization" of acid exposure was not achieved, no corresponding changes were recognized. It can therefore be concluded that without dose adjustment and perhaps pH control as a therapeutic outcome measure some medical therapies seem to be inadequate with regard to acid suppression and also have the potential to inadequately control reflux of duodenal content [44,47]. The consequence of this may be continued noxious impact on the esophageal mucosa with maintained metaplastic and dysplastic drive. A number of case reports and non-randomized open label studies have indeed suggested that regression of Barrett's esophagus can be accomplished by medical antireflux treatment. However, many studies have not been able to confirm or repeat these observations. However, in a recent randomized double blind study[50] 68 patients with acid reflux and proven Barrett's esophagus were included and patients were treated with either omeprazole 40 mg twice daily or with mild acid suppression with ranitidine 150 mg twice daily for 24 months. Although symptoms were ameliorated in both groups there was a small but statistically significant regression of Barrett's esophagus only in the omeprazole group both in length and area (Figure 1).

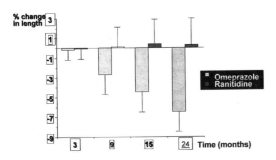

Figure 1. The extent of columnar lined esophagus during omeprazole or ranitidine treatment of Barrett's esophagus (after 50).

The regression was, however, small and the total area of Barrett's esophagus was reduced by only 8% by the end of the two years treatment. Measurement of length is, however, exposed to the risk of underestimating regression if the highest point of the z-line is taken as reference for the measurement or alternatively overestimate regression if the lowest point of the z-line is taken as such. Furthermore, counting of islands may be biased by fusion of island during the regression thus causing its underestimation. In addition the significance of squamous islands may be limited since it is known that in about one third of biopsies taken from these columnar metaplasia was still present now underlying the squamous epithelium[51]. Weinstein and co-workers recently[52] reported a randomized trial comparing 40 mg omeprazole twice daily with ranitidine showing no significant effect during a similar time period as studied above. However, the omeprazole treated group exhibited a statistically significant decrease in the total area and an increase in the number of

islands during the first year without such notable changes during the second year. In a well documented prospective, open single study Sharma and co-workers treated patients with 60 mg of lanzoprazole daily during an average of 5.7 years. Thirteen patients underwent control pH monitoring and only 8 of them had normal result with a mean pH<4 of 0.8% whereas the other 5 still had abnormal acid exposure[42]. These authors observed no significant decrease in the length of Barrett's esophagus although they found a small mean decrease of 0.6 cm in the group with normalization of acid exposure. It can therefore be concluded that regression of columnar metaplasia or normalization of acid exposure on high dose medical therapy, is quantitatively and qualitatively small. Therefore, at this time the clinical significance of this regression is to be qualified as of doubtful clinical significance and these findings do highlight the search for other ways to induce regression. These data do, however, indicate that effective measures to control acid reflux constitute an important basis for prevention of further dysplastic and neoplastic progression. The period of follow-up is apparently pivotal in assessing various therapies capacity and potential to induce regression of Barrett's epithelium. Medical studies have usually applied a relatively short follow-up period and it may be that long periods of treatment are required to encourage regression. This contrasts to most surgical series and in fact regression has been observed in some but not all studies evaluating the effect of anti-reflux surgery. It might well be that antireflux surgery is more likely to be effective in inducing regression since, if successful, reflux should postoperatively be virtually abolished[53]. There are, however, specific methodological problems since the length of Barrett's esophagus, as determined by the measurement of landmarks, may be influenced by surgery per se. In particular, the position of the end of the tubular esophagus may be shifted by the fundoplication and approximation of the crura and this may give false impression of regression. In a carefully conducted study Sagar and co-workers[54] thus observed that regression tended not to be observed at the time of the first and second postoperative endoscopy but rather after more than 2 years had elapsed. The median length of Barrett's esophagus in patients in whom regression occurred was similar before operation and one year afterwards, but there was a steady decline between the measurements recorded at 2 and 7 years after operation. It is well recognized that the absence of heartburn and regurgitation does not exclude significant gastro-esophageal reflux and that sensitivity to reflux varies between patients. A patient who is asymptomatic after antireflux surgery is therefore not necessarily protected against continued reflux and the possibility of persistence of the malignant process. Data have been presented to show that a late progression of Barrett's esophagus may be associated with failures of the surgical procedures to control reflux, observations which may have importance for the design of long term follow up strategies[54]. It can be concluded that long term follow up of patients with Barrett's esophagus after antireflux surgery has shown that both regression and progression of columnar lined epithelium may occur and that conditions favoring regression includes good symptomatic response and effective and maintained control of reflux[55]. Very few authors have reported on the development of Barrett's metaplasia after surgical antireflux procedures. A review over studies on patients having endoscopic follow-up after antireflux surgery, found no study that specifically addressed postoperative development of Barrett's esophagus. Most studies have concentrated on the healing of the esophagitis or commented on and recorded the length of the postoperative metaplastic mucosa that was known to be present before surgery. Taking into consideration the limitations in the validity of the surgical data it must be concluded that the development of Barrett's esophagus seems to be exceedingly rare in patients who have had an effective antireflux repair. On the other hand, some circumstantial information is available to indicate that ongoing mucosal injury during suboptimal acid suppression therapy may be harmful. A population of 138 patients with GORD were studied retrospectively with the focus on prior medical treatment, duration of reflux symptoms, former endoscopic findings, grade of esophagitis before treatment and the development of Barrett's metaplasia while on intermittent or continuous medical acid suppression therapy, Thirty-four percent of patients on intermittent acid suppression medication developed Barrett's metaplasia

although they did not seem to have it before the institution of medical therapy. The median duration of medical treatment in those who developed Barrett's metaplasia was 7 years ranging from 5 months to 20 years[56-58].

4. DOES ANTIREFLUX SURGERY PREVENT FROM DYSPLASIA AND CANCER?

This key question can not be addressed directly based on the obvious methodological issues and difficulties which have to be taken into account. The optimal design of a prospective clinical trial to answer a similar question would require: pre-entry characterization and mapping of both the underlying disease in general and the Barrett's epithelium in particular. Application of proper definition of anatomical, endoscopic landmarks and rigid protocols for tissue sampling, Furthermore a similar clinical protocol requires a long term follow up (>5years, but probably 10 years) with repeated endoscopies and biopsy taking to which must be added objective assessment of the level of reflux control both in the short and long term perspective (minimum standard being, ambulatory 24h pH monitoring). Although ethical difficulties emerge there is always a need for proper controls either in the form of a no therapy arm or a medical therapy group in which focus is focusing only on acid reflux control. The issue of controls is relevant not the least when studying comparatively rare and slow events and processes such as the development of dysplasia and neoplasia in Barrett's esophagus. Presently we are inclined to conclude that no studies are available in the literature which fulfils even some of these basic requirements. Despite these shortcomings there are still important pieces of information which can be extracted from relevant surgical studies and also from an ongoing head-to-head comparison between antireflux surgery and long term treatment of gastroesophageal reflux disease with omeprazole. Compilation of data from surgical series up to February year 2000 reveal 15 publications in the English language literature including 515 cases operated on and followed after antireflux repairs (Table 1).

TABLE 1. Review of the literature over the potential for antireflux surgery to prevent the occurrence of dysplasia and cancer in Barrett's esophagus

Number of publications	15
Number of patients evaluated	515 (range 1 –152)
Follow up period (mean range)	5.0 (1-18) years
Number of patients followed > 5 years	253 (range 0 – 152)
Objective assessment of reflux control (endoscopy ± 24 hour pH monitoring)	438

There was, however, a considerable variability in the length of follow up ranging from 1 to 18 years with a mean of 5 years[3,51,54,59-70]. There are two points which require attention and that is the fact that only 253 patients had been followed >5 years after the antireflux operation and that 438 out of the 515 patients had, at any time during the postoperative period, undergone an investigation to objectively assess the level of reflux control (endoscopy ± 24h pH monitoring). In fact only exceptionally objective data were available on reflux control many years (>5 years) after the antireflux repair (see below). This causes of course some concern depending on the lack of precision of symptom analysis in Barrett's cases as a measure of reflux control (see above).

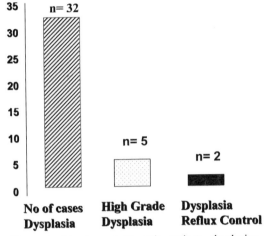

Figure 2. Number of Barrett's patients developing dysplasia in the columnar epithelium after antireflux surgery. Literature review year 2000.

In figure 2 are collected the number of cases in whom dysplasia were revealed in biopsies from the columnar lined esophagus during postoperative follow-up of these patients. One important fact is that only 5 cases of high grade dysplasia have been documented which is probably far fewer than the expected rate in a corresponding non-treated cohort of Barrett's patients. Even more importantly, only 2 cases of dysplasia (both low grade) have been found during follow-up of patients after documented well functioning antireflux repairs when studied in 5 or more years after the operation[60]. One recent study[59] has presented results which have a special bearing on the interpretation of this data base. Csendes and co-workers included 152 non-complicated and complicated Barrett's patients into a randomized trial comparing 2 types of antireflux operations and submitted these patients to a careful and extensive follow-up protocol during 100 months. Dysplasia occurred in 15 patients after a mean of 8.7 years, but exclusively only in those who experienced a surgical failure and

recurrent reflux . The two patients with low grade dysplasia and documented reflux control had the diagnosis established after 5 years very close to the finding of a site with invasive carcinoma within the columnar epithelium. It seems therefore justified to conclude that the occurrence of dysplasia in Barrett's esophagus is rare after antireflux surgery and presents itself at a rate which seems to be definitely lower than the expected one extracted from other non surgically treated cohorts of Barrett's patients. If we then sharpen the criteria to include only those in whom reflux control was maintained, no single case of high grade dysplasia has been convincingly presented. An ongoing randomized trial comparing omeprazole and antireflux surgery in the long term of GORD disease has recently presented 3 and 5 year follow-up data[71,72]. As yet no single case of high grade dysplasia has occurred among the some 50 Barrett's cases treated. In this respect it needs to be mentioned that the protocol allowed dose adjustment of omeprazole in case of symptom relapse up to a daily dose at 40 – 60 mg. Neither at 3 nor at 5 years after induction of therapy was it possible to detect any difference in the point prevalence of columnar lined esophagus between the two study groups. Coming to the delicate question of direct cancer prevention, additional methodological problems emerge. Although we need to clarify the eventual reversibility of the step from high grade dysplasia to neoplasia, a reasonable working hypothesis would presently be that this process is irreversible. Furthermore, it can be concluded that this process is slow. The immediate implications of this valid assumption is that when assessing the occurrence of cancer after induction of effective therapy, a certain time must elapse before de novo neoplasia can be accepted as being casually related or affected by the instituted therapy. Referring again to the previously quoted paper by Csendes and co-workers[59], adenocarcinoma developed in their series after, on an average, 6.9 years of follow-up, again only in those responding less favorably to antireflux surgery. On reviewing the surgical literature, 23 cases of adenocarcinoma could subsequently be found during the follow-up after an antireflux repair. As seen in figure 3, the majority of cases were diagnosed 5 years or less after the operation. More importantly, however, is that in those patients where an objective assessment of reflux control had been carried out, only 7 patients developed an invasive carcinoma. All except one of these latter patients had a cancer diagnosed within 5 years of the operation. In fact only one Barrett's case can be found in the

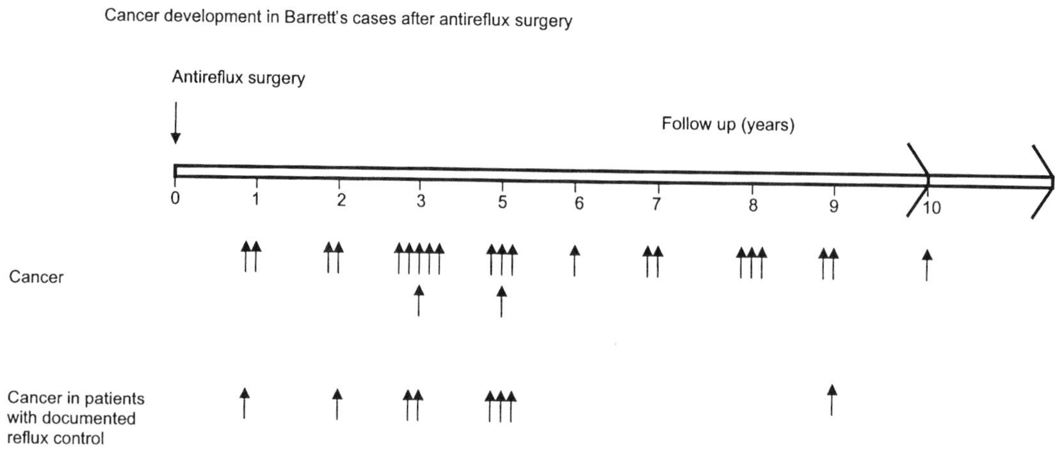

Cancer development in Barrett's cases after antireflux surgery

Figure 3 Cancer development in patient with Barrett's esophagus after antireflux surgery.

surgical literature where an adenocarcinoma has developed > 5 years after a well functioning antireflux operation[60]. It is therefore pertinent to conclude that circumstantial evidence suggests a beneficial effect of chronic and complete reflux control by a fundoplication operation, on the risk for cancer development in patients with Barrett's esophagus. However, still the most important indication for these operations in Barrett's esophagus patients is to effectively and durably control symptoms but future studies have to define the design of endoscopic follow-up strategies after successful antireflux operations.

REFERENCES

1. Cameron AJ, Ott BJ, Payne WS. The incidence of adenocarcinoma in columnar lined (Barrett's) esophagus. N Engl J Med 1985;313:857-9.
2. Haggit RC, Tryzelaar J, Ellis FH, Colcher H. Adenocarcinoma complicating columnar epithelium-lined (Barrett's) esophagus. Am Soc Cl Pathol 1978;70:1-5.
3. Skinner DB, Walther BC, Riddell RH, Schmidt H, Iascone C, DeMeester TR. Barrett's esophagus. Comparison of benign and malignant cases. Ann Surg 1983:554-65.
4. Hameeteman W, Tytgat GN, Houthoff HJ, van den Tweel JG. Barrett's esophagus: Development of dysplasia and adenocarcinoma. Gastroenterology 1989;96:1249-56.
5. Streitz JM Jr, Andrews CW Jr, Ellis FH Jr. Endoscopic surveillance of Barrett's esophagus. Does it help? J Thoac Cardiovasc Surg 1993;105(3):383-7.
6. Peters JH, Clark GW, Ireland AP, Chandrasoma P, Smyrk TC, DeMeester TR. Outcome of adenocarcinoma arising in Barrett's esophagus in endoscopically surveyed and nonsurveyed patients. J Thorac Cardiovasc Surg 1994;108:813-21.
7. Clark GW, Dreuw B, Burdiles P. The importance of endoscopic surveillance in the detection of early Barrett's adenocarcinoma. Gastroenterology 1993;104:392.
8. Spechler SJ, Goyal RK. Cancer surveillance in Barrett's esophagus: What is the end point? Gastroenterology 1994;106 (1):275-7.
9. van Sandick JW, van Lanschot JJB, Kuiken BW, Tytgat GNJ, Offerhaus GJA, Obertorp H. Impact of endoscopic biopsy surveillance of Barrett's carcinoma. Gut 1998:43:216-22.
10. Reid BJ, Haggitt RC, Rubin CE, Rabinovitsch PS. Barrett's esophagus. Correlation between flow cytometri and histology in detection of patients at risk for adenocarcinoma. Gastroenterol 1987;93:1-11.
11. Rabinovitsch PS, Reid BJ, Haggitt RC, Norwood TH, Rubin CE. Progression to cancer in Barrett's esophagus is associated with genomic instability. Laboratory Investigation 1988;60:65-71.
12. Nowell PC. The clonal evolution of tumor cell populations. Science 1976 Oct 1;194:23-8.
13. Raskind WH, Norwood T, Levine DS, Haggitt RC, Rabinovitsch PS, Reid BJ. Persistent clonal areas and clonal expansion in Barrett's esophagus. Cancer Research 1992;52:2946-50.
14. Lane DP, Benchimol S. p53 oncogene or antioncogene? Genes Dev 1990;4:1-8
15. Levine MS, Carolione D, Thompson JJ, Kressel HY, Laufer I, Herlinger H. Adenocarcinoma of the esophagus: relationship to Barrett mucosa. Radiology 1984;150(2):305-9.
16. McArdle JE, Lewin KJ, Randall G, Weinstein W. Distribution of dysplasias and early invasive carcinoma in Barrett's esophagus. Hum Pathol 1992;23:479-82.
17. Iftikhar SY, James PD, Steele RJC et al. Length of Barrett's esophagus: an important factor in the development of dysplasia and adenocarcinoma. Gut 1992; 33:1155-8.
18. Menke Pluymers MBE, Hop WCJ, Dees J et al. Risk factors for the development of an adenocarcinoma in columnar lined (Barrett) esopahgus. Cancer 1993;72:1155-8.
19. Spechler SJ, Robbins AH, Rubins HB, Vincent ME, Heeren T, Doos WG, Colton T, Schimmel EM. Adenocarcinoma and Barrett's esophagus. An overrated risk? Gastroenterology 1984;87:927-33.
20. Iftikhar SY, James PD, Steele RJ, Hardcastle JD, Atkinson M. Length of Barrett's esophagus: An important factor in the development of dysplasia and adenocarcinoma. Gut 1992;33(9): 1155-8.
21. Pera M, Trastek VF, Carpenter HA, Allen MS, Deschamps C, Pairolero PC. Barrett's esophagus with high-grade dysplasia: An indication for

esophagectomy? Ann Thorac Surg 1992;54(2):199-204.

22. Altorki NK, Sunagawa M, Little AG, Skinner DB. High-grade dysplasia in the columnar-lined esophagus. Am J Surg 1991;161:97-9.

23. Rice TW, Falk GW, Achkar E, Petras RE. Surgical management of high-grade dysplasia in Barrett's esophagus. Am J Gastroenterol 1993;88(11):1832-6.

24. Schmidt HG, Riddell RH, Walther B, Skinner DB, Riemann JF. Dysplasia in Barrett's esophagus. J Cancer Res Clin Oncol 1985;110(2):145-52.

25. Reid BJ, Haggitt RC, Rubin CE, Roth G, Surawicz CM, Van Belle G, Lewin K, Weinstein WM, Antonioli DA, Goldman H: Observer variation in the diagnosis of dysplasia in Barrett's esophagus. Hum Pathol 1988;19:166-78.

26. Prevo LJ, Sanchez CA, Galipeau PC, Reid BJ. p53-mutant clones and field effects in Barrett's esophagus. Cancer Res 1999(19);4784-7.

27. Reid BJ, Levine DS, Longton G, Blount PL, Rabinovitch PS. Predictors of progression to cancer in Barrett's esophagus baseline histology and flow cytometry indetify low and high risk patients subsets. Am J Gastroenterol 2000;95(7):1669-76.

28. DeMeester SR, Campos GMR, DeMeester TR, Bremner CG, Hagen JA, Peters JH, Crookes PF. The impact of an antireflux procedure on intestinal metaplasia of the cardia. Ann Surg 1998;228 (4):547-56.

29. Clark GW, Ireland AP, Peters JH, Chandrasoma P, DeMeester TR, Bremner CG. Short-segment Barrett's esophagus: A prevalent complication of gastresophageal reflux disease with malignant potential. J Gastrointest Surg 1997;1:113-22.

30. Zhang F, Subbaramaiah K, Altorki N, Dannenberg AJ. Dihydroxy bile acids activate the transcription of cyclooxygenase -2. J Bio Chem 1998;273:2424-8.

31. DeMeester TR. The surgical management of Barrett's esophagus and mucosal ablation. In: Barrett's esophagus. An update. Ed. Peracchia A, Bonavina L. EDRA Medical Publishing New Media 1990:79-92.

32. Fitzgerald RC, Omary MB, Triadafilopoulos G. Dynamic effects of acid on Barrett's esophagus: an ex vivo proliferation and differentiation model. J Clin Invest 1996;98:2120-8.

33. Ouatu-Lascar R, Fitzgerald RC, Triadafilopoulos G. Differentiation and proliferation in Barrett's esophagus and the effects of acid suppression. Gastroenterology 1999;117:327-35.

34. Peters FTM, Ganesh S, Kuipers EJ, De Jager-Krikken A, Karrenbeld A, Harms G et al. Epithelial cell proliferative activity of Barrett's esophagus. Methodology and correlation with traditional cancer risk markers. Dig Dis Sci 1998;43:1501-6.

35. Devière J, Buset M, Dumonceau J et al. Regression of Barrett's epithelium with omeprazole. N Engl J Med 1989;320:1497-8.

36. Ottenjann R, Heidt H. Regression der Zylinderepithel – Metaplasie bei Barrett-Esophagus. Dtsch Med Wochenschr 1990;115;916-17.

37. Gore S, Healey CJ, Sutton R et al. Regression of columnar lined (Barrett's) esophagus with continuous omeprazole therapy. Aliment Pharmacol Ther 1993;7:623-8.

38. Neuman CS, Iqbal TH, Cooper BT. Long term continuous omeprazole treatment of patients with Barrett's esophagus. Aliment Pharmacol Ther 1995;9:451-4.

39. Malesci A, Savarino V, Zentilin P et al. Partial regression of Barrett's esophagus by long-term therapy with high-dose omeprazole. Gastrointest Endosc 1996;44:700-5.

40. Shaffer RT, Francis J, Carrougher JG et al. Effect of omeprazole on Barrett's epithelium after 3 years of therapy (abstract). Gastroenterology 1996;110:A255.

41. Caldwell MTP, Byrne PJ, Walsh TN et al. A randomised trial on the effect of acid suppression on regression of Barrett's esophagus (abstract). Gastroenterology 1996;110:A74

42. Sharma P, Sampliner RE, Camargo E. Normalization of esophageal pH with high-dose proton pump inhibitor therapy does not result in regression of Barrett's esophagus. Am J Gastroenterol 1997;92:582-5.

43. Sharma P, Morales TG, Bhattacharyya A et al. Squamous islands in Barrett's esophagus: what lies underneath? Am J Gastroenterol 1998;93:332-5.

44. Katzka DA, Castell DO. Successful elimination of reflux symptoms does not ensure adequate control of acid reflux in Barrett's esophagus. Am J Gastroenterol 1994;89:989-91.

45. Ouatu-Lascar R, Triadafilopoulos G. Complete elimination of reflux symptoms does not guarantee normalization of intraesophageal acid reflux in patients with Barrett's esopgagus. Am J Gastroenterol 1998;93:711-6.

46. Kuo B, Castell DO. Optimal dosing of omeprazole 40 mg daily: effects on gastric and esophageal pH and serum gastrin in healthy controls. Am J Gastroenterol 1996;91:1532-8.

47. Ortiz A, Martínez de Haro LF, Parrilla P, Molina J, Bermejo J, Munitiz V. 24-h pH monitoring is necessary to assess acid reflux suppression in patients with Barrett's esophagus undergoing treatment with proton pump inhibitors. Br J Surg 1999;86:1472-4.

48. Johnson D, Winters C, Spurling T et al. Esophageal acid sensitivity in Barrett's esophagus. J Clin Gastroenterol 1987;9:23-7.

49. Peghini PL, Katz PO, Castell DO. Ranitidine controls nocturnal gastric acid breakthrough on omeprazole: a controlled study in normal subjects. Gastroenterology 1998;115:1335-9.

50. Peters FTM, Ganesh S, Kuipers EJ, WJ Sluiter WJ, Klinkenberg-Knol EC, Lamers CBH, Kleibeuker JH. Endoscopic regression of Barrett's esophagus during omeprazole treatment. A randomised double blind study. Gut 1999;45:489 –94.

51. Low DE, Levine DS, Dail DH, Kozarek RA. Histological and anatomic changes in Barrett's esophagus after antireflux surgery. Am J Gastroenterol 1999;94:80-85.

52. Weinstein WM, Lieberman DA. Lewin KJ et al. Omeprazole-induced regression of Barrett's esophagus : a 2 year, randomized, controlled double blind trial. Gastroenterology 1996;110:A294.

53. Stein HJ, Kauer WKH, Feussner H, Siewert JR. Bile reflux benign and malignant Barrett's esophagus: effect of Medical acid suppression and Nissen fundoplication. J Gastrointest Surg 1998;2:333-41.

54. Sagar PM, Ackroyd R, Hosie KB, Pattersson JE, Stoddard CJ, Kingsnorth AN. Regression and progression of Barrett's esophagus after antireflux surgery. Br J Surg 1995;82:806-10.

55. DeMeester TR, Peters JH, Bremner CG, Chandrasoma P. Biology of gastresophageal reflux disease: Pathophysiology relating to medical and surgical treatment. Annual Review of Medicine 1999;50:469-506.

56. Isolauri J, Loustarinen M, Isolauri E et al. Natural course of gastroesophageal reflux disease 17 – 22 year follow up of 60 patients. Am J Gastroenterology 1997;92:37-41.

57. Whetscher GJ, Profanter C, Gadenstätter M et al. Medical treatment of gastro-esophageal reflux disease does not prevent the development of Barrett's

metaplasia and poor esophageal body motility. Langenbecks Arch Chir 1997;382:95-9.

58. Isolauri J, Loustarinen M, Viljakka M, Isolauro E, Keyrilainen O, Karvonen AL. Long-term comparison of antireflux surgery versus conservative therapy for reflux esophagitis. Ann Surg 1997;225:295-9.

59. Csendes A, Braghetto I, Burdiles P, Puente G, Korn O, Diasz JC, Maluenda F. Long term results of classic antireflux surgery in 152 patients with Barrett's esophagus: Clinical, radiologic, endoscopic, manometric, and acid reflux test analysis before and late after operation. Surgery 1998;123:545-57.

60. Håkansson HO, Johnsson F, Johansson J, Kjellen G, Walther B. Development of adenocarcinoma in Barrett's esophagus. Development of adenocarcinoma in Barrett's esophagus after successful antireflux surgery. Eur J Surg 1996;163:469-47.

61. Ortiz A, Martinez de Haro LF, Parrilla P, Morales G, Molina J, Bermejo J, Liron R and Aguilar J. Conservative treatment versus antireflux surgery in Barrett's esophagus: long-term results of a prospective study. Br J Surg 1996;83:274-78

62. Katz D, Rothstein R, Schned A, Dunn J, Seaver K, Antonioli D. The development of dysplasia and adenocarcinoma during endoscopic surveillance of Barret esophagus. Am J Gastroenterol 1998;93:536-41.

63. Williamson WA, Ellis FHE, Gibb SP, Shahian DM, Aretz T. Effect of antireflux operation on Barrett's mucosa. Ann Thorac Surg 1990;49:537-42.

64. Starnes VA, Adkins RB, Ballinger JF, Sawyers JL. Barrett's esophagus. A surgical entity. Arch Surg 1984;119:563-7.

65. Naef AP, Savary M, Ozzello L. Columnar-lined lower esophagus: An acquired lesion with malignant predisposition. Report on 140 cases of Barrett's esophagus with 12 adenocarcinomas. J Thorac Cardiovasc Surg 1975;70:826-35.

66 McDonald ML, Trastek VF, Allen M. Deschamps C, Pairolero PC. Barrett's esophagus: Does an antireflux procedure reduce the need of endoscopic surveillance? J Thorac Cardiovasc Surg 1996;111:1135-40.

67. Hamilton SR, Hutcheon DF, Ravich WJ, Cameron JL, Paulsson M. Adenocarcinoma in Barrett's esophagus after elimination of gastresophageal reflux. Gastroenterol 1984;86:356-9.

68. Attwood SEA, Barlow AP, Norris TL, Watson A. Barrett's esophagus: effect of antireflux surgery on symptom control and development of complications. Br J Surg 1992;79:1050-3.

69. Pearson FG, Cooper JD, Pattersson GA, Prakash D. Peptic ulcer in acquired columnar lined esophagus. Results of surgical treatment. Ann Thorac Surg 1987;43:241-4.

70. Csendes A, Burdiles P, Korn O, Braghetto I, Huertas C, Maluenda F, Diaz J, Rojas J. Late subjective and objective results of a prospective randomised study comparing total fundoplication versus calibration of the cardia with posterior gastropexy. Analysis of 164 patients. Br J Surg, 2000 in press.

71. Lundell L, Miettinen P, Myrvold H et al. Long-term management of gastroesophageal reflux disease with omeprazole or open antireflux surgery: results of a prospective, randomized clinical trial. The Nordic GORD Study Group. Eur J Gastroenterol Hepatol 2000;12(8):879-87.

72. Lundell L, Miettinen P, Myrvold et al. Continued (5 year) follow-up of a randomised clinical study comparing antireflux surgery and omeprazole in gastresophageal reflux disease. J Am Coll Surg 2000, in press.

4.2 PREVENTION OF CANCER IN BARRETT'S BY ABLATION.

James P Byrne and Stephen EA Attwood

1. INTRODUCTION

The problem of cancer in patients with Barrett's is well described in the foregoing chapters of this book. It is clear that the outcomes of treatment for established carcinoma of the esophagus are very poor. Reliance on surveillance programs to achieve adequate early detection of cancer followed by submission of a patient to the major surgery required for esophageal resection is neither an attractive option, nor one of proven value. A potentially attractive alternative is to attempt to prevent the development of carcinoma by the destruction of the Barrett's epithelium in a reflux controlled environment, and to stimulate the regrowth of a normal squamous lining. Prevention of cancer offers the greatest opportunity for improvements in both survival and quality of life of patients with Barrett's esophagus. This chapter will describe techniques that have either been used or are being developed for the ablation of Barrett's epithelium with the intention of cancer prevention. The importance of reflux control, characteristics of the neo-squamous epithelium, current issues/controversies in Barrett's ablation and future strategies in Barrett's ablation will also be explored.

2. THEORY

2.1. BACKGROUND

The risk of cancer in Barrett's esophagus is between 30-200 times that of the normal population. Cancer risk is related to length of Barrett's segment, ulcer, stricture, male gender, smoking, and alcohol consumption. Gastroesophageal reflux disease has recently been shown to be independently associated with a high risk of esophageal adenocarcinoma[1], and Barrett's esophagus is associated with the anatomical and physiological features of end-stage gastroesophageal disease. As well as abnormal gastroesophageal reflux, there is also increased reflux of bile into the stomach and esophagus of patients with Barrett's. Increased cellular injury is associated with combined exposure to acid and bile compared with acid alone. It is not clear what the relative contributions of continuing cellular injury from (duodeno) gastroesophageal reflux and inherent genomic instability in the metaplastic lining of Barrett's esophagus might be. Consequently it is not known what the best method of preventing malignant degeneration might be. Would simple modulation of reflux composition to make it less damaging to cells reduce cancer risk? Is elimination of metaplastic mucosa required to protect against cancer? Or is a combination of the two necessary? There is no hard evidence that the cancer risk in Barrett's is reduced by either medical or surgical treatment of the associated gastro-esophageal reflux disease. Lifestyle changes may improve risks associated with smoking and alcohol, and adequate medical control of gastro-esophageal reflux may allow healing of ulcers and strictures. Obviously in a condition characterized by an irregular proximal border with tongues of columnar epithelium, length is not necessarily an accurate reflection of surface area. Despite this, several studies emphasize the importance of extent of the Barrett's segment in predicting dysplasia and adenocarcinoma [2-4] with Menke-Pluymers[5] describing relative risk of 1.7 with doubling of length. Several studies have sought a possible relationship between control of GOR and alteration in the extent of columnar lining. Neither standard doses of proton pump inhibitor(PPI), doses titrated to normalize lower esophageal acid exposure[6], or very high dose(Omeprazole 80mg/day)[7] have had a significant effect on the length of columnar mucosa. Peters' double blind randomized study[7] did demonstrate a very small (<10%) but statistically significant reduction in surface area of Barrett's epithelium on high dose acid suppression, but failed to demonstrate any reduction in length of the Barrett's segment. Anti reflux surgery has been followed by both progression and regression of Barrett's[2,8]. Difficulties in accurate measurement comparisons before and after surgery are recognized, and all regressions had 5cm or less of columnar lined esophagus. Progression was associated with abnormal acid exposure following surgery (i.e. failed anti-reflux surgery), and eight of nine patients with

H.W. Tilanus and S.E.A. Attwood (eds.), Barrett's Esophagus, 239–258.

progression had continuing reflux symptoms. Medical measures are employed to modulate volume and composition of the esophageal refluxate in the vast majority of patients with Barrett's. These clearly do have an effect on the volume and composition of esophageal refluxate[9], but cancers still develop in patients with Barrett's whilst on powerful acid suppressive therapy. Effective acid suppression does not appear to prevent the development of Barrett's cancers as these are seen both in patients with squamous islands of epithelium, suggesting adequate control of acid, and those without squamous islands. Medical treatment of gastro-esophageal reflux neither eliminates Barrett's epithelium nor the risk of malignant degeneration. A much smaller proportion of patients with Barrett's have surgical control of gastroesophageal reflux, although this may be increasing as the evidence for the effectiveness of surgery compared with medical management of gastroesophageal reflux disease and Barrett's[10] becomes more widely recognized. Successful antireflux surgery may reduce the subsequent risk of cancer, and cancers observed in series of surgically treated patients with Barrett's all seem to occur in treatment failures[2,8,10]. Studies of antireflux surgery in Barrett's published to date have only involved small numbers of patients and cancer prevention has not been a defined study endpoint. Randomized controlled study will be required to compare surgical and medical management of Barrett's in the prevention of esophageal adenocarcinoma. In 1988 Gillen[11] described a canine model of reflux esophagitis which strongly supported the concept of Barrett's metaplasia as arising from a multipotential stem cell. Denuding injury to the esophageal epithelium followed by increased exposure to gastric acid resulted in regeneration of columnar epithelium analogous to Barrett's, whereas in those animals not exposed to acid, there was regrowth of the normal squamous lining. This work led to the hypothesis that removal of Barrett's epithelium in an environment where acid exposure is controlled may allow differentiation of stem cells and lead to regrowth of the normal squamous lining. This hypothesis was confirmed by Li et al[12] who injured the mucosa in the squamous lined canine esophagus. When injury was followed by increased gastroesophageal reflux columnar rather than squamous lining was regenerated in 7 of 10 animals. 6 animals then underwent an anti-reflux procedure at 3 months and were started on Omeprazole. Healing of the esophageal

mucosa with replacement by columnar mucosa occurred in all 6 animals. Interspersed with the columnar mucosa, however, were small islands of squamous epithelium that appeared to be in continuity with the squamous cells in the distal portion of the esophageal glands. This confirmed that the response to esophageal injury is influenced by the luminal environment in the esophagus. Li's work has in turn led to an alternative strategy to reduce cancer risk in Barrett's. Destruction of the abnormal esophageal lining in a reflux controlled environment should encourage replacement of columnar epithelium by the normal squamous lining. By elimination or reduction in numbers of metaplastic cells susceptible to malignant transformation it should be possible to respectively prevent or significantly reduce the risk of developing esophageal adenocarcinoma. Ablative therapies that have been employed or have future potential in Barrett's esophagus are described below. Several issues related to modulation of cancer risk with ablative therapy are as yet unclear. The importance of adequate surgical/medical control of gastroesophageal reflux seems self evident but evidence for this is at best only circumstantial to date even for non-ablated Barrett's. The mechanism of cancer risk in Barrett's is not known. Will given percentage reductions in surface area of metaplastic cells yield an equivalent reduction in malignant risk? It may be that the total number of metaplastic cells in the lower esophagus is the most important factor in predicting malignant risk. Alternatively direct exposure of metaplastic cells to refluxate may be an important factor in carcinogenesis in which case a covering of squamous epithelium over metaplastic cells might be expected to confer a worthwhile reduction in malignant risk. The limited available published evidence will be discussed.

3. TECHNIQUES OF ABLATION

All ablative techniques apply energy to the metaplastic Barrett's mucosa and this destroys or physically removes the mucosal layer of the esophagus. Following elimination of the Barrett's lining, if gastroesophageal reflux is controlled effectively, regenerated epithelium is squamous in nature.

3.1 AIMS OF ABLATIVE TREATMENT

Remove/destroy all cells that have potential for malignant transformation, and then promote regrowth of the normal squamous lining. Maintain an environment that discourages regrowth of Barrett's epithelium.

The long-term aim is to reduce the risk of patients with Barrett's developing esophageal adenocarcinoma.

3.2 OBJECTIVES OF ABLATIVE THERAPY

1. Effective removal of metaplastic cells
2. Replacement with normal squamous epithelium
3. Safety for patients
4. Safety for attendant medical staff
5. Ease of learning and performing technique
6. Equipment inexpensive to purchase/ operate

Thermal
    Laser
    Multipolar electrocoagulation
    Argon Beam Plasma Coagulation
    Heater Probe
    Cryotherapy
Photochemical
    Photodynamic Therapy
Mechanical
    Endoscopic Mucosal Resection
    CUSA

Figure 1. Techniques for ablation of Barrett's epithelium

4. THERMAL ABLATION

4.1 LASER

Lasers have been used in medical practice for more than thirty years as a means of delivering energy to tissues in open surgery. Development of fiberoptic probes which may be passed along the instrument channel of an endoscope have allowed endoscopic application of laser energy described in the treatment of superficial esophageal cancer by Fujimaki[13] in 1986. An important issue in use of laser energy for Barrett's ablation is depth of injury. Depth of injury is related primarily to the wavelength of laser light source and secondarily intensity of the light beam, whilst the pulse duration dictates the total energy delivered (Table 1). Laser ablation is a non contact technique which allows delivery of a narrow area of injury to the esophageal mucosa. A critical factor in the use of laser is the relative difficulty in application, in that tangential application is not possible. This makes laser ablation time consuming and

requires a high endoscopic skill level for safe application.

In 1993 Berenson[14] described regrowth of squamous epithelium in Barrett's esophagus following argon laser ablation of small patches of epithelium in Barrett's esophagus. Squamous regrowth over the ablated patches not only occurred where columnar segment was contiguous with squamous epithelium but also de novo in the middle of areas of columnar epithelium. This supported the existence of a pluripotential stem cell in the esophageal mucosa of humans. Sampliner then described squamous re-epithelialisation in a patient with a 3.5cm Barrett's segment in 1993 after ablation with Nd:YAG laser[15].

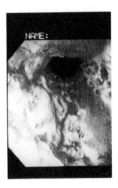

Figure 2. Endoscopic appearance of Barrett's segment after ablation with Argon beam plasma coagulation.
2a. Ablation applied in longitudinal strips with intervening bridges of Barrett's mucosa.

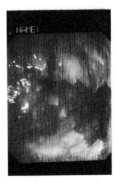

2b. One months after initial treatment before ablation of mucosal columns.

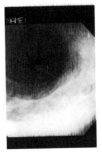

2c. Completion of treatment, 3 months after initial therapy.

Table 1 Laser wavelength and depth of injury

	Wavelength(nm)	Depth of injury
Nd YAG	1064	4mm
KTP(doubled frequency NdYAG)	532	1mm
Argon	514	1mm

Brandt[16] described transient replacement of a 1.5cm tongue of columnar epithelium by squamous epithelium six weeks after ablation with Nd:YAG laser. Two months later there was both endoscopic and histologic recurrence of columnar mucosa.

Investigation confirmed increased acid exposure in the lower esophagus despite adequate symptomatic control of gastroesophageal reflux. Repeat laser ablation on an increased dose of acid suppression was followed by durable squamous re-epithelialisation[16], highlighting the importance of adequate control of gastroesophageal reflux in permitting squamous regrowth.

Luman[18] has published the only randomized-controlled trial of ablation in Barrett's esophagus in a small study of eight patients, four of whom underwent ablation. Nd:YAG laser was used at a power setting of 25 watts with energy administered in one second pulses, delivering a median of 636 joules. Patients had up to three sessions performed at 4-6 weekly intervals. Laser ablation had no effect on the Barretts segment in this study and squamous regrowth did not occur. The reason(s) for these treatment failures are not known. Nd: YAG laser causes tissue injury to a depth of 4mm, and it may be that failure occurred because of overpenetration of the epithelium, with destruction of stem cells that inhabit the superficial layers. Squamous epithelium inhabits the superficial third of ducts, originating at the junction of the superficial and middle thirds. Damage at too deep a level may therefore fail to encourage regrowth of the squamous lining. The technique of ablation may be a second contributory factor, as ablation was commenced at the esophagogastric junction and continued in a retrograde fashion towards the squamo-columnar junction, potentially leaving ablated areas totally surrounded by columnar mucosa.

Against a background of stem cell destruction and an ab-sence of contiguous squamous epithelium to allow creeping growth of squamous cells, if ablated areas were surrounded by columnar epithelium it is possible that proliferation of Barrett's cells overwhelmed proliferation of squamous epithelium causing treatment failure.

In 1995, Ertan[19] described ablation of a more extensive 14cm Barrett's segment associated with a carcinoma using Nd:YAG laser, with squamous replacement occurring in the proximal 3cm following ablation. The whole of the Barrett's segment was not treated.

Salo reported a case control study in patients with Barrett's after anti-reflux surgery[20], where patients had laser ablation with Nd:YAG. Columnar epithelium of median length 4cm was eliminated endoscopically and histologically after a mean of 4 sessions. In 1999, Sharma et al reported use of Nd:YAG laser in conjunction with MPEC at a mean power setting of 30 watts using a continuous free beam method of ablation[21]. Patients again had cancers in their Barrett's segments. Complete endoscopic ablation of columnar lining was achieved in 5 of 6 patients over a mean length of nearly 6cm. Barham et al[22], in 1997 published the most comprehensive study to date of laser ablation as a means of preventing cancer in Barrett's uncomplicated by either dysplasia or cancer. Sixteen patients underwent a median of three treatments, and in thirteen complete replacement of the columnar mucosa by squamous lining was observed. KTP laser was employed at 20 watts setting, with ablation of 30% of esophageal circumference per session. Unfortunately columnar segment length has not been reported in this study. Work (published) by the same group in abstract form only studied thermal injury in the esophagus produced by laser and demonstrated that application of point burns at 20watts for one second generated mucosal esophageal temperatures of 65C, compared with 21C at the external surface. Gossner in 1999 described the use of Nd:YAG KTP laser at 12-18 watts setting and 300-1000 joules per session applied hemicircumferentially in 10 patients with dysplasia or early cancers[23]. Replacement of columnar epithelium was achieved in all patients. Proton pump inhibitor had been titrated to normalize 24-hour pH studies in order to maintain an acid free environment. The columnar segment was 3cm or more in only 3 of these patients. In conclusion, laser ablation is effective in achieving squamous regrowth of the columnar segment, although many of the published studies are in patients with dysplasia/cancer and or those with columnar segments of less than 3cm. The published work suggests that laser is safe, with no reported perforations. To date Salo[21] and Barham[22] are the only groups to have confirmed the utility of laser ablation in patients with Barrett's uncomplicated by dysplasia or cancer. Salo's work is of note in that all ablated patients had previously undergone antireflux surgery. (Table 2)

4.1.2. Multipolar electro coagulation
a)   Gold Probe
b)   Probe in action

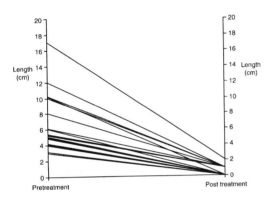

Figure 3. Outcome of Argon Beam plasma coagulation in 34 patients with Barrett's esophagus. Reproduced with permission Byrne et al. Am J Gastroenterol 1998;10:1010-5
3a. Length of Barrett segment before and after treatment with ABPC3b. Number of treatments required to ablate

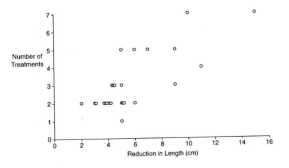

3b. Number of treatments required to ablate Barrett's segments and achieve reduction in extent of the Barrett's.

With multipolar electrocoagulation(MPEC) heat is created on completion of the electrical circuit between the electrodes of a bipolar probe. A wire with two 7 or 10 French gold electrodes at the tip is passed along the instrument channel at flexible endoscopy. 10-20 Watts of energy is delivered to the esophageal mucosa, and is applied until a white coagulum develops. Treatment has been described over 2-3cm hemicircumferential and circumferential lengths[24], with applications repeated at one week intervals. Sampliner originally described ablation of Barrett's with MPEC in 10 patients in a pilot study in 1996[25], with titration of proton pump inhibitor dose to normalize esophageal exposure to acid. Hemicircumferential ablation was performed with the non ablated esophagus acting as a control. These patients have now been followed up for a median of 36 months without development of a cancer or endoscopic recurrence of the Barrett's mucosa[26].

Montes[27] performed MPEC in 14 patients with Barrett's esophagus after antireflux surgery with complete endoscopic and histologic replacement of Barrett's by squamous lining. Kovacs[24] has published the largest series of 27 Barrett's patients treated with MPEC. 2-3cm segments of epithelium were treated at each session, and a median of 2 sessions was required to complete treatment. It should be noted that the median length of columnar segment was 3cm and that only 15/27 patients actually had a true Barrett's segment of at least 3cm. Furthermore, success of ablation with MPEC was clearly related to length of the Barrett's segment with complete reversal in 91% (21/23) of patients with Barrett's 2-4 cm in length, compared with only 25% (1/4) when the Barrett's segment was 5cm or longer. Like argon beam plasma coagulation, MPEC has the advantage that it may be applied tangential to orientation of the flexible endoscope. Sharma and Sampliner have described MPEC employed as an adjunctive ablative endoscopic technique in conjunction with laser. In a series of six patients with early Barrett's adenocarcinomas MPEC successfully ablated areas inaccessible to treatment with laser[21]. MPEC appears to be safe, with no reports of perforation in the literature. There has been no significant study on depth of injury with MPEC, although use has not been associated with stricture formation, suggesting that injury is mucosal rather than involving the deeper layers. The equipment is relatively inexpensive to purchase, being based on a standard electrosurgical generator, and the main

TABLE 2. Results of laser ablation of Barrett's esophagus

	Total no. of patients	<3cm Benign Columnar epithelium	>3cm Benign Barrett's	LGD	HGD	Carcinoma	Reduction in >3cm Barrett's segments
Sampliner[25] Sharma[28]	11	4	7	0	0	0	Complete resolution
Montes [29]	1	0	1	0	0	0	Complete resolution
Montes[27]	14	0	14	0	0	0	Complete resolution
Kovacs[24]	27	12	15	0	0	0	Complete resolution in 9

TABLE 3. MPEC ablation of Barrett's

	Total no. of patients	<3cm Benign Columnar epithelium	>3cm Benign Barrett's	LGD	HGD	Carcinoma	Reduction in >3cm Barrett's segments
Barham [22] 1997	16	0	16	0	0	0	Resolution in those completing treatment
Ertan[19] 1995	1	0	0	0	1	0	To treated areas complete
Gossner[23] 1999	10	0	0	4	4	2	Complete resolution
Brandt[16] 1992	1	1	0	0	0	0	Temporary resolution
Luman[18] 1996	8 (2 arms 4 pts: RCT)	0	4	0	0	0	Nil
Berenson[14] 1993	10	1	9	0	0	0	Resolution in treated areas. incomplete ablation
Salo[20] 1998	17: (6 pts controls)	11 pts no discrimination on length grouds 1-11cm		0	0	0	Near complete resolution
Sharma[21] 1999	6	0	0	0	0	6	Resolution in 2/6, cancer in 1/6
Sampliner[15] 1993	1	0	1	0	0	0	50%:Hemicircumferential application

expense is related to the purchase of disposable electrodes.

4.1.3 Argon Beam Plasma coagulation

Argon beam plasma coagulation is an electrosurgical technique that has been used in open surgery for many years, and is particularly useful for application of energy to large areas of tissue, as in liver surgery. Argon gas is delivered along a flexible tube by means of a pump at a rate of 1 - 4 liters/minute. This tube has been developed to fit along the instrument channel of an endoscope, and in the lumen is a wire carrying current from a standard electrosurgical generator. Energy is delivered to tissue by a stream of argon gas that is ionized as it passes this high frequency electrode at the end of the tube. The ionized argon gas carries a current that is completed with release of energy upon tissue contact.

Argon beam plasma coagulation has theoretical advantages over some other forms of energy delivery. As ionized particles carry ablative energy, tangential application of energy is possible. Secondly, as continued delivery of energy is dependent upon completion of an electrical circuit, formation of an electrically insulating eschar after ablation may help limit the depth of injury to mucosa.

ABPC has now been described in over 150 patients with Barrett's esophagus making it the most frequently used modality. For this reason we shall describe in some detail the practical approach to endoscopic ablation using ABPC. Standard endoscopy equipment and facilities are required, and it is preferable although not essential to use a twin channel operating endoscope as this permits aspiration of insufflated argon gas without withdrawal of

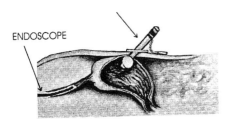

Figure 4. Placement of operating gastrostomy port for laparoscopic application of CUSA. Reproduced with permission Bremner et al. Surg Endoscopy 1998;12:342-7

the argon probe during the ablation session. Ablation is performed by non-contact application of the argon probe, which should be kept 1-3mm away from the surface to be ablated. No evidence exists as to the optimal approach to endoscopic ablation, differing techniques have been described: circumferential[30], hemicircumferential[31,32], and longitudinal[33,34]. Our initial preference was to perform ablations in longitudinal strips during withdrawal of endoscope and argon probe but with preservation of an intact mucosal bridge between ablated areas in order to avoid the potential risk of stricture formation. Van Laethem employed circumferential ablative technique and described troublesome stricture in 2/31 patients requiring 2 and 3 dilatations. Latterly, we have also ablated the full circumference of the esophagus, with a deep ulcer in one case and this has dampened our enthusiasm for this approach. We have had no problems with stricture formation to date. We find it practically more convenient to ablate longitudinal strips of epithelium as the endoscope is withdrawn.

With ABPC it is important to avoid over-insufflation of Argon gas into the stomach, as gaseous distension of the stomach and upper small intestine may produce severe discomfort and retching. The combination of retching and esophageal movement with normal respiration may make ablation difficult at least and dangerous at worst, especially if combined with inadequate sedation. Perforation has been reported with endoscopic ABPC and this appears to have been related to esophageal instrumentation rather than deep tissue injury caused by tissue ablation[34]. Provided the patient is kept comfortable and adequately

sedated, we have found Argon to be safe and have had no perforation or other significant complications in our last 300 endoscopic applications. In our experience patients frequently experience some retrosternal discomfort lasting up to 72 hours after the procedure, although this lasted up to three weeks in 2/31 patients from Van Laethem's study. Provided patients are counselled adequately pre-procedure, and prescribed adequate analgesia together with antacid suspension such as Mucaine Gel, post ablation symptoms are minimal. Other reported complications of ABPC include bleeding sufficient to require transfusion in 1/31 patients[33], and dysphagia[31].

Haemotoporphyrin derivative
Sodium porfimer
m-THPC
5-ALA

Figure 5 Photosensitisers available for use in PDT of Barrett's esophagus

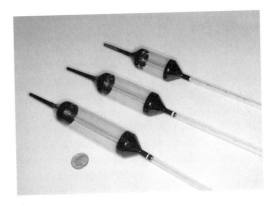

Figure 6 Balloon diffusers of 3,5 and 7 cm in length developed for photodynamic therapy of Barrett's esophagus by Panjehpour et al. Reproduced with permission Panjehpour et al. Gastrointest Clin N America 2000;12(3):513-32

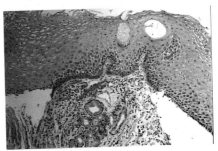

Figure 7. Histological patterns of squamous regrowth after ablation. Figure 7a. Normal glandular structure underlying squamous epithelium

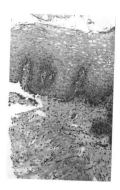

Figure 7b. Scarring of lamina propria deep to neo-squamous epithelium after ABPC

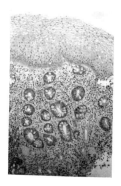

Figure 7c. Goblet cells and extensive intestinal metaplasia under neo-squamous epithelium after ABPC

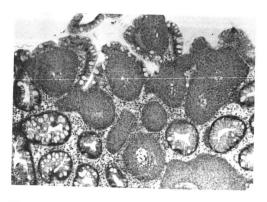

Figure 7d
Spectacular squamous re-epithelialisation within Barrett'

4.1.4 Heater probe

A heater probe that may be passed along the instrument channel of an endoscope is manufactured by Olympus. A group in Athens has used 2.4mm diameter probe delivering 5-10 joule pulses of energy (Total mean energy delivered 933.8 range 100-3300J) in the ablation of Barrett's epithelium[38]. This study described antegrade application of ablation, commencing at the proximal margin of the columnar segment. Complete ablation of the Barrett's epithelium was attempted at each session. In the 36 reported treatments there were no major treatment related complications, and the procedure is described as straightforward to perform. Some patients suffered mild retrosternal discomfort, and there was one case of acute pain associated with an ulcer that subsequently healed.

Only 5 of 13 patients had 3cm or more columnar lining in the lower esophagus, and only 2 of the 13 patients had circumferential Barrett's over the extent of epithelium described. 8 patients simply had 2 or 2.5cm tongues of columnar epithelium. In those with columnar segments 3cm or more in length, a reduction in length of approximately 1cm per ablative session was achieved. Total squamous covering of the columnar segment was described for all patients. Of the five patients with columnar segments >3cm in length, follow up endoscopic biopsy revealed intestinal metaplasia underlying squamous epithelium at only 2 of 20 'normal' endoscopic examinations.

4.1.5 Cryotherapy

Contact cryotherapy involving direct tissue contact with a solid probe has previously been described in the esophagus twenty years ago[39]. As originally described this method of tissue ablation was associated with significant tissue injury and mucosal temperatures as low as – 140 Centigrade, and these low temperatures were associated with a significant risk of complications including esophageal perforation. Johnston et al[40] have since developed an alternative method for delivery of controlled hypothermic tissue injury, utilizing the cryotherapeutic properties of nitrogen gas. A probe has been developed which passes along the instrument channel of the endoscope and delivers cold nitrogen gas in a spray. During application of cryotherapy,

TABLE 4. Argon Beam ablation of Barrett's esophagus

	Total no. of patients	<3cm Benign Columnar epithelium	>3cm Benign Barrett's	LGD	HGD	Carcinoma	Reduction in >3cm Barrett's segments
Byrne[34]	30	0	23	4	3	0	All less than 3cm after treatment
Mork[31]	15	4	11	0	0	0	Complete in 9/10 (1 lost)
Martin[35]	26	Unclear: segments 2-10cm in length all grouped together		0	0	0	Complete resolution 11, partial 11, none 1
v.Laethem[33]	31	0	26	5	0	0	Resolution in 28/31(90%)
Orth[36]	13	0	0	0	5	0	Complete response
Du Moulin[30]	2	0	2	0	0	0	Complete response
Grade[32]	9	3	6	0	0	0	Complete response
May[37]	3	3	0	0	0	3	Complete response

TABLE 5. Heater probe in ablation of Barrett's esophagus

	Total no. of patients	<3cm Benign Columnar epithelium	>3cm Benign Barrett's	LGD	HGD	Carcinoma	Reduction in >3cm Barrett's segments
Michopoulos[38]	13	8	5	0	0	0	Complete resolution

the tip of the probe is maintained at a distance of 0.5 to 1cm away from mucosa, and applied to the lower 2-3cm of the esophagus. Two consecutive phases are described in association with application of the spray. Firstly there is a flushing phase, the time taken until appearance of cryoburn. Cryoburn is found to appear in animals within 30 seconds of initiation, coinciding with a drop in mucosal temperature to between 0 and minus 10 Centigrade. The second phase is known as the cryoburn time, and is the duration of exposure of the esophagus to continuing thermal injury. Johnston studied the effects of exposure to cold nitrogen gas for less than 30 seconds and for 30 – 60 seconds. Cryotherapy was performed either hemicircumferentially or circumferentially. Esophagi from ablated animals were than analyzed at 28 days following necropsy. 27%(3/11) of the high dose cryotherapy animals developed strictures and 54% had transmural inflammation at 28 days post procedure compared with no strictures and transmural inflammation in 18%(2/11) for the low dose cryotherapy group. Interestingly, following spray cryotherapy, mucosa thawed within 60 seconds of thermal injury. In this small study development of stricture or severe inflammation appeared associated with circumferential injury rather than duration of cryoburn. The authors plan to use this technique in humans, and results are awaited with interest.
Technique appears relatively safe and application appears straightforward, if possibly

difficult to target; suggesting that ablation over a 3cm length may be performed in under 30 seconds. The spray applicator, gas and gas delivery system should be relatively cheap to purchase.

4.2 MECHANICAL ABLATION

4.2.1 Endoscopic mucosal resection
Endoscopic mucosal resection has not been used in management of non-dysplastic Barrett's to date, but is an effective method for removing mucosa from the esophagus. Several techniques have been described for mucosal resection, usually in the context of early esophageal and gastric neoplasms. Standard endoscopic techniques are used and a twin channel operating endoscope is passed. Prior to resection, hydrodissection with or without adrenaline as a haemostatic adjunct may be used to develop a submucosal plane and so facilitate resection. The different methods described for resection are as follows:
1. Lift and cut Martin[41]
2. Suck and cut [42,43]
3. Snare mucosectomy[44]
It is interesting to note that the only adenocarcinoma to arise post ABPC ablation of a non dysplastic Barrett's[45] was excised at endoscopic mucosal resection rather than esophagectomy, and that this was apparently at the insistence of the patient rather than the surgeon. There is as yet no published literature on the use of primary EMR in either dysplastic or non-dysplastic Barrett's esophagus.

4.2.2 CUSA

Ultrasonic energy is well established as an irrigation/aspiration system for removal of cellular debris in liver and brain resections, with CUSA originally developed for use in ophthalmic surgery. CUSA acts primarily by means of cavitation at a relatively low frequency of 23kHz. Ultrasonic power cutting machines such as the harmonic scalpel operate at the higher frequency of 55.5kHz, and are dependent on energy liberated by deformation and secondary heat generation as well as cavitation. Intracellular cavitation makes CUSA highly effective in the removal of parenchymal tissue with a high water content such as the metaplastic cells constituting the esophageal lining in Barrett's esophagus. Free extracellular water is also rapidly vaporized which opens up tissue planes. Varying the amplitude of the signal varies the amount of energy transmitted to the tissues. This technique has been developed and evaluated by Bremner et al[46] in Los Angeles.

The ultrasonic probe is a rigid tube 30cm long, and application via flexible endoscopic techniques is not therefore currently feasible. The probe may however be applied laparoscopically if passed through a gastrostomy port.

Pilot studies in a pig model have determined the depth and extent of injury associated with differing settings on the CUSA machine, and defined the optimal power. Complete removal of the lower esophageal epithelium, with preservation of the muscularis mucosa and no injury to either submucosa or muscularis propria was seen in the animals treated. Further operative studies have confirmed feasibility of synchronous antireflux surgery, and ultrasound ablation.

The procedure is potentially very safe providing the energy is delivered to the esophageal mucosa, and to date there have been no treatment related complications. The obvious limitation is the requirement for access to the esophageal mucosa via a gastrostomy port. In the human this would require competence in more advanced laparoscopic skills such as endoscopic suturing. The opening of an abdominal viscus may also be associated with increased operative risk compared with other endoluminal modalities such as laser, MPEC, PDT and Argon Beam.

Ablative technique appears to be straightforward, and has the advantage that all of the esophageal mucosa may be ablated at one session, synchronously with antireflux surgery. Furthermore, aspiration of the ablated cells will allow cytological analysis of the Barrett's mucosa, this is not possible with other destructive ablation modalities. The results of studies using this technique in humans are eagerly awaited.

4.3 PHOTOCHEMICAL ABLATION

4.3.1 Photodynamic therapy

Photodynamic therapy is a form of chemical ablation where a photochemical reaction occurs in tissues previously administered a photosensitiser. Energy is delivered from a source of light energy, usually laser, allowing oxygen free radicals to be released. Oxygen free radicals are highly reactive and cytotoxic, destroying vital cell structures such as mitochondria. The degree of injury depends firstly on delivery of energy to the tissue being ablated and secondly the presence of photosensitize in the tissue to be ablated. The wavelength and intensity of the laser light source are therefore of critical importance. A factor of particular importance in determining energy delivery in the esophagus is the collapsible/distensible nature of the organ. This may lead to uneven delivery of light energy to the esophageal mucosa and has prompted the development of light diffusers that distend the esophagus and permit more even delivery of ablative energy. Different photosensitisers have varying cell tissue penetrations into Barrett's epithelium, and side effect profiles.

Photosensitisers

The ideal photosensitiser has a pure and stable composition, no dark toxicity, a strong absorption peak in the red spectrum of light as this gives the greatest tissue penetration, is an efficient generator of free radicals and causes minimum photosensitivity. Haematoporphyrin derivative was used for much of the development work with PDT. Sodium porfimer(Photofrin) is a partly purified commercial derivative. Unfortunately porfimer sodium has some drawbacks including poor photochemical properties because of a small absorption peak in the red region of the spectrum, needing long treatment times and higher levels of energy delivery(100 J/cm^2). Cutaneous photosensitivity may be a problem for up to 3 months post administration of sensitiser. A major problem relates to the lack of tissue selectivity which means that injury is not confined to the mucosal and submucosal layers and strictures may occur as a consequence of scarring after injury to the muscle layers. Because of this, PDT induced strictures are frequently relatively refractory and difficult to treat compared with peptic esophageal strictures that generally affect mucosa and submucosa only.

Metatetrahydroxyphenyl chlorin(m-THPC)

m-THPC is chemically pure and stable with a strong peak absorption at 652nm meaning lower doses of light energy of approximately 10 J/cm^2 are required. This is about 10% of the energy required for ablation with sodium porfimer. In the small series of patients treated to date with early bronchial and esophageal cancers, photosensitivity lasts one week or less[47]. With m-THPC it was also suggested that green light may be more useful than red as there is less tissue penetration than with red and the muscle damage/perforations seen with red light would be less likely to occur. m-THPC in ablation of Barrett's esophagus has been described as second line photodynamic therapy by Gossner et al[48] (m-THPL achieved remission in 3/5 patiens with early cancer who had unsuccessful treatment with 5-ALA) m-THPC has not been reported in Barrett's uncomplicated by dysplasia or cancer.

5-Aminolaevulinic acid(5-ALA)

This is a naturally occurring precursor of heme, whose production is normally controlled by negative feedback inhibition depending on heme concentration. Following exogenous administration of 5-ALA the natural regulatory process is bypassed and the heme synthesis pathway becomes overloaded. 5-ALA's most important property is its relative tissue selectivity for mucosa. This means that PDT damage does not affect the muscularis propria and the high incidence of refractory strictures seen with porfimer sodium has not been observed. Even ALA however is not entirely without risk, and nausea and hepatotoxicity due to first pass metabolism of the drug limit the maximum oral dose to 60mg/kg. The pharmacokinetics of 5-ALA as a photosensitiser in Barrett's ablation have been studied by Ackroyd[49] who has shown peak concentrations are achieved in esophageal tissue 4 hours post administration and that a dose of 30mg/kg gives near equivalent tissue concentration at this time whilst limiting sytemic side effects of sensitiser. It may be possible to enhance the effect of 5-ALA by using ALA esters, adding an iron chelator to inhibit conversion of PPIX to heme, or fractionating the light dose.

Balloon Diffusers

To address the issue of evenly targeted delivery of energy in the esophageal lumen, a balloon delivery system has been developed by Overholt et al[50].

Diffusers either 3,5 or 7cm in length are passed into the esophagus over a guide-wire. The diffuser balloon is then inflated to a pressure of 20-25mmHg at the appropriate position in the esophagus. Inflation of the balloon to this pressure eliminates the mucosal folds and ridges, and therefore permits an even delivery of light to the esophageal mucosa. A laser diffuser of the appropriate length is then passed into the centering channel of the balloon and delivery of light may then take place. More recently, Gossner[51] has described the successful application of a through endoscope diffuser system with a choice of balloon sizes up to 10cm in length. This system has the advantage that diffuser balloons may now be positioned under direct vision, which may make application of PDT a more reliable technique.

Overholt has published several papers in the use of PDT in Barrett's patients with associated high-grade dysplasia or early cancer[52-54], and the results of his experiences in one hundred patients have been summarised[55]. Intravenous sodium porfimer was administered 48 hours preoperatively and light delivered at 100-250 joules/cm. Total ablation of Barrett's was attempted at each session, and an overall 75-80% reduction in surface area of Barrett's epithelium was noted. Complete elimination of Barrett's mucosa was achieved in 43 patients, although the vast majority of these (35/43) required adjunctive Nd:YAG laser treatment after PDT to achieve this. At this stage, persisting areas of IM were thought in part to be due to folding of mucosa due to inadequate distension of the esophagus. Given the relatively poor photochemical properties of porfimer sodium it is unsurprising that strictures developed in 34% (34/100) of patients. Of the 34 strictures in a hundred patients, 11 were severe, requiring multiple dilatations. Small unilateral or bilateral pleural effusions were noted in the majority of patients on post procedure X rays, and two of these required thoracocentesis. Four patients had significant delayed photosensitivity reactions between one week and 2 months post PDT.

Gossner[48] evaluated PDT with 5-ALA in 32 patients with Barrett's esophagus complicated by high-grade dysplasia or early mucosal cancers. Whilst squamous re-epithelialisation was not a primary outcome measure in this

TABLE 6. Photodynamic therapy in Barrett's esophagus

	Total no. of patients	<3cm Benign Columnar epithelium	>3cm Benign Barrett's	LGD	HGD	Carcinoma	Reduction in >3cm Barrett's segments
Overholt[55]	100	0	0	14	73	13	75-80% reduction in length
Laukka[58]	5						
Barr[57]	5	0	0	0	5	0	Squamous re-epithelialisation
Orth[36]	13	0	0	0	6	2	Resolution in HGD

study partial re-epithelialisation was described in 21/32 patients, with underlying intestinal metaplasia but no dysplasia in 2 of these. In view of the complication rate in PDT, Laukka[56] explored low dose PDT with administration of 0.5mg/kg of photosensitiser. Unfortunately there was failure of re-epithelialisation in this study.

Barr has described successful ablation of dysplastic Barrett's segments with oral 5-ALA in 5 patients.[57]. Persisting areas of metaplastic cells were however noted (within and deep to neo-squamous epithelium).

Several techniques may be effective in achieving ablation of Barrett's columnar epithelium, as described above. However, the total literature to date of ablation in non-dysplastic Barrett's includes less than two hundred patients, with less than one hundred and fifty patient years of follow up. Clearly a great deal more prospective study will be required before the justification for an ablative approach to non-dysplastic Barrett's can be considered proven.

5. CHILDREN

Barrett's is present in up to 10% of children with reflux disease and may arise spontaneously or in association with other developmental abnormalities. In a child with otherwise normal life expectancy, lifelong Barrett's cancer risk might be expected to be very high. Garcia Montes et al[29] provide the only report of Barrett's ablation in a pediatric patient to date. Multipolar electrocoagulation was used via a B.I.C.A.P. probe following antireflux surgery in a 14 year old girl with a 5cm Barrett's segment, with apparent success. Barrett's cancers however very rarely develop before the age of 40 years even in a population exposed to severe gastroesophageal reflux disease as children. Beddow recently reported a series of children with Barrett's, and suggests that surveillance under the age of sixteen is unnecessary[59]. There is no evidence at all to support an ablative approach to Barrett's esophagus in children at present. A program of endoscopic surveillance performed at appropriate intervals followed by ablation at the age of 40 years or more seems a more pragmatic approach. It may well be that if Barrett's ablation is proven to reduce malignant risk in Barrett's, the optimal technique will be more apparent in ten to twenty years time than it is currently.

6. DEPTH OF INJURY

It is essential to define the depth of tissue injury required for ablative therapies as this is likely to be critical in determining the long term success of therapy. Inadequate tissue penetration may lead to incomplete ablation of metaplastic cells having a malignant potential. Excessively deep injury may be associated with injury to the stem cells in the necks of the submucous glands which may be necessary for squamous regrowth. Deep injury may therefore inhibit regrowth of squamous epithelium from stem cells in the esophageal epithelium, although regrowth may still occur by means of direct growth across from surrounding squamous epithelium. Excessively deep injury may obviously cause perforation and may also contribute to the later complications of submucosal scarring and stricture. A mechanical technique such as CUSA has the advantage that tissue disruption occurs at the interface of mucosa and submucosa, so in theory all metaplastic cells may be physically removed.

Ackroyd has assessed the thickness of squamous and metaplastic esophageal epithelium as 0.5mm by studying paraffin embedded biopsies[60]. Allowing for tissue shrinkage due to fixing and processing of approximately 20%, he estimated the likely in-

TABLE 7. Overall results of endoscopic ablation of benign Barrett's columnar segments 3cm or greater in extent, with no dysplasia/neoplasia.
*These studies did not discriminate between Barrett's segments more or less than 3cm in length. † A subsequent case report from this group has identified a cancer in this group of patients, but this has not been included in the final column as the total number of years follow up for this cohort of patients has not been reported.

	Reference	Number of patients reported in study	Patients with ablation of > 3cm columnar lining Benign Barrett's	Median Follow up	Patient years of follow up	Carcinomas / total number of patient years in >3cm benign Barrett's post ablation
Laser	Barham 22	16	16	13; 3-18 months	11.4	0/35
	Luman 18	4	4	Exclude as Rx failed		
	Berenson 14	10	9	Exclude as he mainly ablated patches only		
	Salo 20	17	11*	26 months	23.8 years	
	Sampliner 15	1	1	Exclude as he only ablated 50%		
MPEC	Sharma 28	11	7	Mean 37 months	21.6	0/47
	Montes 29	1	1	12 months	1	
	Montes 27	14	14	21.6 months	25.2	
	Kovacs 24	27	15	Nil	Nil	
Argon	Byrne 34	30	23	Median 9 months	17.25	0/45
	Mork 31	15	11	Mean 8.9 months	7.5	
	Martin 35	26	26*	Nil	Nil	
	Van Laethem 33	31	26†	17; 1 year 14; 3 months	20.5	
	Du Moulin 30	2	2	Nil	Nil	
	Grade 32	9	6	Nil	Nil	
Heat Probe	Michopoulos 38	13	5	21 months	9	0/9
Photodynamic therapy	Laukka 58	5	5			

vivo epithelial thickness to be 0.6mm. Argon laser and Nd:YAG laser cause tissue injury to a depth of approximately 1mm. KTP laser with a shorter wavelength causes tissue injury to 4mm although it has not been noted to cause problems with stricture. This deeper injury may however inhibit regrowth of squamous cells, as the stem cells in the neck of normal esophageal glands may be destroyed with this technique. Argon beam plasma coagulation injury is limited to 1-2mm, because of the electrically insulating properties of the eschar formed during coagulation. Tissue injury deep to the mucosa is unnecessary to prevent cancer, and may lead to scarring and fibrosis with stricture if the muscular layers are involved. In photodynamic therapy there is almost as much uptake of sensitiser in normal stromal tissue as in Barrett's epithelium[49], and it is this non-specific uptake which is likely to account for the diffuse injury and high stricture rate following photodynamic therapy[55]. Because these strictures are due to transmural injury they are frequently difficult to manage, requiring repeated dilation.

7. REFLUX CONTROL

It appears that adequate control of gastroesophageal reflux is important in the development and subsequent durability of neo-squamous epithelium. Brandt et al presented the earliest evidence suggesting that control of gastro-esophageal reflux was necessary for durable re-epithelialisation. They described transient Barrett's regression and re-epithelialisation with squamous cells after ablation with laser[16], although after six months without acid suppression therapy, the columnar lining recurred in the ablated area. Repeat treatment in the same patient was accompanied by long term acid suppression therapy and a durable neo-squamous epithelium[17]. There have been several other reports of ablative failures upon withdrawal of acid suppression and consequent loss of control of gastroesophageal reflux. Acid suppression was withdrawn in four patients after successful Barrett's ablative therapy in Michopoulos' study[38] and Barrett's recurred in two patients with initial 5 and 6cm columnar segments, although it did not in two who initially had 2 and 2.5cm columnar segments. This is consistent with a study of regression of columnar lined esophagus whilst on proton pump inhibitor that described regression in 5/35 with 1-2cm columnar segments and 2/64 with >3cm Barrett's segments[61].

7.1 PROTON PUMP INHIBITOR

The level of medical acid suppression required promoting regrowth of squamous lining after ablation is not known. Sampliner described titration of acid suppression dosage to achieve normalization of esophageal pH prior to MPEC ablation[15]. Kovacs used high dose acid suppression (Lansoprazole 30mg b.d.) in patients undergoing Barrett's ablation and found that success or failure of ablative therapy was not related to normalization of abnormal lower esophageal acid exposure[24]. Many Barrett's ablation studies use high dose proton pump inhibitor to control acid reflux at a standard dose of Omeprazole 20mg b.d. or Lansoprazole 30mg b.d. We have used standard proton pump inhibitor therapy at a normal therapeutic dose. This regime of acid suppression is adequate to ensure re-epithelialisation with squamous epithelium in most patients. In patients with initial failure of re-epithelialisation, we have found that further ablation in conjunction with higher dose acid suppression(20mg b.d. Omeprazole) normally results in successful squamous regrowth[34].

It seems therefore that adequate acid suppression is important to achieve initial regrowth of squamous epithelium, and that a *relatively* anacid environment is required for this to be maintained. It is not clear what level of acid suppression is required for the patient undergoing Barrett's ablation. Standard doses of proton pump inhibitor appear adequate in many patients for initial regrowth of squamous epithelium after ablation, although a proportion do require high dose acid suppression. Limited acid exposure in the lower esophagus does not appear to predict success or failure of ablative therapy. The higher rate of treatment failure in longer Barrett's segments may be related to more severe gastroesophageal reflux disease, and suggests that greater acid suppression may be required in these patients.

A pragmatic approach to PPI therapy in Barrett's ablation may therefore be to employ standard treatment dose for shorter columnar segments (<5cm), provided that careful clinical review confirms adequate symptom control. In longer segments or with inadequate symptom control, it may be appropriate to treat with higher dose PPI during ablative therapy. Should symptoms persist on high dose PPI, pH studies whilst on treatment will assess the adequacy of acid suppression. Patients who require long-term high dose acid suppression, or in whom symptoms are inadequately controlled should be considered for anti-reflux surgery.

7.2 ANTI REFLUX SURGERY

In expert hands laparoscopic surgery is associated with a good durable symptomatic outcome in 95% or more of patients, and has the advantage over medical treatment that gastroesophageal reflux is eliminated. There is as yet no hard evidence that antireflux surgery in non-ablated Barrett's protects against malignant degeneration because no published surgical study has yet addressed this issue with cancer prevention as a primary outcome measure. It is therefore not surprising that no literature exists comparing antireflux surgery with medical treatment in patients undergoing ablation in the long term prevention of cancer.

Anti-reflux surgery may be an attractive therapeutic option in combination with ablation, as gastro-esophageal reflux is eliminated, rather than modulated in composition and reduced in volume as happens with medical therapy. There is good evidence of a harmful role for excessive duodenogastroesophageal(DGER) reflux of bile and pancreatic juices, with evidence that DGER is elevated in Barrett's esophagus. Two series of patients who have all had antireflux surgery followed by ablation with laser[20] or MPEC[27] have been published to date. Both series have relatively small numbers of patients and short follow up.

By elimination of DGER, antireflux surgery may provide a more favorable environment for regeneration of squamous epithelium, a suggestion supported by the observation of occasional difficulties in obtaining squamous regrowth with inadequate medically controlled reflux. Anti- reflux surgery may also encourage a more durable and stable regrowth of squamous epithelium which is unaffected by continuing exposure to duodeno-gastro-esophageal refluxate.

8. REPLACEMENT OF COLUMNAR EPITHELIUM WITH A SQUAMOUS LINING

8.1 LENGTH

The length of Barrett's segment, both before and after treatment is likely to be of critical importance in determining risk of cancer and reduction of this risk. Measurement of length of the Barrett's segment before and after treatment is also likely to be an important measure of the success of any form of ablative therapy, and may be one way in which ablative therapies are compared with each other. It is recognized that routine endoscopic assessment of Barrett's segment length is unreliable with significant inter- and intra-observer differences on differing occasions. Despite this, the length of Barrett's segment may be an important determinant of ablation success. Kovacs[24] found that ablation of longer length Barrett's segments was less likely to result in total removal of epithelium. Complete success with MPEC was achieved in 21/23patients with a segment 2-4cm in length compared with only one of four patients with 5cm or more.

It seems likely, however, that simple measurement of Barrett's segment will be insufficient to allow comparison of reductions in malignant risk within and between current and future studies. This is because there appear to be significant differences in risk of malignant degeneration between series of Barrett's esophagus from 1 in 70 to 1 in 442. It is possible that these differences are a reflection of differences in endoscopic assessment of Barrett's length, especially measurement of tongues of columnar epithelium rather than circumferential. Another possible explanation for such widely varying estimates of malignant risk is differences in definition of Barrett's esophagus. Some authorities regard the presence of any columnar epithelium in the lower esophagus as being diagnostic of Barrett's, whilst others regard only those segments 3cm or more in extent as meriting the label Barrett's esophagus. These differences will lead to great difficulty in interpretation of the literature until they are resolved. It may therefore be more appropriate to consider other techniques for the endoscopic assessment of Barrett's after ablation and these are considered below.

8.2 SURFACE AREA

If malignant risk is related to the number of cells exposed to luminal injury, then surface area of columnar metaplasia may be a much more accurate reflection of malignant risk than length of the columnar segment. This may be particularly relevant with shorter lengths of Barrett's segment when 2 or 3 tongues of columnar epithelium rather than circumferential involvement are frequently present over 30-40% of the Barrett's segment. At present it is possible but difficult to obtain accurate measurements of surface area[7].

Surface area may be important on the following counts:

a. Pre-ablation measurement of area indicates preablation risk
b. Post ablation measurement of area indicates degree of treatment success
c. Future estimates of the importance of relative vs. absolute reduction in surface area after ablation may be made.
d. If surface area measurement could be standardized it would improve comparison between patients and institutions of risks of degeneration.

Surface area of columnar mucosa after ablation may be the most important parameter to define subsequent malignant risk.

8.3 PERSISTENCE OF COLUMNAR EPITHELIUM

Columnar epithelium may persist after ablation because of treatment failure in the context of an inadequate ablative injury or poor control of gastro-esophageal reflux. Columnar epithelium may also persist as islands within neo-squamous epithelium or as islands deep to the neo-squamous lining. All three types of persistent columnar mucosa may have potential for malignant degeneration but it is intestinal metaplasia underlying an apparently normal neo-squamous epithelium that gives rise to greatest concern. This is because of the possibility that malignant degeneration may occur but be difficult to recognize endoscopically as the appearances are obscured by the neo-squamous epithelium.

Intestinal metaplasia underlying apparently normal neo-squamous epithelium has been a consistent finding in all follow up studies where this has been sought and a rigorous post ablation biopsy protocol followed[22,28,33,34,62].

The frequency with which underlying intestinal metaplasia is found varies between 25 and 50% of cases post ablation. It is however, critically important to recognize that glandular epithelium underlying squamous epithelium is a normal finding in esophageal mucosa. Only the presence of intestinal metaplasia should be regarded as abnormal. In our series of patients we found metaplasia underlying neo-squamous epithelium in 30% of patients. A further 27% had glandular tissue deep to the neo squamous epithelium but no intestinal metaplasia as defined by the presence of acid mucins. The precise distribution of underlying metaplastic cells is not yet clear: they may be an invariable accompaniment to ablative therapy and present in all patients if

sought with sufficient vigor. Alternatively they may signify a failure in the ablative technique being employed or be a temporary phenomenon which disappears over time if a reflux free environment is maintained. Indeed, Sharma et al[28] suggest that metaplasia is a variable feature over time in individual patients after Barrett's ablation. Millimeter scale assessment of the neo-squamous epithelium suggested that metaplastic glands lay underneath 0.4%, 2% and 8% of the total squamous epithelium surface area in 3 patients with persistent underlying IM. This study represents a serious attempt to define the morphology of regrown squamous epithelium.

Concerns that areas of intestinal metaplasia underlying apparently normal squamous epithelium may harbor malignancy after ablation of Barrett's have been confirmed in only one case report to date. Eighteen months after argon beam plasma coagulation ablation, an irregular area of squamous mucosa was noted in one patient from Van Laethem's series[33] just above the squamocolumnar junction. Endoscopic mucosal resection confirmed this to be an intramucosal adenocarcinoma underlying squamous epithelium[45]. Van Laethem adhered to a strict biopsy protocol before and during ablative treatment. It seems unlikely that this cancer was present ab initio, and more likely that it developed deep to the neo-squamous lining. The importance of buried metaplastic epithelium as a risk factor for development of adenocarcinoma will only be defined through prospective study and long term follow up of large numbers of ablated patients.

We suspect that one of the mechanisms for squamous epithelium overlying intestinal metaplasia is because following ablation, squamous epithelium grows from the ablated area onto the Barrett's segment, and the precise origin of the neo-squamous epithelium has yet to be determined.

8.4 MALIGNANT POTENTIAL OF NEO-SQUAMOUS EPITHELIAN

Michopoulos[38] assessed expression of p53 and cerbB2 pre and post ablation to assess whether elevated levels may predispose to a poor response to ablation. The neosquamous epithelium expressed cerbb2 and/or p53 in only one of 13 patients after Barrett's ablation: low-grade dysplasia was also seen in this patient alone. No relation was identified between response to ablation and levels of these markers. This work gives some indication that the regrown epithelium may be stable. Garewal[64] et al have also studied p53 levels, Ki 67, and ornithine decarboxylase in ablated Barrett's, normal squamous epithelium and non ablated Barrett's with squamous islands. Neo-squamous epithelium was found to be biologically similar to normal squamous epithelium, in contrast with squamous islands in acid suppressed Barrett's which expressed abnormal levels of these biological markers.

8.5 ASSESSMENT

Accurate endoscopic assessment is critical both before and after ablation of Barrett's epithelium. A number of qualitative techniques have been described to assist with this assessment particularly in delineating areas of unsuspected intestinal metaplasia.

Qualitative methods have been described by Guelrud [63]and Barham[22] using acetic acid to supplement information derived from endoscopic assessment of Barrett's post ablation. 5-10ml of 1.5% acetic acid is sprayed onto the distal esophagus, and then irrigated with 50ml tap water. Areas of IM are demonstrated as velvety and red with a villiform pattern and a white rimmed border. Guelrud[63] found that this technique demonstrated areas of previously unsuspected IM in 11 patients out of 21 who were undergoing ablative therapy for Barrett's. His paper does not make clear what the size of these areas were or whether they were areas of metaplasia in the context of other areas of IM or not. Michopoulos[38] has used methylene blue to stain for intestinal metaplasia post ablation. 5-10ml 0.5% sprayed onto distal esophagus, then irrigated with 120-240 ml water, selectively staining areas of persisting metaplasia blue even after thorough irrigation with water.

9. SHORT SEGMENT BARRETT'S

Another chapter discusses short segments of columnar epithelium or short segment Barrett's in depth. It is widely recognized that many adenocarcinomas may arise in short segments of columnar epithelium at the esophagogastric junction, and that many patients presenting with adenocarcinoma of the esophagus do so without a previous diagnosis of Barrett's esophagus. However the risk of developing a carcinoma in short segments of Barrett's is not yet fully defined, and the available published literature suggests it is much less than for longer Barrett's segments.

Many of the studies of Barrett's ablation described in this chapter include large numbers of patients with short segments or tongues of columnar epithelium 2cm or less in length. Variations in criteria for ablation and publication represent a serious weakness in much of the current literature.

We frequently were left with 1-2cm of columnar epithelium in the lower esophagus after ablation of longer Barrett's segments[34]. Whether these small areas of columnar epithelium are associated with a high risk of malignant degeneration as compared with 'spontaneous' short segment Barrett's is not clear

10. MOTILITY

Esophageal function is frequently abnormal in patients with Barrett's esophagus, although the pathophysiology of this is unclear. Esophageal injury consequent upon exposure to gastroesophageal reflux over many years undoubtedly occurs. Abnormal esophageal function may be related either to this ongoing injury or be a reflection of primary neuromuscular deficit. It is clearly important that esophageal motility and clearance is not further impaired after ablation of benign Barrett's esophagus. Kovacs[24] et al performed epithelial ablation with multipolar electrocoagulation and studied esophageal manometry before, during and upon completion of ablative therapy. Using a standard station pull through technique they measured lower esophageal sphincter pressure, maximum amplitude with wet swallows and recorded simultaneous and non propagated swallows. Apart from a small reduction in the percentage of non propagated contractions there was no difference in motility during or following ablative therapy.

Fass investigated esophageal sensitivity of the neo-squamous epithelium after MPEC ablation with a modified Bernstein acid perfusion test[65]. After complete reversal of Barrett's mucosa, patients demonstrated similar sensory perception as a group of patients with erosive esophagitis, but increased sensitivity compared with untreated Barrett's mucosa.

It seems likely that the depth of injury may be crucial in preventing injury to the myenteric nerves and hence avoiding further impairment of esophageal motility. Laser, MPEC, and Argon beam plasma coagulation all have superficial tissue penetration, and would therefore not be expected to have any lasting effect on motility. Photodynamic therapy however, is frequently associated with a deeper level of tissue injury and diffuse strictures that may be refractory to dilatation as they involve the full thickness of the esophageal wall. In theory these diffuse strictures may either directly involve the myenteric plexus or be responsible for secondary effects on motility. The effect of PDT on esophageal motility has not yet been studied.

11. FUTURE STRATEGIES

Ablation has not yet been shown to have any effect on malignant risk or mortality in a group of patients with Barrett's esophagus. Future studies will need to address the issues listed below.

---

1. Reduction in malignant risk
2. Reduction in mortality
3. Method of GOR control
4. Completeness of ablation
5. Surface continuity
6. Depth. of injury
7. Islands of columnar epithelium within squamous epithelium
8. Columnar epithelium at OG junction: conversion of Barrett's to short segment Barrett's
9. Underlying metaplastic cells
   ?Protected from lumen
   ? more susceptible to malignancy
10. Normality of neo squamous epithelium

Figure 8. Unresolved issues in Barrett's ablation.

11.1 REDUCTION IN INCIDENCE OF AND MORTALITY FROM ESOPHAGEAL CARCINOMA.

Ablation of Barrett's has an underlying principle of esophageal carcinoma prevention rather than early detection as in other national screening and surveillance programs for cervical, breast, and colon cancer. Multi center prospective randomized controlled trial is required to prove any effect of Barrett's ablation on subsequent cancer development. Such a study would be a major undertaking needing long term financial support if it were to be successful.

It could be assumed that ablation of Barrett's reduced the risk of cancer development from 1% per annum in non ablated patients to 0.1% in ablated patients. The most simple trial would require five hundred patients in each arm and follow up of 10 years to have an 80% chance of demonstrating a 10-fold reduction in risk at the 5% significance level. This trial would not be able to consider the relative

merits of ablation plus medical versus surgical control of gastroesophageal reflux in the prevention of cancer. Such a trial would require recruitment of several hundred more patients.

The complexity and cost of any study that might prove the case for Barrett's ablation combined with lack of any direct commercial value of such a study means government funding will be needed to prove a role for ablation in the prevention of cancer.

11.2 IMPROVEMENT OF UNDERSTANDING OF DETERMINANTS FOR SUBSEQUENT MALIGNANT DEGENERATION

Risk of cancer development in Barrett's is known to be multi-factorial, and it seems likely that this will also be the case in ablated Barrett's. Possible added determinants of risk in ablated Barrett's include:

1. Relative reduction in surface area
2. Absolute area of columnar epithelium persisting after ablation.
3. Original surface area
4. Glandular epithelium buried beneat squamous lining
    - Presence
    - Total number or surface area of buried cells
5. Degree of gastroesophageal reflux
6. Method of reflux control
    Standard dose PPI
    Titrated dose PPI
    Antireflux surgery

11.3 TAILORING OF BARRETT'S MANAGEMENT/ABLATION TO INDIVIDUAL RISK PROFILES.

Development of decision matrices may permit prediction of an individual's risk of malignant degeneration and give predictive estimates of risk and benefit for differing strategies in an individual patient[3]. In this way a forty year old male with a 12cm Barrett's segment may be given a number of management options including antireflux surgery, ablation and medical treatment as at present, but with additional information of the likely risks/benefits for individual courses of treatment.

REFERENCES

1. Lagergren J, Bergstrom R, Lindgren A, Nyren O. Symptomatic gastro-esophageal reflux as a risk factor for esophageal adenocarcinoma.N Engl J Med 1999;340(11):825-31.

2. Attwood SEA, Barlow AP, Norris TL, Watson A. Barrett's oesophagus: effect of anti-reflux surgery on symptom control and development of complications. Br J Surg 1992; 79(10):1050-3.

3. Weston AP, Badr AS, Hassanein RS. Prospective multivariate analysis of clinical, endoscopic, and histological factors predictive of the development of Barrett's multifocal high-grade dysplasia or adenocarcinoma. Am J Gastroenterol 1999 ;94 (12) : 3413-9.

4. Iftikhar SY, James PD, Steele RJ, Hardcastle JD, Atkinson M. Length of Barrett's oesopahgus: an important factor in the development of dysplasia and adenocarcinoma. Gut 1992; 33(9):1155-8.

5. Menke-Pluymers MB, Hop WC, Dees J, van Blankenstein M, Tilanus HW. Risk factors for the development of an adenocarcinoma in columnar-lined (Barrett) esophagus. The Rotterdam Esophageal Tumor Study Group. Cancer 1992; 72(4):1155-8.

6. Sharma P, Sampliner RE, Camargo E. Normalization of esophageal pH with high-dose proton pump inhibitor therapy does not result in regression of Barrett's esophagus. Am J Gastroenterol 1997;92(4):582-5.

7. Peters FT, Ganesh S, Kuipers EJ, Sluiter WJ, Klinkenberg-Knol EC, Lamers CB, et al. Endoscopic regression of Barrett's esophagus during omeprazole treatment; a randomised double blind study. Gut 1999;45(4):489-94.

8. Sagar PM, Ackroyd R, Hosie KB, Patterson JE, Stoddard CJ, Kingsnorth AN. Regression and progression of Barrett's esophagus after anit-reflux surgery. Br J Surg 1995; 82:806-10.

9. Marshall RE, Anggiansah A, Manifold DK, Owen WA, Owen WJ. Effect of omeprazole 20 mg twice daily on duodenogastric and gastro-esophageal bile reflux in Barrett's esophagus. Gut 1998;43(5):603-6.

10. Ortiz A, Martinez de Haro LF, Parrilla P, Morales G, Molina J, Bermejo J, et al. Conservative treatment versus antireflux surgery in Barrett's esophagus: long-term results of a prospective study. Br J Surg 1996;83(2):274-8.

11. Gillen P, Keeling P, Byrne PJ, West AB, Hennessy TP. Experimental columnar metaplasia in the canine esophagus. Br J Surg 1996; 75(2):113-5.

12. Li H, Walsh TN, G OD, Gillen P, Byrne PJ, Hennessy TP. Mechanisms of columnar metaplasia and squamous regeneration in experimental Barrett's esophagus. Surgery 1994;115(2):176-81.

13. Fujimaki M, Nakayama K. Endoscopic laser treatment of superficial esophageal cancer. Seminars in Surg Oncol 1986; 2:248-56.

14. Berenson MM, Johnson TD,Markowitz NR, Buchi KN, Samowitz WS. Restoration of squamous mucosa after ablation of Barrett's esophageal epithelium.Gastroenterol 1993: 104:1686-91.

15. Sampliner RE, Hixson LJ, Fennerty MB, Garewal HS. Regression of Barrett's esophagus by laser ablation in an anacid environment. Digest Dis Sc 1993;38(2):365-8.

16. Brandt LJ, Kauvar DR. Laser induced transient regression of Barrett's epithelium. Gastrointest Endosc 1992; 38(5):619-22.

17. Brandt LJ, Blansky RL, Kauvar DR. Repeat laser therapy of recurrent Barrett's epithelium: success with anacidity. Gastrointestinal Endoscopy 1995;41:267.

18. Luman W, Lessels AM, Palmer KR. Failure of Nd-YAG photocoagulation therapy as treatment for Barrett's esophagus--a pilot study. Eur J Gastroenterol & Hepatol 1996;8(7):627-30.

19. Ertan A, Zimmerman M, Younes M. Esophageal adenocarcinoma associated with Barrett's esophagus: Long-term management with laser ablation. Am J Gastroenterol 1995;90(12):2201-3.

20. Salo JA, Salminen JT, Kiviluoto TA, Nemlander AT, Ramo OJ, Farkkila MA, et al. Treatment of Barrett's esophagus by endoscopic laser ablation and antireflux surgery. Ann Surg 1998;227(1):40-4.

21. Sharma P, Jaffe PE, Bhattacharyya A, Sampliner RE. Laser and multipolar electrocoagulation ablation of early Barrett's adenocarcinoma: long-term follow-up. Gastrointest Endosc 1999;49(4 Pt 1):442-6.

22. Barham CP, Jones RL, Biddlestone LR, Hardwick RH, Shepherd NA, Barr H. Photothermal laser ablation of Barrett's esophagus: endoscopic and histological evidence of squamous re-epithelialisation. Gut 1997;41(3):281-4.

23. Gossner L, May A, Stolte M, Seitz G, Hahn EG, Ell C. KTP laser destruction of dysplasia and early cancer in columnar-lined Barrett's esophagus. Gastrointest Endosc 1999; 49(1):8-12.

24. Kovacs BJ, Chen YK, Lewis TD, DeGuzman LJ, Thompson KS. Successful reversal of Barrett's esophagus with multipolar electrocoagulation despite inadequate acid suppression. Gastrointest Endosc 1999;49(5):547-53.

25. Sampliner RE, Fennerty B, Garewal HS. (1996).Reversal of Barrett's esophagus with acid suppression and multipolar electrocoagulation: preliminary results. Gastrointest Endosc1996;44(5):532-5.

26. Sampliner RE. Barrett's esophagus: electrocoagulation. Gastrointest Endosc 1999;49(3 Pt 2):S17-9.

27. Montes CG, Brandalise NA, Deliza R, Novais de Magalhaes AF, Ferraz JG. Antireflux surgery followed by bipolar electrocoagulation in the treatment of Barrett's esophagus. Gastrointest Endosc 1999;50(2):173-7.

28. Sharma P, Bhattacharyya A, Garewal HS, Sampliner RE. Durability of new squamous epithelium after endoscopic reversal of Barrett's esophagus. Gastrointest Endosc 1999; 50(2):159-64.

29. Garcia Montes C, Brandalise NA, Deliza R, Servidoni MF, Ferraz JG, Magalhaes AF. Regression of childhood Barrett's esophageal mucosa by antireflux surgery and bipolar electrocoagulation. J Pediatr Surg 1998;33(5):747-9.

30. Dumoulin FL, Terjung B, Neubrand M, Scheurlen C, Fischer HP, Sauerbruch T. Treatment of Barrett's esophagus by endoscopic argon plasma coagulation. Endoscopy 1997;29(8):751-3.

31. Mork H, Barth T, Kreipe HH, Kraus M, Al-Taie O, Jakob F, et al. Reconstitution of squamous epithelium in Barrett's esophagus with endoscopic argon plasma coagulation: a prospective study. Scand J Gastroenterol 1998;33(11):1130-4.

32. Grade AJ, Shah IA, Medlin SM, Ramirez FC. The efficacy and safety of argon plasma coagulation therapy in Barrett's esophagus. Gastrointestinal Endoscopy;50(1):18-22.

33. Van Laethem JL, Cremer M, Peny MO, Delhaye M, Deviere J. Eradication of Barrett's mucosa with argon plasma coagulation and acid suppression: immediate and mid term results. Gut 1998;43(6):747-51.

34. Byrne JP, Armstrong GR, Attwood SE. Restoration of the normal squamous lining in Barrett's esophagus by argon beam plasma coagulation. Am J of Gastroenterol 1998; 93(10):1810-5.

35. Martin WR, Jakobs R, Spiethoff A, Maass S, Riemann JF. Treatment of Barrett esophagus with argon plasma coagulation with acid suppression--a prospective study. Zeitschrift fur Gastroenterologie 1999; 37(9):779-84.

36. Orth K, Stanescu A, Ruck A, Russ D, Beger HG. Photodynamic ablation and argon-plasma coagulation of premalignant and early-stage malignant lesions of the esophagus--an alternative to surgery?. Chirurg 1999; 70(4):431-8.

37. May A, Gossner L, Gunter E, Stolte M, Ell C. Local treatment of early cancer in short Barrett's esophagus by means of argon plasma coagulation: initial experience. Endoscopy 1999;31(6):497-500.

38. Michopoulos S, Tsibouris P, Bouzakis H, Sotiropoulou M, Kralios N. Complete regression of Barrett's esophagus with heat probe thermocoagulation: mid-term results. Gastrointestinal Endoscopy 1999;50(2):165-72.

39. Rodgers BM, McDonald AP, Tarbert JL, Donnelly WH. Morphologic and functional effects of esophageal cryotherapy. J Thorac Cardiovasc Surg;77:543-9.

40. Johnston CM, Schoenfeld LP, Mysore JV, Dubois A. Endoscopic spray cryotherapy: a new technique for mucosal ablation in the esophagus. Gastrointestinal Endoscopy 1999;50(1):86-92.

41. Martin TR, Onstad GR, Silvis AL. Lift and cut biopsy technique for submucosal samplings. Gastrointestinal Endoscopy 1976;23:29-30.

42. Inoue H, Endo M. .Endoscopic mucosal resection using a transparent tube. Surgical Endoscopy 1990;4:189-201.

43. 43. Sakai P, Filho FM, Iryia K. An endoscopic technique for resection of small gastrointestinal carcinomas. Gastrointest Endosc 1996; 44:65-8.

44. Soehendra N, Binmoeller KF, Bohnacker S, Seitz U, Brand B, Thonke F, et al. Endoscopic snare mucosectomy in the esophagus without any additional equipment: A simple technique for resection of flat early cancer. Endoscopy 1997;29:380-3.

45. Van Laethem JL, Peny MO, Salmon I, Cremer M, Deiere J. Intramucosal adenocarcinoma arising under squamous re-epithelialisation of Barrett's esophagus. Gut 2000;46:574-7.

46. Bremner RM, Mason RJ, Bremner CG, DeMeester TR, Chandrasoma P, Peters JH, et al. Ultrasonic epithelial ablation of the lower esophagus without stricture formation. A new technique for Barrett's ablation. Surgical Endoscopy 1998;12(4):342-6; discussion 346-7.

47. Grosjean P, Savary J-F, Mizeetet J. Tetra(m-hydroxyphenyl) chlorin clinical photodynamic therapy of early esophageal and bronchial cancers. Laser Med. Sci 1996;11:227-35.

48. Gossner L, Stolte M, Sroka R, Rick K, May A, Hahn EG, et al. Photodynamic ablation of high-grade dysplasia and early cancer in Barrett's esophagus by means of 5-aminolevulinic acid. Gastroenterology 1998;114(3):448-55.

49. Ackroyd R, Brown N, Vernon D, Roberts D, Stephenson T, Marcus S, et al. (1999).5-Aminolevulinic acid photosensitization of dysplastic Barrett's esophagus: a pharmacokinetic study. Photochem/Photobiol 1999; 70(4):656-62.

50. Panjhepour M, Overholt BF, DeNovo R, Sneed R, Petersen MG. Centring balloon to improve esophageal photodynamic therapy. Lasers Surg. Med 1992;12:631-8.

51. Gossner L, May A, Sroka R, Ell C. A new long-range through-the-scope balloon applicator for photodynamic therapy in the esophagus and cardia. Endoscopy 1999; 31(5):370-6.

52. Overholt BF, Panjehpour M. Photodynamic therapy for Barrett's esophagus: clinical update. Am J Gastroenterol 1996;91(9):1719-23.

53. Overholt BF, Panjehpour M. Barrett's esophagus: photodynamic therapy for ablation of dysplasia, reduction of specialised mucosa, and treatment of superficial esophageal cancer. Gastrointest Cancer 1995;42(1):64-70.

54. Overholt BF, Panjehpour M. Photodynamic therapy in Barrett's esophagus. Journal of Clin Laser Med Surg 1996; 14(5):245-9.

55. Overholt BF, Panjehpour M, Haydek JM. Photodynamic therapy for Barrett's esophagus: follow-up in 100 patients. Gastrointestinal Endoscopy1999;49(1):1-7.

56. Laukka MA, Wang KK. Initial results using low dose photodynamic therapy in treatment of Barrett's esophagus. Gastrointest Endosc 1995;42:59-63.

57. Barr H, Shepherd NA, Dix A, Roberts DJ, Tan WC, Krasner N. Eradication of high-grade dysplasia in columnar-lined (Barrett's) esophagus by photodynamic therapy with endogenously generated protoporphyrin IX [see comments]. Lancet 1996; 348(9027):584-5.

58. Laukka MA, Wang KK. Initial results using low-dose photodynamic therapy in the treatment of Barrett's esophagus. Gastrointestinal Endoscopy 1995;42(1):59-63.

59. Beddow EC, Wilcox DT, Drake DP, Pierro A, Kiely EM, Spitz L. Surveillance of Barrett's esophagus in children. J Pediatr Surg 1999;34(1):88-90

60. Ackroyd R, Brown NJ, Stephenson TJ, Stoddard CJ, Reed MW. Ablation treatment for Barrett's esophagus: what depth of tissue destruction is needed? J Clin Pathol 1999;52(7):509-12.

61. Weston AP, Badr AS, Hassanein RS. Prospective multivariate analysis of factors predictive of complete regression of Barrett's esophagus. Am J Gastroenterol 1999;94(12):3420-6.

62. Biddlestone LR, Barham CP, Wilkinson SP, Barr H, Shepherd NA. The histopathology of treated Barrett's esophagus: squamous reepithelialization after acid suppression and laser and photodynamic therapy. American J Surg Pathol 1998;22(2):239-45.

63. Guelrud M, Herrera I. Acetic acid improves identification of remnant islands of Barrett's epithelium after endoscopic therapy. Gastrointest Endosc 1998;47(6):512-5.

64. Garewal H, Ramsey L, Sharma P, Kraus K, Sampliner R, Fass R. Biomarker studies in reversed Barrett's esophagus. Am J Gastroenterol 1999; 94(10):2829-33.

65. Fass R, Yalam JM, Camargo L, Johnson C, Garewal HS, Sampliner RE. Increased esophageal chemoreceptor sensitivity to acid in patients after successful reversal of Barrett's esophagus. Dig Dis & Sci 1997;42(9):1853-8.

4.3 THE ROLE OF ABLATION IN THE MANAGEMENT OF HIGH-GRADE DYSPLASIA

Hugh Barr

1. INTRODUCTION

The sequence of events involved in neoplastic progression of Barrett's esophagus from normal squamous epithelium, through the intestinal metaplastic phenotype, low and high-grade dysplasia and on to invasive and finally metastatic adenocarcinoma are not fully understood. It is still therefore a hypothesis, to say that cancer in columnar-lined esophagus progresses through a multi-step process initiated by chronic reflux oesophagitis[1]. There is an increasing understanding of the molecular events that occur during the progression to cancer[2,3]. It was hoped that this increased understanding of molecular events and molecular markers would ultimately lead to identification of the patients with an epithelium that is in danger of malignant degeneration. It had been suggested that p53 would be such a marker. The detection of mutant p53 protein in Barrett's esophagus and cancer is now well documented. It is not present in non-dysplastic epithelium, but is seen in 9% of specimens indefinite for or with low-grade dysplasia, 55% of those with high-grade dysplasia, and 87% of carcinomas[4]. It did appear that p53 would be a useful prognostic marker. Patients with low-grade dysplasia who expressed p53 were likely to progress to high-grade dysplasia or indeed carcinoma. Those that show no expression were less likely to undergo further malignant degeneration[5]. Thus the subgroup of patients with low or indefinite dysplasia and p53 expression should be followed with a more rigorous surveillance regimen. However, it must be emphasized that not all esophageal adenocarcinomas express p53, and patients without expression have progressed to cancer[4]. Other molecular and histological markers are being sought to identify patients at high risk of malignant transformation. Analysis of the DNA content using flow cytometry has shown that columnar epithelium demonstrating aneuploidy or increase in the G2/tetraploidy fraction has an increased of malignant progression[6]. Another critical event in the neoplastic progression is loss of cell adhesion with aberrant expression of adhesion molecules. Most notably there is reduced expression of e-cadherin with localization of catenins, to the nucleus as the mucosa becomes more malignant[2].

Currently we are dependent on the histological diagnosis of dysplasia to indicate that the patient is at risk for malignant transformation. The assessment of dysplasia is fraught with difficulties both of definition and precise diagnosis. Even with experienced pathologists there has been only an 86% inter-observer agreement over the diagnosis of high-grade dysplasia. For the diagnosis of dysplasia or low grade-dysplasia the agreement was only 58% and 75% respectively[7]. This confusing situation has been addressed by histopathologists by the greater use of second opinions and joint surgical and pathological conferences. It should now be mandatory to confirm a diagnosis of dysplasia with at least one other expert parthologist[8]. If there is any doubt-repeated endoscopy and biopsy must be performed.

There are several questions regarding both high-grade dysplasia as an indicator for an "at risk" patient or as a marker for coexisting adenocarcinoma. We need therefore to examine the problem of a missed cancer in a patient with high-grade dysplasia, the natural history of high-grade dysplasia and the choice of therapy or surveillance for the management of patients with high-grade dysplasia.

2. THE NATURAL HISTORY OF HIGH-GRADE DYSPLASIA

It would be a gross presumption to say that we fully understand the natural history of dysplasia and in particular high-grade dysplasia. We must inform our decision making with as much information as we can glean from the literature. Several important attempts have been made to examine the progress and time sequence of carcinogenesis from high-grade dysplasia. An important influence on therapy has been the finding that many patients with high-grade dysplasia have co-existent cancer found after surgical excision of the esophagus[9-25] (Table 1). These data have indicated that there is a strong argument to end surveillance following the detection of dysplasia and intervene with radical surgery. The problem has always been the profound morbidity and mortality associated with esophagectomy. Some patients have died after a prophylactic operation[25].

259

H.W. Tilanus and S.E.A. Attwood (eds.), Barrett's Esophagus, 259–272.
© 2001 *Kluwer Academic Publishers. Printed in the Netherlands.*

TABLE 1. Summary of studies of patients undergoing esophageal resection for high-grade dysplasia and the incidence of occult cancer found in the esophageal specimen.

Studies	Number of studies	Patients with high-grade dysplasia	Number of Cancers
pre 1990	6 [9-14]	15	5
post 1990	11 [15-25]	155	61

TABLE 2. Summary of longitudinal studies of high-grade dysplasia that remain stable or progress to invasive cancer

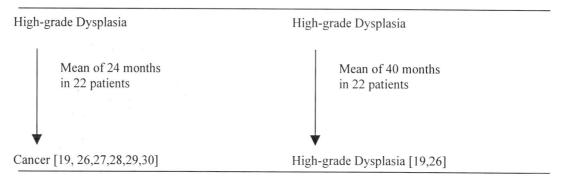

Clinicians worried about this radical approach have instituted rigorous biopsy protocols and have increased the accuracy of pre-operative diagnosis[19]. There is also a worry about "the biopsy cured cancer". These are patients in whom after esophagectomy no residual invasive cancer is found on detailed histological examination. The question remains could these patients have been cured with less radical method, without subjecting them to life threatening surgery. We are also unsure as to whether some of these biopsies could represent a false positive. Following the detection of high grade dysplasia, how long before the mucosa will progress to an invasive cancer? Is it certain that all patients will develop cancer if left untreated? Can high-grade dysplasia ever spontaneously regress, or following control of the reflux disease? Table 2 is a summary of some longitudinal studies that give some indication of the time sequences involved in the progression or non-progression of high-grade dysplasia.

The question as to whether high-grade dysplasia ever regresses remains unanswered. Some authors have documented that high-grade dysplasia has appeared to resolve, particularly when proton pump inhibitor therapy is effective at suppressing acid[31]. This report is very intriguing since the deterioration in proliferation indices associated with dysplasia[3] can be halted. The molecular evidence is that effective acid suppression favors differentiation and decreases proliferation[31]. There is also clinical evidence

that with prolonged continuous treatment with omeprazole, certain histological parameters of Barrett's esophagus are improved. There is a decrease in the length of the Barrett's segment with an increase in the number of squamous islands. There is also a reduction in the proportion of sulphomucin-rich intestinal metaplasia[32]. A randomized double blind study has confirmed that profound acid suppression with a proton pump inhibitor leading to elimination of acid reflux induces a partial regression of the columnar-lined segment[33]. As regards dysplasia we must remain cautious, since there are problems of sampling error. Longer-term follow-up is clearly required. There is concern that the molecular events in some patients may have proceeded to a state where malignant invasion is inevitable. Certainly patients with indefinite and low-grade dysplasia have been shown to revert to metaplasia[26]. There are clear problems of the histological differentiation of inflammation and low-grade dysplasia. Controversy also remains as to whether surgery is effective in causing regression of Barrett's esophagus or halting progression. One study of 56 patients has demonstrated that the mean length of affected esophagus was reduced from 8cms to 4cms after fundoplication in 24 patients, nine patients showed progression of disease, 23 patients showed no change and one patient developed an invasive carcinoma[34]. Overall there appears to be no clear evidence of regression or reduction of neoplastic transformation after anti-reflux surgery, although the rate of progression may be reduced[35]. There is therefore a clear role for minimally invasive methods to attempt to reverse the malignant transformation of high-grade dysplasia in Barrett's esophagus.

3. THEORETICAL AND BIOLOGICAL CONSIDERATIONS FOR ABLATION OF BARRETT'S DYSPLASIA

In order to eradicate dysplasia and Barrett's metaplasia certain parameters must be understood to allow safe destruction and safe healing. First, to what depth should the destruction reach? There is one histopathological report with precise measurements of metaplastic columnar epithelium. These authors report measurement of 100 fixed specimens of Barrett's esophagus and squamous esophageal mucosa[36]. This study is highly informative and demonstrates that columnar-lined epithelium is minimally thicker at 0.5mm (range 0.39-0.59mm) than normal squamous mucosa at 0.49 (range 0.42-0.58mm). It must be remembered that fixing tissue will produce a 10% shrinkage and a further 10% reduction occurs during processing. Overall shrinkage of 20% occurs. If these are accounted for the mean thickness of Barrett's mucosa is approximately 0.6mm. Our measurements of snap frozen fresh freshly excised esophageal tissue using optical coherence topography has recorded a depth of between 0.45-0.5mm[37]. Although this is the depth of metaplastic tissue it is important to know if dysplasia is thicker. There is no definite data on this but initial observations suggest that it is slightly thicker and it is certainly optical denser[37]. Although we have some idea of the depth of the pathological process, we still are unsure as to whether this is the depth that destruction should be attained. Are there critical stem cells that must be destroyed?

The second question that must be addressed is the nature of the injury. Ablation therapy is a form of mucosal injury, which may differ from the original mucosal injury following chemical destruction as a result of gastro-esophageal reflux, in temporal characteristics. Therefore it is vital to examine the mechanisms of regeneration after reflux; and after the more acute ablation of the surface mucosa. In particular we must know what structures must be preserved to allow neo-squamous regeneration after control of acid reflux. The latter question is of crucial importance and has been addressed in a series of elegant animal studies[38,42]. In a canine model of gastro-esophageal reflux, columnar-lined esophagus could be induced, and was thought to be associated with re-growth from the proximal columnar lined portion of the deep esophageal glands. The columnar epithelium was often continuous with the columnar lined portions of these ducts. After full reflux control, an acute injury to the esophageal mucosa was still associated with regeneration by columnar cells, but on occasion squamous epithelium re-grew and formed distinct islands. These squamous cells appeared to arise from the distal squamous portion of the esophageal gland ducts. It had been shown previously that columnar epithelium is unlikely to have migrated from the columnar cells in the cardia[39]. It was postulated that stems cells possibly in the esophageal gland duct have a multi-potentiality for cell differentiation and could produce columnar or squamous cells depending on environmental conditions. Thus the adaptive response to injury under conditions of reflux was to produce columnar epithelium as occurs in the generation of Barrett's esophagus. Squamous re-epithelialization could be encouraged by full reflux control. There have been some recent important studies of a rodent model of Barrett's-like esophagus. These suggest that the ductal epithelium may not be so crucial since the rat does not have deep esophageal glands. It is therefore likely that the multi-potential stem cells are not only located in the duct epithelium but reside in the basal layer of the squamous and the regenerative columnar villi epithelium[3,41,44]. It is essential to examine the injury response following mucosal injury caused by an ablation therapy, since neo-squamous epithelium forms if the reflux is controlled[43]. It is important to note that the proliferation rate of columnar cells is five times that of squamous[40]. Thus it would seem that on turnover criteria columnar cells should always predominant. It appears that the depth of the mucosal injury may be crucial to the type of regeneration[38]. It has been suggested but not established that for squamous cells to predominate, as well as environmental control of reflux being essential, some part of the distal squamous lined esophageal gland duct must survive. Since this duct is the most distal portion and thus the part most likely to destroyed by ablation techniques, the empirical evidence does not support this hypothesis. Certainly multi-potential stem cells must survive to regenerate the epithelium but at present the site and source of these cells is unknown, and they may reside deeper in the esophageal duct.

4. THEORETICAL CONSIDERATIONS FOR THE METHOD OF ABLATION

At present the methods for mucosal ablation through the endoscope are dependent on photodynamic, thermal or mechanical destruction. It is possible that acute cytotoxic local methods may start to prove useful, either by spraying or direct injection therapy. It has to be stated that most of the data on the development of techniques for the mucosal ablation of Barrett's esophagus has been empirical. The principles of treatment are:

1. To destroy all the abnormal epithelium and allow regeneration of the mucosa in an environment where the precipitating cause (acid/alkaline/biliary reflux) has been controlled.

The constraints of treatment are:

1   These patients may be completely asymptomatic and healthy. Those with heartburn are often symptomatically controlled by proton pump inhibitors.
2. Only a proportion of patients with columnar lined esophagus will develop invasive carcinoma.
3. "Primum nil nocere"/ "first do no harm". Any method that causes perforation, bleeding or serious complications risks the patients life are clearly unacceptable. Less serious complications are also not acceptable to asymptomatic patients.

5. PHOTOTERMAL AND THERMAL METHODS

The destruction of the mucosal surface using heat can be achieved electrically with multi-polar electrocoagulation applied directly to the surface or by conducting the electrical energy through a plasma of argon gas (APC). Photothermal ablation can be achieved using laser irradiation.

On theoretical grounds the potassium titanyl phosphate laser (KTP) laser has tissue penetration characteristics that should allow safe thermal treatment of dysplastic columnar lined esophagus. This photothermal laser ablation is non-specific; targeting dysplastic, metaplastic and normal tissue equally. This may be of little consequence providing the depth of damage does not risk perforation and healing occurs without fibrosis and risk of stricture formation.

Three lasers have been compared for the thermal destruction of superficial areas of non-dysplastic mucosa in the esophagus. A thermal imaging system was used to measure the depth of penetration and the thermal profile in tissue produced using each laser at various powers and energy. The purpose was to find parameters of between than $60\text{-}100^{\circ}C$ (coagulative necrosis + vaporisation) on the luminal (mucosal) surface with less than $37^{\circ}C$ (no risk of full thickness necrosis) on the external surface. The main purpose was to find the laser that would produce damage to the surface mucosa but spare deeper tissue. Patient safety considerations were absolutely paramount, and risk of full thickness damage/perforation avoided at all costs. The three lasers investigated were the Neodymium Yttrium Aluminium Garnet-Nd: YAG (1064nm), KTP (532nm) and the diode (805nm). Mounted sections of freshly excised human esophageal tissue were irradiated on a purpose made jig. The imaging system examined the superficial and deep surface, and looked at the thermal profile. The thermal images were stored and thermal plots analyzed. It is certain that in living tissue the thermal relaxation time of the tissue will be reduced because of blood flow. Thus the temperatures in-vivo are unlikely to be rise as much.

Irradiation with the KTP laser, power 15-20W for a 1 second pulse produced mucosal temperatures of greater than 65°C with a temperature of 21°C on the outer surface of the esophagus. It was extremely difficult to generate high temperatures on the external surface of the esophagus using the KTP laser. The diode laser (25W for 5 seconds) could produce surface temperatures of 90°C but with external temperature of 38°C. The Nd: YAG laser tended to produce worrying temperatures through to the external surface at energy levels that were sufficient to produce thermal destruction on the mucosa[45]. For the clinical application of photodestruction with acid suppression for the eradication of non-dysplastic Barrett's esophagus the KTP laser was chosen as the safest and the one most likely to produce intense superficial destruction only[46]. Others have used different laser and in particular the Nd: YAG[47-51,54]. Multi-polar electrocoagulation depends on the heating effect of a current passing between electrodes in contact with the tissue. This method is hard to control and be sure of the depth of damage[56]. Argon Beam Plasma coagulation (APC) is also an electro-surgical technique. Electrical energy is transferred to the tissue by means of an ionized, electrically conducting plasma of argon gas, delivered at between 1 and 3 liters a minute[64]. Both these methods are considerably cheaper than photothermal laser methods[52,53]. The APC has certain theoretical safety advantages. The current causing very high temperatures on the surface produces a zone of revitalization, surrounded by zones of coagulation, desiccation and tissue shrinkage. As soon as the area on the surface loses electrical conductivity as a result of desiccation, the plasma beam has to change direction in order to remain electrically conductive[105]. Therefore the depth effect should be limited and full thickness necrosis and perforation unlikely to occur. This is confirmed by thermal camera experiments using the APC, which have shown that it is extremely unlikely to produce full thickness thermal injury. A continuous pulse of over 20 seconds applied to the excised esophagus was necessary to produce any increase in the thermal profile on the outer aspect, and it was necessary to apply the device directly to the surface[53]. The immediate high power density at the mucosal surface produces little transmission through the esophageal wall.

6. PHOTODYNAMIC THERAPY

Photodynamic therapy (PDT) is an interesting new technique with the potential for selective destruction of cancers. It is based on the systemic administration of certain photosensitizing agents that are retained with some selectively in rapidly proliferating and malignant tissue. When exposed to appropriate wavelength laser light a cytotoxic reaction occurs causing cellular destruction. In extra-cranial tissues the maximum tumor:normal ratio that can be obtained with a variety of photosensitizing agents is 2-3:1. Investigation of photodynamic therapy in experimental gastrointestinal neoplasms has demonstrated important biological advantages. Full thickness intestinal damage produced by photodynamic

therapy unlike thermal damage does not reduce the mechanical strength of the bowel or cause perforation, because the sub-mucosal collagen is preserved. In addition selective necrosis of small areas (less than 2mm) is possible[55] with preservation of adjacent non-malignant structures. It is clear that this process is limited to small areas of tissue.

The most commonly used method of photodynamic therapy is to administer a photosensitiser usually intravenously and allow retention in the tissue for 48 hours prior to irradiation with appropriate wavelength light usually from a laser. The exogenously administered photosensitisers tend to accumulate in tumor stroma and in the sub-mucosal layer of the gastrointestinal tract[57]. This may be of little relevance if all the mucosa above is destroyed but does risk deeper damage.

The problem of targeting the photosensitiser to the dysplastic mucosa, and avoiding systemic photosensitization may be overcome by using endogenous photosensitization. Following an excess administration of 5-aminolaevulinic acid (5-ALA), a precursor of haem, an intracellular accumulation of the photosensitiser protoporphyrin IX (PpIX) is induced[58]. The synthesis of 5-ALA from glycine and succinyl-CoA is the first step in porphyrin biosynthesis and ultimately haem. This pathway is tightly regulated by end product inhibition. If excess endogenous 5-ALA is administered then this regulation is bypassed and an intracellular accumulation of the photosensitiser protoporphyrin IX (PpIX) is induced (Figure 1).

Glycine + Succinyl CoA

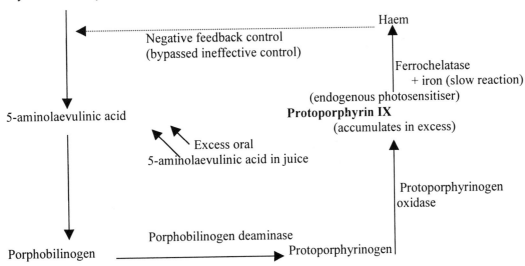

Figure 1. The biochemical mechanism of endogenous photosensitization following the administration of 5 aminolaevulinic acid to generate protoporphyrin IX.

TABLE 3. Studies of photodynamic therapy in patients treated for intestinal tumors where a measure has been made of the depth of necrosis.

Photosensitiser	Dose mg/kg	Light Joules/cm2	Depth of Necrosis mm	Ref
Exogenous				
Dihaematoporphyrin ether	2	191	6	59
Haematoporphyrin Derivative	2.5	100-150	6	60
Endogenous PpIX				
5-aminolaevulinic acid	60	150	2	61
5-aminolaevulinic acid	60-75	150	<2	62

The level of photosensitization is minimized to a few hours and the 5-ALA can be administered orally. The photosensitiser is activated in tissue using 630nm laser light from an appropriate light source, such as a KTP pumped dye laser. The choice of photosensitiser is crucial to achieve the depth of necrosis that is required. The use of an exogenous photosensitiser such as Photofrin or any derivative of di-haematoporphyrin ester/ether will produce damage up to 6mm. Photodynamic therapy to generate PpIX following oral administration of ALA will only produce necrosis to a depth of 2mm (Table 3).

These measurements are particularly crucial if one is concerned that treatment may not destroy an occult cancer or where there is nodularity and the suspicion of an invasive cancer either clinically (Figure 2) or following endoscopic ultrasound evaluation.

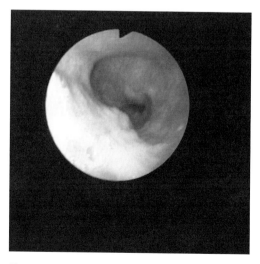

Figure 2. Endoscopic picture of dysplastic Barrett's esophagus with a small nodular area of early invasive cancer. This patient was unsuitable for surgical resection and was treated with photodynamic therapy using Photofrin

7. MECHANICAL

It is possible to resect tissue through the flexible or the rigid endoscope. Most methods have concentrated on endoscopic mucosal resection (EMR) at flexible endoscopy under sedation. The great advantage of these techniques is that histology is available for complete analysis. EMR is very effective if a mucosal abnormality is visible and can be removed with complete clearance. It would seem that it could be more difficult to treat an extensive field change with areas of occult high-grade dysplasia. In addition it may not adequately treat the full metaplastic field. There are essentially two methods that can be employed in the treatment of high-grade dysplasia in Barrett's esophagus. Both depend on the creation of a pseudopolyp either by peri or intralesional injection of saline or by suction. The area of abnormality is then removed with snare diathermy and the specimen retrieved for histological analysis[63]. Direct mechanical abrasion of the area of abnormality can also be particularly effective and ultrasonic dissectors are now common place in other surgical applications and this technique is being actively investigated[65].

8. RESULTS

8.1 ALA PHOTODYNAMIC THERAPY

Photodynamic therapy following endogenous photosensitization with 5-ALA has been reported for the treatment of high-grade dysplasia in Barrett's esophagus. There is extensive data on the uptake and distribution of photosensitisers in gastrointestinal mucosa. In experimental Barrett's like esophagus protoporphyrin IX was generated in the epithelial cells whether squamous or columnar, with maximum levels occurring 3 hours after oral or intravenous injection. The uptake in the mucosa was 3.5 times greater than in the muscularis, and there was little difference between oral or parenteral administration of the 5-ALA[42,72]. These experimental studies have also supplied important reasons for the mucosal localization of PpIX. The muscularis contains more iron and has a reduced activity of one of the rate controlling enzymes. porphobilinogen deaminase[42]. Clinical studies of the PpIX distribution following oral 5-ALA have confirmed the mucosal accumulation relative to surrounding tissues [70,73]. There was little difference in accumulation when the oral dose was increased from 60mg/kg to 75mg/kg and carcinomatous tissue produced PpIX in similar quantities to dysplastic and metaplastic epithelium[73].

Following the accumulation of PpIX, a photodynamic action will only occur following light irradiation. Initially all treatment parameters were empirically selected An elegant study in an experimental model of Barrett's-like esophagus

has confirmed that the most appropriate time for light irradiation is 2-3 hours after 5-ALA administration[74]. This time interval appears critical to achieve mucosal destruction while sparing esophageal function.

There have been two major clinical studies of 5-ALA photodynamic therapy for the ablation of high-grade dysplasia. Both have demonstrated eradication of the dysplasia and one series demonstrated the successful eradication of T1 tumors that were less than 2mm in depth. A prospective randomized trial of the treatment of low-grade dysplasia using ALA and irradiation with green light rather than the usual 630nm red light has again confirmed how effective this treatment is in reversing dysplasia/metaplasia. Healing proceeded with the regeneration of neosquamous epithelium[75]. A variation of 5-ALA photodynamic therapy involves the direct endoscopic spraying of the agent combined with sodium bicarbonate as a mucolytic onto dysplastic Barrett's esophagus. A period of time is allowed for local absorption and then the area is irradiated with light. The response following this technique was variable with 2 of 9 patients failing to show any response[76].

8.2   EXOGENOUS   PHOTODYNAMIC THERAPY

The use of photodynamic therapy for early cancer and high-grade dysplasia has been examined in some detail. Great encouragement for this technique was received when Sibille et al published a large series of patients with early   squamous   cell   carcinoma   and adenocarcinoma   treated   with haematoporphyrin derivative photodynamic therapy [77]. These patients had co-morbid disease and were considered unsuitable for surgery. Sixty-one patients were staged using endosonography as uT1 and 27 patients had uT2 tumors. The 5-year disease specific survival was 74%. The complete response rate was not different between patients treated with photodynamic therapy alone or with a combination of chemotherapy, radiotherapy and photodynamic therapy. This gave a clear indication that if the cancer was local to the esophagus, then a local therapy could eradicate the disease and lead to prolonged survival. This group provided a rationale for the endoscopic treatment of small superficial cancers[78]. Radical surgical therapy appeared to be an excessive response if the disease was only millimeters in size. Vital provisos are that the disease had to be accurately staged and treated. The development of optical biopsy techniques   including   optical   coherence tomography are making accurate preoperative staging possible[79]. There is now consistent data demonstrating   the   effectiveness   of   the Photofrin   (QLT,   Vancouver)   for   the eradication of early adenocarcinoma arising from Barrett's esophagus[80]. The method of treatment has been adapted from the treatment of large areas of Barrett's metaplasia with or without high-grade dysplasia. Forty-eight hours after the administration of 2mg/kg of Photofrin, light from a laser at 630nm is delivered at endoscopy to the esophagus. A diffuser or a windowed centring balloon allows more accurate and even light dosimetry[81]. The length of the light delivering device can be 3,5,7cms. At present it is not recommended that more than 7cms of Barrett's esophagus treated at one session[66]. The power density used is 400 mW/cm2 to provide an energy density of 100 to 250 J/cm2 from the diffuser to the mucosa. Treatment can be performed on an outpatient basis and patients must all received profound acid suppression with proton pump inhibitor therapy. Direct sunlight must be avoided for a period of 4-6weeks. This clearly a more aggressive therapy than ALA photodynamic therapy, and the level of damage is deeper (Table 3) and surrounding tissues may be affected. Most patients develop small unilateral or bilateral pleural effusions. Occasionally   the   patient   required   a thoracentesis. Coetaneous photosensitivity can be a significant problem up to 2 months after photosensitization. The major concern has been the incidence of esophageal stricture. Approximately 30% developed significant stenosis   that   responded   to   endoscopic

TABLE 4. Photodynamic therapy for high-grade dysplasia

A. Exogenous photodynamic therapy for high-grade dysplasia

Number of patients	Follow-up months	Outcome following PDT				Ref
		Cancer	Dysplasia HG	LG	No metaplasia	
73	19(4-84)	0	7	8	32	66
3	6-84	0	0			67
7	6-54	1	1		3	68
6		0	1		2	69

B. Endogenous (5-ALA) photodynamic therapy for high-grade dysplasia

5	26-44	0	0		1	70
10	1-11	0	0		0	61

esophageal dilatation. The results of Photofrin photodynamic therapy are very encouraging, with 75-80% of the Barrett's mucosa being converted to neosquamous mucosa. Complete eradication of all metaplastic epithelium occurred in 43 of 100 patients. Dysplasia disappeared in 78 of 100 patients, although 11 developed dysplasia during follow-up and required repeat treatment. Thirteen patients were treated for early cancer (T1-12 patients; T2-1 patient), and in ten the tumor was eradicated. It is important again to emphasize that the patients must remain under surveillance and repeated treatment will be necessary in some to treat residual or recurrent areas of dysplasia and metaplasia. Usually the areas are rather patchy and are best treated using thermal ablation using a laser or the APC.

8.3 THERMAL AND PHOTOTHERMAL THERAPY

There is less data available on the treatment of dysplastic epithelium with thermal destruction. The treatment and regression of metaplastic epithelium is now widely reported. It is still difficult to say whether the nature of the device to deliver the thermal injury is important or not. The use of multi-polar electrocoagulation and acid suppression is very effective[82-86]. The treatment of over 50 patients has been reported in full or in abstract. Most patients did not have dysplasia, and the metaplasia was usually completely eradicated if acid suppression was adequate.
The use of the endoscopic APC has a more recent history and again is very effective. Two perforations and one death occurred using this device. Both these perforations occurred early in one series and it is believed that they happened when the instrument was pushed through the esophageal wall[52]. On theoretical and experimental grounds it would be surprising if they were related to thermal injury, since our data indicates that the thermal profile and injury is highly localised[53,105]. The authors have concluded that the perforations were either related to advancing the endoscope with the device protruding, or a sudden violent movement against the device when the patients coughs or strains. These two suggestions are entirely appropriate. In our experience the APC can generate a lot gas and distension that may induce coughing in some patients. The forward view can also be compromised with debris. Experience and great care are required. The APC must be withdrawn into the endoscope before advancing. Careful suction and clearance of debris is vital before firing. Regression of the columnar-lined esophagus may not be complete and one patient with low-grade dysplasia has been shown to progress to high-grade dysplasia 12 months after APC therapy[87]. Some patients fail to demonstrate any improvement[88]. In a large series of 27 patients who have completed treatment, two patterns of neo-squamous replacement have been identified. In 70% there is no persistence of the metaplasia but in 30% the metaplasia is buried under a new covering of squamous epithelium[52]. The conclusion at present is that APC therapy can be recommended for the destruction of high-grade dysplasia as an alternative to esophageal resection. The patient surveillance must not stop and repeated endoscopy and biopsy are essential.[52].

The laser is a very effective photothermal instrument. We have predominantly used the KTP laser on theoretical grounds[43,45,46]. Other groups who have used this device have also found it to be highly effective and safe[71]. Treatment is very easy and 2-4 sessions are required to complete therapy. We have found buried metaplasia to be a potential problem in some patients. In our series some 24 post-treatment biopsies were identified by the endoscopist as being from an area that had undergone squamous re-epithelisation. Histology confirmed the presence of squamous epithelium, but surprisingly three showed only glandular mucosa. Thus the endoscopic appearance following treatment can be misinterpreted. Histology is mandatory to confirm neo-squamous re-epithelialization. Eight biopsies of the 21 containing squamous epithelium also contained buried metaplastic glandular mucosa [43]. This problem of buried glands is now confirmed by others with two of ten patients treated with the KTP laser showing buried specialized glandular mucosa under the restored squamous epithelium[72]. No complications have occurred in these two series. Both the argon ion[89] and the Nd:YAG laser[90,91] have been used for photothermal ablation, and were among the first devices to demonstrate effective mucosal destruction with squamous re-epithelialization. One small-randomized study of 8 patients has failed to show any effect using the Nd:YAG laser[92]. The reason for the absence of response in the treated patients is not clear. The authors speculated that their method of laser therapy from gastro-esophageal junction moving proximally as for obstructing tumor therapy may have been responsible. The ablated area remained surrounded by metaplastic columnar epithelium. They suggest that therapy should be from the squamo-columnar junction downwards. It has been suggested that the squamous re-epithelialization occur from contiguous squamous epithelium. These investigators also suggest that the likelihood of achieving complete squamous re-epithelialization increases with the amount of adjacent squamous epithelium[89]. Many using the APC have started distal and withdrawn the scope, they do not comment as to whether they reached the squamo-columnar junction in each patient[52]. They treated areas of 2-4cms in length. It is also possible that the depth of injury with the Nd:YAG laser being greater than the argon or KTP laser may not be ideal to allow stem cells to be preserved and proliferate to heal the mucosa. Others have reported some patients failing to respond to Nd:YAG therapy[93]. There is always a concern that some patients receive inadequate reflux control. Nd:YAG therapy combined with antireflux surgery was effective 6-52 months after treatment[49]. The complication rate following Nd:YAG laser therapy appears more significant than following the use of the KTP laser. This was anticipated from the experimental data. Following the treatment of 15 patients there have been one perforation and one esophageal stricture[93].

8.4. HISTOPATHOLOGY FOLLOWING ABLATION THERAPY

Ablation of high-grade dysplasia offers therapeutic options to those unsuitable or unwilling to contemplate radical surgical excision. It may also become the treatment of choice for dysplasia in the future. The data is clearly incomplete, but there is at least one multi-center randomized study in progress to compare Photofrin photodynamic therapy against proton pump therapy and surveillance. There are many questions that remain. What is the ideal method of destruction? What is the ideal method of reflux control.

TABLE 5. Thermal therapy for high-grade dysplasia

Number of patients (+therapy)	Follow-up months	Outcome following Thermal Therapy			Ref
		Cancer	Dysplasia HG LG	No residual metaplasia	
4 (KTP)	13(9-15)0	0	0	3	71
4 (KTP)	6(5-36)	1 (SCC)	0	0	
3 (APC) (one death)	12	0	0	0	52

KTP= potassium titanyl phosphate laser,
APC= argon plasma coagulator,
SCC= squamous cell carcinoma

How confident can we be in the ultimate prevention of mortality[94-96]. Perhaps the most vital question remaining addresses this latter issue. Will mucosal ablation therapy and reflux control for metaplastic and dysplastic Barrett's esophagus prevent esophageal cancer and premature death?

There is concern that many patients have only partial ablation and that this may be an inadequate end point[97]. It is therefore important to assess in some detail the histopathological outcomes, and collate experience from other diseases and treatments [43]. The finding of endoscopically unsuspected glandular mucosa both superficially and buried under the neo-squamous epithelium means all these treated patients must receive life long biopsy surveillance according to protocol. There are several patterns of squamous regeneration. First there is the formation of squamous islands associated with openings of esophageal squamous gland ducts, the superficial parts of which are lined with squamous epithelium. This feature is often seen to occur in patients treated with long-term proton pump therapy. Secondly, following ablation and reflux control, long stretches of squamous epithelium are seen, frequently overlying Barrett's mucosa (Figure 3).

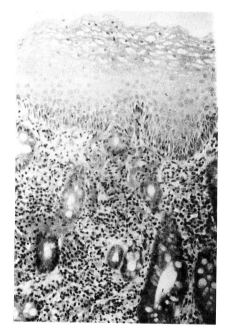

Figure 3. Neo-squamous epithelium overlying glands, 6 months after KTP laser ablation of metaplastic Barrett's esophagus.

A third phenomenon is seen with apparent squamous metaplasia within Barrett's glandular mucosa. This latter appearance suggests the existence of a pluri-potential stem cell within the columnar mucosa, which is capable of differentiation along a squamous lineage under the correct environmental conditions. The presence of buried columnar epithelium has been seen following antireflux surgery[98], long term proton pump inhibitors[99], and also following treatment with H2 receptor antagonists[100]. There appear to be three mechanisms for the squamous re-epithelialization: encroachment from adjacent squamous epithelium, squamous metaplasia within the Barrett's mucosa itself from pluripotential stem cells, and re-growth from squamous lined ducts of the esophageal mucus gland. The concern that the cancer risk is only reduced and not abolished is appropriate and a further compelling argument that treatment may need to be repeated and surveillance must continue. This treatment may only be 'weeding the garden' or 'mowing the grass'. We have one patient with dysplasia who developed a squamous cell carcinoma in the neo-squamous epithelium 36 months after KTP laser ablation of the dysplasia. It appears that the risk of neoplastic progression may not be confined to the buried concealed metaplastic dysplastic glands, but also occurs in the neo-squamous epithelium. The oncogenic pluri-potential stem cells may have survived and produced malignant squamous cell lineage's. The phenotypic expression has been altered but not the malignant genotype. It is highly appropriate to suggest that pathological follow-up should include molecular diagnostics[2,3,96]. It will be extremely important to see if a neoplastic marker such as p53 where to disappear, and persistence would draw attention to incomplete end points of treatment.

9. CONCLUSIONS

High-grade dysplasia is a precursor of invasive carcinoma and is often associated with coexistent early invasive adenocarcinoma. It appears that in some patients high-grade may remain a stable phenotype for a period of time without progression to invasive cancer. Therapy for these patients must be informed by these data. Radical surgical excision is still appropriate therapy for many patients. There are certain groups in whom surgery may be the initial preferred option. If the disease is widespread in young fit patients then the outcome from surgery is likely to be favorable and the patient completely cured. However, few patients fall into this category, and the decision on surgery or continued surveillance is difficult. The introduction of mucosal ablation offers the possibility of treating these patients without the fearful operative morbidity and mortality of surgical resection. It must be remembered that high-grade dysplasia is a mucosal, microscopic disease. It is hardly a triumph to remove the complete esophagus for a few microscopic nests of potentially malignantly invasive cells. This presupposes that staging is accurate[19] and that an invasive cancer has not been missed. The accuracy of optical biopsy [79,101,106] is improving, and ultrasound also allows accurate preoperative staging[102.] There is now wide experience of local therapy both in the stomach[102] and the squamous lining of the esophagus and tracheobronchial tree[103,104], indicating that local mucosal resection or ablation can produce prolonged control and possible cure of early superficial malignant disease [101]. Most of the squamous cancers treated with local ablative therapy are detected following screening of patients who have had a curative resection for cancer. These patients are usually unsuitable for further radical resection of lung or esophagus and the experience indicates that the disease is controlled[103]. It seems clear that the detection of high-grade dysplasia should now be an indication for full staging and ablation of the mucosal disease, with full reflux control and continued surveillance of the ablated segment.

The choice of ablation method is not clear. More widespread use of endoscopic mucosal

resection applied to the esophagus should be encouraged since we can obtain the full histological specimen[103]. The technique at present is only suitable for small areas and it would be daunting to treat a long metaplastic Barrett's segment with multi-focal high-grade dysplasia. Our preferred method is to use photodynamic therapy with 5-ALA as the photosensitiser in these circumstances. The use of a more potent photosensitiser such as Photofrin or the newer mTHPC (meta-tetra (hydroxyphenyl) chlorin-Foscan) is an attractive option if there is concern that there may be areas of early invasive cancer. Thermal ablation with the laser or more usually the APC is also effective in these circumstances. The APC is particularly useful for areas remaining after PDT or for smaller lengths of Barrett's esophagus. It is again emphasized that the endpoint of ablation therapy is not the production of neo-squamous epithelium. Further surveillance is always necessary. These patients remain with an unstable epithelium with buried glands and are still at risk. We hope and speculate that this risk has been considerably reduced. We are in the process of life long follow-up of all our patients treated with ablation therapy for high-grade dysplasia.

REFERENCES

1. Haggitt RC. Barrett's esophagus, dysplasia and adenocarcinoma. Hum Pathol 1994;25:982-93.
2. Bailey T, Biddlestone L, Shepherd N, Barr H, Warner P, Jankowski J. Altered cadherin and catenin complexes in the Barrett's esophagus-dysplasia-adenocarcinoma sequence. Am J Pathol 1998;152:1-10.
3. Whittles CE, Biddlestone LR, Burton A, Barr H, Jankowski JAZ, Warner PJ, Shepherd NA. Apoptotic and proliferative activity in Neoplastic progression of Barrett's esophagus: acompartive study. J Pathol 1999;187:535-40.
4. Younes M, Lebovitz RM, Lechago LV, Lechago J. p53 protein accumulation in Barrett's metaplasia, dysplasia and carcinoma follow-up study. Gastroenterology 1993;105:1637-42.
5. Younes M, Ertan A, Lechago LV et al. p53 protein accumulation is a specific marker of malignant potential in Barrett's metaplasia .Dig Dis Sci 1997;42:697-701.
6. Menke-Pluymers MBE, Mulder AH, Hop WC, van Blankenstein M, Tilanus HW. Dysplasia and aneuploidy as markers of malignant degeneration in Barrett's esophagus. The Rotterdam Oesophageal Tumour Study Group Gut 1994;35:1348-51.
7. Reid BJ. Observer variation in the diagnosis of dysplasia in Barrett's esophagus. Hum Pathol 1988;19:166-78.
8. Dent J, Bremmer CG, Collen MJ et al. Working party report to World Congress of Gastroenterology, Sydney 1990: Barrett's esophagus J Gastroenterol Hepatol 1991;6:1-22.
9. Schmidt HG, Riddell RH, Walther B et al. Dysplasia in Barrett's esophagus. J Cancer res Clin Oncol 1985;110:145-52.
10. Womack C, Harvey L. Columnar epithelial esophagus or Barrett's esophagus: mucin histochemistry, dysplasia, and invasive adenocarcinoma. J Clin Pathol 1985;38:477-8.
11. Lee RG. Dysplasia in barrett's esophagus a clinicopathologic study of six patients. Am J Surg Pathol 1985;9:845-52.
12. Reid BJ, Weinstein NM, Lewin KJ et al. Endoscopic biopsy can detect HGD or early adenocarcinoma in Barrett's esophagus without grossly recognizable neoplastic lesions. Gastroenterology 1988;94:81-90.
13. Hamilton SR, Smith RR. The relationship between columnar epithelial dysplasia and invasive adenocarcinoma arising in Barrett's esophagus. Am J Clin Pathol 1987;85:301-12.
14. Garewal HS, Sampliner RE, Steinbronn K. Increase in ornithine decarboxylase activity associated with development of dysplasia in Barrett's esophagus. Dig Dis Sci 1989;34:312-4.
15. Altorki NK, Sunagawa M, Little AG, Skinner DB. High-grade dysplasia in the columnar-lined esophagus. Am J Surg 1991; 611;97-9.
16. Pera M, Trastek VF, Carpenter HA, Allen MS, Deschamps C, Pairolero PC. Barrett's esophagus with high-grade dysplasia: an indication for esophagectomy? Ann Thorac Surg 1992;54:199-204
17. Rice TW, Falk GW, Achkar E, Petras RE. Surgical management of high-grade dysplasia in Barrett's esophagus. Am J Surg 1997;174:1832-6.

18. Steitz JM Jr, Andrews CW Jr, Ellis FH. Endoscopic surveillance of Barrett's esophagus. Does it help? J Thorac cardiovasc Surg 1993;105:383-8.

19. Levine DS, Haggitt RC, Blount PL, Rabinovitch PS, Rusch VW, Reid BJ. An endoscopic biopsy protocol can differentiate high-grade dysplasia from early adenocarcinoma in Barrett's esophagus. Gastroenterology 1993;105:40-50.

20. Peters JH, Clark GW, Ireland AP, Chandrasoma P, Smyrk TC, DeMeester DR. Outcome of adenocarcinoma in Barrett's esophagus inendoscopically surveyed and non-surveyed patients. J Thorac cardiovasc Surg 1994;108:813-21.

21. Edwards MJ, Gable DR, Lentsch AB, Richardson JD.The rationale for esophagectomy as the optimal therapy for Barrett's esophagus with high-grade dysplasia. Ann Surg 1996;223:585-9.

22. Collard JM, Romagnoli R. Hermans BP, Malaise J. Radical esophageal resection for adenocarcinoma arising in Barrett's esophagus. Am J Surg 1997;174:307-11.

23. Heitmeller RF, redmond M, Hamilton SR. Barrett's esophagus with high-grade dysplasia. An indication for prophylactic esophagectomy. Ann Surg 1996;224:66-71.

24. Ferguson MK, Naunheim KS. Resection for Barrett's mucosa with high-grade dysplasia: implications for prophylactic photodynamic therapy. J Thorac Cardiovasc Surg 1997;114:824-9.

25. Cameron AJ, Carpenter HA. Barrett's esophagus, high-grade dysplasia, and early adenocarcinoma: a pathological study. Am J Gastroenterol 1997;92:586-91.

26. Miros M, Kerlin P, Walker N. Only patients with dysplasia progress to adenocarcinoma in Barrett's esophagus. Gut 1991;32:1441-6.

27. Robertson CS, Mayberry, Nicholson DA, James PD, Atkinson M. Value of endoscopic surveillance in the detection of neoplastic Change in Barrett's esophagus. Br J Surg 1988; 75:760-3.

28. Hameeteman W, Tytgat GN, Houthoff HF, Van Den Tweel JG. Barrett's esophagus: development and adenocarcinoma. Gastroenterology 1989; 96:1249-56.

29. Reid BJ, Blount PL, Rubin CE, Levine DS, Haggitt RC, Rabinovitch PS. Flow-cytometric and histological progression to malignancy in Barrett's esophagus: prospective endoscopic surveillance of a cohort. Gastroenterology 1992; 102:1212-9.

30. Pera M, Trastek VF, Carpenter HA, Allen MS, Deschamps C, Pairolero PC. Barrett's esophagus with high-grade dysplasia: an indication for esophagectomy? Ann Thorac Surg 1992;54:199-204.

31. Ouata-Lascar R, Fitzgerald RC, Triadafilopoulos G. Differentiation and proliferation in Barrett's esophagus and the effects of acid suppression. Gastroenterology 1999;117:327-35.

32. Gore S, Healey CJ, Sutton R, Eyre-Brook IA, Gear MWL, Shepherd NA, Wilkinson SP. Regression of columnar lined (Barrett's) esophagus with continuous omeprazole therapy. Aliment Pharmacol Ther 1993;7:623-8.

33. Peters FTM, Ganesh S, Kuipers EJ, Sluiter WJ, Klinkenberg-Knol EC, Lamers CBHW, Kleibeuker JH. Endoscopic regression of Barrett's esophagus during omeprazole treatment; a randomised double blind study. Gut 199;45:489-4.

34. Sagar PM, Ackroyd R, Hosie KB, Patterson JE, Stoddard CJ, Kingsnorth AN. Regression and progression of Barrett's esophagus after antireflux surgery. Br J Surg 1995;82:806-10.

35. Ortiz A, Martinez de Haro LF, Parrilla P, Moralers G, Molina J, Bermejo J et al. Conservative treatment versus antireflux surgery in Barrett's esophagus: long-term results of a prospective study. Br J Surg 1996;83:274-8.

36. Ackroyd R, Brown NJ, Stephenson TJ, Stoddard CJ, Reed MW. Ablation treatment for Barrett esophagus: what depth of tissue destruction is needed. J Clin Pathol 1999;52:509-12.

37. Bamford K, James J, Barr H, Tatam R. Electromagnetic simulation of laser-induced fluorescence in bronchial tissue and predicted optical scattering behaviour"Optical and Imaging Techniques for Biomonitoring IV(SPIE Proceedings) 1998;3567:18-28.

38. Li H, Walsh TN, O'Dowd G, Gillen P, Byrne PJ, Hennessy TPJ. Mechanisms of columnar metaplasia and squamous regeneration in experimental Barrett's esophagus. Surgery 1994;115:176-181.

39. Gillen P, Keeling P, Byrne PJ, West AB, Hennessy TPJ. Experimental columnar metaplasia in the canine esophagus. Br J Surg 1988;75:113-5.

40. Herbst JJ, Berenson MM, McCloskey D, Wiser WC. Cell proliferation in esophageal columnar epithelium (Barrett's esophagus). Gastroenterology 1978;75:683-7.

41. Jankowski J .Molecular events in Barrett's Metaplasia. Gastroenterology 1993;104:1235.

42. Van den Boogert J, Houtsmuller AB, De Rooij FWM, De Bruin RWF, Siersema PD, Van Hillegersberg R. Kinetics, localization, and mechanism of 5-aminolaevulinic acid-induced porphyrin accumulation in normal and Barrett's-like rat esophagus. Lasers Surg Med 1999;24:3-13.

43. Biddlestone LR, Barham CP, Wilkinson SP, Barr H, Shepherd NA. The histopathology of treated Barrett's esophagus. Am J Surg Pathol 1998;22:239-45.

44. Van den Boogert J, Van Hillegersberg R, De Bruin RWF, Van Velthuysen MLF, Tilanus HW. A rat model for Barrett's esophagus and prospects for photodynamic therapy. Eur J Gastroenterol and Hepatol 1997;9:A53.

45. Dix AJ, & Barr H. Photothermal Ablation of metaplastic Columnar-lined (Barrett's) esophagus, experimental studies for safe endoscopic laser therapy. Progress in Biomedical Optics(SPIE Proceedings).1996; 2922:275-80.

46. Barham CP, Jones RL, Biddlestone LR, Hardwick RH, Shepherd NA, Barr H. Photothermal laser ablation of Barrett's esophagus: endoscopic and histological evidence of squamous re-epithelialization. Gut 1997;41:281-4.

47. Sampliner RE, Hixson LJ, Fennerty MB et al. Regression of Barrett's esophagus by laser ablation in an antacid environment. Dig Dis Sci 1993;38:365-8.

48. Lumen W, Lessels AM, Palmer KR. Failure of Nd-YAG photocoagulation therapy as treatment for Barrett's esophagus-A pilot study. Eur J Gastroenterol and Hepatol 1996;8:627-30.

49. Salo JA, Saliminen JT, Kiviluoto TA et al. Treatment of Barrett's esophagus by endoscopic laser and ablation antireflux surgery. Ann Surg 1998;227:40-4.

50. Krevsky B, Horwitz B, Cohen S et al. Long-term effects of acid suppression on Nd:YAG laser treated Barrett's esophagus: Ongoing studies. Gastroenterology 1998;114:A188.

51. Brandt LJ, Kauvar DR. Laser-induced transient regression of Barrett's epithelium Gastrointest Endosc 1992;38:619-22.

52. Byrne JP, Armstrong GR, Attwood SEA Restoration of the normal squamous lining in Barrett's esophagus by argon beam plasma coagulation. Am J Gastroenterol 1998;93:1810-5.

53. Barham CP, Shepherd N, Barr H. Regression of Barrett's epithelium using Argon Gas coagulation and acid suppression. Gut 1996;39:T114.

54. Fremond L, Bouche O, Diebold M-D. Demange L. Zeitoun P. Thiefin Regression partielle d'un endobrachyoesophage en dysplasie de haut grade avec adenocarcinome apres photocoagulation et endocurietherapie sous traitement antisecretoire. Gastroenterol Clin Biol 1995;19:112-6..

55. Barr H., Tralau CJ, Boulos P.B, Krasner N, Clark CG and Bown. SG. Selective destruction of dimethyl-hydrazine rat colon cancer using phthalocyanine photodynamic therapy. Gastroenterology, 1990; 98:1532-53.

56. Sampliner RE, Fennerty B, Garewai HS. Reversal of Barrett's esophagus with acid suppression and multipolar electrocoagulation: preliminary results gastrointest Endosc 1996;44:523-5.

57. Barr H, Tralau CJ, MacRobert AJ, Morrison I, Phillips D, Bown SG. Fluorescence photometric Techniques for determination of microscopic tissue distribution of phthalocyanine photosensitisers for photodynamic therapy. Las Med Sci 1988;3:81-6.

58. Grant WE, Hopper C, MacRobert AJ, Speight PM, Bown SG. Photodynamic therapy of oral cancer: photosensitisation with systemic aminolaevulinic acid .Lancet 1993;342:147-8.

59. Heier SK, Rothman KA, Heier LM, Rosenthal WS. Photodynamic therapy for obstructing esophageal cancer: light dosimetry and a randomized comparison with Nd:YAG laser therapy . Gastroenterology 1995;109:63-72.

60. Barr H, Krasner N, Boulos PB, Chatlani PT, Bown SG. Photodynamic therapy for colorectal cancer: a quantitative pilot study. Br J Surg 1990;77:93-6.

61. Gossner L, Stolte M, Stroke R et al. Photodynamic therapy of high-grade dysplasia and early stage carcinomas by means of 5-aminolaevulinic acid. Gastroenterology 1998;114: 447-55.

62. Barr H, Tan WC, Shepherd NA. Photodynamic therapy (PDT) using 5-aminolaevulinic acid (5-ALA) for oesophageal adenocarcinoma associated with Barrett's metaplasia. Lasers Med Sci. 1997;4-9.

63. Soehendra H, Binmoeller KF, Bohnacker S et al. Endoscopic snare mucosectomy in the esophagus without any additional equipment: A simple technique for resection of flat early cancer. Endoscopy 1997;29:380-3.

64. Farin G, Grund KE. Technology of argon plasma coagulation with particular reference to endoscopic applications. Endosc Surg 1994;2:71-7.

65. Bremmer RM, Mason RJ, Bremner CG et al. Ultrasonic epithelial ablation of the lower esophagus without stricture formation. A new technique for Barrett's ablation. Surg Endosc 1998;12:342-6.

66. Overholt BF, Panjepour M, Haydek JM. Photodynamic therapy for barett's esophagus:follow-up in 100 patients. Gastrointest Endosc 1999;49:1-7.

67. Spinelli P, Dal Fante M, Mancici A et al. Endoscopic photodynamic therapy of early cancer and severe dysplasia of the esophagus. In Spinelli P, Dal Fante M, Marchesini R, eds. Photodynamic therapy and biomedical lasers Amsterdam: Elsevier Science Inc 1992:262-5.

68. Overholt BF, Panjepour M. Photodynamic therapy in Barrett's esophagus: Reduction of specialized mucosa, ablation of dysplasia, and treatment of superficial esophageal cancer. Semin Surg Oncol 1995,11:372-6.

69. Wang KK, WongKeeSong LM, Nourbakhsh et al. Can consistent tissue necrosis be achieved during photodynamic therapy for high-grade dysplasia or cancer within Barrett's esophagus? Gastroenterology 1997;112:A676.

70. Barr H, Shepherd NA, .Dix A, Roberts DJH, Tan WC, Krasner N. Eradication of high grade dysplasia in columnar-lined (Barrett's) esophagus using

71. Gossner L. May A, Stolte M, Seitz G, Hahn EG, Ell C. KTP laser destruction of dysplasia and early cancer in columnar-lined Barrett's esophagus. Gastrointest Endosc 1999;49:8-12.

72. Van den Boogert J, Van Hillegersberg R, De Rooij FWM, De Bruin RWF, Edixhoven-Bosdijk A, Houtsmuller AB, Siersema PD, Wilson JHP, Tilanus HW. 5-aminolaevulinic acid-induced protoporphyrin accumulation in tissues: pharmacokinetics after oral or intravenous administration. J Photochemistry and Photobiology B: Biology 1998;44,29-8.

73. TanWC, Fulljames C, Stone N, Dix AJ, Shepherd NA Roberts DJH, Brown Krasner N, Barr H. Photodynamic therapy using 5-aminolaevulinic acid for oesophageal adenocarcinoma associated with Barrett's metaplasia. J Photochemistry and Photobiology B: Biology 1999;45, in press.

74. Van den Boogert J, Van Hillegersberg R, Van Staveren HJ, De Bruin RWF, Siersema PD, Tilanus HW. Timing of illumination is essential for effective and safe photodynamic therapy: a study in the normal rat esophagus. Br J Cancer 1999;79:825-30.

75. Ackroyd R, Davis MF, Stephenson TJ et al. Photodynamic therapy for Barrett's esophagus: A prospective randomised trial. Endoscopy 1997;29:E17.

76. Ortner M, Zumbusch K, Liebetruth J et al. Photodynamic therapy in Barrett's esophagus after local administration of 5-aminolaevulinic acid. Gastroenterology 1997;112:A633.

77. Sibille A, Lambert R, Souquet JP, Sabben G, Descos F. Long-term survival after photodynamic therapy for esophageal cancer. Gastroenterology 1997;112:A633.

78. Wang KK, Geller A. Photodynamic therapy for early esophageal cancers: Light versus surgical might. Gastroenterology 1995;108:593-607.

79. Barr H, Dix AJ, Stone N Optical. Spectroscopy for the Early Diagnosis of Gastrointestinal Malignancy Lasers Med Sci, 1998;13:3-13.

80. Overholt B, Panjehpour M, Tefftellar E. Photodynamic therapy for the treatment of early carcinoma in Barrett's esophagus. Gastrointest Endosc 1993;39:73-6.

81. Panjehpour M, Overholt BF, DeNovo R, Sneed R, Petersen MG. Centering balloon to improve esophageal photodynamic therapy. Lasers Surg Med 1992;12:631-8.

82. McBride MA. Vanagunas AA, Breshnan JP et al. Combined endoscopic thermal coagulation with high dose omeprazole therapy in complicated heterotopic gastric mucosa of the esophagus. Am J Gastroenterol 1995;11:2029-31.

83. Sampliner RE, Fennerty MB, Garewal HS. Reversal of Barrett's esophagus with acid suppression and multipolar electrocoagulation: Preliminary results. Gastrointest Endosc 1996;44:532-5.

84. Guelrud M, Herrera I. Multipolar electrocoagulation in the treatment of Barrett's esophagus. Gastrointest Endosc 1997;45:AB69.

85. Jackson FW, Husson M, Lipschultz W et al. Eradication of Barrett's epithelium with multipolar electrocautery. Gastrointest Endosc 1997;45:AB71.

86. Kovacs BJ, Chen YK, Lewis TD et al. Reversal of Barrett's esophagus with multipolar electrocoagulation: Is acid suppression important? Gastroitest Endosc 1997;45:AB72

87. Maass S, Martin WR, Spietff A et al.. Barrett's esophagus with severe dysplasia in argon beam therapy Z Gastroenterol 1998;36:301-6.

88. Martin WR, Benz C, Jakobs R et al. Argon plasma coagulation (APC) in patients with Barrett's esophagus. Gastroenterology 1998;114:A217.

89. Berenson MM, Johnson TD, Markowitz NR et al. Restoration of squamous mucosa after ablation of Barrett's esophageal epithelium. Gastroenterology 1993;104:16868-91.

90. Brandt LJ, Kauver DR. Laser-induced transient regression of Barrett's epithelium. Gastrointest Endosc 1992;38:619-22.

91. Sampliner RE, Hixson LJ, Fennerty MB et al. Regression of Barrett's esophagus by laser ablation in an antacid environment. Dig Dis Sci 1993;38:365-3.

92. Luman W, Lessels AM, Palmer KR Failure of Nd-YAG photocoagulation therapy as treatment for Barrett's esophagus-a pilot study. Eur J gastroenterol Hepathol 1996;8:627-30.

93. Krevsky B, Horwitz B, Cohen S et al. Long-term effects of acid suppression on Nd:YAG laser treated Barrett's esophagus: Ongoing studies. Gastroenterology 1998;114:A188.

94. Caestecker JS de. Endoscopic ablation of Barrett's epithelium Eur J Gastroenterol Hepatol 1996;8:620-1.

95. Lightdale CJ. Ablation therapy for Barrett's esophagus: Is it time to choose our weapons. Gastrointest Endosc 1999;49:122-5.

96. Berenson MM.. Ablation therapy of Barrett's esophagus: measures of success and failure. Am J Gastroenterol 1998;93:1794-5.

97. Sampliner RE, Fass R Partial regression of Barrett's esophagus-an inadequate endpoint. Am J Gastroenterol 1993;88:2092-4.

98. Skinner DB, Walther BC, Riddell RH, Schmidt H, Iascone C, DeMeester TR. Barrett's esophagus. Comparison of benign and malignant cases. Ann Surg 1983;198:554-66.

99. Riddell RH. The biopsy diagnosis of gastroesophageal reflux disease,"carditis", and Barrett's esophagus and sequelae of therapy. Am J Surg Pathol 1996;20(suppl):31-50.

100. Sampliner RE, Steinbronn K, Garewal HS, Riddell RH. Squamous mucosa overlying columnar epithelium in Barrett's esophagus in the absence of anti-reflux surgery. Am J Gastroenterol 1988;83:510-512.

101. Barr H. Gastrointestinal tumours: let there be light. Lancet 1998; 352:1242-4.

102. Ell C, Gossner L, May A et al. Photodynamic ablation of early cancers of the stomach by means of mTHPC and laser irradiation: preliminary clinical experience. Gut 1998;43:345-9.

103. Grosjean P, Monnier P. Photodynamic therapy and mucosectomy for early squamous cell carcinomas in the esophagus and tracheobronchial tree. Eur J Surg Oncol 1998;24:234.

104. Hayata Y, Kato H, Furuse K, Kusunoki Y, Suzuki S, Minura S. Photodynamic therapy of 168 early stage cancers of the lung and the esophagus: a Japanese multicentre study. Lasers Med Sci 1996;11:255-9.

105. Grund KE, Straub T, Farin G. New haemostatic techniques: Argon plasma coagulation. Bailliere's Clinical Gastroenterology 1999; 13: 67-84.

106. Haringsma J, Tytgat GNJ. Fluoresescence and autofluoresescence. Bailliere's Clinical Gastroenterology 1999;13:10.

4.4. SURGICAL TREATMENT OF HIGH-GRADE DYSPLASIA AND SUPERFICIAL CARCINOMA.

Mirjam B. de Jong and Hugo W. Tilanus

1. INTRODUCTION

The recent rise of the incidence of adenocarcinomas of the esophagus and the squamocolumnar junction has resulted in an intense and renewed interest in its precursor lesions like reflux esophagitis, metaplasia and dysplasia. The understanding of these sequential steps to invasive carcinoma resulted in a growing awareness regarding the detection of Barrett's esophagus and initiated some large surveillance programs for patients with this condition. As the large majority of adenocarcinomas is detected at a symptomatic and an advanced stage, the results of treatment are dismal even after surgery.

Identification of high-risk groups, surveillance of progressive disease and timely optimal treatment are the only possible ways to improve the results in selected cases.

Patients with dysplasia in Barrett's esophagus represent such relative high-risk group, which is worthwhile to offer follow-up for the possible progression to invasive carcinoma.

The diagnosis and treatment of progressing and non-progressing dysplasia in Barrett's esophagus is highly controversial as is the estimated time needed to develop from low to high-grade dysplasia. Some authors believe in vigorous screening protocols for all patients with Barrett's epithelium, others argue that only a small minority of patients progresses to high grade dysplasia and that even in this so called high-risk group a substantial number of patients eventually dies of other causes. The pros and cons of various regimens are ample discussed elsewhere in this book.

2. LYMPHATIC DRAINAGE

The reason for this debate is the observation that carcinomas of the esophagus show already lymph node metastases in their earliest stages. Lymph node metastasis (N) and the depth of tumor invasion (T) are two of the most important prognostic factors in patients with esophageal carcinoma. The presence of lymph node metastases and increasing T both greatly reduce survival. There also is a close relationship between these two factors. So it is possible to predict the probability of regional lymph node metastasis from an assessment of the pathological diagnosis of adenocarcinoma, a less than well-differentiated histology and

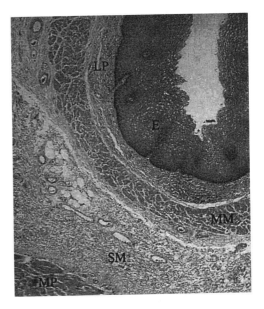

Figure 1. Photomicrograph (40x) illustrating the esophageal wall structure with small lymph vessels in the submucosa. E = Epithelium, LP = Lamina Propria, MM = Muscularis Mucosa, SM = Submucosa, MP = Muscularis Propria.

most importantly, increasing dept of tumor invasion. The recognition that carcinomas invading the submucosa show already lymph node metastases in up to 50% of patients is contrary to carcinomas confined to the mucosa only. This had lead to a refinement of the TNM classification in T1a carcinomas confined to the mucosa only and T1b carcinomas that invade the submucosa[1]. T1a carcinomas very rarely show lymph node involvement whereas T1b carcinomas in resected specimens harbor lymph node involvement in up to 16-50% of patients. The explanation for this phenomenon becomes clear when we look at the lymphatic drainage of the esophageal wall (Figure 1).

Unlike other hollow organs of the digestive tract, in the esophageal mucosa small lymph vessels are already seen just below the basement membrane of the mucosa. They pierce the lamina propria and the submucosa and form a dense longitudinal network outside the submucosa draining to N1 and N2 lymph nodes. Other lymph vessels drain perpendicularly through the muscularis propria into the peri-esophageal lymphatic system or even directly to the lymphatic system and to the venous circulation[2].

H.W. Tilanus and S.E.A. Attwood (eds.), Barrett's Esophagus, 273–280.

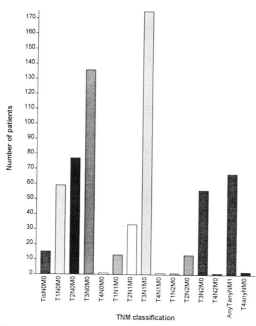

Figure 2. Distribution of TNM classification of all operated patients diagnosed with adenocarcinoma during 1978 – 2000 at the Erasmus university Medical Center.

So there are 2 factors which explain the occurrence of earlylymphatic metastases at stage T1b: firstly, the presence of an extensive submucosal plexus and secondly, the abundant 3-way lymphatic drainage to local and distal lymph nodes. In this light, early detection and treatment of high-grade dysplasia and early carcinomas is, in case of the esophagus, even more important than elsewhere in the digestive tract.

Patients operated for early stages of adenocarcinoma are a small minority. At the Erasmus University Medical Center Rotterdam it was 11% of the total number of patients with adenocarcinoma. Regarding the TNM-stage distribution there seems to be an increase in the lower stage carcinomas, but still T3N1M0 is the most diagnosed tumor stage.

In current series high-grade dysplasia is diagnosed in 3% of all operated adenocarcinomas

3. ANTI-REFLUX SURGERY FOR ASYMPTOMATIC BARRETT'S ESOPHAGUS.

The role of anti-reflux surgery in patients with symptomatic reflux refractory to proton pump inhibitors and/or H.Pylori eradication is well established. Especially in patients with insufficiency of the lower esophageal sphincter, restoration of a high-pressure zone by anti-reflux surgery results in long term relief of symptoms. Anti-reflux surgery for patient with intestinal metaplasia in asymptomatic Barrett's esophagus is more controversial. In theory, restoration of the normal lower esophageal sphincter function by anti-reflux surgery leading to prevention of reflux should stop the ongoing injury of the esophageal epithelium and in an ideal situation results in restoration of normal squamous epithelium. This is however not clearly documented in the current literature. Some authors report the development of islands of squamous epithelium returning into the columnar lined esophagus but the presence of metaplastic epithelium underneath these islands is also reported. The key-question remains if the natural history of Barrett's esophagus i.e. the potential to malignant degeneration, is changed by anti-reflux surgery[3,4]. In our series of adenocarcinomas of the distal esophagus and the gastro-esophageal junction there are patients who developed a carcinoma 5-10 years after anti-reflux surgery[5]. A few studies were especially focussed on the outcome of Barrett's esophagus after antireflux surgery. In one series 92% of 37 patients were followed endoscopically after anti-reflux surgery. Only four of these patients had partial regression of columnar lined epithelium, which was replaced by squamous epithelium, but 2 patients progressed to high-grade dysplasia and carcinoma[6]. Another cohort of patients with combined gastro-esophageal reflux disease and Barrett's esophagus had regression in 24 of 56 patients after anti-reflux surgery but 9 showed progression[7]. Additionally, the last authors concluded that results of anti-reflux surgery are superior in terms of regression of Barrett's epithelium when a vagotomy is added to the procedure.

When medical and surgical treatment are prospectively compared in a randomized fashion, after a median follow-up of 5 years, the results of anti-reflux surgery are superior regarding the decrease of the length of the segment of columnar lined epithelium. Progression was more seen in medically treated patients than in patients after anti-reflux surgery. Two patients developed high-grade dysplasia, one in either group. Both were resected and both showed early carcinoma in the resection specimen[8]. In a series by DeMeester of 35 patients none developed dysplasia or carcinoma after anti-reflux surgery during a follow up of 3 year but the pre-operative existing dysplasia remained unaltered in 10 patients[9]. One of the largest retrospective series today, published by Czendes, shows more sobering results[10]. 152 patients with Barret's esophagus underwent either a posterior gastropexy with so-called calibration of the cardia (n=130), or a 360°

Nissen fundoplication (n=22). In all cases a highly selective vagotomy was added. They were divided in 2 groups: patients with complicated Barrett's esophagus like ulcer or stricture or patients with uncomplicated Barrett's esophagus. The late follow-up of 100 months demonstrated a high percentage of failures among non-complicated BE (54%) and an even higher figure in patients with complicated BE (64%). In this series 15 patients developed low-grade dysplasia and 4 patients an adenocarcinoma at 8 years of follow-up. These results are important regarding the large patient cohort and the long follow-up. It reminds us to the fact that anti-reflux surgery can fail especially many years after operation and secondly that Barrett's esophagus remains a dynamic instead of a static condition. ` Continued long-term endoscopic and histologic follow-up is required in all patients with Barrett's esophagus even after successful anti-reflux surgery[11]. Until further data are available there seems no role for anti-reflux surgery in asymptomatic Barrett's esophagus.

4. SURGERY FOR HIGH-GRADE DYSPLASIA.

The definition and the diagnosis of high-grade dysplasia of intestinalized mucosa in Barrett's esophagus are two very important factors with regard to the correct estimation of the possibility of concurrent adenocarcinoma. The most used definition of high-grade dysplasia is according to Riddel et al adapted from the classification of dysplasia in ulcerative colitis[12] and has been simplified from earlier classifications of those used elsewhere in the gastrointestinal tract[13]. The category of patients positive for dysplasia is divided into low and high-grade, depending on the extent of the cytological architectural changes; the moderate grade has been abolished to eliminate uncertainty in patient management. Reid et al. discovered a considerable inter-observer variability among 8 experienced pathologists but there was agreement in 88% of cases when distinguishing high-grade dysplasia and intramucosal carcinoma which was better than in all other grades[14]. It seems unnecessary and clinically impossible to distinguish high-grade dysplasia from carcinoma in situ and the last classification has now been abolished.

Using the above-mentioned criteria, there is an up to 70% chance of the presence of intra- or sub-mucosal carcinoma in the pathology of resection specimens of the esophagus when surgery is performed for high-grade dysplasia only. Looking at the results of authors with a personal experience of 10 patients or more they show a wide variety of 12-73% adenocarcinomas in patients primarily resected for high-grade dysplasia[15-21] (Table 1). In only 3 series the TNM-staging is given. 50%-75% of these small numbers is stage I, 20% stage II and just 5% stage III. So lymph node metastases are rare in patients with adenocarcinoma who underwent resection for high-grade dysplasia.

TABLE 1. Collective series of patients with adenocarcinoma resected for high-grade dysplasia arising in Barrett's esophagus

Name	Year	No. of patients	No. With adenocarcinoma in resected specimen. (%)
Schnell[15]	1989	43	21 (49%)
Pera[16]	1992	18	9 (50%)
Rice[17]	1993	16	6 (38%)
Wright[18]	1994	15	7 (47%)
Edwards[19]	1996	11	8 (73%)
Heitmiller[20]	1996	30	13 (43%)
Cameron and Carpenter[21]	1997	19	2 (11%)
Current series	2001	17	2 (12%)
Total	1989-2001	169	68 (40%)

4.1 OWN RESULTS

We performed an esophageal resection and reconstruction in 17 patients with high-grade dysplasia in repeated biopsies. Among those 17 patients were 3 female patients. The average age of both groups was 65 years. Prolonged gastro-esophageal reflux symptoms were present in 6 patients. There was a documented previous history of Barrett's esophagus in 10 patients. All patients underwent transhiatal resection of the esophagus and stomach tube reconstruction with colonic interposition in 1 patient. There were no postoperative deaths.

Two patients (12%) were found to have invasive adenocarcinoma in the resected esophagus, whereas 14 patients (82%) were found to have high-grade dysplasia only and 1 patient (6%) had low-grade dysplasia but showed again high-grade dysplasia in the re-evaluated biopsy (Figure 3).

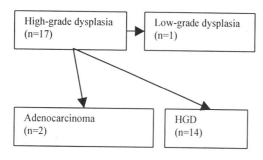

Figure 3: Distribution of diagnosis of patients resected for high-grade dysplasia.

Surprisingly, both patients with adenocarcinoma had a T2N0M0 carcinoma. Preoperative symptoms and postoperative complications are given in Table 2. Both patients with adenocarcinoma are still alive. Concluding from our results we can say that it is safe and possibly justified to perform surgery for high-grade dysplasia.

5. SURGICAL TREATMENT OF SUPERFICIAL CARCINOMA.

Once intestinal metaplasia in Barrett's esophagus under surveillance progresses to high-grade dysplasia, or when high-grade dysplasia is detected at first presentation, surgical treatment is recommended in otherwise healthy patients. Even a Barrett's esophagus, in which the columnar epithelium shows no abnormalities like nodules or ulceration, can harbor early carcinoma mostly restricted to the mucosa. In a selected series of Nigro et al. these occult lesions were analyzed in 33 referred patients.

TABLE 2.   Patients Characteristics of patients with high-grade dysplasia in biopsy.

	(n=17)
Age	65
Sex (M/F)	13/3
Symptoms	
- reflux	6 (35%)
- weight loss	3 (18%)
Hiatal hernia	11 (65%)
Surgical complications	
- bleeding	1 (6%)
- anast. leak.	2 (12%)
- rec. paresis	1 (6%)
Non surgical complications	8 (47%)
Late surgical complications	
- stenosis	4 (24%)
- weight loss	2 (12%)
PO mortality	-

Twenty-three patients showed high-grade dysplasia at first presentation and 10 had early adenocarcinoma with no endoscopically visible lesion in the Barrett's segment[22]. From the 23 patients, 9 showed occult adenocarcinoma at repeated biopsy. All patients underwent esophageal resection: transhiatally in the high-grade dysplasia patients and transthoracic in the carcinoma patients. In the resection specimens of the first group another 6 adenocarcinomas were detected. These 25 occult adenocarcinomas harbored 22 T1mucosal lesions, 3 T1submucosal lesions one of which had a positive lymph node.

Figures regarding the prevalence of occult adenocarcinoma are scarce and vary between 33% for T1a tumors to 10% for T1b tumors[23]. In this light the aforementioned series is exceptional with regard to the high percentage of carcinomas compared to the current literature but nevertheless we can conclude that even "normal" appearing columnar lined epithelium is no guarantee for the absence of carcinoma. Furthermore, when occult adenocarcinoma is detected, it is detected mostly at a T1a stage with lymph node metastases in less than 4% of the total group of patients with a T1 adenocarcinoma.

In our view, especially in these patients there is a place for transhiatal esophagectomy without intrathoracic lymph node dissection.

TABLE 3. Positive lymph nodes in relation to mucosal and submucosal tumor invasion.

Name	Year	T1a	N+ (%)	T1b	N+ (%)
Holscher[24]	1997	10	- (-)	31	5 (16)
Ruol[25]	1997	4	- (-)	22	8 (36)
Rice[26]	1998	38	1 (3)	27	6 (22)
Nigro[27]	1999	15	1 (7)	12	6 (50)
van Sandick[23]	2000	12	- (-)	20	6 (30)
Current series	2000	24	- (-)	47	12 (26)

Moreover when we take a closer look at the T1 patients from larger series of patients resected for adenocarcinoma we can conclude that patients with T1a carcinomas have very seldom lymph node metastases and patients with T1b have lymph node metastases in 16% - 50%[23-27] (Table 3).

5.1 OWN RESULTS

From our own series of resected specimens we collected a group of 71 patients with a T1 adenocarcinoma diagnosed during 1982 - 1999. 58 patients were found to have a T1N0M0 adenocarcinoma (group 1), whereas 12 patients (17%) were found to have a T1N1M0 adenocarcinoma (group 2). Only one patient had a T1N2M0 tumor (Figure 4).

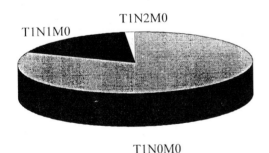

Figure 4. Piechart of TNM distribution of all operated patients with a T1 tumor diagnosed during 1982 – 1999.

Among those patients were 58 male patients and 13 female patients. The average age of both groups was 63 years. Prolonged gastro-esophageal reflux symptoms were present in 15 (26%) group 1 patients and 2 (17 %) group 2 patients. There was a history of Barrett's disease in 27 (47%) group 1 patients and 6 (50%) group 2 patients. All patients underwent esophageal resection. In group 1 there were 5 (9%) postoperative deaths, 3 died from a non-surgical complication and 2 from a surgical

complication. There was one (8%) postoperative death in group 2 due to non-surgical complications. Twenty-one (36%) group 1 patients had surgical complications, 2 had postoperative bleeding, 6 patients had anastomotic leakage, 9 patients had paresis of the recurrent laryngeal nerve, 2 developed a thoracic duct lesion. Six group 2 patients had surgical complications, 1 had postoperative bleeding, 3 showed anastomotic leakage and 1 developed a thoracic duct lesion.

There were 16 (28%) group 1 patients with late surgical complications and 2 (17%) group 2 patients. Thirteen (22%) group 1 patients had stenosis and 2 group 2 patients.

Finally 18 group 1 patients died after a mean follow-up of 50 Months. Nine group 2 patients died after a mean follow-up of 17.5 months (Table 4).

When we compare the survival from the three groups, high-grade dysplasia, T1N0M0 and T1N1M0 group we see that patients with high-grade dysplasia or a T1N0M0 tumor have a better survival than patients with positive lymph nodes (Figure 5).

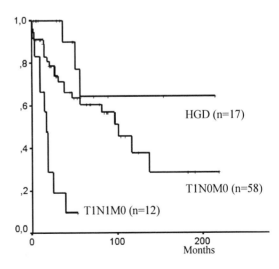

Figure 5. Kaplan Meier Survival Plot of patients with preoperative high-grade dysplasia , T1N0M0 en T1N1M0 adenocarcinoma.

TABLE 4. Patients Characteristics.
Group 1 = T1N0M0 and group 2 = T1N1M0
patients diagnosed during 1982 – 1999

	Group 1 (n=58)	Group 2 n=12
Age	63	63
Sex (M/F	48/10	9/3
Symptoms		
- reflux	15 (26%)	2 (17%)
-weight loss	7 (12%)	-
Hiatal hernia	36 (62%)	5 (42%)
BE	27 (47%)	6 (50%)
Achalasia	-	-
Surgical complications		
- bleeding	2 (3%)	1 (8%)
- anast. leak	6 (10%)	3 (25%)
- rec. n. paresis	9 (16%)	-
- chylothorax	2 (3%)	1 (8%)
Non-surgical complications	21 (36 %)	7 (58%)
Late surgical complications	16 (28%)	2 (17%)
PO mortality	5 (9%)	1(8%)
Late survival	40 (69%)	3 (25%)

6. INTESTINAL METAPLASIA OF THE DISTAL ESOPHAGUS AND THE GASTRO-ESOPHAGEAL JUNCTION.

Intestinal metaplasia of either a short segment of columnar lined epithelium of the distal esophagus or the gastro-esophageal junction is being identified with increasing frequency and therefore asks for a separate discussion[28]. The prevalence of this condition varies between 7% and 20%[29]. It is still unclear whether these conditions are pathogenetically related entities but there is increasing evidence that both are related to a risk of neoplastic changes in both distal esophagus and gastro-esophageal junction[30]. Dysplasia is reported with a prevalence of 8%-9% and also adenocarcinoma is described[31]. These adenocarcinomas are associated with short segments of columnar lined epithelium of the esophagus of less than 3 cm[32].
Van Sandick et al., in a careful study, compared 23 patients with intestinal metaplasia of the gastro-esophageal junction (IM-OGJ) and 14 patients with intestinal metaplasia of a columnar lined distal

esophagus (IM-CLE)[33]. Distinctive features of IM-CLE confirmed it's association with gastro-esophageal reflux while, in contrast, IM-OGJ significantly was associated with intestinal metaplasia in other parts of the stomach. They concluded that IM-OGJ and IM-CLE should be regarded as two separate entities and that the malignant potential of the former condition is lower. Nevertheless it is not impossible that cardial metaplasia is an earlier precursor lesion and also related to gastro-esophageal reflux but that it is more dynamic in its expression. Support for this view is found in a study from DeMeester et al. who compared anti-reflux surgery for both IM-OGJ and IM-CLE in patients with gastro-esophageal reflux disease. They state that IM-OGJ is an acquired condition because it is never seen in individuals under 20 years of age and that it is possibly related to reflux. When detected in the presence of reflux it is invariable inflamed and called "carditis". In this condition it harbors intestinal metaplasia in 10%-15% of patients. After anti-reflux surgery the group of patients with IM-OGJ showed regression of the intestinal metaplasia in 75% of patients whereas regression in patients with IM-CLE was negligible[34].
The role of surgery in patients with uncomplicated intestinal metaplasia of the gastro-esophageal junction is not clear. When concurrent gastro-esophageal reflux disease is present anti-reflux can offer relief of symptoms with a possible beneficial effect on the "carditis" and regression of metaplasia. As the possibility of potential degeneration until now is not clear, asymptomatic intestinal metaplasia of the cardia without "carditis" and without synchronous intestinal metaplasia in adjacent columnar lined epithelium of the esophagus is not an indication for surgical treatment.

7. CONCLUSION

In patients with dysplasia in Barrett's esophagus, two expert pathologists should confirm the grade of the dysplasia. The diagnosis should be confirmed in several biopsies in order to rule out the "biopsy-cured" high-grade dysplasia. In case of high-grade dysplasia resection of the esophagus should be offered to otherwise healthy patients. As upper mediastinal lymph node metastases are a rare finding in distal adenocarcinomas, intrathoracic lymph node dissection seems of no influence on survival[35]. Moreover, some patients die after prophylactic esophagectomy for high-grade dysplasia without any sign of carcinoma in the resection-specimen; a situation which should be avoided at all cost[21].

A lymph node dissection of the celiac trunk and its branches does not increase the morbidity and is advised in order to increase the long-term survival of only the small group of patients showing lymph node metastases in their resection specimen. In conclusion, when 10 patients with high-grade dysplasia undergo an esophageal resection, 4 or 5 patients show an adenocarcinoma of the esophagus. Three of these have a T1 tumor confined to the mucosa without lymph node metastases, one is a T1-carcinoma growing into the submucosa with a N1 positive node and one tumor is more advanced. In the light of these figures a restricted approach to the extend of the lymph node dissection seems rational.

REFERENCES

1. Goseki N, Koike M, Yoshida M. Histopathologic characteristics of early stage esophageal carcinoma. A comparative study with gastric carcinoma. Cancer 1992;69:1088-93.

2. Rice TW. Superficial oesophageal carcinoma: is there a need for three-field lymphadenectomy? The Lancet 1999;354:79204.

3. Low DE, Levine DS, Dail DH, Kozarek RA. Histological and anatomic changes in Barrett's esophagus after antireflux surgery. Am J Gastroenterol 1999:94(1):80-5.

4. Chen LQ, Nastos D, Hu CY, Chughtai TS, Taillefer R, Ferraro P, Duranceau AC. Results of the Collis-Nissen gastroplasty in patients with Barrett's esophagus. Ann Thorac Surg 1999;68:1014-21.

5. Wijnhoven BPL, Siersema PD, Hop WC, Dekken van H, Tilanus HW. Adenocarcinomas of the distal oesophagus and gastric cardia are one clinical entity. Br J Surg 1999;86(4):529-35.

6. Williamson WA, Ellis FH Jr, Gibb SP, Shahian DM, Aretz HT. Effect of antireflux operation on Barrett's mucosa. Ann Thorac Surg 1990;49:537-42.

7. Sagar PM, Ackroyd R, Hosie KB, Patterson JE, Stoddard CJ, Kingsnorth AN. Regression and progression of Barrett's oesophagus after antireflux surgery. Br J Surg 1995;82:806-10.

8. Ortiz A, Martinez de Haro L, Parilla P, et al. Conservative treatment versus antireflux surgery in Barrett's oesophagus: long-term results of a prospective study. Br J Surg 1996;83:274-8.

9. DeMeester TR, Attwood SE, Smyrk TC, Therkildsen DH, Hiner RA. Surgical therapy in Barrett's esophagus. Ann Surg 1990;212:528-40.

10. Csendes A, Braghetto I, Burdiles P, Puente G, Korn O, Diaz JC, Maluenda F. Long-term results of classic antireflux surgery in 152 patients with Barrett's esophagus: Clinical, radiologic, endoscopic, manometric, and acid reflux test analysis before and late after operation. Surgery 1998;123(6):645-57,

11. Clark GWB, DeMeester TR. Surgical Mamagement of Barrett's esophagus. Ann Chir et Gynaecol 1995;84:139-44.

12. Riddel RH, Goldman H, Ransohoff DF et al. Dysplasia in inflammatory bowel disease: standardized classification with provisional clinical applications. Hum Pathol 1983;14(11):931-68.

13. Morson BC, Sobin LH, Grundmann E, Johansen A, Nagayo T, Serck-Hanssen A. Precancerous conditions and epithelial dysplasia in the stomach. J Clin Pathol 1980;33:711-21.

14. Reid BJ, Haggit RC, Rubin CE et al. Observer variation in the diagnosis of dysplasia in Barrett's esophagus. Hum Pathol 1988;19:166-78.

15. Schnell T, Sontag S, Chejfec G, Chintam R, O'Connel S, Kurucar C. High grade dysplasia in Barrett's esophagus: a report of experience in 43 patients.Gastroenterol 1989;96(suppl):A452 (abstract).

16. Pera M, Trastek VF, Carpenter HA, Allen MS, Deschamps C, Pairolero PC. Barrett's esophagus with high-grade dysplasia: and indication for esophagectomy? Ann Thoracic Surg 1992;54:199-204.

17. Rice TW, Falk GW, Achkar E, Petras RE. Surgical management of high grade dysplasia in Barrett's esophagus. Am J Gastroenterol 1993;88:1832-6.

18. Wright TA, Myskow MW, Nash J, Gray M, Kingsnorth AN. High grade dysplasia in Barrett's esophagus. How should it be managed? GUT 1995;35(suppl2):S22(abstract).

19. Edwards MJ, Gable DR, Lentsch B, Richardson JD. The rationale for esophagectomy as the optimal therapy for Barrett's esophagus with high-grade dysplasia. Ann Surg 1996;223(5):585-91.

20. Heitmiller RF, Redmond M, Hamilton SR. Barrett's esophagus with high-grade dysplasia. An indication for prophylactic esophagectomy. Ann Surg 1996;224(1):66-71.

21. Cameron AJ, Carpenter HA. Barrett's esophagus, high-grade dysplasia, and early adenocarcinoma: a pathological study. Am J Gatroenterol 1997;92(4):586-91.

22. Nigro JJ, Hagen JA, DeMeester TR, DeMeester SR, Theisen J, Peters JH, Kiyabu M. Occult esophageal adenocarcinoma. Extent of disease and implications for effective therapy. Ann Surg 1999;230(3):433-40.

23. Sandick van J, Lanschot van J, Kate ten FJ, Offerhaus GJ, Fockens P, Tytgat G, Obertop H. Pathology of early invasive adenocarcinoma of the esophagus or esophagogastric junction: Implications for therapeutic decision making. Cancer 2000;88(11):2429-37.

24. Hölscher AH, Bollschweiler E, Schneider P.M, Siewert JR. Early adenocarcinoma in Barrett's esophagus. Br J Surg 1997;84:1470-3.

25. Ruol A, Merigliano S, Baldan N, Santi S, Petrin GF, Bonavina L, Ancona E, Peracchia A. Prevalence, management and outcome of early adenocarcinoma (pT1) of the esophago-gastric junction. Dis Esophagus 1997; 10(3): 190-5.

26. Rice TW, Zuccaro G, Adelstein DJ, Rybicki LA, Blackstone EH, Goldblum JR. Esophageal carcinoma: dept of tumor invasion is predictive of regional lymph node status. Ann Thorac Surg 1998;65:787-92.

27. Nigro JJ, Hagen JA, DeMeester TR, DeMeester SR, Peters JH, Oberg S et al. Prevalence and location of nodal metastases in distal esophageal adenocarcinoma confined to the wall: implications for therapy. J Thorac and Cardiovasc Surg 1999;117(1):1625.

28. Spechler SJ. The columnar lined oesophagus: a riddle wrapped in a mystery inside an enigma. GUT 1997;41:710-11.

29. Trudgill NJ, Suvarna SK, Kapur KC et al. Intestinal metaplasia at the squamocolumnar junction in patients attending for diagnostic gastroscopy. GUT 1997;41:585-9.

30. Menke-Pluymers MBE, Hop WCJ, Dees J et al. Risk factors for the development of an adenocarcinoma in columnar lined (Barrett) esophagus. Cancer 1993;72:1155-8.

31. Sharma P, Morales TG, Bhattacharyya A et al. Dysplasia in short segment Barrett's esophagus: a prospective 3-year follow-up. Am J Gastroenterol 1997;2:2012-16.
32. Cameron AJ, Lomboy CT, Pera M et al. Adenocarcinoma of the esophagogastric junction and Barrett's esophagus. Gastroenterol 1995;109:1541-6.
33. Sandick van JW. Early detection and surgical treatment of adenocarcinoma of the esophagus or oesophageal gastric junction. Thesis. Amsterdam University , The Netherlands, 1999.
34. DeMeester SR, Campos GMR, DeMeester TR, Bremner CG, Hagen JA, Peters JH, Crookes PF. The impact of an antireflux procedure on intestinal metaplasia of the cardia. Ann Surg 1998;228(4):547-56.
35. Siewert JR, Stein HJ, Sendler A, Fink U. Surgical resection for cancer of the cardia. Semin Surg Oncol 1999;17(2):125-31.

5.1 EPIDEMIOLOGY OF BARRETT'S ESOPHAGUS AND ADENOCARCINOMA

Alan J. Cameron

1. INTRODUCTION

Norman Barrett described the columnar lined esophagus in 1950[1]. In another paper written in 1957[2] he acknowledged the opinion of Allison and Johnstone[3] that the condition represented an acquired disorder, associated with reflux. There is no useful information about its epidemiology before the widespread use of flexible endoscopy in the last quarter of the twentieth century.

1.1 DEFINITIONS

For the purpose of this review, the following arbitrary definitions will be used. Barrett's esophagus (BE) will imply the classical long segment of columnar epithelium in the lower esophagus, usually referring to 3 cm or longer when measured. Essentially all the older literature refers to this type. Short segment Barrett's esophagus (SSBE) refers to segments or tongues of visible columnar epithelium with intestinal metaplasia of less than 3 cm length. Intestinal metaplasia of the cardia refers to the histological finding of intestinal metaplasia below a normally located squamocolumnar junction. This will not be classified as Barrett's esophagus. Adenocarcinoma of the esophagus refers to tumors in which the center of the tumor, or the main bulk of the tumor, is in the esophagus. Adenocarcinoma of the cardia refers to tumors that extend across the esophagogastric junction, involving both the lower esophagus and the proximal stomach. In practice, the distinction between adenocarcinoma arising in these 2 sites is often arbitrary.

1.2 PREVALENCE OF BE IN PATIENTS HAVING ENDOSCOPY

The prevalence of Barrett's esophagus in consecutive patients having endoscopy for any clinical indication was reviewed by Philips and Wong[4]. Usually the age, sex distribution, and the indication for the endoscopy were not recorded in these older reports. In multiple series, BE was found in 0.3-2% of cases, with a median of about 1%. In an Italian multicenter study, 0.74% of 14,898 patients having endoscopy had BE[5]. In a report from Olmsted County, Minnesota,[6] we found a consistent BE prevalence of about 1% in patients having endoscopy over 25 years (Figure 1).

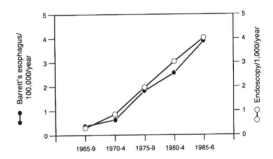

Figure 1. Increasing incidence of diagnosed Barrett's esophagus in Olmsted County, USA, which occurred in parallel with the increasing utilization of upper gastrointestinal endoscopy in the same population. From: Cameron 1990[6] (with permisson)

1.3 PREVALENCE OF BE IN PATIENTS WITH REFLUX SYMPTOMS

Heartburn and acid reflux are common complaints. It is estimated that 15-20% of the adult Western population has heartburn at least once per week [7-10], and about 7% have daily heartburn. BE is believed to be the result of reflux damage to the normal squamous esophageal lining, and most patients with BE have reflux symptoms. Therefore, patients with reflux symptoms should have a higher prevalence of BE than unselected patients undergoing diagnostic endoscopy, and this has been shown. In older retrospective reports, 8-20% of patients with reflux symptoms had BE[11]. The first prospective study of BE in reflux patients was that of Winters et al[12]. They found a 3 cm or longer BE in 12% of 97 patients. Only 6 of these (6%) had intestinal metaplasia on biopsy, and the diagnosis of BE may be questioned in the absence of metaplasia. Mann et al[13] in a similar study found BE in 11% of patients with reflux symptoms. Again, only 7% of the total had intestinal metaplasia confirmed.

H.W. Tilanus and S.E.A. Attwood (eds.), Barrett's Esophagus, 281–290.

Note that both these studies were in male populations, and the prevalence of BE was later shown to be higher in males than in females. In a prospective study of patients of both sexes with heartburn occurring at least weekly, who had never had a previous endoscopy, we found BE in 7 of 200 (3.5%) cases[14].

1.4 AGE AND GENDER DIFFERENCES

BE is an acquired disorder, and its prevalence increases with age. True BE with goblet cell metaplasia is a rare occurrence in children[15]. In a study of 377 patients with BE found in some 51,000 patients having upper gastrointestinal endoscopy at the Mayo Clinic over 20 years, the prevalence was very low in childhood, and increased up to about age 60 (Figure 2)

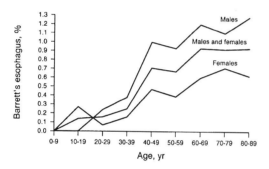

Figure 2. The proportion of patients having endoscopy at Mayo Clinic for any indication, who had Barrett's esophagus, increased with age. Barrett's esophagus was more prevalent in males than females. From Cameron 1992[16] (with permission).

About half the maximum prevalence was reached by about age 40, and the author suggested that was the approximate mean age of developing the condition. The mean age of diagnosing BE in that series was 63 years. It was proposed that the BE found in a patient of that age had probably been present, although not detected, for a mean of perhaps 20-25 years.

In the above report, including patients studied between 1976 and 1989, BE was found to be twice as prevalent in males compared to females. In the large multicenter Italian study [5], with patients enrolled from 1987-1989, BE was 2.6 times more common in males than in females having endoscopy. Two more recent reports showed a greater male preponderance. The data of Hirota et al[17] shows a male/female ratio of 5.5/1. We recently updated our prevalence data

in Olmsted County residents. The numbers of males and females having endoscopy were almost equal, but the prevalence of diagnosed BE in county residents in January 1998 was 148 per 100,000 population in males, 4.1 times greater than the prevalence of 36 per 100,000 in females. It is possible that the male predominance in prevalence of BE has increased over the years.

1.5 GEOGRAPHY AND RACE

BE is frequently described in Western countries, but is apparently rare in other areas, for example Japan, although this may be changing[18]. In South Africa, BE was much more often found in whites than in blacks[19]. In an American study[17], BE was found in 6.5% of 611 white patients having endoscopy, compared to 0 of 200 African Americans.

1.6 PREVALENCE IN PATIENTS WITH AND WITHOUT REFLUX SYMPTOMS

As discussed above, BE is more prevalent in patients with gastroesophageal reflux symptoms (about 5%) than in patients having endoscopy for all clinical indications (about 1%). However, some patients with BE do not have heartburn or acid reflux. Patients presenting with symptoms caused by an adenocarcinoma of the esophagus are often found on endoscopy to have a previously undiagnosed BE in which the adenocarcinoma arose. Some of these patients will admit to a long preceding history of reflux symptoms, but others do not give such a history. In 5 series of patients with adenocarcinoma and BE found simultaneously, a history of preceding reflux symptoms was obtained in 52%[20], 54%[21], 59%[22], 61%[23], 62%[24], and 65%[25] of cases.

1.7 PROGRESSION AND REGRESSION OF BE

Once a patient has acquired a BE, the columnar lined esophagus is unlikely either to regress or to increase in length. We showed[16] that the mean length of BE in patients aged from the 20s to the 80s was the same, 6-7cm. In 21 patients that we followed by endoscopy for a mean of 7.3 years, the length of BE remained the same. Therefore, for population prevalence data, we assume that a patient with a previous diagnosis of BE still has the condition, even if no recent endoscopy has been done.

1.8 INDIRECT ESTIMATION OF POPULATION BE PREVALENCE

Assume that 20% of the population have frequent reflux symptoms, and that 5% of persons with such symptoms have a BE. This suggests that 1% of the population (of older adults) has a symptomatic BE. Assume that 40% of persons with BE do not have reflux symptoms. This would give a total estimate for BE, in those with and without symptoms, that 1.67 % of the older adult population has a BE. This is only an estimate, but shows that BE is not a rare disorder in the general population.

1.9 POPULATION PREVALENCE OF BE.

Information is limited because not many population-wide studies of all patients having endoscopy are available. However, this type of study has been reported by our group at the Mayo Clinic. The Clinic is located in Rochester, Minnesota, which is in Olmsted County, which has a population just over 100,000. For research purposes, we are able to review the records of essentially all residents of the county, including the endoscopic reports from the only two medical groups that perform endoscopy in the county, Mayo Clinic and Olmsted Medical Group.
The clinically diagnosed prevalence of BE included those patients with endoscopic and biopsy findings of BE, established previously, who were still resident in the county. As of January 1, 1987, the clinically diagnosed prevalence of BE, adjusted to correspond to the age and sex distribution of the general US white population, was 22.6 per 100,000[6]. By January 1, 1998, the clinically diagnosed prevalence of BE in the county had increased almost fourfold to 80.3 per 100,000. We believed that the increased prevalence was mainly because the increased use of endoscopy resulted in more cases being detected[26].
In our study, comparing 1965-9 with 1995-7, the number of new cases of BE diagnosed per 100,000 population per year increased from 0.37 to 10.5, a 28 times increase. Over the same years, the number of upper endoscopic examinations performed on county residents increased from 65 to 1461 per 100,000 population per year, a 22 times increase.
A different opinion was given by Prach et al[27]. In a brief report from Dundee, Scotland, they found that the incidence of new diagnosis of BE increased from 1 per 100,000 population in

1980-81 to 48 per 100,000 per year in 1992-93. They found that the rate of BE detection increased over the same years from 1.4 to 42.7 (16.5 if only cases with histologic confirmation were included) per 1000 endoscopic examinations performed. They believed there had been a true increase in the incidence of BE.

1.10 PREVALENCE OF BE AT AUTOPSY

One autopsy study with the specific aim of finding the prevalence of BE has been reported[6]. In this study, we arranged for the esophagus and upper part of the stomach to be removed as a single piece in consecutive Mayo Clinic autopsies. The specimens thus obtained were examined later the same day by an endoscopist, and histological sections made whenever the squamocolumnar junction appeared to be above the gastroesophageal junction. We found 7 cases of BE in 733 consecutive unselected autopsies. At the time of this study, the age and sex adjusted prevalence of BE in Olmsted County residents, based on autopsy, was estimated as 376 per 100,000 population.

1.11 WHAT IS THE "TRUE" PREVALENCE OF BE?

As discussed above, indirect estimates of population prevalence based on the prevalence of reflux symptoms and on the frequency of BE in patients gave an estimate of 1.67 cases of BE per 100 population for adults. The estimate for patients having endoscopy for any clinical indication was about 1%, similar to our finding of BE in about 1 % of persons having autopsy. Each of these methods of estimating the population prevalence gives a reasonably similar result for the prevalence in the older population. However, BE is rare in children and young adults. The writer suggests that the true prevalence of BE is about 1 in 100 older (over age 60) persons, or about 1 in 250 persons in the general population including all ages. This implies that there are about 1 million persons in the US with BE, of whom a majority are males.

1.12 COMPARISON OF "TRUE" AND CLINICALLY DIAGNOSED PREVALENCE.

Our autopsy study [6] gave an estimate of 376 cases per 100, 000 population in Olmsted County. This was about 20 times greater than the clinically diagnosed prevalence of 22.6 per 100,000 in the county at that time. In our 1990 paper, we concluded that the majority of cases of BE in the population had not been detected. By 1998 the clinically diagnosed prevalence of BE in our county had increased to 80.3 per 100,000. If we assume (and this is only an assumption) that the true prevalence of BE had not changed in the previous 11 years, then we may have now diagnosed about 1 in 5 of the actual cases of BE in our county, rather than the 1 in 20 estimated in 1987.

There is other data indicating that a majority of cases of BE in the general population do not know that they have this condition. In a study of 196 patients with adenocarcinoma of the esophagus or cardia[28], only 5% had a BE diagnosed prior to the onset of symptoms related to the tumor. In another study of 189 patients with adenocarcinoma of the esophagus[29], 62% had a BE diagnosed at the same time as the cancer. These findings accord with general clinical experience. These facts suggest that many patients with BE are never diagnosed unless they develop a carcinoma.

1.13 SIGNIFICANCE OF THE DIFFERENCE BETWEEN THE "TRUE" AND THE CLINICALLY DIAGNOSED PREVALENCE

The above information indicates that most individuals with BE in the population have not been recognized, even in our county with its exceptional medical facilities. Most cases are not under surveillance for early detection of dysplasia or early adenocarcinoma. Thus, present efforts to reduce the population death rate from BE related cancer will only have a limited impact.

We have not considered a general population screening program to find new cases of BE to be a realistic proposition. We have no plans to perform endoscopy in the 15-20% of the population that have reflux symptoms every week, which might detect about 60% of the cases of BE in the population. In a population of 100,000 this would involve doing screening endoscopy in many thousands of persons, with the possible benefit of preventing about 2 cancer deaths per year. There are more efficient uses of medical resources.

1.14 SHORT SEGMENTS AND TONGUES OF BE

Most of the epithelium in a long BE consists of intestinal metaplasia containing goblet cells. When the endoscopist finds a segment or tongues

of red lining in the lower esophagus, less than 3 cm long, and biopsy shows intestinal metaplasia, SSBE is diagnosed. Adenocarcinomas may be found in a background of SSBE[30].

Population based information on the incidence and prevalence of SSBE is limited. In Olmsted County, we did not record this diagnosis before 1989. Earlier cases that would now be classified as SSBE were seen but not indexed as such. After 1989 we made a clinical diagnosis of SSBE with increasing frequency. By 1998, the prevalence of SSBE in the county was 33 per 100,000 with a 2:1 male predominance. The number of new cases of SSBE found per year had risen by 1997 to about the same as that of long segment BE. As with BE, we assume that most cases of SSBE in the population are undetected because they have not had endoscopy.

The endoscopic and biopsy diagnosis of SSBE is less specific than that of BE, so prevalence data on SSBE has to be interpreted cautiously. The writer has found that in many cases it is impossible to determine whether small upward extensions of the squamocolumnar junction for 1-2 cm seen at endoscopy represent normal variations the Z-line or SSBE. The finding of intestinal metaplasia on biopsy in such cases does not prove SSBE, because intestinal metaplasia of the cardia is common in patients with no visible evidence of BE of any length.

1.15 GENETIC FACTORS AND BE

Families are reported in which multiple members have BE, sometimes with associated esophageal adenocarcinoma[31,32,33]. Other members of these kindreds had reflux disease without BE. The authors suggested that in these families there might be an inherited predisposition to reflux, which led to development of BE in some cases. As cases were found in consecutive generations, in both sexes, an autosomal dominant inheritance was postulated. In 2 recent reports, it was shown that first degree family members of patients with BE were more likely to have at least weekly reflux symptoms than controls, with odds ratios of 2.2[34] and 4.8[35]. At the time of writing, the prevalence of BE in relatives of BE patients had not been reported.

1.16 INTESTINAL METAPLASIA OF THE CARDIA

In 1994 Spechler[36] reported 142 consecutive patients, without endoscopic evidence of BE, in whom biopsies were taken routinely from the squamocolumnar junction. Histological evidence of intestinal metaplasia was found in 18%, and was equally common in those with or without symptoms of gastroesophageal reflux. This finding has been confirmed many times. Intestinal metaplasia at the cardia was found in 6%[17], 7%[37], 10%[38], 18%[39], 23%[40], and in 36%[41] of cases having gastroscopy. The finding of intestinal metaplasia of the cardia, unlike long segment BE, was of similar prevalence in males and females. The prevalence increased with age, suggesting that it was an acquired condition[14,38].

There are no population based studies on the prevalence of this condition, and no follow up studies of such patients, but the practical conclusion seems clear. If about 1 in 5 of the older population has intestinal metaplasia at the cardia, then the risk of any individual with that finding developing an adenocarcinoma must be extremely remote.

1.17 RISK OF ADENOCARCINOMA AND DEATH IN BE

In 1995 Tytgat[42] reviewed 18 series in which patients with a long segment BE were followed to determine the risk of later development of adenocarcinoma. The risk for a patient with BE to develop esophageal cancer in 3 of these series was 30-52 times greater than for the general population. Cancers were diagnosed at a median rate of about 1 case per 100 patient-years of follow-up. However, these reports, often based on a short follow-up with the chance of including early prevalent cancers as incidence cases, may overestimate the cancer risk. More recent reports with longer follow-up found 1 cancer per 180[43] and 1 cancer per 208[44] patient-years.

Cancers in patients with BE are not always fatal. Van der Burgh[43] found that 79 patients with BE and no cancer at the time of diagnosis of BE died of various causes over a mean 9.3 year follow-up; 5 of 79 had developed esophageal cancer, but only 2 of these actually died from the cancer. Therefore, in that report, only 2.5% of deaths in patients with BE were due to esophageal cancer. The authors concluded that their patients would not have benefited from a surveillance program. Adenocarcinomas may be associated with short tongues or segments of intestinal metaplasia[30]. At present there is insufficient data to show the cancer risk for patients with short segments.

2. ADENOCARCINOMA

2.1 CHANGING DISTRIBUTION OF GASTRIC ADENOCARCINOMA

While the incidence of carcinoma of the distal stomach has generally been declining in Western countries, the incidence of carcinoma of the cardia has increased. This changing pattern of distribution of gastric carcinoma was observed by Golematis et al in Greece[45]. Comparing 1976-81 with 1982-87, the proportion of carcinomas involving the cardia rose from 9.8% to 21.7%. In Boston, Antonioli and Goldman[46] found that carcinomas of the cardia represented 0% of 31 gastric cancer cases seen from 1938-1942 but rose to 27% of 62 gastric cancers seen 1975-1978. In a population based study from Oxfordshire, Rios-Castellanos et al[47] compared the incidence rates for different locations of gastric carcinomas in 1960-1964 with 1984-1988. The incidence of antral cancers fell from 10 to 4.5 per 100,000 while cardia cancers rose from 2.8 to 5.2 per 100,000. Note that the distinction between adenocarcinoma of the cardia (esophagogastric junction) and adenocarcinoma is often difficult, and that there has been a parallel increase in the incidence of both these cancers.

2.2 ADENOCARCINOMAS REPRESENT AN INCREASING PROPORTION OF ESOPHA-GEAL CANCERS

The esophagus is normally lined with squamous epithelium, and until about 1970 most esophageal cancers were squamous cell carcinomas. In 1955 Puestow et al[48] found only 0.8% of 603 esophageal cancers to be adenocarcinomas, and in 1968 Turnbull and Goodner[49] reported 2.4% of adenocarcinomas in 1859 esophageal cancers. Then there occurred a dramatic change. For example, in surgical series, Rahamian and Cham in 1993[50] reported 60% of 298 and Putnam et al in 1994[51] reported 68% of 221 esophageal cancers to be adenocarcinomas.

2.3 POPULATION BASED STUDIES OF ADENOCARCINOMA INCIDENCE

Population based studies provide the most useful information of cancer incidence. Multiple such population based reports have shown a large increase in the incidence of adenocarcinoma of the esophagus and esophagogastric junction in the last 30 years in North America, Western

Europe and Australia [52,53,54,55,56] (Figure 3). In contrast, although data is scanty, adenocarcinoma seems relatively rare in Japan and other Pacific Rim countries.

Blot et al[52] provided information from the National Cancer Institute's Surveillance, Epidemiology, and End Results (SEER) program, covering cancer registries for about 10% of the US population. Combining adenocarcinoma of the esophagus and esophagogastric junction, as similar trends in incidence were noted for both locations, between

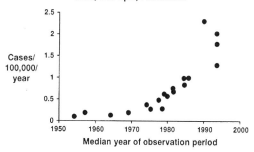

Incidence of Adenocarcinoma of Esophagus
U.S., Europe, Australia

Figure 3. Population-based studies from Western countries show a marked increase in the incidence of adenocarcinoma of the esophagus.

1976 and 1987 the incidence of these cancers increased by 4% to 10% per year in men. The authors stated that this was a greater increase than for any other cancer type. In a further NCI report[54], the incidence of adenocarcinoma of the esophagus in US white males rose over 350% from 0.7 during 1974-1976 to 3.2 per 100,000 during 1992-1994. Over the same interval, the incidence of squamous carcinoma fell from 3.4 to 2.2 per 100,000.

The author and his colleagues have recently updated Mayo Clinic data published earlier[53] from Olmsted County, Minnesota. Comparing 1965-74 with 1990-1997, the incidence of esophageal adenocarcinoma rose from 0.2 per 100,000 to 2.0, a tenfold increase. The incidence of adenocarcinoma of the esophagogastric junction rose to a similar extent, from 0.2 to 2.3 per 100,000 over the same years. Bytzer et al[55] reported from the Danish cancer registry a similar eight-fold increase in esophageal adenocarcinoma from 0.3 to 2.3 per 100,000 between 1970 and 1990. The increases are large in terms of percentage changes, but these are still uncommon malignancies compared to cancer of the colon, lung, breast and prostate. The cause of

the dramatic increase in esophageal and cardia adenocarcinoma incidence is not clear.

2.4 RACE, SEX AND RAGE

Multiple reports confirm that adenocarcinoma of the esophagus and cardia more often occur in white males[57]. In the SEER data, the adenocarcinoma incidence rates 1988-90 were 2.5 per 100,000 for American white males, 0.6 for black males, 0.3 for white females and 0.2 for black females. The sex and race differences are unexplained.

Most patients with adenocarcinoma of the esophagus are older individuals. In 1988 Yang and Davies[58] reported the incidence in men to be 0.1 age 30-39, 0.6 age 40-49, 1.8 age 50-59, 3.9 age 60-69, and 3.9 age 70-79.

2.5 ADENOCARCINOMA AND GASTRO-ESOPHAGEAL REFLUX DISEASE

Two reports have investigated the direct association between reflux and adenocarcinoma, rather than the presumed sequence of reflux disease leading to BE and BE leading later to adenocarcinoma.

Chow et al[28] reviewed the medical records of 196 patients with adenocarcinoma of the esophagus or cardia compared with 196 matched controls in California. The patients had a mean of 17 years of previous medical records available for review by investigators who were blinded as to the diagnosis (case or control). Only 9 patients and no controls had a previous diagnosis of BE. The patients with adenocarcinoma had reflux related histories more often than controls. After adjusting for race, smoking and obesity, the adenocarcinoma risk was increased (odds ratio significant) by factors of 2.1 for a history of reflux, 4.0 for hiatal hernia, and 5.2 for esophagitis or esophageal ulcer. There was no evidence of any increased risk from taking H2 antagonist or anticholinergic drugs.

Lagergren et al[29] interviewed 189 patients with esophageal adenocarcinoma and 262 with cardia adenocarcinoma, comprising 85% of the eligible patients in Sweden 1995-97. 820 population-based controls and 167 patients with squamous esophageal carcinoma were also interviewed. The methodology was different from that of Chow et al., in that reliance was placed on a history of reflux symptoms. Whilst this could be less specific than results of tests for reflux, many persons with reflux symptoms do not consult a physician and in those, the medical record would

TABLE 1. Smoking and adenocarcinoma; summary of case-control studies

Author	Adenoca location	Cases, n	Smoking: Odds Ratio vs controls
Kabat 1993[59]	Esoph and cardia	122	2.3 (95% CI, 1.4-3.9)
Brown 1994[60]	Esoph and cardia	174	2.1 (1.2-3.8)
Vaughan 1995[61]	Esoph and cardia	298	3.4 (1.4-8.0) (>80 pack years)
Zhang 1996[62]	Esoph and cardia	95	1.5 (0.7-3.0)
Gammon 1997[63]	Esophagus	293	2.2 (1.4-3.3)
	Cardia	261	2.6 (1.7-4.0)
Lagergren 1999[64]	Esophagus	189	1.6 (0.9-2.7)
	Cardia	262	4.5 (2.9-7.1)

TABLE 2. Obesity and adenocarcinoma; summary of case-control studies

Author	Adenoca location	Cases, n	Obesity: Odds Ratio vs non-obese
Vaughan 1995[61]	Esophagus	133	2.5 (1.2-5.0)
	Cardia	165	1.6 (0.8-3.0)
Zhang 1996[62]	Esoph and cardia	95	0.93 (0.83-1.03)
Chow 1998[65]	Esophagus	292	5.4 (2.4-12.0)
	Cardia	261	2.1 (1.1-4.1)
Lagergren 1999[66]	Esophagus	189	16.2 (6.3-41.4)
	Cardia	262	4.3 (2.1-8.7)

not reflect the reflux complaints. Lagergren et al found a strong and progressive correlation between reflux symptoms and adenocarcinoma. The esophageal adenocarcinoma risk was 7.7 times increased in persons with heartburn or acid reflux occurring at least once per week. For those with severe symptoms of 20 or more years duration, the risk was 43.5 times increased for esophageal adenocarcinoma, but only 4.4 times increased for cardia adenocarcinoma. There was no correlation between squamous carcinoma and reflux, the odds ratio being 1.1. The authors concluded that there was a strong and probably causal relation between reflux and esophageal adenocarcinoma. In 62% of their patients with esophageal adenocarcinoma, a BE was present, but the association with reflux was as strong for those patients in whom no BE was found. It is likely BE was originally present in many of these, as esophageal cancers can grow over and conceal the underlying BE in which they arose[24].

2.6 RISK FACTORS OTHER THAN REFLUX FOR ADENOCARCINOMA

Epidemiologic studies have addressed the important questions of possible environmental causes of esophageal and cardia adenocarcinoma. These studies have generally used a case-control design, with regression analysis for confounding factors. Earlier studies usually combined cancers in the 2 locations. Often, but not always, factors

associated with esophageal adenocarcinoma are also associated with cardia cancers. Most studies show a positive correlation between smoking and adenocarcinoma in both locations. The association is not as strong as with squamous cell carcinomas. Of interest, the risk for adenocarcinoma appears not to diminish with stopping smoking for up to 30 years, that is, ex-smokers continue to have an increased risk. Gammon et al interpreted their data as showing that 41% of all esophageal and cardia adenocarcinomas might be caused by smoking (attributable risk estimate). These results suggest that obesity is a factor in the etiology of esophageal adenocarcinoma and to a lesser extent cardia adenocarcinoma. Chow et al[65] interpreted their data to show obesity might account for 33% of esophageal and 22% of cardia cancers. While the cause of the increased incidence of adenocarcinomas in recent decades is not clear, the increase in obesity may be a factor. In the US, the proportion of adults who were obese (body mass index 30 or above) rose from 12.0% in 1991 to 17.9% in 1998[67].

2.7 ALCOHOL

In 6 case-control studies, 3 studies[59,60,61] showed a modest correlation between heavy alcohol intake and adenocarcinoma and 3 other studies, including the 2 largest,[62,63,64] showed no correlation. Alcohol is a major factor in the development of squamous cell carcinoma of the esophagus, but is of little importance in adenocarcinomas of the esophagus and cardia.

2.8 OTHER FACTORS

The prevalence of infection with H pylori is declining in the US. Chow et al[68] et al found an inverse relation between infection with cagA strains of this organism and adenocarcinomas of esophagus and cardia. If confirmed, this could indicate a possible protective effect of the organism that might possibly contribute to the rising incidence of adenocarcinoma.

A correlation between adenocarcinoma and lower income and education has been observed[60,63]. This could operate through differences in dietary habits, for example. Kabat et al[59] found adenocarcinomas correlating with a

high dietary fat intake, OR 2.9 (1.5-5.6), and with a low intake of dietary fiber, OR 3.2 (1.5-7). The predilection of adenocarcinomas of the esophagus and cardia for males is not understood. Lagergren and Nyren[69] followed over 100,000 Swedish men with prostate carcinoma, most of whom were taking estrogens. The prevalence of esophageal adenocarcinoma in this group was the same as in the general population, showing no protective effect from estrogen medication.

It does not appear, despite earlier fears, that medications increase the risk of adenocarcinoma. Chow et al[28] found no association with the use of H2 antagonists or anticholinergic drugs. Vaughan et al[70] found no correlation with the use of drugs that relaxed the lower esophageal sphincter, in particular with calcium channel blockers.

REFERENCES

1. Barrett NR. Chronic peptic ulcer of the oesophagus and "esophagitis". Br J Surg 1950; 38: 175-182.
2. Barrett NR. The lower esophagus lined by columnar epithelium. Surgery 1957; 41: 88-1894.
3. Allison PR, Johnstone AS. Oesophagus lined with gastric mucous membrane. Thorax 1953; 8: 87-93.
4. Philips RW, Wong RKH. Barrett's esophagus: Natural history, incidence, etiology, and complications. Gastroenterol Clin N Am 1991; 20: 791.
5. Gruppo Operativo per lo studio delle precancerosi dell esophago (GOSPE): Barrett's esophagus: epidemiological and clinical results of a multicentric survey. Int J Cancer 1991;48: 364.
6. Cameron AJ, Zinsmeister AR, Ballard DJ, Carney JA. Prevalence of columnar-lined (Barrett's) esophagus. Comparison of population-based clinical and autopsy findings. Gastroenterology 1990; 99: 918-922.
7. Nebel OT, Fornes MF, Castell DO. Symptomatic gastresophageal reflux: incidence and precipitating factors. Dig Dis Sci 1976; 21: 953-956.
8. Locke GR III, Talley NJ, Fett SR, Zinsmeister AR, Melton LJ III. Prevalence and clinical spectrum of gastroesophageal reflux: a population based study in Olmsted County, Minnesota. Gastroenterology 1997; 112: 1448-1456.
9. Thompson WG, Heaton KW. Heartburn and globus in apparently healthy people. Canad Med Ass J 1982; 126: 46-48.
10. Isolauri J, Laippala P. Prevalence of symptoms suggestive of gastroesophageal reflux in an adult population. Ann Med 1995;27: 67-70.
11. Spechler SJ, Goyal RK. Barrett's esophagus. N Engl J Med 1986; 315: 362-371.
12. Winters C, Spurling TJ, Chobanian SJ, Curtis DJ, Esposito RL, Hacker JF, Johnson DA, Cruess DF, Cotelingam JD, Gurney MS, Cattau EL. Barrett's esophagus. A prevalent, occult complication of gastroesophageal reflux disease. Gastroenterology 1987; 92: 118-124.
13. Mann NS, Tsai MF, Nair PK. Barrett's esophagus in patients with symptomatic reflux esophagitis. Am J Gastroenterol 1989; 84: 1494-1496.
14. Cameron AJ, Kamath PS, Carpenter HA. Prevalence of Barrett's esophagus and intestinal metaplasia at the esophagogastric junction. Gastroenterology 1997; 112: A82.
15. Hassall E. Barrett's esophagus: congenital or acquired? Am J Gastroenterol 1993; 88:819-824.
16. Cameron AJ, Lomboy CT. Barrett's esophagus: age, prevalence and the extent of columnar epithelium. Gastroenterology 1992; 103: 1241-1245.
17. Hirota WK, Loughney TM, Lazas DJ, Maydonovitch CL, Rholl V, Wong RKH. Specialized intestinal metaplasia, dysplasia and cancer of the esophagus and esophagogastric junction: prevalence and clinical data. Gastroenterology 1999; 116: 277-285.
18. Shoji T, Hongo M, Fukudo S, Handa M, Inaba H, Kano M, Narita H, Tamura D. Increasing incidence of Barrett's esophagus and Barrett's carcinoma in Japan. Gastroenterology 1999; 116: A 312.
19. Mason RJ, Bremner CG. The columnar-lined (Barrett's) oesophagus in black patients. S Afr J Surg 1998; 36: 61-62.
20. Williamson WA, Ellis FH, Gibb SP, Shahian DM, Aretz HT, Heatley GJ, Watkins E. Barrett's esophagus. Prevalence and incidence of adenocarcinoma. Arch Int Med 1991; 151: 2212-2216.
21. Van Sandick JW, Van Lanschot JJB, Kuiken BW, Tytgat GNJ, Offerhaus GJA, Obertop H. Impact of endoscopic biopsy surveillance of Barrett's oesophagus on pathological stage and clinical outcome of Barrett's carcinoma. Gut 1998; 43: 216-222.
22. Harle IA, Finley RJ, Belsheim M, Bondy DC, Booth M, Lloyd D, McDonald JWD, Sullivan S, Valberg LS, Watson WC, Frei JV, Slinger R, Troster M, Meads GE, Duff JH. Management of adenocarcinoma in columnar-lined esophagus. Ann ThoracSurg 1985;40:330-335.
23. Sanfey H, Hamilton SR, Smith RRL, Cameron JL. Carcinoma arising in Barrett's esophagus. Surg Gynecol Obstet 1985; 161: 570-4.
24. Cameron AJ, Ott BJ, Payne WS. The incidence of adenocarcinoma in columnar-lined (Barrett's) esophagus. N Engl J Med 1985; 313: 857-859.
25. Menke-Pluymers MBE, Schoute NW, Mulder AH, Hop WCJ, Van Blankenstein M, Tilanus HW. Outcome of surgical treatment of adenocarcinoma in Barrett's oesophagus. Gut 1992; 33: 1454-1458.

26. Conio M, Cameron AJ, Romero Y, Branch CD, Schleck CD, Burgart LJ, Zinsmeister AR, Locke GR III. Barrett's esophagus and adenocarcinoma. Prevalence and incidence in Olmsted County, Minnesota. Gastroenterology 1999; 116: A384.

27. Prach AJ, MacDonald TA, Hopwood DA, Johnston DA. Increasing incidence of Barrett's oesophagus: education, enthusiasm, or epidemiology? Lancet 1997; 350: 933.

28. Chow WC, Finkle WD, McLaughlin JK, Frankl H, Ziel HK, Fraumeni JF. The relation of gastroesophageal reflux disease and its treatment to adenocarcinomas of the esophagus and gastric cardia. JAMA 1995; 274: 474-7.

29. .Lagergren J, Bergstrom R, Lindgren A, Nyren O. Symptomatic gastroesophageal reflux as a risk factor for esophageal adenocarcinoma. N Engl J Med 1999; 340: 825-831.

30. Schnell TG, Sontag SJ, Chejfec G. Adenocarcinomas arising in tongues or short segments of Barrett's esophagus. Dig Dis Sci 1992; 37: 137-143.

31. Crabb DW, Berk MA, Hall TR, Conneally PM, Biegel AA, Lehman GA. Familial gastroesophageal reflux and development of Barrett's esophagus. Ann Int Med 1985; 103: 52-54.

32. Jochem VJ, Fuerst PA, Fromkes JJ. Familial Barrett's esophagus associated with adenocarcinoma. Gastroenterology 1992; 102: 1400-1402.

33. Fahmy N, King JF. Barrett's esophagus: an acquired condition with genetic predisposition. Am J Gastroenterol 1993; 88: 1262-1265.

34. Romero Y, Cameron AJ, Locke III GR, Schaid DJ, Slezak JM, Branch CD, Melton III LJ. Familial aggregation of gastroesophageal reflux in patients with Barrett's esophagus and esophageal adenocarcinoma. Gastroenterology 1997; 113: 1449-1456.

35. Trudgill NJ, Kapur KC, Riley AS. Familial clustering of reflux symptoms. Am J Gastroenterol 1999; 94:1172-1178.

36. Spechler SJ, Zeroogian JM, Antonioli DA, Wang HH, Goyal RK. Prevalence of metaplasia at the gastro-oesophageal junction. Lancet 1994; 344: 1533-1536.

37. Johnson MH, Hammond AS, Laskin W, Jones DM. The prevalence and clinical chararteristics of short segments of specialized intestinal metaplasia in the distal esophagus at routine endoscopy. Am J Gastroenterol 1996; 91: 1507-1511.

38. Voutilanen M, Farkkila M, Juhola M, Nuorva K, Mauranen K, Mantynen T, Kunnamo I, Mecklin J-P, Sipponen P. Specialized columnar epithelium of the esophagogastric junction: prevalence and associations. Am J Gastroenterol 1999; 94: 913-918.

39. Trudgill NJ, Suvarna SK, Kapur KC, Riley SA. Intestinal metaplasia at the squamocolumnar junction in patients attending for diagnostic endoscopy. Gut 1997; 41: 585-589.

40. Morales T, Sampliner RE, Bhattacharyya A. Intestinal metaplasia of the gastric cardia. Am J Gastroenterol 1997; 92: 414-418.

41. Nandurkar S, Talley NJ, Martin CJ, Ng THK, Adams S. Short segment Barrett's esophagus: prevalence, diagnosis and associations. Gut 1997; 40: 710-715.

42. Tytgat GNJ. Does endoscopic surveillance in esophageal columnar metaplasia have any real value? Endoscopy 1995; 27: 19-26.

43. Van der Burgh A, Dees J, Hop WCJ, et al. Oesophageal cancer is an uncommon cause of death in patients with Barrett's esophagus. Gut 1996; 39: 5-8.

44. Drewitz DJ, Sampliner RE, Garewal HS. The incidence of adenocarcinoma in Barrett's esophagus: a prospective study of 170 patients followed 4.8 years. Am J Gastroenterol 1997; 92: 212-215.

45. Golematis B, Tzardis P, Hatzikostas P, Papadimitriou K, Haritopoulos N. Changing pattern of distribution of carcinoma of the stomach. Br J Surg 1990; 77: 63-64.

46. Antonioli DA, Goldman H. Changes in the location and type of gastric adenocarcinoma. Cancer 1982; 50: 775-781

47. Rios-Castellanos E, Sitas F, Shepherd NA, Jewell DP. Changing pattern of gastric cancer in Oxfordshire. Gut 1992; 33: 1312-1317.

48. Puestow CB, Gillesby WJ, Guynn VL. Cancer of the esophagus. Arch Surg 1955; 70: 662-668.

49. Turnbull ADM, Goodner JT. Primary adenocarcinoma of the esophagus. Cancer 1968; 22: 915-918.

50. Rahamim J, Cham CW. Oesophagogastrectomy for carcinoma of the oesophagus and cardia. Br J Surg 1993; 80: 1305-1309.

51. Putnam JB, Suell DM, McMurtrey MJ, Ryan MB, Walsh GL, Natarajan G, Roth JA. Comparison of three techniques of esophagectomy within a residency training program. Ann Thorac Surg 1994; 57: 319-325.

52. Blot WJ, Devesa SS, Kneller RW, Fraumeni JF Jr. Rising incidence of adenocarcinoma of the esophagus and gastric cardia. JAMA 1991; 265: 1287-1289.

53. Pera M, Cameron AJ, Trastek VF, Carpenter HA, Zinsmeister AR. Increasing incidence of adenocarcinoma of the esophagus and esophagogastric junction. Gastroenterology 1993; 104: 510-513.

54. Devesa SS, Blot WJ, Fraumeni JF. Changing patterns in the incidence of esophageal and gastric carcinoma in the United States. Cancer 1998; 83: 2049-53.

55. Bytzer P, Christensen PB, Damkier P, Vinding K, Seersholm N. Adenocarcinoma of the esophagus and Barrett's esophagus: a population-based study. Am J Gastroenterol 1999; 94: 86-91.

56. Lord RVN, Law MG, Ward RL, Giles GG, Thomas RJS, Thursfield V. Rising incidence of oesophageal adenocarcinoma in men in Australia. J Gastroent Hepatol 1998; 13: 356-362.

57. Rogers EL, Goldkind SF, Iseri OA, Bustin M, Goldkind L, Hamilton SR, Smith RRL. Adenocarcinoma of the lower esophagus. A disease primarily of white men with Barrett's esophagus. J Clin Gastroenterol 1986; 8: 613-618.

58. Yang PC, Davis S. Incidence of cancer of the esophagus in the US by histologic type. Cancer 1988; 61: 612-617.

59. Kabat GC, Ng SKC, Wynder EL. Tobacco, alcohol intake, and diet in relation to adenocarcinoma of the esophagus and gastric cardia. Cancer Causes and Control 1993; 4: 123-132.

60. Brown LM, Silverman DT, Pottern LM, Schoenberg JB, Greenberg RS, Swanson GM, Liff JM, Schwartz AG, Hayes RB, Blot WJ, Hoover RN. Cancer Causes and Control 1994; 5: 333-340.

61. Vaughan TL, Davis S, Kristal A, Thomas DB. Obesity, alcohol, and tobacco as risk factors for cancers of the esophagus and gastric cardia: adenocarcinomas versus squamous cell carcinoma. Cancer Epidemiology Biomarkers and Prevention 1995; 4: 85-92.

62. Zhang ZF, Kurtz RC, Sun M, Karpeh M, Yu GP, Gargon N, Fein JS, Georgopoulos SK, Harlap S. Adenocarcinomas of the esophagus and gastric cardia: medical conditions, tobacco, alcohol, and socioeconomic factors. Cancer Epidemiol Biomarkers and Prevention 1996; 5: 761-768.

63. Gammon MD, Schoenberg JB, Ahsan H, Risch HA, Vaughan WJ, Chow WH, Rotterdam H, West AB, Dubrow R, Stanford JL, Mayne ST, Farrow DC, Niwa

S, Blot WJ, Fraumeni JF.   Tobacco, alcohol and socioeconomic status and adenocarcinoma of the esophagus and gastric cardia.   J Natl. Cancer Inst 1997; 89: 1277-1284.

64. Lagergren J, Bergstrom R, Lindgren A, Nyren O. The role of tobacco, snuff, and alcohol use in the etiology of esophageal and gastric cardia cancer.   Ph D thesis, Karolinska Institute, Stockholm, 1999.

65. Chow WH, Blot WJ, Vaughan WJ, Risch HA, Gammon MD, Stanford JL, Dubrow R, Schoenberg JB, Mayne ST, Farrow DC, Ahsan H, West AB, Rotterdam H, Niwa S, Fraumeni JF. Body mass index and risk of adenocarcinomas of the esophagus and gastric cardia. . J Natl. Cancer Inst 1998; 90: 150-155.

66. Lagergren J, Bergstrom R, Nyren O.   Association between body mass and adenocarcinoma of the esophagus and gastric cardia. Ann Int Med 1999; 130: 883-890.

67. Mokdad AL, Serdula MK, Dietz WH, Bowman BA, Marks JS, Koplan JP.   The spread of the obesity epidemic in the United States, 1991-1998.

68. Chow WH, Blaser MJ, Blot WJ, Gammon MD, Vaughan TL, Risch HA, Perez-Perez GI, Schoenberg JB, Stanford JL, Rotterdam H, West AB, Fraumeni JF. An inverse relationship between cagA strains of Helicobacter pylori infection and risk of esophageal and gastric cardia adenocarcinoma.   Cancer Res 1998; 58: 588-590.

69. Lagergren J, Nyren O. Do sex hormones play a role in the etiology of esophageal adenocarcinoma? A new hypothesis tested in a population-based cohort of prostate cancer patients. Cancer Epidemiol Biomarkers and Prevention 1998; 7: 913-915.

70. Vaughan TL, Farrow DC, Hansten PD, Chow WH, Gammon MD, Risch HA, Stanford JL, Schoenberg JB, Mayne ST, Rotterdam H, Dubrow R, Ahsan H, West AB, Blot WJ, Fraumeni JF. Risk of esophageal and gastric adenocarcinomas in relation to use of calcium channel blockers, asthma drugs, and other medications that promote gastroesophageal reflux.   Cancer Epidemiol Biomarkers and Prevention 1998; 7: 749-75

5.2 ADENOCARCINOMA IN BARRETT'S ESOPHAGUS: SIGNS, SYMPTOMS AND ENDOSCOPIC APPEARANCE

Gary W. Falk

1. INTRODUCTION

The incidence of adenocarcinoma of the esophagus has increased at a rate greater than that for any other cancer over the last 20 years. Whereas early adenocarcinoma is clinically silent but imminently curable, advanced cancer classically presents with progressive dysphagia to solids and liquids and is generally incurable. This chapter will review the clinical and endoscopic findings of esophageal adenocarcinoma.

2. SYMPTOMS

The clinical presentation of esophageal adenocarcinoma is highly variable for both early and advanced cancer. Early carcinoma is characterized by disease limited to the mucosa or submucosa without lymph node metastases[1] whereas advanced disease includes all tumors invading into the muscularis propria and beyond[1,2]. Early cancer typically has no symptoms. It is usually found incidently in patients undergoing endoscopy for symptoms of gastroesophageal reflux disease (GERD) or dyspepsia, as well as in patients with known Barrett's esophagus already enrolled in an endoscopic surveillance program. The difficulty in finding Barrett's esophagus, the precursor lesion of esophageal adenocarcinoma, is that symptoms are typically no different than those encountered in GERD patients without Barrett's esophagus, namely heartburn and acid regurgitation[3]. Furthermore, dysphagia, the classic symptom of esophageal cancer, may be encountered in some patients with reflux esophagitis in the absence of a peptic stricture and in Barrett's esophagus uncomplicated by cancer[4,5]. A recent landmark epidemiologic study found that frequent, severe, long-lasting symptoms of GERD are associated with an increased risk of developing esophageal adenocarcinoma[6].

However, finding at risk individuals is hampered by two problems. First, GERD is a common clinical condition. For example, weekly heartburn and/or acid regurgitation is present in 20% of the population of Olmsted County, Minnesota[7]. Second, Barrett's esophagus patients have an impaired sensitivity to esophageal acid perfusion[12,14]. This has led to the observation that most patients with esophageal adenocarcinoma are not known to have Barrett's esophagus prior to their diagnosis and as such are not enrolled in a surveillance program[10,11].

In a recent Danish cancer registry study, Bytzer et al. found 578 cases of esophageal adenocarcinoma of whom only 7 patients (1.3%) were previously enrolled in an endoscopic surveillance program[10]. The symptoms of advanced cancer are insidious in onset and often no different than the classic symptoms of GERD. The classic clinical presentation of advanced adenocarcinoma is progressive dysphagia, first to solids and then to liquids accompanied by weight loss. The clinical presentation of 524 patients with esophageal adenocarcinoma in the Danish Cancer Registry is shown in Table 1.

TABLE 1. Presenting Symptoms of 524 Patients with Esophageal Adenocarcinoma from the Danish Cancer Registry

Presenting Symptoms	Number (%)
Dysphagia	413 (79%)
Heartburn	105 (20%)
Pain	225 (43%)
Weight loss	336 (64%)

Modified from Bytzer P et al. Adenocarcinoma of the esophagus and Barrett's esophagus: a population-based study. Am J Gastroenterol 1999;94:86-91.

Unfortunately, the tumor is quite large before it compromises the lumen sufficiently to cause dysphagia. Typically, the critical lumen size for persistent solid food dysphagia is 13 mm[12].

H.W. Tilanus and S.E.A. Attwood (eds.), Barrett's Esophagus, 291–295.
© 2001 *Kluwer Academic Publishers. Printed in the Netherlands.*

Dysphagia may be insidious in onset and may be sensed initially as a transient delay in the passage of a food bolus. As dysphagia progresses, patients will modify their eating habits by chewing food more carefully and eating more slowly. This is then followed by modification of the diet by first eating softer foods and later switching to semisolids and liquids. The typical delay from onset of dysphagia to diagnosis is 3 months or more[10,13,14]. In case series of adenocarcinoma patients, dysphagia is described in 20% to 95% of patients at presentation, with the majority of series on the order of 60% to 75%[10,11,13-16]. Weight loss often accompanies dysphagia and is caused by a combination of decreased oral intake and tumor related cachexia. While a history of heartburn is a key epidemiological risk factor for esophageal cancer[6], it is described by only 20% of patients in the Danish esophageal cancer registry study by Bytzer et al[10]. However, other series report a history of reflux symptoms in 50% to 90% of patients[5,11,14-18]. Gastrointestinal bleeding is a less common presentation of esophageal cancer. This may range from occult bleeding with iron deficiency anemia to hematemesis and melena. Other symptoms of advanced esophageal adenocarcinoma include odynophagia, chest pain and epigastric pain.

Even in advanced cancer, a prior history of Barrett's esophagus is uncommon. Barrett's esophagus was previously diagnosed in only 6 of 112 adenocarcinoma patients (5%) in a case series from Rotterdam[11] and 7 of 524 patients (1.3%) in the Danish cancer registry study[10].

3. PHYSICAL EXAMINATION

The physical examination rarely if ever provides clues to the diagnosis of esophageal adenocarcinoma[13,19]. The prototypical esophageal adenocarcinoma patient is a middle-aged or older white male[11,20,21]. Occasionally, there may be evidence of cachexia or tumor metastases at sites such as supraclavicular lymph nodes or the liver. The physical examination is otherwise typically unremarkable and offers little clue to the diagnosis and extent of disease[13].

4. ENDOSCOPIC APPEARANCE

Early cancer has a subtle endoscopic appearance in marked contrast to the obvious endoscopic abnormalities encountered in patients with advanced cancer. Early carcinoma can be subdivided into three distinct subtypes based on the tumor's height relative to the adjacent noncancerous epithelium[22] (Figure 1).

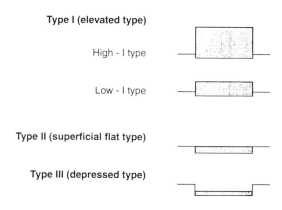

Figure 1.   Classification system for early esophageal adenocarcinoma. Modified from Nishimaki T, Holscher AH, Schuler M, Bollschweiler E, Becker K, Siewert JR. Histopathologic characteristics of early adenocarcinoma in Barrett's esophagus. Cancer 1991;68:1731-6, with permission.

While this system is not widely used in the literature, it provides a useful framework to approach these lesions in a systematic manner. Type I lesions (high ≥ 3 mm in height; low < 3 mm in height) are elevated or protruding and often have a polyploid appearance (Figure 2).

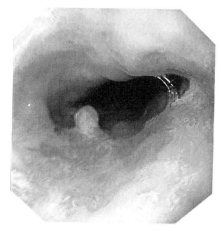

Figure 2. Early elevated (type I) adenocarcinoma in Barrett's esophagus.

Type II lesions, the superficial flat type, are the most difficult to detect endoscopically. These lesions include slightly elevated plaques, verrucous thickening and subtle mucosal color changes. The type III excavated or depressed lesions, have the appearance of an erosion or an ulcer in the

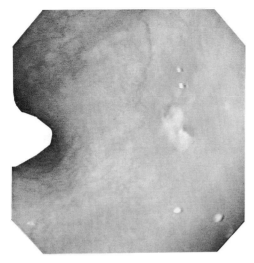

Figure 3. Early depressed (type III) adenocarcinoma in an erosion in Barrett's esophagus

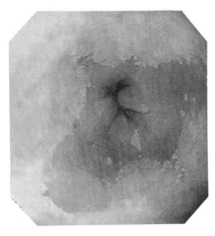

Figure 4. Early adenocarcinoma in a unremarkable segment of Barrett's esophagus. There are no mucosal lesions yet this patient had intramucosal carcinoma.

Barrett's segment and are endoscopically indistinguishable from a benign appearing Barrett's ulcer or erosion (Figure 3). The other finding of early cancer in Barrett's esophagus is a bland nondescript Barrett's segment where surveillance biopsies surreptitiously detect cancer (Figure 4). This has been described by multiple authors, especially in patients with high-grade dysplasia who underwent esophagectomy[23,24,25]. Systematic esophagectomy mapping studies by Cameron et al. demonstrated just how focal dysplasia and superficial cancer may be[25]. In 30 esophagectomy specimens from patients undergoing surgery for either high-grade dysplasia or early invasive adenocarcinoma with no endoscopic evidence of cancer, the median surface area of total Barrett's esophagus was 32 cm^2; low-grade dysplasia 13 cm^2; high-grade dysplasia 1.3 cm^2; and adenocarcinoma 1.1 cm^2 (Figure 5).

The three smallest cancers had surface areas of 0.02, 0.3 and 0.4 cm^2. Invasive adenocarcinoma was associated with either focal or extensive areas of high-grade dysplasia. Thus, detection of adenocarcinoma in Barrett's patients with high-grade dysplasia may be akin to looking for a "needle in a haystack." It should come as no surprise that unsuspected carcinoma can be found in up to 73% of resected specimens when esophagectomy is done for high-grade dysplasia[23]. Subtle mucosal abnormalities such as ulcers, erosions, nodularity, friability, and strictures are often encountered in patients with high-grade dysplasia. Unfortunately, these findings do not necessarily predict which patients will have cancer at esophagectomy[23-26] (Figure 6).

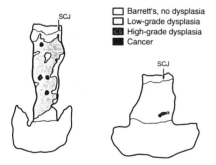

Figure 5. Surface area involved with Barrett's esophagus, low-grade dysplasia, high-grade dysplasia and adenocarcinoma in 30 patients without obvious carcinoma undergoing resection for high-grade dysplasia or superficial adenocarcinoma. From Cameron AJ, Carpenter HA. Barrett's esophagus, high-grade dysplasia and early adenocarcinoma: a pathological study. Am J Gastroenterol 1997;92:586-91, with permission.

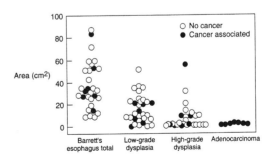

Figure 6. Histological maps of the esophagus and proximal stomach in two resection cases with adenocarcinoma. Note the small focus of adenocarcinoma in both cases. From Cameron AJ, Carpenter HA. Barrett's esophagus, high-grade dysplasia and early adenocarcinoma: a pathological study. Am J Gastroenterol 1997;92:586-91, with permission

Thus, the concept of dysplasia associated mass or lesion (DALM) used in ulcerative colitis surveillance programs is not necessarily applicable to Barrett's

esophagus. Current guidelines suggest performing endoscopic surveillance in Barrett's esophagus patients in an effort to detect cancer in an early and potentially curable stage[27]. It is recommended that systematic four quadrant biopsies are obtained at 2 cm intervals once inflammation related to GERD is controlled with antisecretory therapy [27]. Mucosal abnormalities, such as ulceration, erosion, plaque, nodule, stricture, or other luminal irregularity in the Barrett's segment, should also be biopsied. The rational for such a comprehensive biopsy program comes from observations that high-grade dysplasia and early carcinoma in Barrett's esophagus often occur in the absence of endoscopic abnormalities and the focal nature of dysplasia as described above. In the future, our ability to detect early cancer may be enhanced by a variety of endoscopic optical technique that have the potential to obtain "light" biopsies of Barrett's esophagus. Candidate techniques include fluorescence spectroscopy, light spectroscopy, optical coherence tomography, light scattering spectroscopy, and light induced fluorescence endoscopy. All of these techniques are based on the principle that benign and malignant tissue have different optical qualities. In theory, these techniques would permit optical sampling of larger areas of the columnar-lined esophagus and improve the efficiency of biopsies by targeting areas thought to harbor dysplasia or cancer. While promising, these techniques need to decrease the overlap encountered between normal mucosa, Barrett's epithelium and all grades of dysplasia[28-30]. Because of the focal nature of dysplasia and cancer, some experts recommend that endoscopic surveillance should utilize a large particle (jumbo) forceps to obtain biopsies. Studies by Levine et al.[24] suggest that this type of systematic biopsy protocol can reliably distinguish patients with high-grade dysplasia alone from those with intramucosal or submucosal adenocarcinoma, thereby avoiding the risk of unnecessary surgery in these patients. However, the generalizability of this labor intensive technique in general clinical practice is questionable, and work by our group failed to confirm these findings[23]. Furthermore, few gastroenterologists in practice use large particle forceps[31]. The endoscopic appearance of advanced cancer is less subtle than that of superficial carcinoma and typically present with an

obvious tumor mass (Figure 7,8). The tumor may be exophytic, polyploid or ulcerated with a broad base. A variable circumference of the esophageal lumen is involved. Central parts of the tumor may be ulcerated and friable and can bleed spontaneously. Esophageal adenocarcinoma may also present as a smooth tapering stricture as well, especially if the tumor diffusely infiltrates the submucosa (Figure 9). Multiple discrete primary tumors may also be encountered. Diagnosis is made by biopsy and cytologic brushing with an accuracy approaching 100%[32].

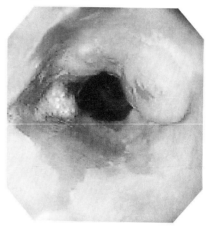

Figure 7. Polypoid mass in the distal esophagus in a patient with advanced adenocarcinoma in Barrett's esophagus.

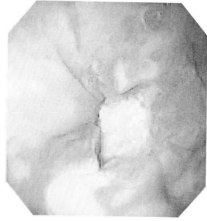

Figure 8. Ulcerating mass in the distal esophagus in a patient with advanced adenocarcinoma in Barrett's esophagus.

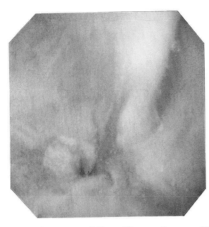

Figure 9. Segment of Barrett's esophagus with bland appearing stricture. Esophageal adenocarcinoma was diagnosed from biopsies and cytology of the stricture.

REFERENCES

1. Tytgat G. Does endoscopic surveillance in esophageal columnar metaplasia (Barrett's esophagus) have any real value? Endoscopy 1995;27:19-26.
2. Sabik JF, Rice TW, Goldblum JR, Koka A, Kirby TJ, Medendorp SV, Adelstein DJ. Superficial esophageal carcinoma. Ann Thorac Surg 1995;60:896-902.
3. Falk GW. Unresolved issues in Barrett's esophagus in the new millennium. Dig Dis 2000;18:27-42.
4. Triadafilopoulos G. Nonobstructive dysphagia in reflux esophagitis. Am J Gastroenterol 1989;84:614-8.
5. Skinner DB, Walther BC, Riddell RH, Schmidt H, Iascone C, DeMeester TR. Barrett's esophagus. Comparison of benign and malignant cases. Ann Surg 1983;198:554-66.
6. Lagergren J, Bergstrom R, Lindgren A, Nyren O. Symptomatic gastroesophageal reflux as a risk factor for esophageal adenocarcinoma. N Engl J Med 1999;340:825-31.
7. Locke GR, Talley NJ, Fett SL, Zinsmeister AR, Melton LJ. Prevalence and clinical spectrum of gastroesophageal reflux: a population-based study in Olmsted County, Minnesota. Gastroenterology 1997;112:1448-56.
8. Johnson DA, Winters C, Spurling TJ, Chobanian SJ, Cattau EL. Esophageal acid sensitivity in Barrett's esophagus. J Clin Gastroenterol 1987;91:23-7.
9. Grade A, Pulliam G, Johnson C, Garewal H, Sampliner RE, Fass R. Reduced chemoreceptor sensitivity in patients with Barrett's esophagus may be related to age and not to the presence of Barrett's epithelium. Am J Gastroenterol 1997;92:2040-3.
10. Bytzer P, Christensen PB, Damkier P, Vinding K, Seersholm N. Adenocarcinoma of the esophagus and Barrett's esophagus: a population-based study. Am J Gastroenterol 1999;94:86-91.
11. Menke-Pluymers MB, Schoute NW, Mulder AH, Hop WC, Van Blankenstein M, Tilanus HW. Outcome of surgical treatment of adenocarcinoma in Barrett's esophagus. Gut 1992;33:1454-8.
12. Boyce HW. Dysphagia. Clinical Update. American Society for Gastrointestinal Endoscopy 1993;1:1-4.
13. Witt TR, Bains MS, Zaman MB, Martini N. Adenocarcinoma in Barrett's esophagus. J Thorac Cardiovasc Surg 1983;85:337-45.
14. Sanfey H, Hamilton SR, Smith RL, Cameron JL. Carcinoma arising in Barrett's esophagus. Surg Gynecol Obstet 1985;161:570-4.
15. Williamson WA, Ellis FH, Gibb SP, Shahian DM, Aretz HT, Heatley GJ, Watkins E. Barrett's esophagus. Prevalence and incidence of adenocarcinoma. Arch Intern Med 1991;151:2212-6.
16. Duhaylongsod FG, Wolfe WG. Barrett's esophagus and adenocarcinoma of the esophagus and gastroesophageal junction. J Thorac Cardiovasc Surg 1991;102:36-42.
17. Heitmiller RF, Redmond M, Hamilton SR. Barrett's esophagus with high-grade dysplasia. An indication for prophylactic esophagectomy. Ann Surg 1996;224:66-71.
18. Lerut T, Coosemans W, Van Raemdonck D, Dillemans B, De Leyn P, Marnette JM, Geboes K. Surgical treatment of Barrett's carcinoma. Correlations between morphologic findings and prognosis. J Thorac Cardiovasc Surg 1994;107:1059-66.
19. Spechler SJ. AGA technical review on treatment of patients with dysphagia caused by benign disorders of the distal esophagus. Gastroenterology 1999;117:233-54.
20. Cameron AJ, Lomboy CT. Barrett's esophagus: age, prevalence, and extent of columnar epithelium. Gastroenterology 1992; 103:1241-5.
21. Hamilton SR, Smith RR, Cameron JL. Prevalence and characteristics of Barrett's esophagus in patients with adenocarcinoma of the esophagus or esophagogastric junction. Hum Pathol 1988;19:942-8.
22. Nishimaki T, Holscher AH, Schuler M, Bollschweiler E, Becker K, Siewert JR. Histopathologic characteristics of early adenocarcinoma in Barrett's esophagus. Cancer 1991;68:1731-6.
23. Falk GW, Rice TW, Goldblum JR, Richter JE. Jumbo biopsy forceps protocol still misses unsuspected cancer in Barrett's esophagus with high-grade dysplasia. Gastrointest Endosc 1999;49:170-6.
24. Levine DS, Haggitt RC, Blount PL, Rabinovitch PS, Rusch VW, Reid BJ. An endoscopic biopsy protocol can differentiate high-grade dysplasia from early adenocarcinoma in Barrett's esophagus. Gastroenterology 1993;105:40-50.
25. Cameron AJ, Carpenter HA. Barrett's esophagus, high-grade dysplasia and early adenocarcinoma: a pathological study. Am J Gastroenterol 1997;92:586-91.
26. Pera M, Trastek VF, Carpenter HA, Allen MS, Deschamps C, Pairolero PC. Barrett's esophagus with high-grade dysplasia: an indication for esophagectomy? Ann Thorac Surg 1992;54:199-204.
27. Sampliner RE. Practice guidelines on the diagnosis, surveillance, and therapy of Barrett's esophagus. Am J Gastroenterol 1998;93:1028-32.
28. Panjehpour M, Overholt BF, Vo-Dinh T, Haggitt RC, Edwards DH, Buckley FP. Endoscopic fluorescence detection of high-grade dysplasia in Barrett's esophagus. Gastroenterology 1996;111:93-101.
29. Von Holstein CS, Nilsson AM, Engels SA, Willen R, Walther B, Svanberg K. Detection of adenocarcinoma in Barrett's oesophagus by means of laser induced fluorescence. Gut 1996;39:711-6.
30. Haringsma J, Prawirodirdjo W, Tytgat GN. Accuracy of fluorescence imaging of dysplasia in Barrett's esophagus. Gastroenterology 1999;116:A418 (Abstract).
31. Falk GW, Ours TM, Richter JE. Practice patterns for surveillance of Barrett's esophagus in the USA. Gastrointest Endosc 2000;52:197-203.
32. Lightdale CJ. Esophageal cancer. Am J Gastroenterol 1999;94:20-9.

5.3 ADENOCARCINOMA IN BARRETT'S ESOPHAGUS - CLASSIFICATION AND STAGING

Arnulf H. Hölscher, Wolfgang Schröder and Stephan P. Mönig

1. DEFINITION AND CLASSIFICATION

The definition and classification of adenocarcinomas of the gastro-esophageal junction is not standardized and the choice of surgical procedures still causes controversial discussion. In contrast to the decreasing frequency of gastric cancer and squamous cell carcinomas of the esophagus authors of various western countries showed an increasing incidence of adenocarcinoma of the esophagus as well as the cardia[1,2,15,31,46]. The reason for this shift is not known. Because of this increasing frequency a precise classification of adenocarcinomas of the gastro-esophageal junction becomes more important for daily surgical routine. This is necessary for planning the extent of resection as well as for the comparability of surgical results from different institutions.

In the present literature the technical term "adenocarcinoma of the gastro-esophageal junction" summarizes different tumor entities. In order to compare different treatment modalities a new classification for carcinomas of the gastro-esophageal junction was introduced in 1987[26,50]. This classification has been widely accepted[10,35]. Alternative classifications will be mentioned in this chapter.

1.1. SURGICAL CLASSIFICATION OF ADENOCARCINOMAS OF THE GASTRO-ESOPHAGEAL JUNCTION TYPE I-III

Carcinomas of the gastro-esophageal junction are designated as those with a tumor center 5 cm oral and aboral of the lower esophageal sphincter. Adenocarcinoma of the distal esophagus and subcardial gastric cancer are only included if they infiltrate the cardia. Following this definition carcinomas of the gastro-esophageal junction can be classified according to their location into three different types (Figure 1):

Type I: Adenocarcinoma of the distal esophagus which infiltrates the gastro-esophageal junction and mostly develops in Barrett's esophagus (Figure 2).

Type II: True carcinomas of the cardia arising from the cardiac mucosa (Figure 3).

Type III: subcardial gastric carcinoma which infiltrates the cardia and the lower esophagus, mostly submucosally (Figure 4).

The assignment of these tumors to the three different types is based on the anatomic localization of the center of the tumor. According to this classification the distribution of the types is summarized in table 1[26].

TABLE 1. Distribution of 445 patients with adenocarcinoma of the gastro-esophageal junction type I-III[26]

Tumor type	n	%
Type I	156	38
Type II	137	28
Type III	152	34
All types	445	

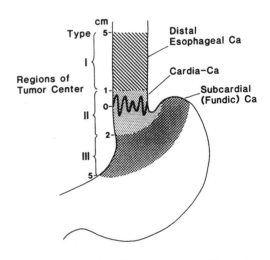

Figure 1: Classification of adenocarcinomas of the gastro-esophageal junction[50].

1.1.1 Type I-adenocarcinoma

The type I-adenocarcinoma represents a distal esophageal cancer and consequently is treated by subtotal esophagectomy (Figure 2 and 5)[6,25]. This can be performed as transhiatal abdomino-cervical esophagectomy especially in carcinomas of the lower esophagus. In case of an extended Barrett's esophagus with carcinoma of the thoracic esophagus right-sided transthoracic en bloc esophagectomy with mediastinal lymphadenectomy is recommended[27].

H.W. Tilanus and S.E.A. Attwood (eds.), Barrett's Esophagus, 297–306.
© 2001 Kluwer Academic Publishers. Printed in the Netherlands.

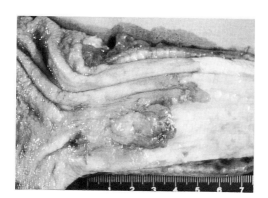

Figure 2. Macroscopic appearance of adenocarcinoma of the distal esophagus (type I)

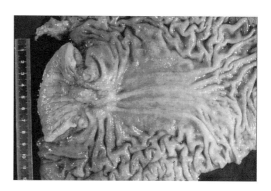

Figure 4. Macroscopic appearance of subcardial gastric cancer (type III)

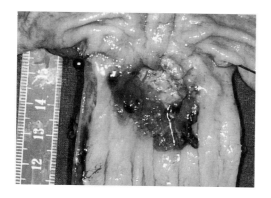

Figure 3. Macroscopic appearance of true carcinoma of the cardia (type II)

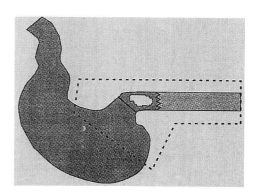

Figure 5.Extent of resection in type I adenocarcinoma of the gastro-esophageal junction: transhiatal / transthoracic esophagectomy.

Both procedures include the resection of the lesser curvature with partial abdominal lymphadenectomy since the majority of lymph node metastases are located along the lesser curvature and the left gastric artery[10,49]. The reconstruction is performed by the formation of a gastric tube which is anastomosed to the cervical esophagus in case of transhiatal resection and to the esophagus in the upper mediastinum in case of a transthoracic resection. In cases of mucosal carcinoma of Barrett' esophagus lymph node metastases are not observed[28]. Therefore, a limited resection of the distal esophagus and cardia with regional lymphadenectomy (Merendino procedure) is justified. An alternative would be

a local resection by endoscopic mucosectomy and ablation of Barrett's mucosa in suitable cases.

1.1.2 Type III-adenocarcinoma

Subcardial adenocarcinoma (type III) is surgically treated by an extended total gastrectomy with transhiatal distal esophageal resection. This comprises a D2-lymphadenectomy and in advanced cases a pancreas preserving splenectomy (Figure 4 and 6). Some Japanese surgeons are now performing a limited operation for early cancer in the upper third of the stomach[19]. In case of a carcinoma which is limited to the mucosa or submucosa without evidence of nodal metastases a proximal gastrectomy without splenectomy and extended lymphadenectomy is considered to be an adequate resection[32]. The prognosis of this approach seems to be similar to that of total gastrectomy[21] and also prevents the patient to develop pernicious anemia. On the other hand, proximal gastrectomy frequently causes gastro-esophageal reflux and, subsequently, results in varying degrees of esophagitis[30,63]. Therefore, a total gastrectomy is recommended by the authors.

(so called "zone splenectomy") in order to achieve radical nodal dissection without increasing the complication rate in the pancreatic region[27,38,39,52]. In cases of mucosal carcinoma of the cardia the Merendino procedure as mentioned for type I is also a possible solution. In cases of very advanced type II carcinoma total esophagogastrectomy may also be necessary[26].

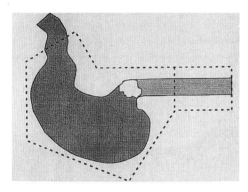

Figure 6. Extent of resection in type III adenocarcinoma of the gastro-esophageal junction: transhiatal extended gastrectomy.

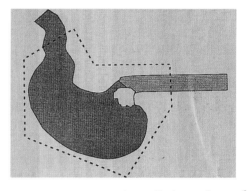

Figure 7. Extent of resection in type II adenocarcinoma of the gastro-esophageal junction: transhiatal extended gastrectomy.

1.1.3 Type II-adenocarcinoma

The extent of resection in type II-adenocarcinoma is still under discussion. It is questionable whether the resection should be extended in the proximal direction that means subtotal esophagectomy as in type I, or in the opposite direction that means extended total gastrectomy as in type III. Because of a lower postoperative morbidity and mortality the authors prefer a transhiatal extended gastrectomy instead of a subtotal esophagectomy (Figure 3 and 7)[26,51]. In order to achieve a good exposure of the cardiac region the approach of choice is an upper transverse laparotomy with a median extension to sternum. The reconstruction of the intestinal passage is done with Roux-Y esophagojejunostomy. Since advanced carcinomas of type II can metastasize to lymph node group 10 and 11 in the upper left abdominal region a splenectomy is recommended in cases of very advanced tumors[26,29,41]. This splenectomy should be performed as a pancreas preserving procedure

1.2 TOPOGRAPHICAL CLASSIFICATION OF ESOPHAGEAL CANCER

Another topographical classification is proposed by Ellis and coworkers[12-14]. Carcinoma of the cardia is defined as a carcinoma arising in the upper third of the stomach and involving the esophagogastric junction and the lower esophagus. Adenocarcinoma in Barrett's esophagus is not included even though it might involve the esophagogastric junction. The surgical procedure recommended for both tumor entities is the resection of the cardia and distal esophagus via a left thoracotomy[15].

2. CLINICAL STAGING

In order to choose the adequate treatment for carcinomas of the gastro-esophageal junction an exact preoperative staging is mandatory[11]. Beside a precise histological diagnosis the staging has to assign the carcinoma to one of the three types of the gastroesphageal junction and has to clarify whether a complete resection of the tumor can be achieved (so called "R0-resection")[55].

Since advanced adenocarcinomas have the same radiographic features as squamous cell carcinomas of the distal esophagus the following description of the clinical staging includes both histological entities.

2.1 TUMOR LOCALIZATION

The best way to assign adenocarcinomas of the gastro-esophageal junction to the different types is by radiological and endoscopic examination.

A thoracic survey radiograph in two planes with contrast visualization of the esophagus and stomach (Thoramat x-ray) is taken to localize the tumor topographically and anatomically, particularly in relation to the diaphragm and the tracheal bifurcation (Figure 8). Esophagogastroscopy must be performed in the prograde as well as retrograde view of the cardia in order to define the localization of the major part of the tumor.

The final matching to one of the three different types has to be done intraoperatively and on the resected specimen. In some cases the preoperative assessment has to be revised.

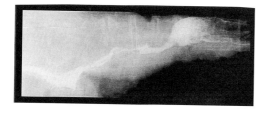

Figure 8. Thoramat x-ray for localization of the tumor.

2.2 T-CATEGORY

The preoperative clinical staging of the T category is primarily based on endoluminal ultrasound (EUS). It is the only radiological examination that is safely able to differentiate between the single layers of the esophageal wall (Figure 9). High frequency probes can even visualize mucosal and submucosal carcinomas with an accuracy of 75 - 80%[53,67]. This technical innovation subsequently resulted in the concept of local resection of mucosal adenocarcinomas of the distal esophagus. A review of the literature clearly demonstrates that the overall accuracy for

endosonography to classify the T-category is higher compared to CT[24,60](table 2).

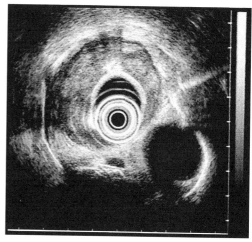

Figure 9. Endoluminal ultrasound demonstrating a locally advanced adenocarcinoma (T3) of the distal esophagus.

As described in other reviews the reported accuracy of EUS compared to histopathology is more than 80% for the T category [5,24]. A limiting factor for EUS is a severe esophageal stenosis which cannot be passed with the instrument. This problem of nontraversable tumors reduces the overall accuracy of EUS in T classification[11,47,62]. However, tumors large enough to cause luminal obstruction are nearly all full thickness (T3) and frequently have mediastinal lymph node metastases (N1) at the time of examination[61]. The problem of nontraversable tumors might be overcome by the use of miniature ultrasonic probes which have a similar accuracy regarding T and N category[4,65].

As CT cannot differentiate the individual layers of the esophageal wall CT is not suitable for precise evaluation of the T category[24]. In contrast to the EUS the assessment of the T category with the computed tomography (CT) predominantly relies on the wall thickness[59]. CT scan typically reveals marked circumferential soft-tissue thickening of the esophageal wall in patients with advanced lesions and can safely diagnose the invasion of adjacent organs (T4 category) such as the mediastinum, the aorta, the tracheobronchial tree and the pericardium.

MRT has shown to have a similar accuracy for T staging compared to the CT since it suffers from the same limitation of not safely identifying the individual layers of the esophageal wall. However, using a new magnetic resonance imaging with an endoluminal surface coil the accuracy rate increases to 83% regarding the depth of tumor invasion[45] and seems comparable to the EUS examination[34].

TABLE 2. Radiological imaging techniques to evaluate the T category

T-category						
Author	Year	Imaging	Patients (n)	Sensitivity	Specificity	Accuracy
Tio[59]	1989	CT	74	-	-	59
		EUS	74	-	-	89
Vilgrain [62]	1990	CT	-	-	-	-
		EUS	46	-	-	73
Botet [3]	1991	CT	42	-	-	60
		EUS	50	-	-	92
Takashima [58]	1991	CT	35	100	82	84
		MR	35	100	86	87
Ziegler [68]	1991	CT	37	-	-	51
		EUS	37	-	-	89
Dittler [11]	1993	EUS	167	86	96	86
Massari [40]	1997	CT	40	-	-	90
		EUS	40	-	-	50
Yamada [66]	1997	MRT	70	-	-	94
Vickers [61]	1998	EUS	50	97	73	92
Hansen [20]	20u0	CT	30	10	90	63

2.3 N-CATEGORY

Standard evaluation of the preoperative nodal status includes endosonography and computed tomography[3,18,24,57]. Precise evaluation of the N status is more difficult than evaluation of the T category and the reported overall accuracy rates are lower[24] (table 3). This is caused by the fact that both EUS and CT lack an exact morphological description of metastatic lymph nodes which correlates with the histopathological findings. Therefore, the classification of lymph nodes as metastatic is primarily based on lymph node size (Figure 10,11 and 12). Morphological studies on esophageal and gastric cancer demonstrated only a poor correlation between lymph node size and metastatic infiltration[42,44,48] Benign lymph nodes preoperatively classified as metastatic may be enlarged due to inflammation. Vice versa, small lymph nodes preoperatively classified as benign may show micrometastatic involvement. Inflammatory changes and micrometastases were the most important causes of false positive and false negative results[42,48]. In addition, a thorough pathologic work-up of the specimens showed that a major portion of the resected metastatic

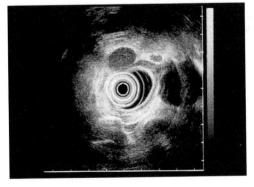

Figure 10. Endoluminal ultrasound demonstrating enlarged periesophageal lymph nodes

and non metastatic lymph nodes are smaller than 5 mm in diameter[42,44,48] These lymph nodes are difficult to detect with EUS or CT at all. Therefore, an accurate preoperative evaluation of the N-category is not possible.

As with the T category a comparison between EUS and CT for N classification demonstrates the superiority of EUS[24,60] (table 3). However, most studies evaluating a radiological examination technique concerning the N category are difficult to interpret since they do not define the type of lymphadenectomy performed and do not exactly correlate the preoperative with the postoperative histopathological findings[3,17,58]. The most reliable criterion for defining the N category is still the accompanying T category[61].

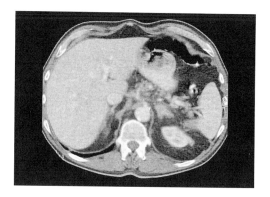

Figure 13. Computed tomography demonstrating smaller lymph nodes at the celiac axis

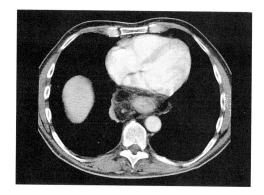

Figure 11. Computed tomography demonstrating a locally advanced carcinoma of the distal esophagus.

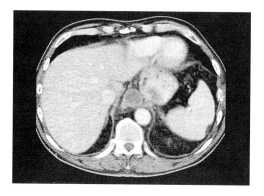

Figure 12. Computed tomography demonstrating enlarged lymph nodes at the celiac axis

2.4 M-CATEGORY

Organs predominantly involved are the liver (32%) and the lung (21%)[24]. Since all other organs are rarely involved preoperative examination should focus on these organs. CT scan of the abdomen and thorax is the standard examination in order to preoperatively classify the M category (Figure 13). In patients with questionable hepatic metastases percutaneous ultrasound and MRI with gadolinium enhancement can help to verify intrahepatic lesions. Recent studies with PET could demonstrate that PET was more accurate than CT in detecting distant metastases[36,37,54].

In cases of advanced adenocarcinoma of the distal esophagus, peritoneal carcinomatosis (M1 per) has to be excluded. This can be best done by video assisted staging laparoscopy which has shown to be more sensitive and accurate compared to EUS, CT and PET[16,22,36,37,56,64].

In lower esophageal carcinoma nodal metastases at the coeliac trunc are classified as M1 lymph. These can be visualized with the EUS and CT which have their methodological limitations as described above. In case of suspicious lymph nodes staging laparoscopy enables opening the lesser sack for direct inspection of the lymph nodes around the celiac axis.

3. PATHOLOGICAL STAGING

Beside the topographical anatomical classification the morphological and histopathological classification is of prognostic relevance. The depth of infiltration of the primary tumor, the nodal status and distant metastasis are classified according to the guidelines of the UICC (table 4 and 5) and are major prognostic factors[23,55]. These guidelines do not propose a separate classification for tumors of the gastro-esophageal junction. Adenocarcinomas of the distal esophagus (type I) are classified as esophageal carcinomas whereas type II and III carcinomas are classified according to the guidelines for gastric cancer.

TABLE 3. Radiological imaging techniques to evaluate the N.category

N-category						
Author	Year	Imaging	Patients (n)	Sensitivity	Specificity	Accuracy
Tio [59]	1989	CT	74	34	88	51
		EUS	74	92	54	80
Vilgrain[62]	1990	CT	44	48	99	94
		EUS	23	84	-	-
Botet[3]	1991	CT	42	-	-	74
		EUS	50	-	-	88
Takashima[58]	1991	CT	35	53	83	65
		MR	35	58	83	68
Ziegler[68]	1991	CT	37	-	-	51
		EUS	37	-	-	69
Dittler[11]	1993	EUS	167	75	70	73
Catalano[7]	1994	EUS	100	89	91	100
Chandawakar[8]	1996	EUS	74	37	90	87
Natsugoe[43]	1996	EUS	37	80	87	86
Flanagan[17]	1997	CT	29	28	73	45
		PET	29	72	82	76
Luketich[36]	1997	PET	35	45	100	48
Massari[40]	1997	CT	23	-	-	39
		EUS	23	-	-	87
Vickers[61]	1998	EUS	50	97	54	86
Kobori[33]	1999	PET	33	-	-	85
Choi[9]	2000	CT	48	-	-	60
		EUS	45	-	-	58
		PET	48	-	-	83
Hansen[20]	2000	CT	30	37	90	57

Table 4A/B. TNM classification and UICC stages of esophageal carcinoma

Esophagus	
T1	Lamina propria, submucosa
T2	Muscularis propria
T3	Adventitia
T4	Adjacent structures
N1	Regional lymph nodes
M1	Distant metastasis
	Tumor of lower thoracic esophagus
M1a	Coeliac nodes
M1b	Other distant metastasis
	Tumor of upper thoracic esophagus
M1a	Cervical nodes
M1b	Other distant metastasis
	Tumor of mid-thoracic esophagus
M1b	Distant metastasis including non-regional lymph nodes

Stage Grouping Esophageal carcinoma			
Stage 0	Tis	N0	M0
Stage I	T1	N0	M0
Stage IIA	T2	N0	M0
	T3	N0	M0
Stage IIB	T1	N1	M0
	T2	N1	M0
Stage III	T3	N1	M0
	T4	Any N	M0
Stage IV	Any T	Any N	M1
Stage IVA	Any T	Any N	M1a
Stage IVB	Any T	Any N	M1b

TABLE 5A/B. TNM classification and UICC stages of gastric carcinoma

Stomach	
T1	Lamina propria, submucosa
T2	Muscularis propria, subserosa
T3	Penetrates serosa
T4	Adjacent structures
N1	1 to 6 nodes
N2	7 to 15 nodes
N3	>15 nodes

Stage Grouping Gastric carcinoma			
Stage 0	Tis	N0	M0
Stage IA	T1	N0	M0
Stage IB	T1	N1	M0
	T2	N0	M0
Stage II	T1	N2	M0
	T2	N1	M0
	T3	N0	M0
Stage IIIA	T2	N2	M0
	T3	N1	M0
	T4	N0	M0
Stage IIIB	T3	N2	M0
Stage IV	T4	N1, N2, N3	M0
	T1, T2, T3	N3	M0
	Any T	Any N	M1

REFERENCES

1. Bollschweiler E, Boettcher K, Hölscher AH, Sasako M, Kinoshita T, Maruyama K, Siewert JR. Is the prognosis between Japanese and German patients with gastric cancer really different? Cancer 1993;71:2918-25.

2. Bollschweiler E, Hölscher AH. Rising incidence of esophageal adenocarcinoma. Dt Ärzteblatt 2000;97:A-1896-1900.

3. Botet JF, Lightdale CJ, Zauber AG, Gerdes H, Winawer SJ, Urmacher C, Brennan MF. Preoperative staging of esophageal and gastric cancer:comparison of endoscopic US and dynamic CT. Radiology 1991;181:419-32.

4. Bowrey DJ, Clark GW, Roberts SA, Maughan TS, Hawthorne AB, Williams GT, Carey PD. Endosonographic staging of 100 consecutive patients with esophageal carcinoma:introduction of the 8-mm-esophagoprobe. Dis Esophagus 1999;12(4):258-63.

5. Boyce HW. Endosonographic staging of esophageal cancer. Cancer Control 1999;6(1):28-35.

6. Bumm R, Hölscher AH, Feussner H, Tachibana M, Bartels H, Siewert JR. Endodissection of the thoracic esophagus. Technique and clinical results in transhiatal esophagectomy. Ann Surg 1991;218(1):97-104.

7. Catalano MF, Sivak MV Jr, Rice T, Gragg LA, Van Dam J. Endosonographic features predictive of lymph node metastasis. Gastrointest Endosc 1994;40(4):442-6.

8. Chandawarkar RY, Kakegawa T, Fujita H, Yamana H, Toh Y, Fujitoh H. Endosonography for preoperative staging of specific nodal groups associated with esophageal cancer. World J Surg 1996;20:700-2.

9. Choi JY, Lee KH, Shim YM, Lee KS, Kim JJ, Kim SE, Kim BT. Improved detection of individual nodal involvement in squamous cell carcinoma of the esophagus by FDG PET. J Nucl Med 2000;41(5):808-15.

10. Clark GWB, Peters JH, Ireland AP, Ehsan A, Hagen JA, Kiyabu MT, Brenner CG, DeMeester TR. Nodal metastasis and sites of recurrence after en bloc esophagectomy for adenocarcinoma. Ann Thorac Surg 1994;58:646-54.

11. Dittler HJ, Siewert JR. Role of Endoscopic Ultrasonography in Esophageal Carcinoma. Endoscopy 1993;25:156-61.

12. Ellis FH. Esophagogastrectomy for carcinoma: technical considerations based on anatomic location of the lesion. Surg Clin North Am 1980;60:265-79.

13. Ellis FH, Maggs PR. Surgery for carcinoma of the lower esophagus and cardia. World J Surg 1981;5(4):527-33.

14. Ellis FH, Gibb SP, Watkins E. Limited esophagogastrectomy for carcinoma of the cardia:indications, technique and results. Ann Surg 1988;208:354-60.

15. Ellis FH, Heatley GJ, Krasna MJ, Williamson WA, Balogh K. Esophagogastrectomy for carcinoma of the esophagus and cardia:a comparison of findings and results after standard resection in three consecutive eight-year intervals with improved staging criteria. J Thorac Cardiovasc Surg 1997;113:836-847.

16. Feussner H, Kraemer SJ, Siewert JR. Staging laparoscopy. Chirurg 1997;68(3):201.

17. Flanagan FL, Dehdashti F, Siegel BA, Trask DD, Sundaresan SR, Patterson GA, Cooper JD. Staging of Esophageal Cancer with 18F-Fluorodeoxyglucose Positron Emission Tomography. AJR 1997;168:417-24.

18. Fukaya T, Honda H, Hayashi T, Kaneko K, Tateshi Y, Ro T, Maehara Y, Tanaka M, Tsuneyoshi M, Masuda K. Lymph-node metastases:efficacy of detection with helical CT in patients with gastric cancer. Radiology 1995;197:705-11.

19. Furukawa H, Hiratsuka M, Imaoka S, Ishikawa O, Kabuto T, Sasaki Y, Kameyama M, Ohigashi H, Nakano H, Yasuda T. Limited surgery for early gastric cancer in cardia. Ann Surg Oncol 1998;5:338-41.

20. Hansen CP, Oskarsson K, Mortensen D. Computed tomography for staging of esophageal cancer. Ann Chir Gynaecol 2000;89(1):14-8.

21. Harrison LE, Karpeh MS, Brennan MF. Total gastrectomy is not necessary for proximal gastric cancer. Surgery 1998;123:127-30.

22. Heath EI, Kaufmann HS, Talamini MA, Wu TT, Wheeler J, Heitmiller RF, Kleinberg L, Ynag SC, Olukayode K, Forastierre AA. The role of laparoscopy in preoperative staging in esophageal cancer. Surg Endosc 2000;14(5):495-9.

23. Hermanek P, Hutter RVP, Sobin LH, Wagner G, Wittekind C. UICC TNM classification of malignant tumors. Berlin 1998:Springer, 4th edition

24. Hölscher AH, Dittler HJ, Siewert JR. Staging of squamous esophageal cancer: accuracy and value. World J Surg 1994;18:312-20.

25. Hölscher AH, Bollschweiler E, Bumm R, Bartels H, Höfler H, Siewert JR (1995) Prognostic factors of resected adenocarcinoma of the esophagus. Surgery 1995;118:845-55.

26. Hölscher AH, Bollschweiler E, Siewert JR. Carcinoma of the gastric cardia. Ann Chir Gynaecol 1995;84:185-192.

27. Hölscher AH, Bollschweiler E, Beckurts KTE, Siewert JR. Radikalitätsausmaß beim Cardiacarcinom – Oesophagektomie oder Gastrektomie? Langenbecks Arch Chir 1996;Suppl II:169-72.

28. Hölscher AH, Bollschweiler E, Schneider PM, Siewert JR. Early adenocarcinoma in Barrett's esohagus. Br J Surg 1997;84:1470-3.

29. Hölscher AH, Bollschweiler E. Ausmaß von Resektion und Lymphadenektomie beim Magenkarzinom – eine anhaltende Kontroverse. Onkologe 1998;4:301-9.

30. Hsu CP, Chen CY, Hsieh YH, Hsia JY, Shai SE, Kao CH. Esophageal reflux after total or proximal gastrectomy in patients with adenocarcinoma of the gastric cardia. Am J Gastroenterol 1997;9:1347-50.

31. Kalish RJ, Clancy PE, Orringer MB, Appelmann HD. Clinical, epidemiologic and morphologic comparison between adenocarcinoma arising in Barrett's esophageal mucosa and in the gastric cardia. Gastroenterology 1984;86:461-7.

32. Kitamura K, Nishida S, Yamamoto K, Ichikawa D, Okamoto K, Taniguchi H, Yamaguchi T, Sawai K, Takahashi T. Lymph node metastasis in gastric cancer in the upper third of the stomach – surgical treatment on the basis of the anatomical distribution of positive node. Hepatogastroenterology 1998;45:281-5.

33. Kobori O, Kirihara Y, Kosaka N, Hara T. Positron emission tomography of esophageal carcinoma using (11)C-choline and (18)F-fluorodeoxyglucose:a novel method of preoperative lymph node staging. Cancer 1999; 86(9):1638-48.

34. Kulling D, Feldman DR, Kay CL, Hoffman BJ, Reed CE, Young JW, Hawes RH. Local staging of esophageal cancer using endoscopic magnetic resonance imaging: prospective comparison with endoscopic ultrasound. Endoscopy 1998;30(9):745-9.

35. Lozach P. Cancers de l'oesophage et du cardia.1995;Ellipses, Paris.

36. Luketich JD, Schauer PR, Meltzer CC, Landreneau RJ, Urso GK, Townsend DW, Ferson PF, Keenan RJ, Belani CP. Role of positron emission tomography in staging esophageal cancer. Ann Thorac Surg 1997;64(3):765-9.

37. Luketich JD, Friedman DM, Weigel TL, Meehan MA, Keenan RJ, Townsend DW, Meltzer CC Evaluation of distant metastases in esophageal cancer:100 consecutive positron emission tomography scans. Ann Thorac Surg 1999;68(4):1133-6.

38. Maruyama K, Sasako M, Kinoshita T, Okajima K. Effectiveness of systematic lymph node dissection in gastric cancer surgery. In:Gastric cancer. Nishi M, Ichikawa H, Nakajima T, Maruyama K, Tahara E (eds.) 1993;Springer Verlag, pp. 293-305.

39. Maruyama k, Sasako M, Kinoshita T, Sano T, Katai H, Okajima K. Pancreas-preserving total gastrectomy for proximal gastric cancer. World J Surg 1995; 19:532-6.

40. Massari M, Cioffi U, De Simone M, Lattuada E, Montorsi M, Segalin A, Bonavina L. Endoscopic ultrasonography for preoperative staging of esophageal carcinoma. Surg Laparosc Endosc 1997;7(2):162-5.

41. Mönig SP, Collet P, Baldus SE, Schmackpfetter K, Schröder W, Thiele J, Dienes HP, Hölscher AW. Splenectomy in priximal gastric cancer: frequency of lymph node metastasis to the splenic hilus. J Surg Oncol 2001;76:89-92.

42. Mönig SP, Zirbes TK, Schröder W, Baldus SE, Lindemann DG, Dienes HP, Hölscher AH (1999) Staging of gastric cancer:correlation of lymph node size and metastatic infiltration. AJR 1999;173:365-7.

43. Natsugoe S, Yoshinaka H, Morinaga T, Shimada M, Baba M, Fukumota, Stein HJ, Aikou T. Ultrasonographic detection of lymph node metastases in superficial carcinoma of the esophagus. Endoscopy 1996;28(8):674-9

44. Noda N, Sasako M, Yamaguchi N, Nakanishi Y. Ignoring small lymph nodes can be a major cause of staging error in gastric cancer. Br J Surg 1998;85:831-4.

45. Ozawa S, Imai Y, Suwa T, Kitajima M What's new in imaging? New magnetic resonance imaging of esophageal cancer using an endoluminal surface coil and antibody-coated magnetite particles. Recent Results Cancer Res 2000;155:73-87.

46. Pera M, Cameron AJ, Tratsek VF, Carpenter HA, Zinsmeister AR.Increasing incidence of adenocarcinoma of the esophagus and esophagogastric junction. Gastroenterology 1993; 104:510-3.

47. Rösch T, Lorenz R, Zenker K et al. Local staging and assessment of resectability in carcinoma of esophagus, stomach and duodenum by endoscopic ultrasonography. Gastrointest Endosc 1992;38:460.

48. Schröder W, Baldus SE, Mönig S, Zirbes TK, Dienes HP, Hölscher AH. Diagnostic impact of lymph node size after 2-field lymphadenectomy in esophageal cancer. Langenbecks Arch Chir 1998;Suppl. 501-3

49. Schröder W, Baldus SE, Mönig S, Zirbes TK, Beckurts TKE, Hölscher AH. Lesser curvature lymph node metastases in squamous cell carcinoma of the esophagus:implications for formation of gastroplasty. World J Surg 2001 (in press)

50. Siewert JR, Hölscher AH, Becker K, Gössner W. Kardiacarcinom:Versuch einer therapeutisch relevanten Klassifikation. Chirurg 1987;58:25-32.

51. Siewert JR, Kestlmeier R, Busch R. Benefits of D2 lymph node dissection for patients with gastric cancer and pN0 and pN1 lymph node metastases. Br J Surg 1996;83:1144-7.

52. Siewert JR, Stein HJ, Böttcher K. Lymphadenektomie bei Tumoren des oberen Gastrointestinaltrakts. Chirurg 1996;67:877-88.

53. Simizu Y, Tsukagoshi H, Nakazato T, Karawazaki M, Sai K, Oikawa Y, Mera K, Hosokawa M, Oohara M, Fujita M. Clinical evaluation of endoscopic ultrasonography (EUS) in the diagnosis of superficial esophageal carcinoma. Rinsho Byori 1995;43(3):221-6

54. Skehan SJ, Brown AL, Thompson M, Young JE, Coates G, Nahmias C. Imaging features of primary and recurrent esophageal cancer at FDG PET. Radiographics 2000; 20(3):713-23.

55. Sobin LH, Wittekind C. Stomach. In:Sobin LH, Wiltekind C, eds. Union Internationale Contre le Cancer (UICC):TNM-Classification of malignant tumors. 5th edition. Wiley & Sons 1997:59-62.

56. Stein HJ, Kraemer SJ, Feussner H, Fink U, Siewert JR. Clinical value of diagnostic laparoscopy with laparoscopic ultrasound in patients with cancer of the esophagus or cardia. J Gastrointest Surg 1997;1(2):167-73.

57. Susman SK, Halvorsen RA, Illescas FF, Cohan RH, Saeed M, Silverman PM, Thompson WM, Meyers WC. Gastric adenocarcinoma: CT versus surgical staging. Radiology 1988;167:335-340.

58. Takashima S, Takeuchi N, Shiozaki H, Kobayashi K, Morimoto S, Ikezoe J, Tomiyama N, Harada K, Shogen K, Kozuka T. Carcinoma of the Esophagus:CT vs MT imaging in determining resectability. AJR 1991;156:297-302.

59. Tio TL, Cohen P, Coene PP, Udding J, Den Hartog Jager FCA, Tytgat GNJ. Endosonography and computed tomography of esophageal carcinoma. Gastroenterology 1989;96:1478-86.

60. Van Dam J. Endosonographic evaluation of the patient with esophageal cancer. Chest1997;112(4 Suppl):184S-190S.

61. Vickers J, Alderson D. Oesophageal cancer staging using endoscopic ultrasonography. Br J Surg 1998;85(7):994-8.

62. Vilgrain V, Mompoint D, Palazzo L, Menu Y, Gayet B, Ollier P, Nahum H, Fekete F. Staging of eseophageal carcinoma:comparison of results with endoscopic sonography and CT. AJR 1990;155:277-81.

63. Wang CY, Hsu HK, Chang HC, Huang MS, Goan YG, Su JM. Reflux esophagitis after proximal subtotal gastrectomy. Chung Hua I Hsueh Tsa Chih 1997;59:348-53.

64. Watt I, Stewart I, Anderson E, Bell G, Anderson JR. Laparoscopy, ultrasound and computed tomography in cancer of the esophagus and gastric cardia:a prospective comparison for detecting intraabdominal metastases. Br J Surg 1989;76:1036

65. Xu GM, Niu YL, Zou XP, Jin ZD, Li ZS. The diagnostic value of transendoscopic miniature ultrasonic probe for esophageal disease. Endoscopy 1998;30 Suppl 1:A28-32

66. Yamada I, Murata Y, Izumi Y, Kawano T, Endo M, Kuroiwa T, Shibuya H. Staging of esophageal carcinoma in vitro with 4.7-T MR imaging. Radiology 1997;204(2):521-6.

67. Yoshikane H, Tsukamoto Y, Niwa Y, Goto H, Hase S, Shimodaira M, Maruta S, Miyata A, Yoshida M. Superficial esophageal carcinoma:evaluation by endoscopic ultrasonography. Am J Gastroenterol 1994;89(5):702-7.

68. Ziegler K, Sanft C, Zeitz M. .Evaluation of endosonography in TN staging of oesophageal cancer. Gut1991; 32: 16-2

5.4 DIAGNOSIS AND IMPLICATIONS OF BONE MARROW MICROMETASTASES

Donal Maguire, Fergus Shanahan and Gerald C. O' Sullivan

1. INTRODUCTION

At presentation cancer is a systemic disease in the majority of patients with malignancy of the esophagus and stomach. This dissemination is represented by either isolated or microaggregates of tumor cells, which have the potential to establish overt metastases, and are not detectable by serological measurements of tumor markers or by radiological imaging. These micrometastases are present in approximately 90% of patients who are subjected to curative excisional surgery and explain the frequent early tumor recurrences after radical resection. At diagnosis, the clinico-pathological stage of primary cancer remains the best predictor of outcome and is the determinant of treatment strategy[1-3]. When disseminated disease is present, cure by excision of the primary is not possible unless effective adjuvant therapies are available. This implies that rigorous detection of metastatic disease is required to ensure optimal treatment. At present detection of sub-clinical disease is not possible as imaging techniques lack the temporal and spatial resolution to discover individual or small groups of disseminated tumor cells[4]. Specifically, in patients with esophagogastric malignancy, ultrasound and CT detects peritoneal or hepatic metastases with a sensitivity of only 21% and 47% respectively[4]. Similarly, the sensitivity and specificity of serum tumor antigens is limited[5,6] and the analysis of primary tumors for DNA content, oncogene mutations, tumor suppressor genes, and proliferative markers does not provide a direct measure of tumor burden or metastatic spread[7]. Despite radical excisional surgery and multimodal therapy, most patients with clinically manifest esophagogastric cancer die from metastatic disease within three years of presentation, even though dissemination was not evident on pre-operative evaluation. This is compelling circumstantial evidence for the existence of a minimal residual state in most of these patients after surgery. Traditionally, these cancers have been thought to spread sequentially in a step-wise manner, directly from mucosa to the esophageal wall, to the regional lymph nodes and finally by systemic dissemination. This paradigm has dominated the clinical care of patients with adenocarcinoma of the gastro-esophageal junction, from pre-operative staging investigations through to attempts at disease control. In the absence of overt metastatic disease, staging investigations have defined the lymph node status as a surrogate indicator of systemic spread, but the majority of patients with node-negative cancer also die of metastases. This indicates the biologically aggressive nature of this disease and clearly suggests that haematogenous dissemination occurs independently of spread by the lymphogenous route. This has recently been confirmed by detection of micrometastases in bone marrow samples from resected rib segments of patients with esophageal adenocarcinoma[8]. Thus, both clinical experience and bone marrow analysis suggest that most patients have residual disease after resection of the primary cancer and the regional lymph nodes and that lymph node status alone is not an accurate marker for systemic spread[9,10]. Because of the ability to detect occult dissemination, by bone marrow analysis, there is also objective evidence that from an early phase of tumor development esophagogastric cancer is a systemic disease[8,11]. The presence of bone marrow micrometastases has been shown to be associated with early treatment failures and a poor prognosis in patients with cancers of breast, lung colon and esophagus. In contrast clearance of metastatic cells from marrow either spontaneously or in response to antibody targeting is associated with improved patient survival. This indicates that these cancer cells in bone marrow are a reflection of systemic disease. We recently demonstrated that 88% of patients, having resections for cure of esophagogastric cancer, have micrometastases in their rib bone marrow. These cells are viable, actively proliferate,

307

H.W. Tilanus and S.E.A. Attwood (eds.), Barrett's Esophagus, 307–315.
© 2001 *Kluwer Academic Publishers. Printed in the Netherlands.*

grow independently in tissue culture and form malignant tumors when injected into immunocompromised mice[8]. Furthermore, these cancer cells are often present in marrow of patients after intensive neoadjuvant chemotherapy and radiation therapy indicating resistance to the treatment. Thus, it is possible to diagnose chemotherapy resistance *in vivo* at a cellular phase and prior to tumor recurrence and there is now a robust system for study of genetic regulation of metastatic cancer cell behavior. Their easy access also provides the clinical investigator an opportunity to study variables in biological behavior (cell cycle control, metastatic cell dormancy, immune escape, angiogenesis, chemo-responsiveness) of minimal residual disease and a resource for development of novel therapies.

2. WHAT IS THE THEORETICAL SIGNIFICANCE OF BONE MARROW METASTASES?

Most cells within the primary tumor are terminally differentiated, and do not possess the intrinsic capabilities necessary to disseminate and propagate. In contrast the presence of viable micrometastatic deposits in tissues implies dissemination of cancer cells with the facility for independent survival and growth[1,2]. These are most likely metastatic stem cells and are the appropriate targets for effective systemic therapy. Such cells have the capability to detach from the primary growth, travel through extracellular matrix and basement membrane into the local microvasculature, survive transit in the circulation, and exit by attaching and extravasating through the endothelium at another site[1,12]. This complex process involves several interdependent steps regulated by cascades of cytokines, chemokines, growth factors and matrix metalloproteinases[13,19]. Thus the finding of malignant epithelial cells in bone marrow indicates metastatic phenotypes with tumorogenic potential[20,21].

3. HOW ARE MICROMETASTASES DETECTED?

Bone marrow is derived from the embryonic mesoderm and therefore does not normally express epithelial cell-specific components. Epithelial-derived malignancies retain expression of many epithelial specific proteins such as cytokeratins (CK's), carcinoembryonic antigen (CEA) and epithelial membrane antigen (EMA). The finding of these markers in the bone marrow indicate the presence of metastatic tumor cells. Strategies that search for cells bearing these markers within marrow include morphological identification by immunohistochemical staining (Figure 1), antibody-based identification by flow cytometry, and genetic identification by reverse transcriptase-polymerase-chain reaction (rt-PCR). While these techniques are sensitive there are several potential sources for measurement error.

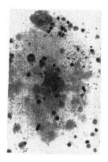

Figure 1. Cluster of tumorcells in a bone marrow aspirate from a patient with esophageal carcinoma. Alkaline phosphatase anti-alkaline phosphatase staining from cytokeratin 18 demonstrates hyperchromatic tumorcells staining positive (center)

3.1 POTENTIAL FOR BONE MARROW SAMPLING ERRORS

There is a variable distribution of tumor cells at different marrow aspiration sites. This introduces potential sampling errors, specifically, false negative detection[24]. Bilateral iliac crest sampling is superior to unilateral analysis[25], and most studies now include both sites to optimize results with minimal added morbidity[26,28]. When triple sampling (left and right iliac crests and sternum) was performed, it increased the frequency of detection of micrometastases from 11% to 28% in patients with beast carcinoma[25]. In patients with esophageal cancers, yields of micrometastases from resected rib segments are superior to those from the iliac crest aspirates in patients undergoing surgery[29]. It is unlikely that the improved detection rates are site-specific, but are due to enhanced quality of undiluted marrow; marrow aspirates are diluted to a variable degree by peripheral blood. A standardized method of assessment and reporting of marrows is necessary, both to allow enumeration and to determine the significance of negative results. Potentially, one could relate the numbers of detected micrometastatic cells to a standard for marrow cells (megakaryocyte or stem cell count). Until such standardization is available a resected segment of rib obtained at thoracotomy, prior to manipulation of the tumor is the 'gold standard' for detecting micrometastases in esophageal cancer.

3.2 MARKERS USED FOR TO DETECT MICROMETASTASES

The epithelial cell protein markers used in detection of micrometastatic disease include cytokeratins, epithelial membrane antigen, carcinoembryonic antigen (CEA) and mucinous-like carcinoma antigen[27-35]. Epithelial membrane antigen and mucinous-like carcinoma antigen are used predominantly for breast cancer patients, while cytokeratins and to a lesser extent CEA are most validated for gastrointestinal malignancies. Cytokeratins constitute the intermediate filaments of epithelial cytoskeleton accounting for almost 85% of the total cellular protein[36,37]. Cytokeratins 8, 18, 19 and 20 are restricted to simple epithelia and are conserved in tumors derived from these[38-40]. Control studies of freshly isolated cells from bone marrow aspirates of patients without epithelial malignancies show that they are neither stained by pancytokeratin nor isotype specific antibodies. False positive imaging rates of less than two percent have been reported [26-31,41-43]. Comparative study of marrow samples stained with either the broad-spectrum monoclonal antibody A45-B/B3, or an antibody directed against cytokeratin 18 (CK18) have demonstrated a 50% down-regulation of CK18 expression in micrometastatic cells in bone marrow aspirates[44]. It appears therefore, that to eliminate false negative results, concurrent staining with a number of anti-cytokeratin antibodies is required. The discriminative value of immunocytochemical staining of bone marrow aspirates for CEA has been disappointing, but reverse transcription polymerase chain reaction (rtPCR) for messenger ribonucleic acid (mRNA) coding for the CEA protein appears to be sensitive and specific for bone marrow micrometastases[45,46]. In these reports, there were no false positive results in marrow from control subjects, while single CEA-expressing tumor cells were reliably detected among $2\text{-}5 \times 10^7$ normal marrow cells.

3.3 IMMUNOCYTOCHEMISTRY/FLOW CYTOMETRY/rtPCR

To detect of metastatic cells in human bone marrow by light microscopy requires both tumor cell specific staining and morphological recognition (Figure 1). Optimum detection requires both enrichment of the nucleated cell component of the marrow by density centrifugation and application of cells to adherent slides by cytospin. However, 1-4 million cells are scanned by light microscopy which makes the process labor intensive and observer dependent. Flow cytometric analysis of immunocytochemically stained marrow for tumor cell contamination allows for automation and enumeration[26,29,47]. Marrow samples pre-treated with fluorescent labeled monoclonal antibody directed against the epithelial cell component are passed through a detection system which can count total cell numbers and cells with adherent antibody[26]. A single tumor cell per 10^5 marrow cells may be detected with accuracy. Detection of messenger ribonucleic acid (mRNA) coding for a specific marker protein, by reverse-transcription polymerase chain reaction (rtPCR) may be the most sensitive approach but awareness of pitfalls in relation to cytokeratin markers of epithelial micrometastases is critical. Essentially the technique detects specific mRNA (coding for the specific epithelial cell protein) but pseudogenes for some cytokeratins including CK18 are present in normal marrow cells[45,48] and amplification occurs in the absence of the specific cytokeratin except for cytokeratin 20[49]. Alternatively, CEA may be better suited to rtPCR methods[45,46]. Detection of single metastatic cells per 2×10^7 bone marrow cells has been reported using rtPCR for CEA message and this was more sensitive than immunostaining for CEA or cytokeratins[45,46]. The most accurate and efficient technique(s) of micrometastases detection will only be determined by comparative study of the different methods using appropriate markers. These studies, combined with follow-up data from patients, measuring disease-free interval/survival are necessary prior to routine clinical application. Our current practice is to sample iliac crest marrow bilaterally and to take marrow from resected rib segment.

4. BIOLOGIC PROPERTIES OF BONE MARROW MICROMETASTASES

4.1 ORIGIN OF MICROMETASTASES

The possibility that cytokeratin-positive micrometastases might not originate from the primary tumor and represent harmless epitheliod reactions has been refuted. Study of patients with prostatic cancers allowed for identification of cells that express a unique well preserved specific marker (prostate specific antigen) in addition to cytokeratins. Prostatic cancer cell deposits in marrow were found to demonstrate similar chromosomal aneusomies to the primary tumor[54] and when double stained for cytokeratin and prostatic-specific antigen (PSA), a significant concordance rate of expression of PSA between primary prostatic carcinoma cells and marrow micrometastases was found[55,56]. These data indicate that cytokeratin positive cells represent cancer cells derived from the primary tumor.

4.2 TUMOROGENICITY, VIABILITY, PROLIFERATIVE POTENTIAL

There remains the possibility that micrometastatic cells might be transient cells (detached from the primary tumor but unable to establish at a secondary site or unable to escape destruction by the immune system). Possibly some micrometastatic cells are in this category as a recent study of bone marrow from patients with esophageal adenocarcinoma before and six months after 'curative' surgery showed that patients were able to clear their marrow of metastatic cells[29]. However, persistence of micrometastatic cells was noted in most and carried a high risk of development of overt metastatic disease within the subsequent months[29]. The viability and proliferative capacity of bone marrow micrometastases has been confirmed *in vitro* using combinations of growth factors in the presence of extracellular matrix proteins[57,58]. Cytokeratin positive cells in the bone marrow of tumor patients also express markers of proliferative activity such as Ki 67 nuclear antigen, receptors for transferrin and epidermal growth factor[25,59]. Micrometastatic cells also have measurable levels of nucleolar antigen p120 (found in G1 and S phase) which is not found in non-malignant hemopoietic cells[60]. We have been able to consistently generate tumor cell lines from marrow of patients with esophageal adenocarcinoma in culture from rib bone marrow which were tumorogenic when transferred to immunodeficient athymic nude mice[8]. Historically, tumorogenicity of bone marrow micrometastases has also been inadvertently uncovered in patients, when autologous bone marrow transplants have been used in the treatment of epithelial malignancies[61,62]. Taken together these data indicate that micrometastatic cells are viable and tumorogenic.

4.3 WHY DO MICROMETASTATIC CELLS SURVIVE IN AN IMMUNOLOGICALLY HOSTILE ENVIRONMENT?

Potentially, isolated and small groups of tumor cells in hemopoietic bone marrow should be accessible to immunological attack but it appears that these cells can survive for long periods[63]. It is likely that metastatic cells deploy the same defensive strategies used by primary tumors to evade the immune system. These include the production of immunosuppressive factors and cytokines to create a local microenvironment immunosuppression as has been clearly documented in esophageal carcinoma[64]. Metastatic tumor cells also express the Fas ligand on their surface and therefore can trigger apoptosis of immune cells on cell-cell contact[65,66]. Binding of leukocytes to tumor cells also involves the expression of intercellular adhesion molecules and altered expression of these in micrometastases may be involved in immune escape. For example the prognosis of patients with micrometastatic non-small cell lung cancer was found to be significantly better if the bone marrow micrometastatic cells expressed the adhesion molecule ICAM-1[67]. Metastatic tumor cells may also effectively camouflage themselves by down-regulation of expression of major histocompatibility complex (MHC) class I antigens for presentation of tumor antigens to the immune system and generation of cytotoxic T cells[68].

5. ROLE OF MICROMETASTASES IN THE MANAGEMENT OF PATIENTS WITH ESOPHAGEAL ADENO-CARCINOMA

There is general acceptance that for chemotherapy or chemoradiotherapy to be effective against esophagogastric cancer it must be given in a neoadjuvant setting, before tumor vascularity and patient fitness are further compromised by extensive excisional surgery. The choice of chemotherapeutic agents needs to be determined by the responses of both the primary tumor and the sensitivity/resistance of disseminated metastatic cells. It is noteworthy that in a recent large-scale clinical trial of fluoruracil and platinum the clinical response rate of the primary tumor was not reflected in improved survival[69]. That this was due to resistance of minimal residual disease or micrometastases to the chemotherapeutic agents has been confirmed by the finding of viable tumor cells in bone marrow of patients who received similar treatment[8]. Perhaps the responsiveness to therapy should be assessed at the level of micrometastases (accessible in bone marrow) rather than by measurements of shrinkage of primary tumors where most of the cells are terminally differentiated and may be induced to die while the metastatic stem cells are chemoresistant and remain viable. To date, improvements in survival from multimodal programs have been modest, with most patients succumbing to metastases[72-74]. Surgical resection remains the standard of care, although more than half the patients are inoperable at presentation[69,70,75]. Access to bone marrow at various stages of treatment permits a diagnosis of subclinical residual disease and assessment of responsiveness to systemic agents. In addition, by clinical correlation with phenotypic and cytogenetic variables, the spectrum of metastatic cell behavior including progression, dormancy or clearance, may be predictable.

6. CANCER DORMANCY

Cancer dormancy is an apparent tumor-free or latent state in which disseminated malignant cells are present but are under growth control by biological mechanisms. Withdrawal or inhibition of these restraining mechanisms leads to overt tumor progression[77]. Historically, the occurrence of metastatic cancer, particularly of breast, melanoma and stomach after more than an apparent tumor-free decade, post curative treatment of the primary tumor is referred to as cancer dormancy[77-79]. Recurrent disease is precipitated by systemic events such as infection, surgery, or immunosuppression suggesting loss of biological control by inhibition of immune containment or by stimulation of pro-tumorogenic mechanisms. It is likely that the transition from dormancy to progressive disease involves to some degree cellular genetic changes, angiogenic stimulation and immune evasion (Figure 2).

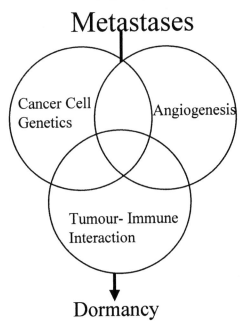

Figure 2. Micrometastases may remain dormant or progress to overt metastatic disease. This process is determined by a number of factors including genetic alterations in the cancer cell which enhance its survival and replication ability, immune escape capability and angiogenic potential of the tumor cells the relative ability to stimulate angiogenesis.

Potentially, the development of ultra-sensitive techniques to detect micro deposits of tumor cell in bone marrow, may allow for precise diagnosis, characterization of the cancer cells and correlation with the clinical course of the patient[8,80-84]. Through bone marrow analysis we have identified a cohort of patients with epithelial micrometastases several months after curative surgery[29]. While the majority of these patients developed overt disease on follow up, a small cohort of long term survivors emerged suggesting dormant disease in some after 'curative' treatment for gastrointestinal cancer. Thus, sequential analysis of bone marrow allows a precise diagnosis of dormancy and study of relevant gene expression and determination of the cell cycle and proliferative status of the metastatic cells.

7. TOWARDS THE CONTROL OF MINIMAL RESIDUAL DISEASE

The control of minimal residual disease is potentially a realizable goal. Repeated access of bone marrow will help define minimal residual disease status, responsiveness to therapy, and provide a source of micrometastases for genetic modification and manufacture of tumor-specific vaccine. Until more specific antitumor drugs are developed, the residual disease burden in most patients can only be controlled by ablation of the primary tumor, and adjuvant biological approaches at general host and metastatic cell level. This will involve the development of strategies aimed at controlling the immunosuppressive and angiogenic responses to surgical trauma and infection. Recent successes in murine models suggest that effective tumor specific vaccines can be developed for even MHC negative cancers without prior antigen isolation[88]. Data from studies utilizing dendritic cells that were primed *in vitro* by fusion with tumor cells or by pulsing with RNA or membrane components have also been encouraging. Genetic modification of tumor cells to secrete GMCSF and to express the B7 co-stimulatory molecule, permit undefined tumor antigen presentation by dendritic cells, and tumor control by specific natural killer cells. The clinical application of these vaccines is now feasible with the culture of metastatic cell lines from bone marrow aspirates.

8. CONCLUSIONS

Conventional methods for assessment of tumor load understage many patients. Bone marrow micrometastases are viable cells with proliferative and tumorgenic potential.

Their presence preoperatively is associated with a poor patient outcome. Persistence of micrometastases following 'curative' surgery indicates minimal residual disease that also carries a poor prognosis, whereas clearance of marrow micrometastases is associated with a favorable outcome. The metastatic process is not haphazard and represents a complex process by which cells invade blood vessels, evade the immune system, may remain dormant for prolonged periods and become re-established as metastases at a distant site. Occult deposits of cells within bone marrow fulfil the criteria required for successful metastases. Bone marrow represents a convenient window on the metastatic process because it is an accessible mesenchymal tissue in which deposits of neoplastic cytokeratin-positive epithelial cells may be identified and quantified by several techniques. Since the outcome of patients with esophagogastric and other cancers is determined by the fate of disseminated micrometastases, it is time to direct attention to the study of these cells. This may offer the best hope for development of rational treatments which can be based on biological control mechanisms of dormancy or clearance. Whether specific immune, anti-angiogenic or chemoradiotherapeutic strategies are adopted, the study of systemic micrometastatic disease in esophageal cancer will be critical for predicting and assessing clinical responsiveness, and is likely to provide valuable insights for management of other solid tumors. Minimal Residual Disease is now accessible and predictive factors such as tumor progression, dormancy, and metastatic cell elimination are amenable to clinical definition. Control of MRD will be a prolonged process and success will demand an ever increasing health care commitment. Halting the transition from MRD to overt metastases whether by cellular elimination or by induction of dormancy will in effect be a cure for cancer for many patients.

REFERENCES

1. Liotta LA, Stetler-Stevensen WG. Tumor invasion and metastases:an imbalance of positive and negative regulation. Cancer Res 1991;51 (suppl):5054-9.
2. Liotta LA, Stegg PS, Stetler-Stevensen WG. Cancer metastases and angiogenesis:an imbalance of positive and negative regulation. Cell 1991;64:327-36.
3. O' Brien MG, Fitzgerald EF, Lee G, Crowley M, Shanahan F, O' Sullivan G. A prospective comparison of laparoscopy and imaging in the staging of esophagogastric cancer before surgery. Am J Gastroenterol 1995;90:2191-4.
4. Posner MR, Mayer RJ. The use of serologic tumor markers in gastrointestinal malignancies.

Hematology/Oncology Clin North America 1994;8:533-53.

5. Pandha HS, Waxman J. Tumor markers. Q J Med 1995;88:233-41.

6. NIH Consensus conference. Adjuvant therapy for patients with colon and rectal cancer. JAMA 1991;264:1444-50.

7. O'Sullivan G, Sheahan D, Clarke A, Stuart R, Walsh T, Kelly J, Kiely MD, Collins JK, Shanahan F. Micrometastases in esophagogastric cancer:high detection rate in resected rib segments. Gastroenterology 1999;116:543-548.

8. Akiyama H, Tsuramaru M, Udagawa H, Kajiyama Y. Systematic lymph node dissection for esophageal cancer - effective or not. Dis Esophagus 1994;7:2-13.

9. Altorki NK, Skinner DB. Occult cervical nodal metastases in esophageal cancer:preliminary results of three field lymphadenectomy. J Thorac Cardiovasc Surg 1997;113:540-4.

10. Sporn MB. The war on cancer. Lancet 1996;347;1377-81.

11. Hart IR, Goode NT, Wilson RE. Molecular aspects of the metastatic cascade Biochem Biophys Acta 1989;989:65-84.

12. Duffy MJ. Cancer metastasis: biological and clinical aspects. Ir J Med Sci 1998;167:4-8.

13. Jiang WG, Hallett MB, Puntis MCA. Motility factors in cancer invasion and metastasis Surgical Research Communications 1994;16:219-37.

14. Matrisian LM The matrix-degrading metalloproteinases Bio Essays 1992;14:455-63.

15. Albelda SM. Role of integrins and other cell adhesion molecules in tumor progression and metastases. Lab Invest 1993;68:4-17.

16. Hynes RO. Integrins:versatility, modulation and signalling in cell adhesion Cell 1992;69:11-25.

17. Banks RE, Gearing AJ, Hemmingway IK, Norfolk DR, Perren TJ, Selby PJ. Circulating intercellular adhesion molecule-1 (ICAM-1), E-selectin and vascular cell adhesion molecule-1 (VCAM-1) in human malignancies Br J Cancer 1993;68:122-4.

18. Gearing AJ, Hemingway I, Pigott R, Hughes J, Rees AJ, Cashman SJ. Soluble forms of vascular adhesion molecules E-selectin, ICAM-1, and VCAM-1:pathological significance Ann NY Acad Sci. 1992;667:324-31.

19. Fidler IJ, Hart IR. Biological diversity in metastatic neoplasms:orgins and implications. Science 1982;217:998-03.

20. Fidler IJ. Metastases:quantative analysis of distribution and fate of tumor emboli labelled with ^{125}I-2-deoxyuridine. J Natl Cancer Inst 1970;45:773-82.

21. Schlimok G, Funke I, Holzmann B, Gottlinger HG, Schmidt G, Hauser H, Swierkot S, Warneke HH, Schneider B, Koprowski H, Riethmuller G. Micrometastatic cancer cells in bone marrow:in vitro detection with anti-cytokeratin and in vivo labelling with anti-17-1-A monoclonal antibodies. Proc Natl Acad Sci USA 1987;84:8672-6.

22. Gatter KC, Alcock C, Heryet A, Mason DY. Clinical importance of analysing malignant tumors of uncertain orgin with immunohistochemical techniques Lancet 1985;1:1302-5.

23. Mansi JL, Berger U, Easton D. Micrometastases in bone marrow patients with primary breast cancer:Evaluation as an early predictor of bone metastases. Br Med J 1987;295:1093-6.

24. Schlimok G, Riethmuller G. Detection, characterization and tumorgenicity of disseminated tumor cells in human bone marrow. Sem Cancer Biol 1990;1:207-15.

25. O' Sullivan GC, Collins JK, O' Brien F, Crowley B, Murphy K, Lee G, Shanahan F. Micrometastases in bone marrow of patients undergoing "curative surgery for gastrointestinal cancer. Gastroenterology 1995;109:1535-40.

26. Schlmok G, Funke I, Holzmann B, Gottlinger G, Schmidt G, Hauser H, Swierkot S, Warnecke HH, Schneider B, Koprowski H. Micrometastatic cancer cells in bone marrow:in vitro detection with anti-cytokeratin and in vivo labelling with anti-17-1A monoclonal antibodies Proc Natl Acad Sci USA 1987;84(23):8672-6.

27. Lindemann F, Schlimok G, Dirschedel P, Witte J, Riethmuller G. Prognostic significance of micrometastatic tumor cells in bone marrow of colorectal cancer patients Lancet 1992;340:685-9.

28. O' Sullivan G, Collins JK, Kelly J, Morgan J, Madden M, Shanahan F Micrometastases:marker of metastatic potential or evidence of residual disease Gut 1997;40:512-5.

29. Pantel K, Aignherr C Kollermann J, Caprano J Reithmüller G, Kollermann MW. Immunocytochemical detection of isolated tumor cells in bone marrow of patients with untreated stage C prostatic cancer. Eur J Cancer 1995;31A(10):1627-32.

30. Tsuchiya A, Sugano K, KImijima I Abe R Immunohistiochemical evaluation of lymph node micrometastases from breast cancer. Acta Oncolog 1996;35(4):425-8.

31. Harbeck N, Untch M, Pache L, Eiermann W Tumor cell detection in bone marrow of breast cancer patients at primary therapy:results of a 3-year median follow-up Br J Cancer 1994;69(3):566-71.

32. Basu D, Singh T, Shinghal RN. Micrometastases in bone marrow in breast cancer. Indian J Patho. Micrbiol 1994;37(2):159-64.

33. Neumaier M Gerhard M, Wagener C Diagnosis of micrometastases by the amplification of tissue-specific genes. Gene 1995;159(1):43-7.

34. Gerhard M, Juhl H, Kalthoff H, Schreiber HW, Wagener C, Neumaier M. Specific detection of carcinoembryonic antigen expressiong tumor cells in bone marrow aspirates by polymerase chain reaction. J Clin Oncol 1994;12(4):725-9.

35. Moll R, Franke WW, Schiller DL, Geiger B, Krepler R. The catalog of human cytokeratins:pattern of expression in normal epithelia, tumors and cultured cells. Cell 1982;31:11-24.

36. Fuchs E. Keratins as biochemical markers of epithelial differentiation. Trends Genet 1988;4:277-81.

37. Badder BL, Frank WW. Cell type-specific and efficient synthesis of human cytokeratin 19 in transgenic mice. Differentiation 1990;45:109-18.

38. Stasiak PC, Lane EB. Sequence of cDNA coding for human cytokeratin 19. Nucleic Acids Res 1987;15:10058.

39. Stasiak PC, Purkis PE, Leigh IM Lane EB. Keratin 19:predicted amino acid sequence and broad tissue distribution suggest it evolved from keratinocyte keratins J Invest Dermatol 1989;92:707-16.

40. Schlimok G, Funke I, Pantel K, Strobel F, Lindemann F, Witte J, Reithmüller G Micrometastatic tumor cells in bone marrow of patients with gastric cancer:methodological aspects of detection and prognostic significance. Eur J Cancer 1991;27(11):1461-5.

41. Knapp AC, Franke WW Spontaneous losses of control of cytokeratin gene expression in transformed non-epithelial human cells occuring at different levels of regulation. Cell 1989;59:67-9.

42. Jarvinen M, Andersson L, Virtanen I. K562 erythroleukaemia cells express cytokeratins 8, 18 and 19 and epithelial membrane antigen that dissapear after induced differentiation. J Cell Physiol 1990;143:310-20.

43. Pantel K, Schlimok G, Angstwurm M, Weckermann D, Schmaus W, Gath H, Passlick B, Izbicki JR, Riethmüller G. Methodological analysis of immunocytochemical screening for disseminated epithelial tumor cells in bone marrow. J Haematotherapy 1994;3(3):165-73.

44. Neumaier M, Gerhard M, Wagener C Diagnosis of micrometastases by the amplification of tissue-specific genes. Gene 1995;159(1):43-7.

45. Gerhard M, Juhl H, Kalthoff H, Schreiber HW, Wagener C, Neumaier M. Specific detection of carcinoembryonic antigen expressing tumor cells in bone marrow aspirates by polymerase chain reaction J Clin Oncol 1994;12(4):725-9.

46. Hussain M, Kurkuraga M, Biggar S, Sakr W, Cummings G, Ensley J. Prostate cancer:flow cytometric methods for detection of bone marrow micrometastases. Cytometry 1996;26:40-6.

47. Traweek ST, Liu J Battifora H. Keratin gene expression in non-epithelial tissues Am J Pathol 1993;142(4):1111-8.

48. Burchill SA, Bradbury MF, Pitman K, Southgate J, Smith B, Selby P. Detection of epithelial cancers in peripheral blood by reverse transciptase-polymerase chain reaction Br J Cancer 1995;71(2):278-81.

49. Chelly J, Concordet JP, Kaplan JC, Khan A. Illegitimate transcription:transcription of any gene in any cell type. Proc Natl Acad Sci USA 1989;86:2617-21.

50. Hochtlen-Vollamar W, Gruber R, Bodenmuller H, Felber E, Lindemann F, Schlimok G, Pantel K, Riethmüller G. Occult epithelial tumor cells detected by an enzyme immunoassay specific for cytokeratin 19. Int J Cancer 1997;70:396-400.

51. Little VR, Lockett SJ, Pallavicini MG. Genotype/phenotype analyses of low frequency tumor cells using computerize image microscopy Cytometry 1996;23:344-57.

52. Muller P, Weckermann D, Reithmüller G, Schlimok G. Detection of genetic alteration in micrometastatic cells in bone marrow of cancer patients by fluorescence in situ hybridization Cancer Genet Cytogenet 1996;88:8-16.

53. Pallavicini MG, Cher ML, Bowers EE, Wessman M, Balouch M, Presti J, Carroll PR. Chromosomal aneusomies in prostate cancer micrometastasis Proc. Am Acad Cancer Res 1995;36:69.

54. Riesenberg R, Oberneder R, Kriegmair M, Epp M, Bitzer U, Hofstetter A, Braun S, Riethmüller G, Pantel K Immunocytochemical double staining of cytokeratin and prostate specific antigen individual prostatic tumor cells Histochemistry 1993;99:61-6.

55. Gallee MPW, VanDer Korput HAGM, VanDerKwast TH, TenKate FJW, Romijn JC, Trapman J Characterization of monoclonal antibodies raised against prostatic cell line PC-82. Prostate 1986;9:33-45.

56. Braun S, Pantel K. Biological characteristics of micrometastatic carcinoma cells in bone marrow. Curr Top Microbiol Immunol 1996;213:163-77.

57. Pantel K, Dickmanns A, Zippelius A, Klein C, Shi J, Hoechtlen-Vollmar W, Schlimok G, Watermann D, Oberneder R, Fanning E Establishment of micrometastatic carcinoma cell lines:a novel source of tumor cell vaccines. JNCI 1995;87:1162-8.

58. Pantel K, Schlimok G, Braun S, Kutter D, Lindmann F, Schaller G, Funke I, Izbicki JR, Reithmüller G Differential expression of proliferation-associated molecules in individual micrometastatic carcinoma cells. JNCI 1993;85(17):1419-24.

59. Braun S, Pantel K Biological characteristics of micrometastatic carcinoma cells in bone marrow. Cur Top Microbiol Immunol 1996;213:163-77.

60. Shpall EJ, Stemmer SM, Bearman SI, Meyers S, Purdy M, Jones RB. New strategies in marrow purging for breast cancer patients receiving high-dose chemotherapy with autologous bone marrow transplantation. Breast Cancer Res Treat 1993;26 (suppl):519-27.

61. Ross AA, Miller GW, Moss TJ, Kahn DG, Warner NE, Sweet DL, Louie KG, Schneidermann E, Pecora AL, Meagher RC. Immunocytochemical detection of toumour cells in bone marrow and peripheral blood stem cell collections from patients with ovarian cancer Bone Marrow Transplant 1995;15:929-33.

62. Riethmüller G, Johnson JP. Monoclonal antibodies in the detection and therapy of micrometastatic epithelial cancer. Curr Opin Immunol 1992;4:647-55.

63. O'Sullivan GC, Corbett AR, Shanahan F, Collins JK. Regional immunosuppression in esophageal squamous cancer: Evidence from functional studies with matched lymph nodes. J Immunology 1996;157:4717-20.

64. O'Connell J, O'Sullivan GC, Collins JK, Shanahan F. The Fas counter attack: Fas-mediated T cell killing by colon cancer cells expressing Fas ligand. J Exp Med 1996;184:1075-82.

65. Bennett MW, O' Connell J, O' Sullivan GC, Brady C, Roche D, Collins JK, Shanahan F The Fas counterattack in vivo:apoptotic depletion of tumor-infiltrating lymphocytes (TIL) associated with Fas ligand (FasL) expression by esophageal carcinoma. J Immunology 1998;1600:5669-75.

66. Passlick B, Izbicki JR, Simmel S, Kubushcok B, Karg O, Habekost M, Thetter O, Schweibeibeer L, Pantel K. Expression of major histocompatibility class I and class II antigens and intercellular adhesion molecile-1 expression on operable non-small cell lung carcinomas. Eur J Cancer 1995;30:376-81.

67. Pantel K, Schlimok G, Kutter D, Schaller G, Genz T, Wiebecke B, Backmann R, Funke I, Riethmüller G. Frequent down regulation of major histocompatibility class I antigen expression on individual micrometastatic carcinoma cells. Cancer Res 1991;51:4712-15.

68. Kelsen DP, Ginsberg R, Pajak TF, Sheahan DG, Gunderson L, Mortimer J, Estes N, Haller DG, Ajani J, Kocha W, Minsky BD, Roth JA.

Chemotherapy followed by surgery compared with surgery alone for localised esophageal cancer. N Engl J Med 1998;339:1979-84.

69. Lighdale CJ. Esophageal Cancer. Am J Gastroenterology 1999;94:20-9.

70. Pera M, Cameron AJ, Trastek VF, Carpenter HA, Zinsmeister AR. Increasing incidence of adenocarcinoma of the esophagus and esophagogastric junction. Gastroenterology 1993;104:510-13.

71. Bytzer P, Christensen PB, Damkier P, Vinding K, Seersholm N. Adenocarcinoma of Esophagus and Barrett's esophagus:a population based study. Am J Gastroenterology 1999;94:86-91.

73 Walsh TN, Noonan N, Hollywood D, Kelly A, Keeling N, Hennessy TPJ. A comparison of multimodal therapy with surgery for esophageal adenocarcinoma. N Engl J Med 1996;335:462-7.

73. Shanahan F, O'Sullivan GC. Progress in treating esophageal adenocarcinoma Gastroenterology 1997;112:1417-8.

74. O'Brien MG, Fitzgerald E, Lee G, Crowley M, Shanahan F, O'Sullivan GC. A prospective comparison of laparoscopy and imaging in the staging of esophagogastric cancer before surgery. Am J Gastroenterology 1995;90(12):2191-219.

75. Pantel K, Dockmanns A, Zippelius A, Klein C, Shi J, Hoechtlen-Vollmar W, Schlimok G, Weckermann D, Oberneder R, Fanning E, Riethmuller G. Establishment of micrometastatic carcinoma cell lines: a novel source of tumor cell vaccines. J Natl Cancer Inst 1995;87:1162-8.

76. Uhr, J.W., Scheuermann, R.H., Street, N. E. and Vitetta, E.S. 1997. Cancer dormancy:opportunities for new therapeutic approaches. Nature Medicine 1997; 3:505-9.

77. Callaway MP and Briggs JC. The incidence of later recurrence (greater than 10 years):An analysis of 536 consecutive cases of cutaneous melanoma. Br J Plast Surg 1989;42:46-9.

78. Henderson JC, Harris JR, Kinne DW, Hellman S. Cancer of the breast. in Cancer:Principles and Practice of Oncology, 3rd edn (eds DeVita VJ, Jr, Hellman S and Rosenberg SA) 1197-1268 (Lippincott, Philadelphia, 1989).

79. Schlimok, G., Funke, I., Bock, B., Schweiber, B., Witte, J., Riethmüller, G. 1990. Epithelial tumor cells in bone marrow of patients with colorectal cancer:immunocytochemical detection, phenotypic characterisation and prognostic significance. JClinical Oncology 8:831-7.

80. Lindemann, F., Shlimok, G., Dirshedl, P., Witte, J. and Reithmüller, G. 1992. Prognostic significance of micrometastatic tumor cells in bone marrow of colorectal cancer patients. Lancet 340:685-9.

81. Cote, R.J., Rosen, P.P., Lesser, M.L., Old, L.J. and Osborne, M.P. 1991. Prediction of early relapse in patients with operable breast cancer by detection of occult bone marrow micrometastases. Journal of Clinical Oncology 9:1749-56.

82. Braun, S., Pantel, K., Muller, P. et al. 2000. Cytokeratin positive cells in the bone marrow and survival of patients with Stage I II or III Breast Cancer. N Engl J Med 342:525-33.

83. Pantel, K., Izbicki, J., Passilick, B., Angstwurm, M., Haussinger, K., Thetter,O. and Riethmüller,G. 1996. Frequency and prognostic significance of micrometastatic tumor cells in bone marrow of patients with non-small-cell lung cancer without overt metastases. Lancet 347:646-3.

84. Uhr, J.W., Scheuermann, R.H., Street, N. E. and Vitetta, E.S. 1997. Cancer dormancy:opportunities for new therapeutic approaches. Nature Medicine 3:505-9.

85. Levy R and Miller RA. Therapy of lymphoma directed at idiotypes. 1990;J Natl Cancer Ins Monogr 10:61-8.

6.1 INDICATIONS AND OUTCOME OF ESOPHAGEAL RESECTION.

Toni Lerut

1. INTRODUCTION

It is now a generally recognized fact that the incidence of adenocarcinoma of the esophagus and gastro-esophageal junction has shown a remarkable increase during recent decades[1,2].

It is well established that the vast majority of adenocarcinomas especially when arising in the lower esophagus and gastro-esophageal junction are associated with areas of intestinal metaplasia i.e. Barrett's esophagus[3].

Adenocarcinoma of the esophagus and GEJ in general is a disease associated with a high mortality despite aggressive therapy. This poor prognosis is mainly due to the fact that patients with these tumors frequently remain asymptomatic until dysphagia develops from obstruction of the lumen, a common symptom in patients with advanced disease. Often the tumor is invading through the wall of the esophagus/cardia and spread of the disease to lymph nodes and/or distant organs has already occurred at the time of diagnosis and/or therapy.

Barrett's esophagus would be only of passing interest were it not for it's association with an increased risk for developing primary adenocarcinoma.

As a result an increasing number of patients especially those patients presenting with an extended zone of biopsy proven metaplasia will be enrolled in a surveillance program.

Such surveillance program is resulting in a growing number of patients that -in contrast with the classic presentation of an advanced stage carcinoma- is presenting with an early stage carcinoma i.e. tumor confined to the mucosa or submucosa. This group of patients offers the most favorable prerequisites for curative therapy[4] an additional reason why Barrett's esophagus remains a fascinating and challenging condition.

2. INDICATION FOR SURGERY

If early detection is one important factor for a favorable outcome complete removal is the second proven pillar contributing to the cure of the disease when treated by surgery.

Therefore staging is of paramount importance whether the patient is presenting with an early or more advanced stage.

Physical examination may reveal distant lymph node metastasis e.g. in the cervical region or other clinical manifestation of organ metastasis. But for most of the patients one has to rely on further technical examinations.

Today a wide variety of investigative techniques are available: Ba swallow, endoscopy and biopsy, CT scan, ultrasound, echo-endoscopy (EUS), Position Emission Tomography scan, staging thoracoscopy, laparoscopy.

3. STAGING

3.1 T-STAGING

Accuracy of CT in assessing tumor infiltration in surrounding structures in particular infiltration of the aorta is about 80%. When esophageal contact exceeds 90% of the aortic circumference over a distance of more than two images invasion is likely. Also the loss of the triangular fat plane between esophagus, aorta and spine is helpful to assess invasion of the aorta. CT scan is less accurate in assessing infiltration of the pericardium because the lack of fat plane between esophagus and pericardium[5,6].

Suspicion of invasion of the tracheobronchial tree is based on displacement or indentation of the posterior wall of either the trachea or bronchus. Accuracy of CT is here 75%.

Endoscopic ultrasonography (EUS) is a more accurate technique in defining the T parameter[7]. Nevertheless a margin of error both false positive and false negative is still around 20 to 30% in the T_1T_2 tumors. Moreover in T_1 tumors it is important to discriminate between the T_{1a} (intramucosal) and T_{1b} (submucosal) infiltration. Indeed in the T_{1b} tumors the likelihood of lymph node invasion is approximately 25 to 50%[8] whereas the incidence of lymph node involvement is almost 0% in T_{1a} tumors. A frequency of 20 megahertz is required to discriminate between these structures[9]. The accuracy of EUS in the diagnosis of infiltration to adjacent anatomical structures ($T_3 - T_4$) is around 80% provided an ability to pass the tumor. The inability to pass a tumor or stenosis ranges between 20 and 40% which of course also restricts the possibility of

H.W. Tilanus and S.E.A. Attwood (eds.), Barrett's Esophagus, 317–324.
© 2001 *Kluwer Academic Publishers. Printed in the Netherlands.*

assessing not only tumors but also lymph node invasion[10,11].

3.2 N-STAGING

Occasionally cervical nodes can be diagnosed by clinical examination (supraclavicular and cervical lymph nodes). CT accuracy in diagnosing invasion of mediastinal lymph nodes is about 60%. The CT criterion for an abnormal node is a transverse axis of 10 mm or greater. In such cases overstaging is to be taken in consideration[12]. EUS accuracy for positive lymph node detection is about 70 to 80%. However EUS has a tendency to overestimate histologic involvement (sensitivity 90%, specificity 60%)[7,6,13]. As a result of these difficulties there is a growing interest for minimal invasive techniques such as thoracoscopy and laparoscopy in the pretreatment staging of esophageal carcinoma. However because of the rather chaotic pattern of lymph node metastasis theoretically both laparoscopic and thoracoscopic staging will be required which is rather time consuming and probably rather a (too?) invasive staging methodology[14].

Recently FDG-PET scan has been introduced as a promising tool in detecting distant lymph nodes metastasis. In a recent study[15] we reported a sensitivity of 77%, a specificity of 90% and an accuracy of 86% for detecting $M+_{Ly}$ in a series of 42 patients with carcinoma of the esophagus and GEJ treated with curative intent.

3.3 M-STAGING

Chest X-ray, liver ultrasound, ultrasound of the neck, CT of the chest and abdomen are performed in order to detect visceral metastasis and distal lymph node metastasis. PET scan (Positron Emission Tomography) is offering additional possibilities in detecting otherwise occult visceral organ metastasis and distant lymph node metastasis in approximately 5 – 10%[16].

4. IMPLICATIONS OF CLINICAL STAGING ON THERAPEUTIC STRATEGY AND INDICATION FOR SURGERY.

4.1 EARLY CARCINOMA.

Much debate persists on the treatment modalities of carcinoma confined to the mucosa i.e. high grade dysplasia – T_1 tumors. Endoscopic ablation by laser technology or by endoscopic mucosectomy has been advocated recently[17,18].

The rationale for this approach is based on the fact that in high grade dysplasia (= carcinoma in situ) there is no lymphatic invasion, while lymph node metastasis in intramucosal (T_{1a}) carcinoma is uncommon[19].

As a consequence reported 5-year survival for high-grade dysplasia and intramucosal carcinoma is ranging between 90-100% both after endoluminal mucosectomy or after esophagectomy. Proponents of esophagectomy however argue that in patients with documented high-grade dysplasia invasive adenocarcinoma is present in other areas of the metaplastic mucosa in approximately 50% of the cases when analyzing the resected specimen[20-22].

For this reason most surgical groups advocate esophagectomy in medically operable patients presenting with high-grade dysplasia.

A second critical issue is whether intramucosal (T_{1a}) carcinoma can be correctly discriminated from submucosal tumor (T_{1b}) before surgery. Certainly 20 mHz echo-endoscopes can be helpful to solve this problem but these endoscopic ultrasonographic systems are not available in most centres[9]. Using conventional EUS a recent analysis of 11 T_{is}-T_1 tumors at our institution revealed 6 T_{1b} tumors on final postresection pathology.

The importance of the (in)ability to discriminate T_{1a} from T_{1b} tumors relates to the reported incidence of 25-50% lymph node involvement in T_{1b} tumors.

Mostly the number of involved lymph nodes is rather limited and most surgeons will argue that this group of patients is benefiting most from surgery with curative intent.

4.2 ADVANCED CARCINOMA

As tumor penetrates deeper into or through the muscular wall of the esophagus the incidence of lymph node involvement will increase. For T_3 tumors the incidence of lymph node involvement is up to 80%[23]. Lymph node involvement is considered to be the most important prognostic factor (4). From these findings different attitudes towards therapeutic strategies emerged.

One concept is based on the fact that lymph node involvement is to be considered as systemic disease and that surgery aiming at removal of more than the primary tumor is not helpful. Many surgeons however agree that complete (R_0) resection of the primary tumor together with its lymphatic drainage may alter the natural cause of the disease and therefore offers the best potential for long term survival.

As the tumor spreads through the esophageal wall chances of obtaining R_0 resection are decreasing. Especially when dealing with T_4 tumors the percentage of complete resection is falling sharply, below 50%[24].

In case of supracarinal tumors it is difficult to discriminate between stage T_3 and T_4, it seems much easier to make this distinction for infracarinal tumors. And provided there is no gross aortic invasion on CT or EUS it has been our experience that in most of the infracarinal tumors a complete R_0 resection is possible in over 90% of our patient material[4].

Nevertheless the results of surgery alone in advanced stages remain disappointing stimulating neo adjuvant chemo- or radiotherapy.

There are few studies available on adenocarcinoma with conflicting data.

The so called Irish trial[25] comparing neo-adjuvant chemoradiation plus surgery versus surgery alone reported marked downstaging in the multimodality arm and a significant survival benefit as compared to surgery alone.

However the study has been heavily criticized because of a number of obvious and serious shortcomings, mainly in the way patients were selected, the poor quality of clinical staging, the lack of data on R_0 resection rate and the unacceptable low survival, 6% at three years in the surgery alone arm[26]. Clearly other studies with better study design are needed before generalizing the use of induction therapy in potentially resectable carcinoma.

In our center induction therapy is advocated in cases of clear clinical T_4 tumors or more recently in patients who present with multiple lymph node metastases in distant compartments ($M+L_y$) as identified by cervical US or more recently on PET scan and confirmed on biopsies. In T_3-T_4 tumors of the GEJ laparoscopic staging is performed to judge the possible invasion into the surrounding structures and to rule out occult peritumoral or minute liver metastasis.

Preliminary data from literature seem to indicate that such a policy is resulting in a survival benefit especially in complete responders (occurring in approximately 20-25% when using chemoradiation, 5-10% when using chemotherapy alone) when compared to historical series[23].

These data are encouraging but at the same time indicate a high failure rate mostly due to progression of disease during treatment or systemic recurrence after completing the treatment. Therefore too liberal indications for induction therapy should be avoided taking into account the well established increase in incidence of morbidity (infection, anastomotic leak, pulmonary complications) and in some series of postoperative mortality.

5. SURGICAL TECHNIQUE

There is controversy about the optimal route and extent of resection for adenocarcinoma of the distal esophagus and GEJ. This controversy is mainly fueled by different opinions regarding lymph node involvement. Some authors like Orringer[27] consider lymph node involvement equal to systemic disease and therefore outcome of treatment being determined at the time of diagnosis.

Removal of the primary tumor aiming at relief of symptoms is the primary goal of resection, systematic removal of involved lymph nodes being judged of no benefit. The operation typically is performed by transhiatal resection restoring continuity by gastric pull up and cervical esophagogastrostomy.

Such operations today can be performed equally using VATS technology[28].

Many others however believe that the natural course of the disease can be influenced by a wide peritumoral or an en bloc dissection combined with meticulous lymphadenectomy of the upper abdominal compartment (so called D_2 lymphadenectomy) and posterior mediastinal lymphadenectomy[29-31].

According to Siewert lymph flow in carcinoma of the distal esophagus and GEJ is mainly directed downwards towards the lymphatic nodes around the coeliac axis. In his analysis lymph node metastases were rarely found in the paratracheal, subcarinal or mid thoracic para-esophageal lymph nodes.

As a result the Munich group favors a "radical" transhiatal lymphadenectomy and en bloc lymphadenectomy of the distal posterior mediastinum and upper abdominal compartment[32].

Our own data analysis from transthoracic resection especially in the more advanced T_3N_+ stage shows a high incidence of lymph node involvement around the subcarinal and aortopulmonary region in both adenocarcinoma of the distal esophagus and GEJ. Moreover systematic resection of the thoracic duct, hard to perform through a transhiatal approach, showed in this subset of patients lymphatic involvement in up to 50% of the distal esophageal[33] tumors. Adding the so-called third field i.e. a bilateral cervical lymphadenectomy showed a 35% and 20% unforeseen lymph node involvement for distal esophageal tumors and GEJ tumors respectively.

As a result our standard approach for adenocarcinoma of the distal esophagus and GEJ is through a left transthoracic approach with inverted T shaped incision of the diaphragm at its periphery (Figure 1).

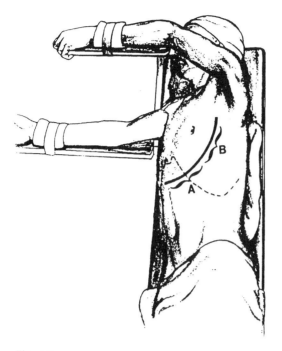

Figure 1a

This approach offers an excellent exposition of both the upper abdominal compartment and posterior mediastinum allowing adequate dissection and lymphadenectomy. In patients without major comorbidity an additional bilateral cervical lymphadenectomy is added.

Beside efforts to perform peritumoral resection as wide as possible experience learns that carcinoma of the esophagus and GEJ have a tendency to extend submucosally in the longitudinal axis and many patients present with multicentric localizations (skip lesions).

In order to decrease the risk of anastomotic recurrences most authors today agree on performing a subtotal esophagectomy for carcinoma of the esophagus and many advocate the same procedure for tumors of the GEJ. For the same oncologic reasons resection of the lesser curvature of the stomach is advocated to obtain a negative distal section plane and to resect potentially positive lymph nodes at the level of the lesser curvature. For tumors extending more than 5 cm towards the stomach as a rule a total gastrectomy will be performed.

While our group prefers a left sided transthoracic approach for infracarinal tumors, others prefer the right sided Ivor Lewis or McKeown type approach.

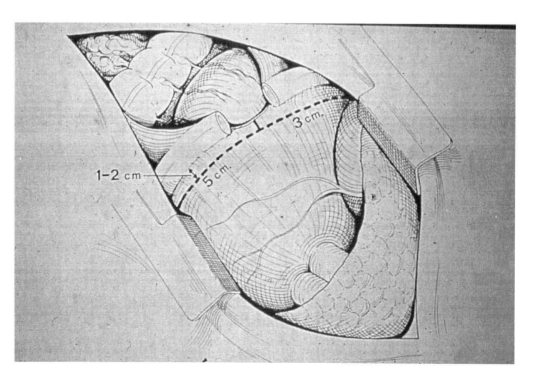

Figure 1 b

6. RESULTS

Over the last two decades important improvement in surgical techniques and pre- and postoperative management have been resulting in a significant decrease in postoperative mortality and morbidity. Today postoperative hospital mortality in centers with large experience is below 5%. Postoperative morbidity is mainly caused by pulmonary complications (infection, atelectasis) in about 25% of the patients. Anastomotic leaks occur in 5 to 10% but rarely result in fatal septic complications especially if anastomosis is performed in the neck. Figure 2 shows the overall survival curve of a series of esophagectomy in 63 patients with a Barrett adenocarcinoma in the tubular esophagus from our own experience. There was no postoperative hospital mortality and overall 1-year survival was 80%, 62.7% at 2 years and 58.2% at 5 years. According to the different pTNM stages 5-year survival for patients with stage 0 or I disease was 100% for stage II 87.5% for stage III 22.2% and for stage IV 0% (Figure 3). Five-year survival of patients without lymph node involvement was 85.3% versus 38.8% for patients with lymph node involvement (p=0.0033). This difference clearly illustrates the importance of lymph node status as a prognostic index (Fig. 4).

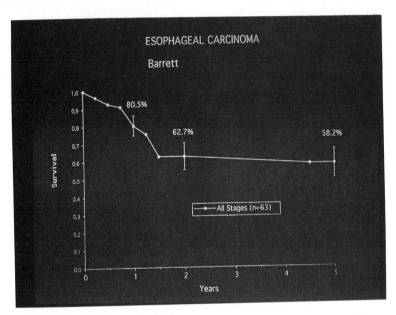

Figure 2

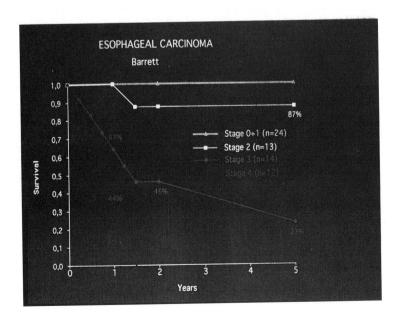

Figure 3

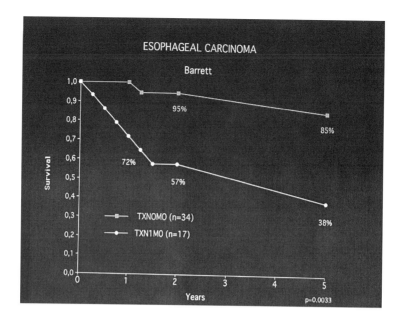

Figure 4

In this respect it is important to notice that 34 patients (54.5%) were under medical surveillance for a related or unrelated upper gastrointestinal condition before diagnosis. Only 9 of these patients (26.5%) had diseased lymph nodes. All stage 0 and 14 of the 17 stage I carcinomas belonged in this group. On the contrary in 32 patients (48.5%) the diagnosis was established during their first medical contact for tumor related symptoms. In this group the percentage of diseases lymph nodes was 78%.

These survival curves are better than the survival curves obtained in adenocarcinoma of the GEJ and squamous cell carcinoma probably reflection the effect of the relative higher number of early carcinomas and a relative lower tumor load even in patients presenting with positive nodes. The latter clearly underlines the effect of extensive lymphadenectomy in patients with a limited number of positive nodes resulting in 5-year survival as high as 38.3%.

Furthermore extensive lymphadenectomy clearly offers prolonged disease free survival and a lesser incidence of locoregional disease. In our own experience with 37 patients treated with 3-field lymphadenectomy 6 (17%) developed recurrence within the operative field. All six patients had stage IV disease because of distant lymph node metastasis

(M_{+Ly}) and a heavy tumor load all with $\geq$ 5 positive lymph nodes. Yet 3 out of the six developed their recurrence at 3 years or later after surgery which is definitely in contrast with the usual finding of locoregional recurrence within the first year post surgery[34]. Locoregional recurrence was below 10% in the series of Altorki (35), Clark (36), Collard (37) whereas Barbier[38] had a 50% locoregional recurrence after transhiatal recurrence and van Lanschot[39] 32%.

Several other groups[4,32,40-42] have reported similar results (Table I). The message from these different series is obvious. Adenocarcinoma arising in Barrett's can be cured by surgical resection when detected at an early stage.

The 100% survival in stage I in some of these series should be the gold standard to which any other regimen such as mucosal ablation and mucosectomy has to be compared.

Similarly for patients with more advanced carcinoma induction therapy should not be used too liberal since it seems that such regimens will not result in a survival patients in potentially resectable tumors.

It is our opinion, together with others, that induction regimens should be reserved only for those patients in whom a complete resection with an adequate safety margin (R_0) appears unlikely.

TABLE I. Results of surgical resection in Barrett adenocarcinoma

	n	MORTALITY RATE	5-YR SURVIVAL
DeMeester[40]	16	6.2%	53%
Streitz[41]	61	3.3%	23%
Lerut[4]	66	0%	58.2%
Siewert[24]	163	37%	44%
Collard[42]	55	0%	59%

REFERENCES

1. Blot WJ: Esophageal cancer trends and risk factors. Semin Oncol 1994;21:403-10.

2. Pera M, Cameron AJ, Trastek VF, Carpenter HA, Zinsmeister AR: Increasing incidence of adencarcinoma of the esophagus and esophagogastric junction. Gastroenterol 1993;104:510-3.

3. Spechler S: Barrett's esophagus. Semin Oncol 1994;2:431-7.

4. Lerut T, Coosemans W, Van Raemdonck D, Dillemans B, De Leyn P, Marnette JM, Geboes K: Surgical treatment of Barrett's carcinoma. Correlations between morphologic findings and prognosis. J Thorac Cardiovas Surg 1994;107:1059-66.

5. Takashima S, Tokeuchi N, Shiozaki H, Kabayashi K, Marimoto S, Ikezoe J: Carcinoma of the esophagus: CT versus MR imaging in determing resectability. AJR 1999;156:297-2.

6. Fekete F, Sauvanet A, Zins M, Berthoux L, Amouyal C: Imaging of cancer of the esophagus: ultrasound endoscopy or computed tomography? Ann Chir 1995;49:573-8.

7. Pham T, Roach E, Falk GL, Chu J, Ngu MC, Jones DB: Staging of oesophageal carcinoma by endoscopic ultrasound: preliminary experience. Aust N Z J Surg 1998;68(3):209-12.

8. Cameron AJ, Carpenter HA: Barrett's esophagus, high grade dysplasia and early adenocarcinoma: a pathological study. Am J Gastroenterol 1992;92:586-91.

9. Natsugoe S, Baba M, Yoshinaka H, Kijima F, Shimada M, Shirao K, Kusano C, Fukomoto T, Mueller J, Aikou T: Mucosal squamous cell carcinoma of the esophagus: a clinicopathologic study of 30 cases. Oncology 1998;55(3):235-41.

10. Lightdale CJ: Diagnosis of esophagogastric tumors. Endoscopy 1996;28:22-6.

11. Ditter HJ, Siewert JR: Role of endoscopic ultrasonography in esophageal carcinoma. Endoscopy 1993;25:156-6.

12. Maerz LL, Deveney CW, Lopez RR, et al: Role of computed tomorgraphic scans in the staging of esophageal and proximal gastric malignancies. Am J Surg 1993;165:558-60.

13. Vickers J: Role of endoscopic ultrasound in the preoperative assessment of patients with oesophageal cancer. Ann R Coll Surg Engl 1998;80(4):233-9.

14. Luketich JD, Schauer P, Landreneau R, et al: Minimally invasive surgical staging is superior to endoscopic ultrasound in detecting lymph node metastasis in esophageal cancer. J Thorac Cardiovasc Surg 1997;114:817-21.

15. Lerut T, Flamen P, Ectyors N, Van Cutsem E, Peeters M, Hiele M, De Weber W, Coosemans W, Decker G, De Leyn P, Deneffe G, Van Raemdonck D, Mortelmans L: Histopathological validation of lymph node staging in cancer of the esophagus and gastro-esophageal junction with FGD-PET scan : a prospective study based on primary surgery with extensive lymphadenectomy. Annals Thorac Surg, 2000, in press.

16. Flamen P, Lerut A. The utility of Positron Emission Tomography (PET) for the staging of patients with potentially operable esophageal carcinoma. J Clin Oncol, 2000, in press.

17. Van Laethem JL, Jagodinski R, Devière R, Cremer M: Argon plasma coagulation (APC) in the treatment of high grade dysplasia or early carcinoma: cure or palliation? Gastrointest Endosc 19987:AB77.

18. Ell C, May A, Gossner L, Pech O, GünterE, Mayer G, Henrich R, Vieth M, Müllmer H, Seitz G, Stolte M: Endoscopic mucosal resection of early cancer and high-grade dysplasia in Barrett's Esophagus. Gastroenterol 2000;118:1-8.

19. Hölscher A, Bollschweiler E, Schneider PM, Siewert JR: Early adenocarcinoma in Barrett's esophagus. Br J Surg 1997;84:1470-3.

20. Peters JH, Clark GW, Ireland AP, et al: Outcome of adenocarcinoma arising in Barrett's esophagus in endoscopically surveyed and nonsurveyed patients. J Thorac Cardiovasc Surg 1994;108:13-822.

21. Altorki NK, Sunagawa M, Little AG, Skinner DB: High-grade dysplasia in columnar –lined esohpagus. Am J Surg 1991;161:97-100.

22. Pera M, Trastek VF, Carpenter HA, et al: Barrett's esophagus with high-grade dysplasia: an indication for esophagectomy? Ann Thorac Surg 1992;54:199-204.

23. Rice TW, Zuccaro G, Adelstein GJ, Rybicki LA, Blackstone EH, Goldblum JR: Esophageal carcinoma : Depth of tumor invasion is predictive of regional lymph node status. Ann Thorac Surg, 1998;787-92.

24. Siewert JR, Stein MJ: Barrett's Cancer: Indications, extent, and results of surgical resection. Semin Surg Oncol 1997:245-52.

25. Walsh TN, Noonan N, Hollywood D, et al: A comparison of multimodal therapy and sugery for esophageal adenocarcinoma. N Engl J Med 1996;335:462-7.

26. Wilke H, Fink U: Mutimodal therapy for adenocarcinalm of the esophagus and esophagogastric junction (Editorial) (Comment in : N Engl J Med 335:462-467) N Engl J Med 1996;335:509-10.

27. Orringer MB: Transhiatal esophagectomy without thoracotomy for carcinoma of the thoracic esophagus. Ann Surg 1984;200:282-8.

28. Collard JM, Lengele B, Otte JB, Kestens PJ: En bloc and standard esophagectomies by thoracoscopy. Ann Thorac Surg 1993;56:675-9.

29. Skinner DB: En bloc resection for neoplasms of the esophagus and cardia. J Thorac Cardiovasc Surg 1983;85:59-71.

30. Lerut T, De Leyn P, Coosemans W, et al: Surgical strategies in esophageal carcinoma with emphasis on radical lymphadenectomy. Ann Surg 1992;16:583-90.

31. Hagen JA, Peters JH, DeMeester TR: Superiority of extended en bloc esophagogastrectomy for carcinoma

of the lower esophagus and cardia. J Thorac Cardiovasc Surg 1993;106:850-9.

32. Hölscher AH, Bollschweiler E, Bumm R, et al: Prognostic factors of resected adenocarcinoma of the esophagus. Surgery 1995;118:845-55.

33. van de Ven C, De Leyn P, Coosemans W, Van Raemdonc D, Lerut T: Three-field lymphadenectomy and pattern of lymph node spread in T3 adenocarcinoma of the distal esophagus and the gastro-esophageal junction. Europ J Cardio-thorac Surg 1999;15:769-73.

34. Lerut T: Esophageal surgery at the end of the millenium. J Thorac Cardiovasc Surg 1998;116:1-20.

35. Altorki NK, Girardi L, Skinner DB: En bloc esophagectomy improves survival for stage III esophageal cancer. J Thorac Cardiovasc Surg 1997;114:948-56.

36. Clark GWB, Peeters JH, Ireland AP, et al: Nodal metastasis and sites of recurrence after en bloc esophagectomy for adenocarcinoma. Ann Thorac Surg 1994;58:646-54.

37. Collard JM, Otte JB, Reynaert MS, Michel LA, Malaise JF, Lengele BG, Hermans BP, Kestens PJ: Extensive lymph node clearance for cancer of the esophagus or cardia: Merits and limits in reference to 5-year absolute survival. Hepato-Gastroent 1995;42:619-27.

38. Barbier PA, Luder PJ, Schupfer G, Becker CD, Wasner H. Quality of life and patterns of recurrence following transhiatal esophagectomy for cancer: results of prospective follow-up n 50 patients. World J Surg 1988;12:270-6.

39. van Lanschot JJ, Tilanus HW, Voormolen MH, van Deelen RA: Recurrence pattern of oesophageal carcinoma after limited resection does not support wide local excision with extensive lymph node dissection. Br J Surg 1994;81:1320-4.

40. DeMeester TR, Attwood SE, Smyrk TC, et al: Surgical therapy in Barrett's esophagus. Ann Surg 1990;212:528-42.

41. Streitz JM, Ellis FH jr, Gibb SP et al: adenocarcinoma in Barrett's esophagus. A clinicopathologic study of 65 cases. Ann Surg 1987;205:557-62.

42. Collard JM, Romagnoli R, Hermans BP, Malaise J: Radical esophageal resection for adenocarcinoma arising in Barrett's esophagus. Am J Surg 1997;174:307-11.

6.2   TRANSHIATAL ESOPHAGECTOMY

Rudolf Bumm and J.Rüdiger Siewert

1. INTRODUCTION

The surgical removal of the thoracic esophagus through the open chest is an invasive operation which usually involves two body cavities and, therefore, lead to a considerable morbidity and mortality in the 50's and 60's. Consequently, the limited short- and long term results led to the opinion that the option "surgery" was only a minor one in the late 70's, and that the central goal of treatment of esophageal adeno- and squamous cell carcinoma was: palliation.

There have been several efforts to avoid thoracotomy in patients with esophageal carcinoma. The concept of transhiatal esophagectomy (THE) was proposed in the early 20th century by Denk[10] in Austria, and the operation was first performed by Turner[36] and in Germany, by Fischer[13]. In recent decades THE was rediscovered by several working groups and made popular by Orringer and Sloan[26,27]. In fact the special anatomy and blood supply of the esophagus allowed routinely for blunt mobilisation of the esophagus by finger-dissection and , for the first time, esophageal resection could be performed in large series with acceptable mortality and morbidity.

However, even in experienced hands THE still had a considerable intraoperative complication rate due to the 'blind' mediastinal dissection. These complications included lesions of the recurrent nerve, the trachea and mediastinal bleedings. In addition, THE was stated to be a non-radical procedure and still primarily a method for palliation. Transthoracic esophagectomy and "En-bloc" resection (TTE) of the thoracic esophagus was introduced by surgeons from the eastern[1,2], later from the western hemisphere[31-33]. For the first time favourable long term results were described for patients with mid- and late stage esophageal carcinoma, and although the Japanese results were never entirely reproduced in the US and Europe, there was, after some time, a marked improvement of long term results in most of the centers dealing with esophageal surgery[25]. There is strong evidence that

this was mainly because radical lymphadenectomy and 'en Bloc' resection was used[9].

In 1990 Buess and coworkers described an endoscopic technique for dissection of the thoracic esophagus from the neck and under direct vision[21,22,5]. In order to improve THE-techniques we modified, evaluated and applied this method clinically. Furthermore, we added regional lymphadenectomy and transhiatal "en bloc" resection of the primary tumor as the standard technique. A similar modification was published by Alderson[3].

In general, we use TTE as the standard procedure for squamous cell carcinoma of the esophagus, and THE is reserved for the treatment of Barrett's carcinoma[30] because it allows for secure resection of the primary tumor and sufficient abdominal and lower mediastinal lymphadenectomy. Esophago-gastrostomy is accomplished via a cervical access. This chapter describes the standard procedure which was, over the years, supplemented by 'en-bloc' resection techniques and endoscopic mediastinal dissection (endodissection).

2. INDICATION FOR SURGERY

All patients with Barrett's carcinoma undergo preoperative staging including endoscopy and endosonography with rebiopsy of the tumor, CT-scan of thorax and abdomen and abdominal ultrasound. Patients undergo a detailed risk analysis including pulmonary, hepatic and renal function tests as well as a cardiologic check-up. An internet-based JAVA applet for calculation of our risk score is available under http://nt1.chir.med.tumuenchen.de/risiko-e.html. Cooperation as well as Karnovsky (general) status are evaluated.

Surgical resection remains the method of choice for treatment of adenocarcinoma of the distal esophagus. The value of prophylactic surgery in cases with dysplasia in the mucosa of the distal esophagus is under evaluation, and general recommendations cannot be made. We see an indication for a 'limited' resection of the distal esophagus

H.W. Tilanus and S.E.A. Attwood (eds.), Barrett's Esophagus, 325–333.

and small gut interposition in cases with high-grade dysplasia in Barrett's epithelium of the esophagus. Patients with advanced tumors (UICC T 3 N+) may be included into neoadjuvant chemotherapy protocols, but this should be strictly done in trials because there are no conclusive results to date whether neoadjuvant treatment is followed by a significant prognostic benefit. In case of extended tumors or limited patient status palliative treatments include laser or stent therapy. In our clinical practice there is to date no place for palliative resections. Surgery should only be attempted if an R0/R1-situation (no macroscopic residual tumor) can be reached.

3. TECHNIQUE

All patients must be informed that in rare cases THE needs to be transformed into TTE when intraoperative staging reveals that the tumor extends into the supracarinal region or when complications such as mediastinal bleeding occur. The operation begins with bringing the patient into a supine position and desinfection of the skin. We usually have two operating teams as outlined in Figure 2.
The esophagus should be intubated with a rigid rubber tube. The abdominal wall, the anterior thorax and the left side of the neck must be completely exposed. The complete operation can be done in 2 ½ to 3 hours in a two team approach in which one (the cervical) team mobilizes the esophagus via a cervical access (Figure 1), combined with mediastinal endodissection and the other (the abdominal) team performs en-bloc resection of the primary with lymphadenectomy and preparation of the gastric tube.

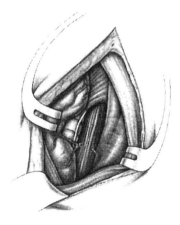

Figure 1. Cervical access showing the carotid artery and jugular vein (right), the esophagus and the left recurrent nerve (source: Breitner Chirurgie des Abdomens 2, Hrsg. J.R. Siewert, München; Wien, Baltimore; Urban und Schwarzenberg 1989 [modified])

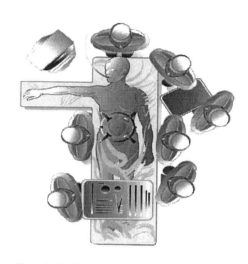

Figure 2. Position of the operating team (source: Bumm)

3.1 CERVICAL PROCEDURE AND ENDODISSECTION

The cervical incision (Figure 1) should be made at the anterior edge of the m.sternocleidomastoideus. The m. omohyoideus is divided by monopolar electrocautery and the inferior thyroid artery is divided between ligatures and the left lobe of the thyroid should be mobilized. The recurrent laryngeal nerve must be identified and carefully preserved during the next steps of the dissection. The nerve is best located at the point where it is undercrossing the inferior thyroid artery. Further dissection of the nerve should be avoided in order to prevent secondary lesions. The cervical esophagus is then circumferentially mobilized by careful blunt / sharp dissection and drawn laterally by help of a silicone tube in order to gain some dissection space between esophagus and trachea. The mediastinal endodissector (Figure 3) is then assembled and inserted into the upper mediastinum. This instrument (Storz Inc., Tuttlingen, Germany) features a tissue dilator at the tip , a 15 degree Hopkins fiberoptical device and a working channel for one 5mm laparascopic instruments. The tissue dilator is anatomically designed so that it can "ride" on the esophageal surface and opens an anterograde dissection space of 2-3 cm in the mediastinum. The tissue dilator of the mediastinoscope can be freely rotated 360 degrees. For full operation the mediastinoscope is connected to a video camera (Storz endocamera), a xenon light source and a flushing / suction device.

It is normal that the first steps of endoscopic dissection of the retrotracheal space are difficult due to the limited initial vision and the anatomical narrowing behind the jugulum.

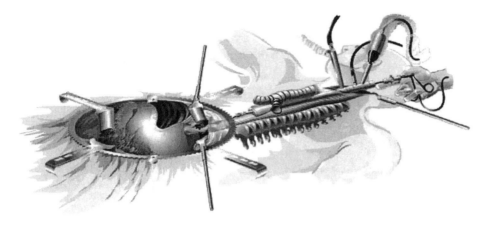

Figure 3. En-Bloc resection of the primary tumor, combined with simultaneous endodissection (source: Bumm)

Microinstruments such as scissors, forceps or a coalgulation / suction instrument can be used through the working channel of the mediastinoscope. The retrotracheal tissues are divided by pushing the tissue with the coagulation / suction device followed by the application of a short "coagulation" impulse. Direct dissection with the scissor is also possible but less recommended due to the risk of damage of mediastinal structures such as the trachea. The anterior surface of the esophagus is subsequently dissected until 2-3 cm below the tracheal bifurcation, which can be easily identified. There should be no attempt to mobilize the primary tumor by endodissection because this should be better-accomplished transhiatally by "en-bloc" techniques. The mediastinoscope is then slowly retracted which offers an excellent view (Figure 3) of the back wall of the trachea and the tracheal bifurcation. Visible lymph nodes can either be removed in total or biopsied. The tissue dilator at the tip of the instrument is then rotated anticlockwise and 90 degrees so that the left surface of the esophagus can be dissected. This is usually easy until the esophagus undercrosses the left main bronchus, where physiological adhesions / ligaments are present. These adhesions must be totally divided. Care has to be taken not to divide the longitudinal muscle layer of the esophagus at this point. The back wall (Figure 4) and the right surface of the esophagus usually presents no major difficulties, and opening of the mediastinal pleura is usually uncritical. Step by step, the esophagus is circumferentially mobilized. It is advisable for the abdominal team (see below) to keep the hiatus closed during mediastinal dissection in order to avoid flooding of the mediastinum by lavage fluids. However, at the end of mediastinal dissection contact

between cervical and abdominal team should be made. The cervical team assists during the phase of en-bloc dissection of the infracarinal esophagus (Figure 3) by providing light and suction from above. This can be helpful especially in large tumors. Finally, the cervical esophagus is divided by a longitudinal stapler device and retracted into the abdominal cavity. The mediastinal procedure is completed by control of hemorrhage and removal of visible lymph nodes for supplementary staging information.

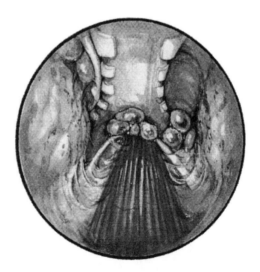

Figure 4. Endodissection: Anterior view with tracheal bifurcation (middle) and mediastinal lymph nodes, left recurrent nerve and anterior surface of the esophagus (below) esophagus (source: Minimally invasive surgery of the foregut. Eds.: J.H. Peters, T.R. DeMeester. Quality Medical Publishing, St. Lois, Missouri, 1994)

3.2 ABDOMINAL PROCEDURE

The abdominal team performs an inverse-"T"-laparotomy where the transverse incision is made approx. 2-3 cm above the umbilicus and the median incision reaches the proc.

xiphoideus. The use of self-holding retractors is mandatory as well as the use of a median ("Stuhler's") retractor. The abdominal approach starts with complete inspection and palpation of the abdomen.

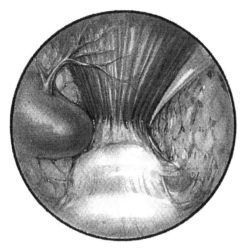

Figure 5. Endodissection: Posterior view with esophageal back wall (up), spine (below) and pleural layers as well as a direct nutritional artery from a bronchial artery (source: Minimally invasive surgery of the foregut. Eds.: J.H. Peters, T.R. DeMeester. Quality Medical Publishing, St. Lois, Missouri, 1994)

The routine replacement for the resected esophagus is a gastric tube and the preparation will be described in the following. The left lobe of the liver is mobilized and both crura of the diaphragm are dissected. The duodenum is well mobilized in an extended "Kocher's" procedure until the anterior surface of the vena cava and the aorta become visible. From this point the interaortocaval lymph nodes become accessible. The gastrocolic ligament is dissected from the colon unless the bursa omentalis is wide open (Figure 6).

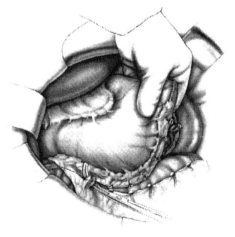

Figure 6. Dissection of the greater curvature. The gastroepiploic artery and vein must be preserved. (source: Breitner Chirurgie des Abdomens 2, Hrsg. J.R. Siewert, München; Wien, Baltimore; Urban und Schwarzenberg 1989)

The lig. gastrolienale are divided between clamps so that the greater curvature of the stomach is entirely mobilized. Extreme care has to be taken to preserve the right gastroepiploic vein and artery (Figure 8). This arcade will serve for the main portion of the blood supply of the gastric tube may not be hurt under any circumstances. Until this step of the operation the hiatus of the diaphragm remains closed so that endoscopic mediastinal dissection is possible. When endodissection is nearly completed the abdominal team widely opens the hiatus by excising portions of the crura of the diaphragm (left adherent to the specimen) and dividing the diaphragmatic vein between clamps. Palpation of the lower mediastinum secures that the primary tumor is located in the infracarinal segment of the esophagus. The periesophageal mediastinal fat and lymphatic tissue are dissected from the pericardium and remains adherent to the specimen in en 'en bloc' fashion. The primary tumor should not be exposed during the operation (Figure 13). Both visceral layers of the pleura may be resected without problems if necessary (Figure 11, 12, 14). In these cases we suggest drainage of both pleural cavities. The azygos vein remains in place and damage and risk of damage to the thoracic duct is minimal. Both vagus truncs are divided. When the specimen is completely mobilized the cervical team divides the cervical esophagus with a linear stapler and the esophagus is retracted into the abdominal cavity. The gastroduodenal artery is demonstrated and serves as a landmark for the abdominal lymphadenectomy. Dissecting from here to central, all lymph nodes along the hepatic artery, the splenic artery and the upper margin of the pancreas are resected (Figure 7). They can also be left adherent to the specimen, but this is not mandatory. Additional lymphadenectomy can be performed by resecting the paraduodenal lymph node and the interaortocaval lymph nodes, but the value of such an extended procedure is unclear.

The left gastric artery and the coronary gastric vein are divided between clamps. The right gastric artery must be preserved for additional blood supply of the gastric tube. The gastric tube should be narrow (approx. 4 cm) and long enough to reach the cervical incision easily. It is formed by three applications of a linear stapler device beginning horizontally and cranial from the "craw's foot" divisions of the vagus nerve (Figure 9). The subsequent stapler applications (Figure 10) should result in a sufficient gastric tube, and the stapler lines are additionally oversewn.

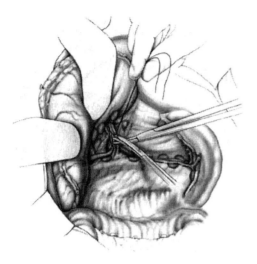

Figure 7. Lymphadenectomy in transhiatal esophagectomy: Dissection of the left gastric artery and the coronary vein as well as suprapancreatic lymph nodes and lymph nodes along the splenic artery (source: Breitner Chirurgie des Abdomens 2, Hrsg. J.R. Siewert, München; Wien, Baltimore; Urban und Schwarzenberg 1989 [modified])

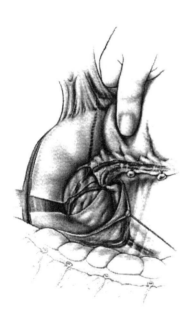

Figure 8. Dissection of the gastroepiploic artery and vein during THE device (source: Breitner Chirurgie des Abdomens 2, Hrsg. J.R. Siewert, München; Wien, Baltimore; Urban und Schwarzenberg 1989 [modified])

Finally, the gastric tube is retracted in the posterior mediastinum to the cervical incision where a esophago-gastrostomy is performed end-to-end or end-to-side by single sutures with absorbable suture-material (f.e. Vicryl ®, Ethicon, USA). The anastomosis can also be performed by a running suture with an absorbable monofilament suture material such as

Monocryl ® (Ethicon Inc., USA) or by circular stapler. As anastomotic fistulas are frequent we only partially close the cervical excision and place an additional drainage into the upper mediastinum, so that treatment of a fistula is uncomplicated .

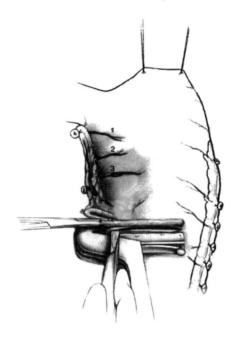

Figure 9. Preperation of the gastric tube: Horizontal application of a linear stapler outgoing from the "crowfoot" angle at the lesser curvature device (source: Breitner Chirurgie des Abdomens 2, Hrsg. J.R. Siewert, München; Wien, Baltimore; Urban und Schwarzenberg 1989 [modified])

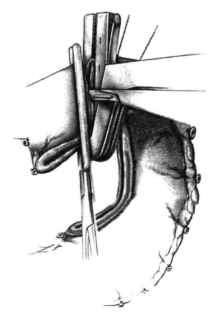

Figure 10. Preparation of the gastric tube II: A narrow gastric tube of sufficient length is made by two applications of a TA 90 linear stapling device (source: Breitner Chirurgie des Abdomens 2, Hrsg. J.R. Siewert, München; Wien, Baltimore; Urban und Schwarzenberg 1989 [modified])

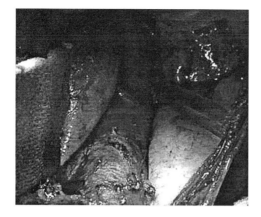

Figure 11. Final transhiatal view from the abdominal position after radical transhiatal esophagectomy (source: Bumm)

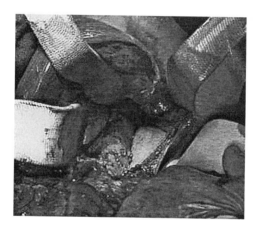

Figure12. Status after "en bloc" resection of an adenocarcinoma of the distal esophagus and partial resection of both crura of the diaphragm. (source: Bumm)

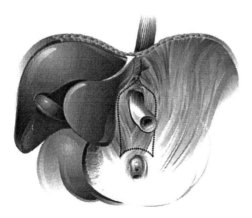

Figure 13. Excision of the crura of the diaphragm and hiatal incision line during transhiatal esophagectomy (source: Bumm)

3.3 MODIFICATIONS

80-90% of all patients can be treated as outlined above. In cases with advanced tumors it is advisable to perform a retrosternal pullthrough to facilitate postoperative

radiation therapy. The retrosternal channel is made by blunt dilation with sponges after digital dissection. Behind the jugulum can be a nasty narrowing which impairs the blood supply of the gastric tube, and in these cases we suggest a partial upper sternotomy. Sometimes the stomach is inaccessible for interposition because of prior surgery or tumor infiltration. In these cases the reconstruction of the gastrointestinal passage is best performed with interpositioning of the transverse colon connected to the ascending branch of the inferior colonic artery.

THE can be a demanding procedure in selected cases. Surgeons performing THE must be capable of converting THE to TTE if intraoperative complications such as bleeding or damage to mediastinal structures occur or if, despite preoperative staging, the tumor cannot be resected transhiatally.

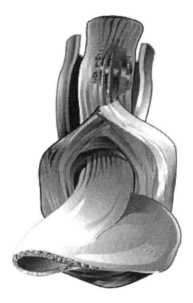

Figure 14. Schematic drawing of tumor in distal esophagus, both pleural layers, crura of the diaphragm and fundus. All should be resected during radical transhiatal esophagectomy (source: Bumm)

3.4 POSTOPERATIVE CARE

After the operation the patients are transferred to the intensive care unit. The tracheal tube is routinely removed early on the first postoperative day, and in patients with good lung function it can be removed during the first hours after the operation. The gastric interponate is armed with a two-lumen gastric tube which can be removed on the third postoperative day. The patient is allowed to swallow from the fourth postoperative day onwards. To avoid aspiration, it is advisable to allow initial swallowing only if a bedside nurse is present.

Uncomplicated cases can be discharged on the 12th to 14th postoperative day.

Vocal cord paralysis occurs in appr. 10 % of all patients and is usually non-permanent. The patients require speech and swallowing training - and must be monitored extremely well during the initial postoperative days to avoid aspiration.

Anastomotic fistulas are frequent but easy to treat. First of all free flow of saliva from the cervical wound must be secured by adequate opening / dilation. Patients are being kept on a liquid diet for the next day. Usually the fistula as well as the cervical wound closes spontaneously during the next 4-5 days. If not, an endoscopy with mild dilation of the anastomosis and placement of a feeding tube should be performed. If there is, endoscopically, a large dehiscence between stump of the esophagus and gastric tube a surgical reintervention with redo of the anastomosis over a large-diameter-T-tube is better then waiting for spontaneous closure.

4. OWN RESULTS

Between 7/1982 and 12/1999 304 patients (n=266 men [87,5 %] and 38 women [14,3 %], median age 60 yrs) underwent THE in our department. The majority of these patients suffered from adenocarcinoma of the esophagus (n=259, 85,2%). The other patients had squamous cell carcinoma (n=32, 10,5%) or other reasons for esophagectomy as f.e. acid ingestion or spontaneous perforation (n=13, 4,3%). 74 patients were included in neoadjuvant treatment protocols prior to esophagectomy (24,3%). The frequency of esophagectomies performed in our department increased over the years. Micro- and macroscopically complete tumor resection (R0-resection according UICC[19] was achieved in 80 % of all patients. There was a 4,9 % (n=15) overall hospital mortality with an overall decreasing tendency over the years and a 37,5 % overall complication rate [excluding minor cervical fistulas] in the total cohort.

A prospective study[10] revealed that addition of ‚en-bloc‘ resection and endodissection techniques (Radical Transhiatal Esophagectomy, RTE) increased short-term as well as long-term results. Patients after RTE suffered from less pulmonary (18.9 vs 27.9 %) and cardiac (2 % vs. 12 %) complications. In addition, we were able to demonstrate a prognostic benefit for patients after RTE over THE (40 % 5-yr survival vs. 20 %[8])

5. SUMMARY

THE is in use in a variety of surgical departments for treatment of adenocarcinoma of the esophagus. To date operative mortality as well as complication rate are acceptable. Survival after THE (Table 1) has increased over time and there is some evidence that application of "en-bloc" resection techniques as well as radical lymphadenectomy are responsible for this. However, studies are very difficult to compare because patient cohorts as well as surgical techniques vary greatly. Concerning adenocarcinoma of the esophagus there is no evidence from a prospective randomized study that TTE is superior over THE in terms of better long term results. This may be caused by a different lymphatic tumor spread in adenocarcinoma of the esophagus, with predominant metastasation into abdominal lymph nodes. We[10] as well as others[16] have shown that upper mediastinal lymph node metastasis in adenocarcinoma of the esophagus are a rare finding. In this light, THE seems the operation of choice for adenocarcinoma of the esophagus.

TABLE 1. Survival after transhiatal esophagectomy (literature review)

Author	Year	N Pat	Interval	Survival (%)	Comments
Hankins [18]	1987	26	1982-86	~40 % 2 yrs	Adeno and squamous cell carcinoma
Mahoney [23]	1987	37		5 % 5 yrs	Adeno only
Barbier [4]	1988	50	1981-86	23 % 3 yrs	Adeno and squamous cell carcinoma; prospective analysis
Finley [12]	1989	98	1980-88	~33 % 2 yrs	Adeno only
Moon [24]	1992	93	1974-90	13 % 5 yrs	Adeno only
Jauch [20]	1992	131	1982-89	20 % 5 yrs	Adeno and squamous cell carcinoma, part of an analysis TTE vs. THE
Tilanus [35]	1992	141	1986-91	~30 % 3 yrs	Retrospective: Adeno and squamous cell carcinoma
Gelfand [13]	1992	160	1979-90	~20 % 5 yrs	
Goldminc [15]	1993	32	1988-91	~25 % 3 yrs	Adeno and squamous cell carcinoma. Randomized study.
Gertsch [15]	1993	100	1981-91	20 % 5 yrs	Adeno and squamous cell carcinoma
Vigneswaran [37]	1993	131	1985-91	~20 % 5 yrs	Adeno and squamous cell carcinoma
Hagen [16]	1993	141	1986-89	~15 % 5 yrs	Adeno and squamous cell carcinoma, retrospective
Orringer [27]	1993	417	1978-93	27 % 5 yrs	Adeno and squamous cell carcinoma
Thomas [34]	1997	164	1979-95	17 % 5 yrs	Retrospektive study, adeno only
Bumm [10]	1997	127	1991-97	40 % 5 yrs	Radical transhiatal esophagectomy, adeno only.
Boyl	1999	65	1991-96	40 % 4 yrs	Adeno and squamous cell carcinoma
Orringer [28]	1999	1085	1976-98	21 % (all) 24 % (adeno) 5 yrs	Largest series available; Adeno- and squamous cell carcinoma
Parshad [29]	1999	78	1982-96	21.3 % 5 yrs	Adeno only

REFERENCES

1. Akiyama H, Tsurumaru M, Kawamura T, Ono Y. Principles of surgical treatment for carcinoma of the esophagus. Ann Surg 1981;194:438-46
2. Akiyama H, Tsurumaru M, Ono Y, Udagawa H, Kajiyama Y. Background for Lymph node dissection for sqamous cell carcinoma of the esophagus. In:Color atlas of surgical anatomy for esophageal cancer (Sato T, Iizuka T, eds.) Tokyo/Berlin/Heidelberg/New York Springer, 1992:9-24
3. Alderson D, Courtney SP, Kennedy RH. Radical transhiatal oesophagectomy under direct vision. Br J Surg 1994;81:404-7
4. Barbier PA, Luder PJ, Schupfer G, Becker CD, Wagner HE:Quality of life and patterns of recurrence following transhiata esophagectomy for cancer:results of a prospective follow-up in 50 patients. World J Surg 12 2 (1988) 270-6
5. Boyle MJ, Franceschi D, Livingstone A:Transhiatal versus transthoracic esophagectomy:complication and survival rates. Am Surg 1999;65(12):1137-41;discussion 1141-2
6. Buess G, Becker HD, Mentges R, Teichmann R, Lenz G. Die endoskopisch-mikrochirurgische Dissektion der Speiseröhre. Chirurg 1990;61:308-11
7. Bumm R, Hölscher AH, Feussner H, Tachibana M, Bartels H, Siewert JR. Endodissection of the thoracic esophagus. Technique and clinical results in transhiatal esophagectomy. Ann Surg 1993;218 1:97-104
8. Bumm R, Hölscher AH, Siewert JR. Transmediastinal endodissection. In:Minimally invasive surgery of the foregut (eds.:Peters JH, DeMeester TR). Quality Medical Publishing Inc. St. lois Missouri 1994;pp 250-61
9. Bumm R, Wong J. More or less surgery for esophageal cancer:Extent of lymphadenectomy for squamous cell esophageal carcinoma:How much is necessary ? Dis Esoph 1994;73: 151-5
10. Bumm R, Feussner H, Bartels H, Stein H, Dittler HJ, Höfler H, Siewert JR. Radical transhiatal esophagectomy with two field lymphadenectomy and endodissektion for distal esophageal adenocarcinoma. World J Surg 1997;21:822-31.
11. Denk W. Zur Radikaloperation des Ösophaguskarzinoms. Zentral Chir 1913;40:1065-9

12. Finley RJ, Grace M, Duff JH:Esophagogastrectomy without thoracotomy for carcinoma of the cardia and the lower part of the esophagus. Surg Gynecol Obstet 1985;160:49-56

13. Fischer AW:Erfolgreiche Entfernung eines Krebses der Speiseröhre nach dem abdominocollaren Durchzugsverfahren.

14. Gelfand GAJ, Finley RJ, Nelems B, Inculet R, Evans KG. Transhiatal esophagectomy for carcinoma of the esophagus and cardia. Arch Surg 1992;127:1164-68

15. Gertsch P, Vauthehey JN, Lustenberger AA, Friedlander-Klar H. Long term results of transhiatal esophagectomy for esophageal carcinoma. A multivariate analysis of prognostic factors. Cancer 1993;27 8:2312-9

16. Goldminc M, Maddern G, LePrise E, Meunier B, Campion JP, Launois B. Esophagectomy by a transhiatal approach or thoracotomy:a prospective randomized trial. Br J Surg 1993;80:367-70

17. Hagen JA, Peters JH, DeMeester TR. Superiority of extended en bloc esophagogastrectomy for carcinoma of the lower esophagus and cardia. J Thorac Cardiovasc Surg 1993;106:850-8

18. Hankins JR, Miller JE, Attar S, McLaughlin JS. Transhiatal esophagectomy for carcinoma of the esophagus:Experience with 26 patients. Ann Thorac Surg 1987;44:123-7

19. Hermanek P, Sobin LH:UICC 87 TNM Classification of Malignant Tumors. 4th ed. Berlin:Springer 1987

20. Jauch KW, Bacha EA, Denecke H, Anthuber M, Schildberg FW:Esophageal carcinoma:prognostic features and comparison between blunt transhiatal and transthoracic resection. Eur J Surg Oncol 1992;18:553-62

21. Kipfmüller K, Buess G, Nahrun M, Bätz W. Die endoskopisch-mikrochirurgische Dissektion der Speiseröhre. Eine tierexperimentelle Studie. Chirurg 1990;61:187-91

22. Kipfmüller K, Duda D, Kessler S, Melzer A, Buess G. Die endoskopische-mikrochirurgische Dissektion der Speiseröhre:ein Beitrag zur Reduzierung pulmonaler Komplikationen nach Ösophagusresektion? Eine vergleichende tierexperimentelle Studie. Langenbecks Arch Chir 1990;375:11-8

23. Mahoney JL, Condon RE. Adenocarcinoma of the esophagus. Ann Surg 1987;205:557-62

24. Moon MR, Schulte WJ, Haasler GB, Condon RE. Transhiatal and transthoracic esophagectomy for adenocarcinoma of the esophagus. Arch Surg 1992;127:951-5

25. Müller JM, Erasmi H, Stelzner M, Zieren U, Pichlmaier H. Surgical therapy of esophageal carcinoma. Br J Surg 1990;77:845-57

26. Orringer MB. Transhiatal esophagectomy without thoracotomy for carcinoma of the thoracic esophagus. Ann Surg 1984;200:282-8

27. Orringer MB:Transhiatal esophagectomy for benign disease. J Thorac Cardiovasc Surg 90 5 (1985) 649-55

28. Orringer MB, Marshall B, Iannettoni MD. Transhiatal esophagectomy:clinical experience and refinements. Ann Surg 1999 Sep;230(3):392-400;discussion 400-3

29. Parshad R, Singh RK, Kumar A, Gupta SD, Chattopadhyay TK Adenocarcinoma of distal esophagus and gastroesophageal junction:long-term results of surgical treatment in a North Indian Center. World J Surg 1999 Mar;23(3):277-83

30. Siewert JR, Hölscher AH, Horvath OP:[Transmediastinal esophagectomy] Transmediastinale Ösophagektomie. Langenbecks Arch Chir 367 3 (1986) 203-13 (Published in German and Russian)

31. Siewert JR, Hölscher AH, Roder J, Bartels H. En bloc Resektion der Speiseröhre beim Ösophaguskarzinom. Langenbecks Arch Chir 1988;373:367-76

32. Skinner DB, Ferguson MK, Soriano, Little AG, Stanszak VM. Selection of operation for esophageal cancer based on staging. Ann Surg 1986;204:391-401

33. Skinner DB. En bloc resection for neoplasms of the esophagus and cardia. J Thorac Cardiovasc Surg 1983;85:59-71

34. Thomas P, Doddoli C, Lienne P, Morati N, Thirion X, Garbe L, Giundellicelli R, Fuentes P:Changing patterns and surgical results in adenocarcinoma of the oesophagus. Br J Surg 1997, 84, 119-25

35. Tilanus HW, Hop WC, Langenhorst BL, van Lanschot JJ:Esophagectomy with or without thoracotomy. Is there any difference? J Thorac Cardiovasc Surg 105 5 (1993) 898-903

36. Turner GG. Excision of the thoracic esophagus for carcinoma with construction of an extrathoracic gullet. Lancet 1933;2:13-5

37. Vigneswaran WT, Trastek VF, Pairolero PC, Deschamps C, Daly RC, Allen MS. Transhiatal esophagectomy for carcinoma of the esophagus. Ann Thorac Surg 1993;56:838-46.

6.3   RESECTION OF ESOPHAGEAL CARCINOMA: THE ROLE OF LYMPH NODE DISSECTION

Jan B.F. Hulscher and Jan J.B. van Lanschot

1. INTRODUCTION

The way lymph node metastases and cancer in general are looked upon has changed significantly over the years.   From the middle of the 20th century cancer was thought of more and more as a disease already disseminated at the time of presentation, and tumor positive lymph nodes were considered metastatic disease.   Lymph node dissection was accordingly not considered curative anymore, but turned into a mere staging procedure. Lymph node metastases had become "indicators, but not governors of survival"[1].

Recently however, it has been shown that optimal loco-regional treatment, might lead to a decrease in locoregional recurrence, an improved disease-free survival and overall survival. For e.g. breast carcinoma, adding locoregional radiotherapy to axillary dissection and chemotherapy, might improve disease-free and overall survival rates[2,3].   In one of these trials a decrease in systemic recurrence was also observed, suggesting that in breast carcinoma locoregional disease may be a potential source for future dissemination[3]. It is not only breast carcinoma that benefits from an improved loco-regional treatment. Total mesorectal excision (TME), with wide excision of the tumor and resection of all regional lymph nodes, for rectal cancer has become the standard practice in many Western countries, leading to improved locoregional control and increased survival-rates[4]. However, it is uncertain whether this is due to an improved lymph node clearance or an increase in the number of patients with microscopically radical resection.   In the same way elective lymph node dissection might improve locoregional control and survival in patients (younger than 60 years of age) with intermediate thickness melanomas[5]. These findings should lead to a reconsideration of the role of lymphnode dissection, which might be an important step in obtaining locoregional control. However, there are limits to the extent of the lymph node dissection. An extended (D2) dissection for gastric carcinoma is propagated by many Japanese surgeons, claiming more favorable outcomes when compared with non-extended resections[6].

However, a recent study from the Netherlands showed that an extended (D2) resection for gastric carcinoma is associated with a significant increase in post-operative morbidity and mortality when compared with limited (D1) resection (43% vs 25% and 10% vs 4% resp.) , while the long-term results were not significantly improved (risk of relapse 37% vs 43%, p=0.22)[7,8].

In the same way the role of lymph node dissection is debated among esophageal surgeons.

Esophageal carcinoma is an aggressive disease with a poor chance of definite cure. Approximately 50% of the patients already present with irresectable local ingrowth and/or distant metastases, thus precluding curative resection. Surgery remains, until today, the best curative option. But even after 'curative surgery' the average five-year survival rates do not exceed 30%[9]. Up to three-quarters of the patients undergoing resection have metastases to the abdominal and/or mediastinal lymph nodes, a factor that also accounts for the dismal prognosis. Many studies focus on the optimal surgical approach, but great controversy exists among esophageal surgeons as to the value of (extended) lymphadenectomy.

Two main strategies for improving the results of surgical therapy for esophageal carcinoma have emerged over the last decades. The first aims to decrease early morbidity and mortality by minimizing surgical trauma. This might be achieved by performing a transhiatal resection, thus avoiding a formal thoracotomy with its alleged (mainly pulmonary) complications. The second aims to improve the long-term cure rates by performing a more radical (transthoracic) resection, accepting a potential increase in early morbidity and mortality. This rests on the belief that in some patients with lymph node metastases cure can be obtained by an aggressive surgical resection of peri-tumoral tissue combined with extended lymph node dissection in abdomen and chest (and possibly also in the neck).

Arguments in favor of more extensive surgery are an improved (if not optimal) staging, and an improved locoregional control leading to a possibly prolonged disease-free survival and perhaps an improved long-term survival as

H.W. Tilanus and S.E.A. Attwood (eds.), Barrett's Esophagus, 335–346.
© 2001 *Kluwer Academic Publishers. Printed in the Netherlands.*

well. Opponents of this strategy object that post-operative morbidity and mortality might be increased, and that the alleged beneficial effects on disease-free survival and/or overall long-term survival have not been proven (yet). Also, the natural protective filter for tumor cells may be removed when an extensive lymph node dissection is performed, and the injury of major surgery may have detrimental immuno-suppressant effects[10].

2. SURGERY FOR ESOPHAGEAL CARCINOMA: AN OUTLINE OF THE DIFFERENT RESECTION FORMS WITH EMPHASIS ON LYMPH NODE DISSECTION

Over the years many resection forms have been developed. The different operative procedures vary mainly in one or more of the following: type of incision, extent of resection, conduit for reconstruction, and type of anastomosis. We will focus on the first two differences: type of incision and extent of resection, which are closely related.

Resections of the esophagus can be (generally) divided into (with increasing complexity): a) transhiatal resection without thoracotomy, b) standard or limited resection, c) radical *en-bloc* resection, d) radical resection with two-field lymphadenectomy and finally e) radical resection with three-field lymphadenectomy.

A) *Transhiatal resection* is a resection through the abdomen and neck[11,12]. The esophagus is approached through a surgically widened hiatus of the diaphragm. Theoretically the avoidance of a formal thoracotomy might decrease peri-operative morbidity and mortality by lessening the physiologic impact of a combined thoracic and abdominal operation. In most patients the esophagus can be dissected under direct vision up to the level of the carina, with *en bloc* removal of the tumor and its adjacent lymph nodes, including nodes near the celiac axis and hepatic and splenic arteries. Opponents of the transhiatal resection emphasize the uncontrolled part of the operation: proximal to the carina the (normal) thoracic esophagus is dissected bluntly, *i.e.* not under direct vision. This might lead to damage to major intrathoracic structures such as trachea, (mainstem) bronchi, thoracic duct, azygos vein or aorta, implying, according to some, a higher per-operative risk when compared with transthoracic resections. It may also cause damage to the tumor itself with the associated tumor spill. A radical lymphadenectomy of all regional thoracic lymph nodes is impossible through a transhiatal incision, although lymph node clearance can be achieved up to (and sometimes including) the subcarinal nodes. Some opponents consider a transhiatal approach therefore a violation of radical oncological surgery, a claim that can also be supported by the assumption that transhiatal resections might limit the yield of tumor-negative dissection margins. Also, lymph node staging might be less effective because not all lymph nodes are dissected. Further details of this operation are provided in the previous chapter.

B) *Standard or limited resection* (as described by Ivor Lewis and Norman Tanner in 1946) implies a combined abdominal/thoracic approach[13,14]. This has been the standard procedure until recently, and internationally many centers still consider this the procedure of first choice. The tumor and peri-esophageal tissue with its adjacent lymph nodes are resected through a right-sided thoracotomy. A margin of at least five centimeters proximally and distally is required. When the tumor is situated in the lower third of the esophagus a left thoracotomy can also be used. The position of the heart limits the extent of the resection and makes the intrathoracic anastomosis more difficult when using a left sided approach. No formal lymph node dissection is performed in chest or abdomen.

C) *Radical en bloc resection* includes a wide excision of the primary tumor (including the azygos vein, thoracic duct, overlying pleura and pericardium) combined with a complete lymph node dissection of the middle and lower third of the posterior mediastinum[15]. Some surgeons perform routinely frozen sections biopsies of the lower paratracheal nodes, portal and retropancreatic nodes (when they are positive a curative operation is deemed impossible) before starting the dissection[15]. The intrathoracic esophagus is removed with an en bloc dissection of the adjacent bronchial, subcarinal, paraesophageal and parahiatal nodes. The block of tissue is bounded superiorly by the upper border of the azygos vein and inferiorly by the superior border of the pancreas. Lateral margins are the right and left mediastinal pleura. Anteriorly the resection is bounded by the membranous portions of the main bronchi and pericardium, while the posterior border is formed by the aorta and vertebral column. The claimed advantage of this type of resection is a better locoregional control without increasing peri-operative morbidity and mortality. This might diminish the number of patients with locoregional recurrence and thus prolong the disease-free interval.

D) *Radical resection with two-field lymphadenectomy* is an *en-bloc* resection combined with a complete lymph node dissection in chest and abdomen. In the two-field dissection all nodes in the posterior mediastinum and upper abdomen are removed. This comprises the paratracheal nodes, the nodes in the aorta-pulmonary window and the subcarinal nodes in the chest and in the abdomen the nodes near the celiac axis, near the splenic and the hepatic artery, and finally the nodes along the lesser curvature and the lesser omentum. Most of the time the anastomosis is, just as in a transhiatal resection, made in the neck, thereby theoretically reducing the risk of local recurrence at the suture line.

E) *Radical resection with three-field lymphadenectomy* adds a formal dissection of the infra-omohyoidal cervical lymph nodes (deep internal, deep external and the deep lateral nodes) to the dissection of the abdominal and mediastinal lymph nodes[16,17]. Although results have been favorable in some (mostly Japanese) studies, most Western centers consider this approach associated with unacceptable morbidity and therefore do not perform this type of resection. Therefore it will not be discussed extensively in this chapter.

3. THE EXTENT OF LYMPH NODE INFILTRATION IN ESOPHAGEAL CARCINOMA

Due to the non-segmental lymph drainage of the esophagus lymph node metastases may occur on distant sites relatively early in the course of disease. Little is known about the preferential spreading pattern of lymph node metastases in adenocarcinoma of the esophagus and/or gastric cardia. Knowledge hereof might be of assistance in deciding upon the optimal surgical approach regarding lymph node dissection. In this paragraph we will discuss the results of a few studies concerning the extent of lymph node metastases.

Both intramucosal (T1im) and submucosal (T1sm) tumors are considered as T1 (early tumors) according to the UICC'97 staging system. However, there is a considerable difference in T1 im and T1 sm tumors when the prevalence of lymph node metastases is concerned. Different studies have shown that lymph node metastases are rare in T1im tumors (0-7%), but increase in incidence when there is submucosal spread (22-50%)[18,19]. We have found lymphatic spread in 30% of the patients with T1sm tumors, while none of the patients with T1 im tumors showed positive lymph nodes[20]. This is in accordance with a recent report by Nigro, which mentions positive lymph nodes in 10% of the patients with occult (not visible on endoscopy) carcinoma of the esophagus[21]. Lymph node metastases therefore occur already early in the course of the disease, as up to 50% of the patients with a T1 tumor already have positive nodes. When there is transmural tumor spread, over three-quarters of the patients have nodal metastases[16,19,22,23,24]. However, there is still a significant number of patients (10-20%) that do not have lymph node metastases despite transmural growth.

Many groups report a higher incidence of distant (not in the same anatomical compartment) lymph node spread in larger tumors with often more than one field positive for lymph node metastases. The distribution of lymph node metastases probably fans out according to the depth of tumor invasion. In distal adenocarcinomas the parahiatal and lesser curvature nodes are often the first to become affected, up to 30% of the patients with submucosal adenocarcinoma show already tumor positivity in these nodes (±15% for both lymph node stations). The parahiatal and lesser curvature nodes can adequately be resected during a transhiatal resection. When there is intramural spread the percentage of patients with positive nodes near the lesser curvature increases from ±15% to ±33.3%. The para-esophageal (±33%), tracheo-bronchial (±10%) and subcarinal nodes (±10%) might also become affected, just as the nodes near the greater curvature (±10%), the left gastric artery (±10%) and the celiac trunc (±10%)[22]. While the subcarinal nodes can often be reached through the widened diaphragm during transhiatal resection, the tracheo-bronchial nodes can not be reached. Some centers routinely perform a lymph node dissection in the abdomen during transhiatal resection, sometimes resecting the lymph nodes near the celiac axis, while others consider positive nodes near the celiac axis distant metastasis and therefore a contraindication for curative surgery. When there is transmural carcinoma the percentage of patients with positive nodes near the celiac axis increases to 30%, while 50% show tumor positivity at the parahiatal and lesser curvature nodes[22].

The number of tumor positive nodes (or the lymph node ratio, *i.e.* the ration of positive to removed nodes) might also be an indicator for distant lymph node metastases. Nigro describes a high risk for distant lymph node metastases when more than four local nodes are affected, while 69% has local lymph node spread only when less than four nodes are tumor positive[25]. The frequency and the extent of nodal metastases therefore apparently increase with greater wall penetration.

Some (mostly) Japanese authors report high incidences of tumor positive cervical lymph nodes after three-field lymphadenectomy, even in tumors located in the distal esophagus. Akiyama *e.g.* describes a ± 30% incidence of positive lymph nodes in patients with a middle or distal carcinoma[16]. In some studies the recurrent nerve node group is most frequently infected: up to 70% of the patients with invaded lymph nodes had positive recurrent nerve nodes regardless of tumor site and depth of invasion[26]. These results are confirmed by a few Western studies: Altorki and Skinner find positive cervical lymph nodes also in 30% of their patients with a distal carcinoma, without a difference between T1 and T3 tumors[27]. This suggests that esophageal carcinoma is a systemic disease from the moment it invades the basement membrane, which is why many (mostly Japanese) surgeons favor a three-field approach, in which a formal lymph node dissection in the neck is carried out together with lymph node clearance in chest and abdomen, claiming survival benefits even when the cervical nodes are positive[26].

4. THE CLINICAL SIGNIFICANCE OF LYMPH NODE DISSECTION

4.1 STAGING AND PROGNOSIS

The pre-operative staging procedures serve to select patients with potentially curable tumors. Positive lymph nodes in the neck and/or irresectable lymph nodes near the celiac axis are often considered metastatic disease for (distal) esophageal carcinoma (M), thus precluding long term survival. Because esophagectomy is generally not considered appropriate as a palliative option, tumor spread in these lymph nodes is considered a contraindication for resection in most Western centers. However, a recent study by Clark et al. showed no significant survival disadvantage for patients with (resectable) celiac node involvement versus patients without celiac node involvement, although the number of patients was small and there seemed to be a tendency to a lower survival[22]. In our center we resect tumor positive lymph nodes near the celiac axis when possible during transhiatal resection and achieved long-term survival

(over 24 months) in 7 of 27 patients with M1 (n) disease when a macroscopically radical resection could be performed[28]. Lymph nodes near the celiac axis that can be resected are therefore probably no absolute contraindication for surgical resection.

Nodal metastasis is correlated with survival. In multivariate analyses R-category (R0=microscopically radical resection, R1=macroscopically radical but microscopically irradical resection, R2=macroscopic tumor remaining) and nodal status are often the predominant prognostic factors[29]. This is confirmed by a recent study from our institution investigating the recurrence pattern after transhiatal resection: radicality and lymph node status were the strongest independent prognostic factors on multivariate analysis[28]. Patients with involved lymph nodes have significantly lower long-term survival rates than patients without nodal spread, which is reflected in the survival analyses of the different TNM-stages (90% stage I, 70% stage II, 30% stage III, 10% stage IV, overall 30%). The relatively high percentage of survivors with stage IV tumors is mainly due to the patients with resectable tumor positive lymph nodes near the celiac axis. Steup et al. even mention 5-year survival rates of 60-70% for patients without celiac nodal involvement versus 10-20% for patients with such nodal involvement (all regarding tumors of the gastro-esophageal junction and the esophagus)[30].

Patients with four or less involved lymph nodes may have a survival advantage over patients with more than four metastatic nodes, which is correlated with the finding that patients with more than four involved nodes have a higher risk of distant positive nodes[21,24]. The extent of nodal metastases is also correlated with survival: patients with involvement of only the abdominal lymph nodes have a survival advantage over patients with metastatic lymph nodes in both abdomen and chest[30]. For squamous cell carcinoma this relationship has also been described: when nodal spread involved two (or three) anatomic compartments, 2- year survival was 0%, versus 29.8% when only one compartment was involved[31]. Other authors argue that it is not (or not only) the absolute amount of positive lymph nodes, but the ratio of removed to positive nodes. This might better reflect the state of disease than the absolute number of positive nodes, especially when one takes in account that the number of lymph nodes removed per patient may vary greatly. This also holds true for transhiatal resections, in which by definition a formal lymph node dissection is not carried out, certainly not in the chest. In a recent analysis of 115 patients undergoing transhiatal resection with curative intent multiple stepwise regression analysis identified the lymph node ratio (with a ratio between positive and removed nodes of >0.30) as the strongest independent predictor of long-term survival[32]. Also after extended transthoracic resection for squamous cell carcinoma, the ratio of invaded to removed mediastinal nodes was (after the presence of residual tumor after resection, R1 and R2) the second most important independent prognostic factor on multivariate analysis[33]. The prognosis for patients with nodal metastases deteriorates when more than 20 - 30 percent of the removed nodes are invaded by tumor. Some authors consider this an indirect argument in favor of more extended lymph node dissections.

This approach also underlies the phenomenon of stage migration. Dissecting more lymph nodes increases the chance of finding a tumor positive node. This influences the tumor stage significantly. TNM-stage (and thus prognosis) is based on the resection specimen with its resected lymph nodes. In transhiatal resections, the lymph node dissection is far from complete: unresected tumor positive lymph nodes may remain, which might lead to understaging. Transhiatal resections might therefore not reflect the true state of disease. When in the same patient a formal lymph node dissection would have been performed, a positive lymph node might have been found, leading to a different TNM-stage (with positive nodes and thus a worse prognosis). When the results of the different resection-forms are compared, this is frequently done on a stage-by-stage basis. Stage migration might seriously hamper this comparison, because patients with the same stage might be staged differently based on extent of the lymph node dissection and the increased possibility of finding a positive node in more extended resections.

Another problem frequently encountered is the sensitivity of routine post-operative pathological staging procedures. Sampling error and the sensitivity of the techniques used might have a large impact on the results. There might also be a large inter-observer variation in the staging of resected specimens. Furthermore, routine pathological (histological) techniques may not be able to identify all (micro)-metastases. A recent German study of the prognostic value of immuno-histochemically identifiable tumor cells in lymph nodes of patients with completely resected (R0) esophageal cancer showed that of 399 lymph nodes tumor-free on routine analyses, 67 (17 percent) showed tumor-cells on immuno-histochemical analysis[34]. The presence of tumor cells not detected on routine histology but demonstrated with immuno-histochemistry was a significant independent prognostic factor, both for disease-free survival and overall survival. In a smaller series this was confirmed by Bonavina et al, who found micrometastases in 33.3% of the patients after resection for adenocarcinoma of the esophagogastric junction considered N0 after routine histology[35]. An impact on survival was also found in this series[35].

However, although there was a significant relation between the presence of immuno-histochemically detected tumor-cells in lymph nodes and relapse with distant metastases, no correlation could be proven between the presence of such cells and local recurrence[34]. The predisposition to have distant metastases among patients with immuno-histochemically detected tumor cells in their lymph nodes suggests that these cells are the consequence of advanced tumors and/or aggressive tumor behavior, rather than indicators of sites of subsequent disease. Lymph node (micro)-metastases may therefore be only indicators, not governors, of survival[1]. The clinical significance of these findings thus remains uncertain. Although in a rat model it has been shown that remaining cells (isolated from human micrometastases as mentioned above) are able to develop into carcinomas, as yet there is no conclusive data that these tumor cells are indeed viable cells in humans. The growth of single tumor cells into overt metastases is also determined by the local environment and the capacity of the cells to respond to it[36]. It is unlikely (due to the short time frame in which recurrence occurs) that lymph node recurrence primarily occurs and hematogenic metastasis from the recurrent lymph nodes to the organs results in distant recurrence. Until more data regarding the biologic behavior of these remaining tumor cells become available, the clinical significance of removing these residual cells by routine extended nodal clearance remains uncertain. The immuno-histochemical techniques currently in use are rather time-consuming and at present (in most hospitals) impossible to be implemented in routine clinical practice.

In conclusion, an extended lymph node dissection does add information regarding the prognosis. The number of tumor positive nodes and the lymph node ratio are independent prognostic factors. Whether the detection of micrometastases will be of use in the routine clinical setting remains to be seen. In the near future more accurate non-invasive staging procedures might become available, such as endosonography with ultrasonographically guided fine needle aspiration and improved helical CT, MRI or PET, making extensive surgery unnecessary for staging only.

4.2 SURGICAL ASPECTS OF LYMPH NODE DISSECTION: TRANSTHORACIC RESECTION VERSUS TRANSHIATAL RESECTION

4.2.1 Early morbidity and mortality

While a formal lymph node dissection of the abdomen can be performed during both transhiatal and transthoracic resections, a formal lymph node dissection in the chest can only be carried out through a thoracotomy. The avoidance of a thoracotomy is one of the alleged advantages of the transhiatal approach. By diminishing the extent of the operation early morbidity and mortality may decrease. This might especially hold true for cardio-pulmonary complications. When the literature of the last decade is analyzed, however, data are conflicting. In the following section we will compare transhiatal and transthoracic resections concentrating on the most important intra- and post-operative complications, early mortality and survival. Because most Western centers do not perform three-field resections, this approach is not included in the analysis.

4.2.2 Intra-operative complications

Opponents of the transhiatal resection claim that this approach carries a high risk of intra-operative complications such as severe hemorrhage due to tearing of major blood vessels or inadvertent injury to the major airways. When the literature is reviewed major mediastinal hemorrhage is rare (0-3%) during transhiatal resection, conversion to a thoracotomy for severe bleeding even more so[11, 37,38,39]. Anatomical studies have revealed that large nutritional arteries branch into an arterial network of minute branches within the peri-esophageal tissue before entering the esophageal wall. When these small vessels are torn, contractive hemostasis, rather than massive bleeding, occurs[40]. When major hemorrhage occurs, it is most often due to tearing of the aorta or azygos vein invaded by tumor. However, this apparently is a rare event. The risk of excessive bleeding can be diminished further by maintaining a plane of dissection immediately on the muscular wall of the esophagus (proximal to the tumor). If the neo-esophagus is situated in the pre-vertebral

position, mediastinal bloodloss is further diminished due to the local tamponade.

The incidence of membranous tracheal lesions is <1%[11,38,39,40,41,42]. There might be a higher incidence of tracheal tears in the middle/upper part of the esophagus, where esophagus and trachea are in close contact, but this has not been demonstrated clearly in larger series[38]. Orringer performed 417 transhiatal resections for cancer including 137 for midthoracic tumors, with an incidence of tracheal lesions of < 1%[11]. Adherence to a dissection plane immediately on the esophageal wall (of the healthy esophagus proximal to the tumor) will minimize the risk of this complication, especially when digital pressure on the posterior part of the trachea is avoided. In those patients who underwent pre-operative radiotherapy or patients with a history of mediastinitis, this plane between the trachea and esophagus may be hardly discernible or obliterated, resulting in a higher incidence of tracheal lesions[41].

4.2.3 Early post-operative complications

Overall patients tend to spend more time on artificial ventilation and in the ICU after transthoracic resection than after transhiatal resection. This is confirmed by interim results of a trial currently in progress, in which patients stayed on the ICU for a median of 2.5 days after transhiatal esophagectomy, while they stayed on the ICU for 6.0 days after transthoracic resections[42]. However, in the three trials published as yet there is no difference in post-operative ICU-stay[37,43,44]. In a recent report Orringer describes patients being extubated in the operating theater after transhiatal resection[11]. Routinely patients do not stay overnight in the intensive care in his series. This is also recommended by some surgeons for transthoracic resections: patients remain in a high care unit after surgery and are extubated in the early post-operative phase[37,45].

Post-operative complication rates vary between 40%-80%, partly depending on the applied criteria. The most important complications are cardio-pulmonary complications, anastomotic leakage, mediastinitis, vocal cord paralysis due to injury to the recurrent laryngeal nerve(s), and chylothorax or – peritoneum. Comparison of cardio-pulmonary complications after transthoracic and transhiatal resections is extremely difficult because most authors do not define these complications precisely. This might be one of the reasons of the wide variance in incidence of these complications. In an interim analysis of a trial comparing transhiatal resection and transthoracic resection with two-field lymphadenectomy we found a significantly higher incidence of pulmonary complications after transthoracic resections (62%) than after transhiatal resections (21%)[42]. One of the alleged advantages of transhiatal surgery is the avoidance of a formal thoracotomy, which should – theoretically – lead to fewer post-operative pulmonary complications. In two (retrospective) comparative studies Tilanus et al. and Paç et al. for instance find a higher incidence of pulmonary complications in the transthoracic group[38,46]. However, in two other reports Stark et al. and Gluck et al. state exactly the opposite, while data from the (small) trials published so far do not show a significant difference[37,43,44,46,47]. Transthoracic resections may be associated with a transient deterioration of pulmonary function during one-lung ventilation in the left-lateral position[44]. With the aid of CPAP the collapsed lung can be prevented from becoming atelectatic, while the administration of low levels of PEEP might improve the deployment of the lung when returning to two-lung ventilation. The relatively low overall incidence of pulmonary complications (when compared with earlier reports) may be the result of improvements in anesthesiologic techniques (such as the administration of a low level of positive pressure ventilation to prevent a total collapse of the lung during transthoracic procedures), peri-operative respiratory care and post-operative pain control. However, due the lack of specific definitions, comparison of the prevalence of pulmonary complications after transhiatal and transthoracic resections remains very difficult.

In the literature the incidence of anastomotic leakage ranges widely: from 3 to 50%. Many authors report a higher incidence of anastomotic leakage when the anastomosis is made cervically, which is the case after all transhiatal resections and after most extended transthoracic resections, as a cervical anastomosis is relatively easy to perform even in transthoracic procedures[38,49,50,51,52,53]. Horstmann even mentions an anastomotic leakage rate of 50% when a cervical anastomosis is performed, versus 10% when an intrathoracic anastomosis is constructed[49]. However, most (cervical) leakages are minor (only seen on the barium swallow) and do not require surgical exploration as they resolve spontaneously 10 to 35 days after operation[38,41,45,50,53]. When surgical drainage is required, opening of the cervical incision will almost always provide sufficient drainage. A cervical anastomosis decreases the risk for mediastinitis or empyema secondary to anastomotic leakage[54].

Vocal cord paralysis due to injury of the recurrent laryngeal nerve is another well-known complication of esophagectomy. Incidences of up to 26% are reported, but most of the time the paralysis disappears within a few months[53]. The performance of a lymph node dissection in the chest may endanger the recurrent nerves, especially when dissecting the nodes in the aorta-pulmonary window or along the recurrent nerves itself. This concerns mainly the left recurrent nerve, as it travels into the chest, turns around the aorta and runs up cranially again. The right recurrent nerve is hardly at risk during transthoracic lymph node dissection because it is at the upper border of the operating field. Both recurrent nerves may also be injured cervically, while dissecting the esophagus. Finally, traction injury to the recurrent nerves may occur during a transhiatal operation while stripping the esophagus. Some comparative studies show a higher incidence of vocal cord paralysis in transhiatal resections. Despite all cautionary methods, such as early division of the vagal nerves to avoid traction injury during the stripping of the esophagus and the avoidance of placement of retractors in the tracheo-esophageal groove, a high incidence of vocal cord paralysis is mentioned by almost all authors after a cervical anastomosis, indicating that the recurrent nerve is mainly at risk during the cervical dissection and the construction of the anastomosis[38,53,54,55]. It is therefore not the transhiatal resection per se, but the cervical anastomosis that puts the recurrent nerve at risk.

4.2.4 In-hospital mortality
Hospital mortality has decreased over the last decades. Earlam describes hospital mortality rates of 29% in the seventies, Müller mentioned 13% in the eighties, while nowadays most high-volume centers are able to keep in-hospital mortality rates well below 5%[9,11,38,52,56,57]. Although most reports do not find significant differences between transthoracic and transhiatal approaches, the literature suggests mortality rates of approximately 9% vs. 6%, favoring the transhiatal approach. This despite the fact that some authors indicate to perform transhiatal resections preferably on older patients with more co-morbidity[58,59]. When reviewing the complications associated with the different resection forms no clear reason for this suggested difference in mortality could be

given, although there is a higher incidence of pulmonary complications after transthoracic resections. Histo-pathologic factors such as tumor type or differentiation probably do not influence in hospital mortality[45,60]. Some authors use location of the tumor as a criterium whether or not to perform a transhiatal resection. Some surgeons prefer a transthiatal resection in tumors located either in the upper or lower thoracic esophagus where they can be dissected under direct vision (in case of an upper thoracic tumor dissection takes [34]place through the neck) or for relatively early middle-third cancers, while others consider at or proximal to the carina a contra-indication for transhiatal resection[38,53]. Most authors did not find a difference in mortality (or morbidity) due to the location of the tumor although selection bias almost certainly plays a role[38,60,61]. In the largest single institute study Orringer even performed 137 transhiatal resections for carcinoma of the upper and middle esophagus without adding substantial mortality[11].

4.2.5 Immunologic aspects of lymph node dissection

All major surgery is accompanied by a depression in cellular immune responses. These changes may in turn be associated with infectious complications in the post-operative phase. Complete dissection of all lymph nodes entails extensive surgery and tissue injury, probably leading to immunosuppression. This in turn might influence post-operative morbidity and mortality but also survival due to its potential influence on tumor growth and host defense mechanisms. In a recent study van Sandick et al. showed that esophageal surgery is associated with a severe post-operative depression of monocyte and T-cell immune responses[62]. They showed severely depressed production of IL-12, IL-10, IFN-γ, IL-2, IL-4 and IL-13 at the first post-operative day. After the initial post-operative decline, the functional depression of monocyte and T-cell immune response persisted significantly longer after transthoracic esophagectomy than after transhiatal resection, reflecting the extent of the surgical trauma[62]. A causative relation between post-operative changes in cellular immune responses and infectious complications could not be established however. Little is known about the prognostic importance of immunologic parameters and the importance of immunologic factors on long-term survival.

4.2.6 Long-term survival, disease free interval and recurrence rates

Opponents of the transhiatal resection claim that it is an inadequate oncological resection because it does not attempt to achieve an oncologically radical resection, as no formal lymphadenectomy is performed. This should become visible in survival curves, disease-free interval and recurrence rates (including the localization of the recurrence) when comparing transhiatal resections with more extended (transthoracic) resections.

Although early postoperative mortality has decreased over the past decades, long-term survival has not improved substantially, when the results of all different surgical procedures are combined. Both after transhiatal resections and transthoracic approaches five-year survival rates of approximately 20% are described, with three-year survival rates of approximately 25%, thereby reflecting the early and aggressive recurrence pattern of esophageal carcinoma and the relatively small impact of the operative procedure performed. In the extensive literature of the past decade only a few authors find a survival benefit for transthoracic (en bloc) resections[58,59,63]. In early esophageal cancer (T0, T1im and T1sm) Bonavina noted an overall five-year survival advantage for patients undergoing transthoracic resections compared with transhiatal excision (66% and 50% resp.)[63]. The incidence of local recurrence was also significantly lower in the patients undergoing transthoracic resection (1/80 vs 5/150, p<0.05). However, when patients were stratified according to the depth of tumor infiltration, this advantage disappeared except for the patients with submucosal tumor spread (T1sm). Although this could be due to selection bias, it might also suggest a beneficial role for lymph node dissection when submucosal spread has been proven or suggested. These results are confirmed by a study by Hagen et al[58]. They also report a clear overall survival benefit for patients undergoing transthoracic en-bloc resection. However, this was a non-randomized study in which patients were allocated to the transhiatal group based on unfavorable tumor characteristics (transmural spread and lymphadenopathy as seen on CT-scan), although there still remained a survival benefit for patients with early or late tumors undergoing transthoracic resection when the groups were stratified according to the post-operative pathology results. Especially those patients with early tumors seem to benefit from the en-bloc approach: 41% five-year survival after en-bloc resection versus 20% after transhiatal resection[58]. However, this study lacks sufficient power, including only 69 patients with squamous cell carcinoma, adenocarcinoma and cardia-carcinoma. Comparison of the results of transthoracic and transhiatal resections is also hampered by the earlier mentioned phenomenon of stage migration: the increased number of resected nodes in transthoracic resections increases the possibility of finding a positive node which might upgrade the tumor stage, which in turn might improve the results when compared stage by stage.

Despite the findings of the reports mentioned above, randomized trials have not been able to show a clear survival benefit of one resection form over the other. Goldminc et al. showed even a survival benefit (although not statistically significant) for patients undergoing transhiatal resection (ca. 30% vs. 15% 3 year survival), while Chu et al. found median survival rates of 16 and 13.5 months after transhiatal and transthoracic resections resp[37,43]. These results are confirmed by many non-randomized comparative studies[38,48,52]. Analysis of the literature of the last decade therefore suggests that overall survival is not clearly improved after transthoracic resections when compared with transhiatal resections. Both transhiatal resections and transthoracic approaches have five-year survival rates of approximately 20%, with three year survival rates of approximately 25%, reflecting the early and aggressive recurrence pattern of esophageal carcinoma.

When local recurrence rates are concerned, most authors were not able to find a difference in recurrence rates between transthoracic and transhiatal resections. In a study especially addressing the recurrence pattern of both transhiatal and standard Ivor Lewis resections, Van Lanschot et al. demonstrated isolated locoregional recurrence in ca. 10% of the patients who underwent a transhiatal or standard transthoracic resection[64]. Locoregional recurrence in combination with tumor elsewhere occurred in ca. 20% of the patients. Therefore, only 1/3 of the patients, at most, might have benefited from more radical local resection, which might have led to an improved cure rate in at most 10%, and might have prolonged the disease-free interval in the other 20%.

In a recent study analyzing the recurrence pattern in 137 patients following transhiatal resections (with a follow-up of at least two years or until death) we found an overall recurrence rate of 55.4%[65]. Isolated locoregional recurrence without distant metastases occurred in 32 patients (23.4%), while systemic disease without locoregional recurrence developed in 21 patients (15.3%). Nineteen patients (13.8%) developed a combination of both locoregional and distant recurrent disease. The median time to recurrence was 11 months. There was no significant difference between recurrence in adenocarcinoma and squamous cell carcinoma, concerning neither localization nor time of recurrence[65].

Our results are quite similar to those of Clark et al. who found (overall) nodal recurrence in 39.5%, systemic recurrence in 39.5% and anastomotic recurrence in 10.5% of the cases after en-bloc resections for adenocarcinoma with a mean follow-up of 16.5 months. However, in his series the percentage of patients with locoregional recurrence only was 13%, as compared with 23.4% in our series. Our overall recurrence rate of 55.4% is comparable with their 52.6%, which suggests that the addition of a wide local excision including a radical lymphatic dissection does not necessarily lead to better results.

A recent abstract addressing the pattern of recurrence following subtotal esophagectomy with two field lymphadenectomy also describes a median time to recurrence of 11 months, with locoregional recurrence occurring in 23% and hematogenous recurrence in 18%, also suggesting that an extended lymph node dissection does not substantially improve locoregional control or disease-free interval. After extended resection, Morita found locoregional recurrence in 31% of the patients, hematogenous metastases in 15% and a combination of both also in 15%, giving an overall recurrence rate of 66%[66].

Most western authors report rather low incidences of upper mediastinal and/or cervical recurrence. In our series only 8% of the patients developed recurrent disease in the neck after transhiatal resection. This corresponds well with numbers cited after transthoracic resection: upper mediastinal and cervical recurrence occurred in 3% and 2% of all patients after an extended transthoracic resection including two-field lymph node dissection[67].

When these data are combined, there seems to be no gross difference in recurrence pattern after transhiatal, transthoracic en-bloc and extended transthoracic resections with two-field (or three-field) lymph node dissection. The same holds true for the disease free interval: most authors report median disease-free intervals of approximately one year.

5. CONCLUSION

Over the last decade there has been much debate about the optimal resection form for esophageal cancer. Main focus of this debate is the theoretical approach to esophageal cancer. In view of the grim prognosis in many patients, should we attempt to improve the early results by decreasing early morbidity and mortality, or should we attempt to improve the long-term results by performing a more radical resection with the dissection of more surrounding tissue and more lymph nodes? Advocates of the first principle propagate the transhiatal resection, claiming less post-operative complications, while advocates of the latter approach discard the transhiatal approach for the alleged violation of basic oncological principles. Despite this ongoing discussion, only three randomized trials have been published, including a total of only 138 patients. The other studies are mostly (retrospective) consecutive case studies, describing the authors' experience with one or several procedures, thereby mostly reflecting the personal preference of the surgeon. Comparison of different series is further hampered because results are not presented in a standardized format, often including different histologic subtypes and tumor stages.

The positive significance of lymph node dissection has therefore not been established yet. Extended lymph node dissection might be of use as a staging procedure, which might become important in the (future) allocation of adjuvant treatment. However, the development of more sophisticated non-invasive diagnostic modalities (EUS-guided fine needle aspiration, PET-scan etc.) might render this function of lymph node dissection obsolete. The prognostic significance of lymph node status including lymph node ratio seems well established, but the question remains whether lymph node status may only be "an indicator and not a governor" of prognosis, as Cady pointed out correctly already in the mid-eighties. There are contradictory data about the benefit of more extended resections for survival. Some authors argue in favor of more extended resections, while others claim that long-term outcome is just as good or even better after transhiatal resections. Others suggest a selective surgical approach based on pre-operative staging results, advocating e.g. the transhiatal approach for early tumors or, conversely, for locally advanced tumors. However, as we have shown in the previous paragraphs, early tumors might display a relatively high prevalence of lymph node metastases. Until the pre-operative staging procedures are able to rule out lymph node metastases, and offer a reliable indication of the intra- or transmural growth of the tumor, the surgical approach should not be dependent on pre-operative staging. When all data of the last decade are compared there seems to be no difference in recurrence pattern, disease-free interval or survival rates, not even when stage is taken into account. As yet there has been no large trial including a sufficient number of patients to compare the long-term results of transhiatal resections with transthoracic resection with two-field lymphadenectomy. Until the results of such a study are known, many institutions regard transthoracic esophagectomy with or without extended lymph node dissection as the standard procedure, reserving the transhiatal resection for patients with more co-morbidity who are physically not able to undergo a thoracotomy. In the Netherlands the transhiatal resection is generally preferred, based on the assumption that it carries less early morbidity and mortality without a decrease in long-term survival, awaiting the results of an ongoing trial comparing transhiatal esophagectomy with transthoracic esophagectomy with two-fields lymph node dissection. However, until the results of this study are known, all evidence linking certain resection forms with specific complications or tumor recurrence remains circumstantial. At present, the choice between transhiatal and transthoracic approaches, and thus the extent of the lymph node dissection, rests on the subjective experience of the surgeon, not on evidence based medicine.

REFERENCES

1. Cady B. Lymph node metastases:indicators, but not governors of survival. Arch Surg 1984;119:1067-72.
2. Overgaard M, Hansen PS, Overgaard J, Rose C, Andersson M, Bach F, Kjaer M, Gadeberg CC, Mouridsen HT, Jensen K-B, Zedeler K. Post-operative radiotherapy in high-risk premenopausal women with breast cancer who receive adjuvant chemotherapy. N Engl J Med 1997;337:949-55.
3. Ragaz J, Jackson SM, Le N, Plenderleith IH, Spinelli JJ, Basco VE, Wilson KS, Knowling MA, Coppin CML, Paradis M, Coldman AJ, Olivotto IA. Adjuvant radiotherapy and chemotherapy in node-positive premenopausal women with breast cancer. N Engl J Med 1997;337:956-62.
4. Havenga K, Enker WE, Norstein J, Moriya Y, Heald RJ, Van Houwelingen HC, Van derVelde CJH. Improved survival and local control after total mesorectal excision or D3 lymphadenectomy in the treatment of primary rectal cancer:an international analysis of 1411 patients. Eur J Surg Oncol 1999;25:368-74.

5. Balch CM, Soong S-j, Bartolluci A, Urist MM, Karakousis CP, Smith TJ, Temple WJ, Ross MI, Jewell WR, Mihm MC, Barnhill RL, Wanebo HJ. Efficacy of an elective regional lymph node dissection of 1 to 4 mm thick melanomas for patients 60 years of age and younger. Ann Surg 1996;224:255-63.

6. Akoh JA, Macintyre IMC. Improving survival in gastric cancer:review of 5-year survival rates in english language publications from 1970. Br J Surg 1992;79:293-9.

7. Bonenkamp JJ, Hermans J, Sasako M, Welvaart K, Plukker JTM, Van Elk P, Obertop H, Gouma DJ, Taat CW, Van Lanschot J, Meyer S, De Graaf PW, Von Meyenfeldt MF, Tilanus H, Van de Velde CJH (for the Dutch gastric cancer group). Randomised comparison of morbidity after D1 and D2 dissection for gastric cancer in 996 Dutch patients. Lancet 1995;345:745-8.

8. Bonenkamp JJ, Hermans J, Sasako M, Van de Velde CJH. Extended lymph-node dissection for gastric cancer. N Engl J Med 1999;340(12):908-14.

9. Müller JM, Erasmi H, Stelzner M, Zieren U, Pichlmaier H. Surgical therapy of oesophageal carcinoma. Br J Surg 1990;77:845-57.

10. Akiyama H. Surgery for Cancer of the Esophagus. Williams and Wilkins 1990, Baltimore, USA

11. Orringer MB, Marshall B, Iannettoni MD. Transhiatal esophagectomy:clinical experience and refinements. Ann Surg 1999;230:392-403.

12. Orringer MB. Transhiatal oesophagectomy. In:Jamieson GC, Debas HT eds. Surgery of the Upper Gastrointestinal Tract. Chapman & Hall Medical, London 1994.

13. Lewis I. The surgical treatment of carcinoma of the oesophagus with special reference to a new operation for growths of the middle third. Br J Surg 1946:34:18-31.

14. Tanner NC. The present position of carcinoma of the oesophagus. Postgrad Med J 1947;23:109-39.

15. Hagen JA, DeMeester TR. En bloc oesophagectomy for cancer of the distal oesophagus, cardia and proximal stomach. In:Jamieson GC, Debas HT eds. Surgery of the upper gastrointestinal tract. Chapman & Hall Medical 1994, London, England.

16. Akiyama H, Tsumumaru M, Udagawa H, Kajiyama Y. Radical lymph node dissection for cancer of the thoracic esophagus. Ann Surg 1994;3:364-73.

17. Nishimaki T, Suzuki T, Suzuki T, Kuwabara S, Hatakeyama K. Outcomes of extended radical esophagectomy for thoracic esophageal cancer. J Am Coll Surg 1998;186:306-12.

18. Nigro JJ, Hagen JA, DeMeester TR, DeMeester SR, Peters JH, Oberg S, Theisen J, Kiyabu M, Crookes PF, Bremner CG. Prevalence and location of nodal metastases in distal esophageal adenocarcinoma confined to the wall:implications for therapy. J Thorac Cardiovasc Surg 1999;17:16-25.

19. Sugimachi K, Ikebe M, Kitamura K, Toh Y, Matsuda H, Kuwano H. Long-term results of esophagectomy for early esophageal carcinoma. Hepato-Gastroenterol 1993;40:203-6.

20. Van Sandick JW, Van Lanschot JJB, Ten Kate FJW, Offerhaus GJA, Fockens P, Tytgat GNJ, Obertop H. Pathology of early invasive adenocarcinoma of the oesophagus or oesophagogastric junction:implications for therapeutic decision making. Cancer, in press.

21. Nigro JJ, Hagen JA, DeMeester TR, DeMeester SR, Theisen J, Peters JH, Miyaby M. Occult esophageal adenocarcinoma. Extent of disease and implications for effective therapy. Ann Surg 1999;230:433-40.

22. Clark GWB, Peters JH, Ireland AP, Ehsan A, Hagen JA, Liyabu MT, Bremner CG, DeMeester TM. Nodal metastasis and sites of recurrence after en bloc esophagectomy for adenocarcinoma. Ann Thorac Surg 1994;58:646-54.

23. Nishimaki T, Tanaka O, Suzuki T, Aizawa K, Hatakeyama K, Muto T. Patterns of lymphatic spread in thoracic esophageal cancer. Cancer 1994;74:4-11.

24. Matsubara T, Ueda M, Nagao N, Takahashi T, Nakajima T, Nishi M. Cervicothoracic approach for total mesoesophageal dissection in cancer of the thoracic esophagus. J Am Coll Surg 1998;187:238-45.

25. Nigro JJ, DeMeester SR, Hagen JA, DeMeesrter TR, Peters JH, Kiyabu M, Campos GMR, Oberg S, Gastal O, Crookes PF, Bremner CG. Node status in transmural esophageal adenocarcinoma and outcome after en bloc esophagectomy. J Thorac Cardiovasc Surg 1999;117:960-8.

26. Matsubara T, Ueda M, Yanagida O, Nakajima T, Nishi M. How extensive should lymph node dissection be for cancer of the thoracic esophagus? J Thorac Cardiovasc Surg 1994;107:1073-8.

27. Altorki NK, Skinner DB. Occult cervical nodal metastasis in esophageal cancer:preliminary results of three-field lymphadenectomy. J Thorac Cardiovasc Surg 1997:113;540-4.

28. Hulscher JBF, Van Sandick JW, Tijssen JGP, Obertop H, Van Lanschot JJB. The recurrence pattern of esophageal carcinoma after transhiatal resection. J Am Coll Surg, in press

29. Siewert JR, Fink U, Beckurts KTE, Roder JD. Surgery of squamous cell carcinoma of the esophagus. Ann Oncol 1994:; (Suppl.3):S1-S7.

30. Steup WH, De Leyn P, Deneffe G, Van Raemdonck D, Coosemans W, Lerut T. tumors of the esophagogastric junction. Long-term survival in relation to the pattern of lymph node metastasis and a critical analysis of the accuracy of pTNM classification. J Thorac Cardiovasc Surg 1996;111:85-95.

31. Abe S, Tachibana M, Shiraishi M, Nakamura T. Lymph node metastasis in resectable esophageal cancer. J Thorac Cardiovasc Surg 1990;100:287-91

32. Van Sandick JW, Van Lanschot JJB, Fockens P, Obertop H. Peri-operative complications and prognostic factors after transhiatal oesophageal resection without thoracotomy for cancer. Thesis, 1999, University of Amsterdam.

33. Roder JD, Busch R, Stein HJ, Fink U, Siewert JR. Ratio of invaded to removed lymph nodes as a predictor of survival in squamous cell carcinoma of the oesophagus. Br J Surg 1994;81:410-3.

34. Izbicki JB, Hosch SB, Pichlmeier U, Rehders A, Busch C, Niendorf A, Passlick B, Broelsch CE, Pantel K. Prognostic value of immunohistochemically identifiable tumor cells in lymph nodes of patients with completely resected esophageal cancer. N Engl J Med 1997;337:118-94.

35. Bonavina L, Ferrero S, Midolo V, Buffa R, Cesana B, Peracchia A. Lymph node micrometastases in patients with adenocarcinoma of the esophagogastric junction. J Gastrointest Surg 1999;3:468-76.

36. Paget S. The distribution of secondary grwoths in cancer of the breast. Lancet 1889;1:571-3.

37. Chu KM, Law SY, Fok M, Wong J. A prospective randomized comparison of transhiatal and transthoracic resection for lower-third esophageal carcinoma. Am J Surg 1997;174:320-4.

38. Tilanus HW, Hop WCJ, Langenhorst BLAM, Van Lanschot JJB. Esophagectomy with or without thoracotomy. J Thorac Cardiovasc Surg 1993;105:898-903.

39. Gupta NM. Oesophagectomy without thoracotomy:first 250 patients. Eur J Surg 1996;162:455-61.

40. Lieberman-Meffert DMI, luescher U, Neff U, Ruedi TP, Allgower M. Esophagectomy without thoracotomy:is there a risk of intramediastinal bleeding? Ann Surg 1987;206:84-92.
41. Daniel TM, Fleisher KJ, Flanagan TL, Tribble CG, Kron IL. Transhiatal esophagectomy:a safe alternative for selected patients. Ann Thorac Surg 1992;54:686-90.
42. Van Sandick JW, Van Lanschot JJB, Tilanus HW, Wijnhoven B, Hennipman A, Obertop H. Transhiatal esophagectomy versus transthoracic esophagectomy with two-fields lymphadenectomy. Interim results of a randomized study. Can J Gastroenterol 1998;12(B):48B.
43. Goldminc M, Maddern G, LePrise E, Meunier B, Campion JP, Launois B. Oesophagectomy by transhiatal approach or thoracotomy:a prospective randomized trial. Br J Surg 1993;80:367-70.
44. Jacobi CA, Zieren HU, Müller M, Pichlmaier H. Surgical therapy of esophageal carcinoma:the influence of surgical approach and esophageal resection on cardiopulmonary function. Eur J Cardiothoracic Surg 1997;11:32-7.
45. Lerut T, DeLeyn P, Coosemans W, Van Raemdonck D, Scheys I, LeSaffre E. Surgical strategies in esophageal carcinoma with emphasis on radical lymphadenectomy. Ann Surg 1992;216:583-90.
46. Paç M, Basoglu A, Koçak H, et al. Transhiatal versus transthoracic esophagectomy for esophageal cancer. J Thorac Cardiovasc Surg 1993;106:205-9.
47. Stark SP, Romberg MS, Pierce GE et al. Transhiatal versus transthoracic esophagectomy for adenocarcinoma of the distal esophagus and cardia. Am J Surg 1996:172;478-82.
48. Gluch L, Smith RC, Bambach CP, Brown AR. Comparison of outcomes following transhiatal or Ivor Lewis esophageactomy for esophageal carcinoma. World J Surg 1999;23:271-6.
49. Horstmann O, Verreet PR, Becker H, Ohmann C, Röher HD. Transhiatal oesophagectomy compared with transthoracic resection and systematic lymphadenectomy for the treatment of oesophageal cancer. Eur J Surg 1995;161:557-67.
50. Moon MR, Schulte WJ, Haasler GB, Condon RE. Transhiatal and transthoracic esophagectomy for adenocarcinoma of the esophagus. Arch Surg 1992;127:951-5.
51. Putnam JB, Suell DM, McMurtey MJ , et al. Comparison of three techniques of esophagectomy within a residency training program. Ann Thorac Surg 1994;7:319-25.
52. Fok M, Law S, Stipa F, Cheng S, Wong J. A comparison of transhiatal and transthoracic resection for oesophageal carcinoma. Endoscopy 1993;25 (Suppl.) 660-3.
53. Jauch KW, Bacha EA, Denecke H, Anthuber M, Schildberg FW. Esophageal carcinoma:prognostic features and comparison between blunt transhiatal dissection and transthoracic resection. Eur J Surg Oncol 1992;18:553-62.
54. McLarty AJ, Deschamps C, Trastek VF, Allen MS, Pairolero PC, Harmsen WS. Esophageal resection for cancer of the esophagus:long-term function and quality of life. Ann Thorac Surg 1997;63:1568-72.
55. Hulscher JBF, Van Sandick JW, DeVriese PP, Van Lanschot JJB, Obertop H. Vocal cord paralysis after subtotal oesophagectomy. Br J Surg, 1999;86:1583-6.
56. Earlam R, Cunha-Melo JR. Oesophageal squamous cell carcinoma:I. a critical review of surgery. Br J Surg 1980;67:381-90.
57. Patti MG, Corvera CU, Glasgow RE, Way LW. A hospital's annual rate of esophagectomy influences the operative mortality rate. J Gastrointest Surg 1998;2:186-92.
58. Hagen JA, Peters JH, DeMeester TR. Superiority of extended en bloc esophagectomy for carcinoma of the lower esophagus and cardia. J Thorac Cardiovasc Surg 1993;106:850-9.
59. Junginger T, Dutkowski P. Selective approach to the treatment of oesophageal cancer. Br J Surg 1996;83:1473-7.
60. Gertsch P, Vauthey JN, Lustenberger AA, Friedlander-Klar. Long-term results of transhiatal esophagectomy for esophageal carcinoma. Cancer 1993;72:2312-9.
61. Bolton JS, Ochsner JL, Abdoh A. Surgical management of esophageal cancer:a decade of change. Ann Surg 1994;219:475-80.
62. Van Sandick JW, Gisbertz SS, Ten Berge IJM, Van der Pouw Kraan TCTM, Out TA, Boermeester MA, Van Lanschot JJB. Relations between preoperative T cell response profile and infectious complication risk in patients undergoing transhiatal or transthoracic oesophagectomy for cancer. In:Van Sandick JW. Early detection and surgical treatment of adenocarcinoma of the oesophagus or oesophagogastric junction. Thesis 1999, University of Amsterdam.
63. Bonavina L. Early oesophageal cancer:results of a European multicentre survey. Br J Surg 1995;82:98-101.
64. Van Lanschot JJB, Tilanus HW, Voormolen MHJ, Van Deelen RAJ. Recurrence pattern of oesophageal carcinoma after limited resection does not support wide local excision with extensive lymph node dissection. Br J Surg 1994;81:1320-3.
65. Hulscher JBF, Van Sandick JW, Tijssen JGP, Obertop H, Van Lanschot JJB. The recurrence pattern of esophageal carcinoma after transhiatal resection. J Am Coll Surg, in press.
66. Morita M, Kuwano H, Ohno S, Furusawa M, Sugimachi K. Characteristics and sequence of the recurrent patterns after curative esophagectomy for squamous cell carcinoma. Surgery 1994;116:1-7.
67. Dresner SM, Wayman J, Shenfine J, Harris A, Hayes N, Griffin SM. The pattern of recurrence following subtotal oesophagectomy with two field lymphadenectomy. Gut 1999;45 (Suppl V):A235.

6.4 VIDEOENDOSCOPIC ESOPHAGECTOMY FOR CANCER

Jean-Marie Collard

1. INTRODUCTION

Various esophageal procedures are now feasible through a few holes in the thoracic or abdominal wall, or through the working channel of an endoluminal endoscope[1] rather than through a large parietal incision. This is the case for antireflux fundoplication[2,3], myotomies[4], enucleation of a benign tumor[5], clippage of the thoracic duct[6], and so on ... The esophagus itself can be removed by so-called minimally invasive approaches that are the right thoracoscopy[7-14], the transcervical mediastinoscopy combined with conventional transhiatal dissection by laparotomy[15-17], and the laparoscopic transhiatal esophagogastric mobilization in combination with conventional cervicotomy for esophageal extraction and esophagogastric anastomosis[18-23]. All those new surgical modalities are not only very attractive because they obviously reduce the parietal damage related to the classic incisions but they constitute also a very appealing technical challenge for the surgeon.

However, concerning esophagectomy, the critical questions are

1. Can the new approaches to the esophagus provide intraoperative conditions of safety similar to those that have existed in conventional surgery for many years ?
2. Are they liable to reduce the risk of postoperative parietal discomfort, respiratory complication, or mortality ?
3. Do they allow fulfilment of the criterias of oncologically radical esophageal surgery ?

2. SURGICAL TECHNIQUE

2.1 EXTENDED EN BLOC ESOPHAGEC-TOMY BY RIGHT THORACOSCOPY

Using a double-lumen intubation system (Carlen's endotracheal tube), and with the patient on his left side, five 1 cm holes are created in the wall of the right side of the chest. The posterior mediastinum is entered through two longitudinal incisions in the right mediastinal pleura, one along the right sympathetic cord and one along the right wall of the trachea in the upper part of the chest, and along the pericardium in the caudal part.

All the right intercostal veins and the distal segment of the left hemiazygous vein going into the right azygous vein are divided between metal clips. The right azygos vein is divided with use of an endo-GIA 30 stapler just above the diaphragm. Care must be taken when removing soft tissues and nodes surrounding the terminal segments of these veins just in front of the spine, so that the initial segments of all the right intercostal arteries remain intact. The thoracic duct is identified for division just above the diaphragm between the descending aorta and the right azygous vein in front of the spine. The segment of the thoracic duct up to where it crosses behind the upper third of the esophagus is included in the bloc. The anterior aspect of the descending aorta is cleared up. This step of the procedure requires careful identification and clippage of two or three very small arteries entering the esophageal wall[24]. The posterior mediastinal bloc is freed from the pericardium, the right pulmonary veins, and the left mediastinal pleura. After identification of the lower aspect of the right main stem bronchus, subcarinal soft tissue and lymph nodes are dissected and removed en bloc. Division of the azygous arch with use of an endo-GIA 30 stapler gives access to the lower part of the trachea, so as to allow clearance of the soft tissue along the membranous wall. The right vagus nerve is divided. The left recurrent nerve may be identified, and the lymph nodes alongside removed. Posteriorly, middle and upper mediastinal dissection leads to division of the left vagus nerve just below the left main stem bronchus, and of one or two large esophageal arteries originating from the aortic arch. The right hemiazygous vein is divided at the apex of the chest either between metal clips or with use of an endo-GIA 30 stapler.

The final result of the procedure is a real skeletonization of the posterior mediastinum. During the whole procedure, the esophageal wall is not visualized, except in the upper third owing to paucity of the surrounding soft tissue at this level. The esophageal bloc is eventually abandoned in the chest. The chest is drained by two tubes inserted through two of the parietal holes. The three other holes are closed. The patient is then placed in the

347

H.W. Tilanus and S.E.A. Attwood (eds.), Barrett's Esophagus, 347–355.
© 2001 *Kluwer Academic Publishers. Printed in the Netherlands.*

recumbent position for laparotomy and cervicotomy. The esophagus is divided at the cervical level and pulled down in the abdomen.

2.2 MINIMAL EN BLOC ESOPHAGEC-TOMY BY RIGHT THORACOSCOPY

When the azygous vessels lie on the spine far away from the descending aorta, *en-bloc* esophagectomy can be made less extensive by maintaining the right azygous and the right hemiazygous veins in place. In such an instance, the initial pleural incision is made between the esophagus and the right azygous vein, the arch of which is however transected using an endo-GIA 30 stapler. Care must be taken to identify the lower segment of the thoracic duct which runs between the aorta and the right azygous vein. The rest of the mediastinal dissection is similar to that described for the extended en bloc esophagectomy.

2.3 ESOPHAGECTOMY WITH LIMITED LYMPH NODE CLEARANCE BY RIGHT THORACOSCOPY

This kind of esophagectomy includes removal of the esophagus tube together with some of the lymph nodes located in its immediate vicinity. In this situation, the dissection is carried out neither flush with the esophageal wall nor close to the wall of the adjacent mediastinal structures such as the trachea, main stem bronchi, or pulmonary veins, but through the mediastinal soft tissue that surrounds the esophagus. Because of the absence of precise anatomical landmarks, bleeding from small vessels within the peri-esophageal soft tissue may make dissection more difficult than that carried out flush with the main mediastinal structures.

2.4 REMOVAL OF THE ESOPHAGUS TUBE BY RIGHT THORACOSCOPY

Removal of the esophagus tube without any attempt to resect peri-esophageal lymph nodes is the easiest technique of thoracoscopic esophagectomy. Unlike the *en-bloc* technique, the procedure requires early identification of the esophageal wall which serves as a reliable landmark at any time. It is also the safest technique because dissection is carried out far away from the vital mediastinal structures. This limited procedure is best indicated in high-grade dysplasia arising in Barrett's esophagus. Indeed, although T1

adenocarcinoma may be disclosed at postoperative examination of the resected specimen, neoplastic spread into peri-esophageal lymph nodes is very unusual[25]. A long caustic stenosis unresponsive to endoscopic dilations constitutes also a good indication for limiting esophageal resection to the esophagus tube. However, in the presence of hard adhesions between the esophagus and the immediately adjacent mediastinal structures after transmural caustic injury, dissection has to be carried out within the fibrotic muscular layers of the esophageal wall, leaving the outermost muscle fibers in place.

2.5 ESOPHAGECTOMY BY TRANS-CERVICAL ENDODISSECTION

This technique was first experimented on the lamb by Kipfmuller[26] and, afterwards, applied to humans by Buess[15,16] and Bumm[17]. The upper thoracic esophagus is approached from a left cervical incision while another surgeon initiates lower peri-esophageal dissection through the diaphragmatic hiatus by conventional laparotomy. The esophagus is dissected off the adjacent mediastinal structures under videoscopy by means of a specifically designed mediastinoscope. The latter contains a central working channel and has a shaped olive at the tip which exposes both the esophageal wall, the soft tissue around and the wall of the adjacent mediastinal structures. Different instruments can be inserted into the working channel, such as a sucker, grasping forceps, insulated scissors as well as insulated forceps for monopolar coagulation. Thus, dissection is carried out flush with the esophageal wall without removing the lymph nodes located in the posterior mediastinum. However, transcervical endodissection of the upper half of the posterior mediastinum in combination with radical resection of the lower half of the esophagus *en-bloc* with all the potentially involved lymph nodes in the lower mediastinum and upper abdomen has been applied to lower-third adenocarcinomas[27]. After completion of the mediastinal endodissection, the esophagus is transected in the neck and pulled down in the abdominal cavity. Digestive continuity is restored by gastric pull-up to the neck.

2.6 LAPAROSCOPIC TRANSHIATAL ESOPHAGECTOMY AND GASTRIC PULL-UP

The hiatus is approached through 4 to 5 1-cm holes in the abdominal wall. Mediastinal dissection is then carried out through the soft tissue around the esophagus tube. Care must be taken not to open either of the two mediastinal pleural sheats in order to prevent CO_2 from spreading into the pleural spaces and subsequent pneumothorax formation. In fact, transmission of the positive abdominal pressure to the mediastinum prepares instrumental dissection in such a way that the soft tissue around the esophagus tube acquires an areolar aspect. After esophageal mobilization has been completed as far as the trachea, the greater curvature of the stomach is dissected off the greater omentum, keeping the gastroepiploic vascular arcade intact. The fundus is then separated from the spleen by division of the short gastric vessels. Lifting of the gastric pouch gives access to the left gastric vessels that are divided either between metal clips or with use of an endo-GIA stapler. The proximal half of the lesser curvature is separated from the rest of the stomach by stapling division of the gastric wall 1 to 3 cm away from the right border of the stomach, so as to create a greater curvature tube based on the right gastroepiploic vessels. However, the subcardial area of the stomach remains attached to the greater curvature tube, so as to allow elevation of the latter in continuity with the esophagus once cervical dissection has been completed. For this, the cervical esophagus is dissected off the trachea through a left cervical incision along the anterior aspect of the sterno-cleido-mastoid muscle. Upper dissection is then carried out from this cervical incision in order to meet the retrotracheal compartment that has already been dissected through the hiatus. Gentle traction on the cervical esophagus allows the elevation of both the esophagus and gastric transplant through the mediastinum. This manœuvre can be facilitated pouching the stomach into the lower mediastinum with use of the laparoscopic forceps under videocontrol in order to prevent the esophageal substitute from twisting. After division of the cervical esophagus and stapling separation of the subcardial area of the stomach from the greater curvature tube, the cervical esophageal stump is anastomosed to the upper end of the gastric transplant.

3. PERSONAL EXPERIENCE OF THORACOSCOPIC ESOPHAGECTOMY

From 1991 to 1993, esophagectomy by right thoracoscopy was attempted on 14 patients as a pilot study. Eleven patients had a cancer of the thoracic esophagus that was not suspected for adhering to adjacent mediastinal structures at preoperative computed tomography scan of the chest, and three patients had a long caustic stenosis that was not suitable for endoscopic dilation. All patients were thin and had no history of previous thoracic surgery. Thoracoscopy was converted into thoracotomy in two patients because of a loss of selectivity in one lung ventilation or injury to a right intercostal artery at its aortic origin. In a third patient, exploratory thoracoscopy disclosed tumor invasion to the lung parenchyma that had not been suspected at preoperative work-up. The esophagus was only by-passed. Eleven esophagectomies (i.e. 9 for cancer and 2 for caustic stenosis) were completed by exclusive thoracoscopy, i.e. four extensive en bloc resections, three minimal en bloc resections, one esophagectomy with more limited lymph node clearance, and three resections of the esophagus only. Overall, there were 9 potentially curative Ro esophageal resections, among which 8 were performed by exclusive thoracoscopy and one by thoracoscopy converted into thoracotomy. Duration of the thoracoscopic time ranged from 240 to 390 minutes for the extensive en bloc resections, from 150 to 225 minutes for the minimal en-bloc resections, and from 180 to 190 minutes for the other procedures. Only one of the eleven patients required blood transfusion to correct preoperative anemia. Digestive continuity was restored using the stomach in all but one patient who had a colonic interposition.

One cancer patient died of postoperative hepatic failure while all the other patients were discharged home. Two patients (one thoracoscopy and one thoracoscopy converted into thoracotomy) developed acute pneumonitis, requiring prolonged antibiotic therapy in one and 3-week assisted ventilation in the other. Two of the eleven patients in whom esophagectomy was completed by thoracoscopy complained of residual chest pain at some of the trocar sites. In one of these two patients, parietal discomfort persisted for the 6 years that preceeded his death of an unrelated cause.

4. FEASIBILITY AND SAFETY

The experiences of videoendoscopic esophageal surgery reported over the current decade show that different kinds of esophagectomy are feasible using one of the aforedescribed so-called minimally invasive approaches. However, these procedures appear to be all the more demanding and time-consuming as the esophagectomy is combined with more extensive lymph node clearance in the posterior mediastinum. So, unlike resections limited to the esophagus tube, en bloc resections carried out close to the vital structures of the posterior mediastinum give the surgeon a feeling of insecurity in spite of routine experience with both conventional and videoendoscopic esophageal surgery and thorough knowledge of the surgical anatomy of the esophagus[24].

There are several reasons for this :

-          the long arm of the thoracoscopic instruments

-          the technical problems related to the functioning of the videoendoscope, the microcamera and the television screen.

-          the need for preventive coagulation of any soft structure prior to its division.

-          the difficulties in reclining the lung parenchyma while dissecting peritracheal soft tissue due to displacement of the Carlen's tube[7,28].

We know indeed that severe intraoperative complications such as injury to the subclavian vessels[9], to a right intercostal artery just as it comes out of the descending aorta[7], or to the membranous wall of the trachea[17,29] can occur during minimally invasive operations, while they are very uncommon in conventional surgery. Prompt management of such technical complications is made difficult by the fact that the surgeon's index finger, which is the most reliable "surgical instrument" in thoracic surgery, is not immediately available to cover the site of laceration until proper repair of the injuried structure can be done. Therefore, the conventional surgical instrumentation must be displayed on a table located inside of the operating room, and the surgeon must not hesitate to open the chest as soon as a major technical complication is suspected or in the absence of optimal conditions for a safe thoracoscopic dissection. In this respect, careful analysis of 13 series of videoendoscopic esophagectomies totalizing 224 patients[11-14,18-22,28-31] published during the last four years indicates that conversion into an open approach was necessary in 20 patients (9 %) because of dense pleural adhesions, incomplete lung collapse, life-threatening technical complication, or locally advanced tumor. In any case, we have to bear in mind that what can be done easily on very selected patients with respect to small tumor size and favourable anatomical status of the chest may not be feasible with acceptable conditions of safety on fat and stout patients operated on for a huge esophageal tumor.

5. POSTOPERATIVE MORTALITY AND MORBIDITY

In the early nineties, i.e. at the time of the videosurgery boom, an extensive review of the literature including more than 46,000 operations[32] had shown that one patient out of eight still experienced a fatal outcome and that one out of three developed a postoperative complication after esophagectomy for cancer in spite of considerable advances in intensive care. We also knew that both mortality and morbidity rates were closely related to the individual experience of resective esophageal surgery in terms of number of cases operated on per year[33], and that a very low mortality could be achieved in specialized centers as a consequence of routine practice of major esophageal procedures and of deep personal investment of all the members of the surgical team at large including surgeons, intensive care physicians, anaesthesiologists, nurses, and physiotherapists[34]. In this setting, great hopes were placed upon the introduction of minimal access techniques of esophagectomy in an attempt to reduce the risk of complication after the operation. We knew however that the very low postoperative mortality achieved by some experienced teams had been obtained irrespective of the parietal incision through which the esophagus had been approached[34] and that the absence any chest wall damage, as is the case with conventional transhiatal esophagectomy, failed to lower the risk of postoperative complication in comparison with transthoracic esophageal resection[35]. Although a learning-curve effect might be advocated, the prohibitive 17 % intra- and postoperative mortality rate reported in 1994 by HOUBEN[36] in a collective series of 40 patients who had undergone esophagectomies by thoracoscopy cast doubt on the idea that the novel approaches to the esophagus could give patients more chance of complete postoperative recovery that did conventional surgery.

TABLE 1. Factors predisposing to postoperative respiratory complications after esophagectomy.

1. Poor initial respiratory condition (tobacco abuse)
2. Weak immunologic barrier (alcohol abuse)
3. Extended mediastinal dissection close to the respiratory airways
4. Peritracheal lymph node clearance leading to lymphatic stasis in lung parenchyma
5. Intraoperative damage to lung parenchyma[28] (manual or instrumental retraction)
6. Injury to the recurrent laryngeal nerves[18,20,29,30]
7. Aspiration of gastric juice due to stasis in the esophageal substitute lumen
8. Sepsis secondary to necrosis of the esophageal substitute or anastomotic leakage
9. Parietal discomfort and pain (drains, incisions, ...)

However, more encouraging reports[11-14,18-22,28-31] were published during the last four years, indicating that a postoperative mortality rate similar to that observed after conventional surgery i.e. ranging from 0 % to 12 % (mean : 3.5 %), could be achieved after videoendoscopic esophagectomy probably because of better knowledge of the videoendoscopic dissection technique. Actually, deaths from injury to one of the vital structures in the posterior mediastinum are now exceptional, the more common cause of death is the development of one of the classic complications of resective esophageal surgery such as respiratory failure[30], anastomotic leak[14,31], or necrosis of the esophageal substitute[17,23]. This confirms that major esophageal surgery addresses patients with a relatively poor general status and includes multiple surgical steps other than esophageal dissection. For instance, the only one of our own patients who was not discharged home after thoracoscopic esophagectomy died of hepatic failure secondary to inadvertent ligation of a single left hepatic artery at the time of the gastric mobilization by conventional laparotomy[7]. Another purposed advantage of minimal access surgery of the esophagus was that it was supposed to reduce the risk of postoperative respiratory complication.

In retrospect however, most of the surgical teams[7-10,12,13,20,28,30,31] have reported respiratory complications after videoendoscopic esophageal resections including acute pneumonitis[7,13,31], atelectasis[20,30,31], purulent pleural effusion[30], pleural effusion in the contralateral pleural cavity[31], persistent air leak[19], or adult respiratory distress syndrome[7,30]. This is not surprising bearing in mind that respiratory complications are multifactorial in origin (Table I), and that again, the absence of damage to the thoracic wall, as is the case with transhiatal

esophagectomy without thoracotomy, has been shown not to lower the risk of respiratory problems[35].

In fact, postoperative parietal discomfort plays an accessory role in the genesis of postoperative respiratory complications after major thoracic procedures, inasmuch as postoperative pain is now easily controlable with use of the modern analgesia techniques including epidural analgesia with drugs like clonidin and morphine[37]. Even, minimal access to the esophagus through a few holes in the chest wall is not necessarily synonymous with minimal parietal damage. This viewpoint supported by the fact that thoracic pain due to compression of one or several of the intercostal nerves by trocars inserted into the chest through narrow interspaces has been reported after thoracoscopic esophagectomy[7,9]. This is also in line with the observation that larger changes in serum cytokine levels occur after thoracoscopic than after conventional transthoracic esophagectomy, probably because of longer operating time and subsequent increase of the surgical stress with the former technique[38]. In spite of the fact that mediastinal dissection is performed under videocontrol, transient or persistent dysphonia has been experienced by patients operated on by laparoscopic transhiatal, transcervical, or thoracoscopic esophagectomy, as a consequence of indavertent injury to recurrent laryngeal nerves[18,20,29,30]. This may account for some of the respiratory complications reported, secondary to difficulties in approximating the vocal cords for coughing or rather, difficulties in maintaining the glottis open, the latter situation requiring temporary tracheostomy[29].

Necrosis of the esophageal substitute is another complication reported after either right thoracoscopy[23] or transcervical mediastinoscopy[17]. In the latter instance, narrowness of the mediastinal channel related to minimal intramediastinal dissection predisposes to compression of the substitute, a condition which is liable to compromise blood supply to the fundus and anastomotic site[39]. In addition, tiredness of the surgeon after a long-lasting endoscopic esophageal procedure may account for the fact that he is no longer in good shape for constructing the esophageal substitute in a meticulous fashion. The same arguments may be advocated to explain the 20 % leakage rate that was reported at the cervical level after videoendoscopic transmediastinal endodissection[17].

6. RADICALITY OF SURGERY

Extended esophageal resection including removal of the esophagus tube with all the lymph nodes and soft tissues in the posterior mediastinum is the corner stone of the radical treatment of cancer of the esophagus[40-42]. The goal of the procedure is to surround some of those neoplastic processes that have already spread into some of the locoregional lymph nodes. The benefit that can be drawn from doing en bloc esophagectomies according to the "no touch" technique with minimal visualization of the esophagus tube itself becomes quite clear when analysing the number of patients who may anticipate 5-year survival in spite of involvement of some of the resectable locoregional lymph nodes. For instance, 5-year survival rate in a personal series of 106 consecutive patients with metastatic lymph nodes who underwent Ro esophageal resection was 31%[41a], an observation that confirms data from Akiyama in Japan who has reported a 28 % survival rate at 5 years in a series of 179 similar patients[42]. The same author also showed that still higher survival rate (i.e. 43 % at 5 years) can be achieved when radical neck dissection is added to the conventional "two-field" dissection[42].

Our own experience shows that extended lymph node clearance in the posterior mediastinum can be done thoracoscopically[7]. This is attested to by the number of lymph nodes seen in the resected specimens(i.e. 21 to 51), and by the fact that survival of the 9 patients (No : n=4; N1 : n =5) who underwent Ro esophageal resection with mediastinal lymph node clearance is similar to that obtained in a series of 204 patients who underwent a similar operation through conventional approaches (Fig. 1). Our data are confirmed by those of Robertson and co-workers[31] who have reported survival rates of 73 % at one year and of 63 % at two years after

thoracoscopically-assisted Ivor-Lewis esophagectomy in 17 consecutive patients.

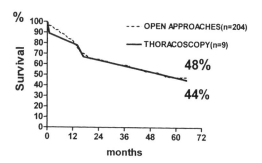

Figure1. Kaplan-Meier's survival curve of 204 consecutive patients who underwent Ro en-bloc esophageal resection with use of conventional approaches (dashed line) and of 9 patients who underwent either Ro en-bloc esophagectomy (n = 8) or Ro resection of the esophagus with closely related lymph nodes (n = 1) by either exclusive thoracoscopy (n = 8) or thoracoscopy converted into thoracotomy (n = 1) (thick line)

As for Dexter and co-workers[11], two-year cancer-specific survival was 33 % in a series of 22 patients in whom 6 to 28 lymph nodes had been removed by right thoracoscopy, laparotomy, and cervicotomy. As for the esophagectomy by combined transcervical endodissection and conventional transhiatal approach, because it does not allow lymph node clearance of the posterior mediastinum, it appears to be a palliative procedure unless the neoplastic process is still confined to the esophageal wall. Buess and co-workers[16] have indeed reported that all their patients but those operated on for a T1 tumor had died before the term of 3 years following the esophagectomy. On the other hand, the rather high 3-year survival rate of 40 % (estimation on figure) achieved in adenocarcinoma patients with metastatic lymph nodes after combined transcervical and transhiatal en bloc esophagectomy is more likely related to very extended lymph node clearance of the lower mediastinum and upper abdomen than to endodissection of the upper-half of the esophagus tube under videocontrol[27].

At evidence, we have to keep in mind that the new approaches to the esophagus are unlikely to improve long-term survival and cure of cancer patients because lymph node clearance cannot be made more extended than what is done by conventional thoracotomy.

TABLE 2. Factors predisposing to parietal neoplastic seeding during a videoendoscopic operation for cancer

1.	Direct contact of the chest wall with the tumor during its extraction (stab incision)
2.	Disruption of the tumor at the time of its extraction through a narrow channel
3.	Contamination of the thoracoscopic instruments during dissection due to direct manipulation of the tumor with grasping forceps
4.	Transtumoral dissection (poorly-delimited lesion)
5.	Leaving pleural washing fluid inside of the chest cavity at the end of the procedure, since it may contain malignant cells[45].
6.	Gas turbulences as well as intracavitary high pressure may contribute to spillage of neoplastic cells (laparoscopic transhiatal esophagectomy)

Rather, port-site neoplastic recurrence that was reported after thoracoscopic esophagectomy[13,43,44] appears to be a novel cause of failure of potentially curative esophageal resection that was unknown until the introduction of videoendoscopic surgery. In fact, although multifactorial in-origin (table 2), parietal neoplastic seeding[46] is probably due to repetitive passage of contaminated surgical instruments through the thoracic holes, since this upsetting complication occurred even though the tumor itself had not been extracted through the port-site concerned.

7. CONCLUSIONS AND PERSPECTIVES

Today, although an oncologically radical esophagectomy can be done by videoendoscopy or video-assisted conventional surgery, esophageal surgeons are much less enthusiastic about removing the esophagus by so-called minimal approaches than they were a few years ago[13,14,28,30,31]. Routine practice of videoendoscopic surgery teaches us that the benefit one can expect from minimal access surgery depends on the ratio of the parietal damage in conventional surgery to the internal damage. In major esophageal surgery, this ratio is not high enough to expect substantial modification of the postoperative course. On the contrary, both exploratory thoracoscopy and laparoscopy[47] appear to be valuable applications of the minimally invasive surgery, that are liable to challenge the classic preoperative investigation methods such as computed tomography scan or ultrasonography which, with time, have been proved to be less contributive than initially claimed and expected. Likewise, conditioning of the fundus to relative ischemia by laparoscopic ligation of the left gastric vessels[48] prior to the esophagectomy is another interesting application of the videoendoscopic surgery technique in an attempt to reduce, as was observed after two-stage esophago-gastrostomy[49], the risk of cervical anastomotic leakage. Actually, over the nineties, esophageal surgeons have learned two important messages. First, minimal access esophageal surgery is unable to lower the risk of postoperative complications after esophageal resection for cancer, and second, combination of the currently available non-surgical therapies to resection of the esophagus does not significantly improve long-term survival rates achieved after exclusive esophagectomy[41]. Real advances in esophageal cancer management will probably come from better understanding of the cancer mechanisms and from subsequent refinements in immunotherapy[50]. For this, a new millennium starts very soon ...

REFERENCES

1. Collard JM. Endoscopic approach to hypopharyngeal diverticulum. In:Minimally invasive surgery of the foregut. JH Peters, TR Demeester, eds. Quality Medical Publishing, Inc. St-Louis, MO;73-82:1994.

2. Weerts JM, Dallemagne B, Hamoir E. et al. Laparoscopic Nissen fundoplication:detailed analysis of 132 patients. Surg Laparosc Endosc 1993;3:357-64.

3. Collard JM, De Gheldere C, De Kock M, Otte JB, Kestens PJ. Laparoscopic antireflux surgery. What is real progress ? Ann. Surg 1994;220:146-54.

4. Collard JM, Lengele B, Malaise J, Otte JB, Kestens PJ. Minimally invasive surgery for achalasia. In:Atlas of video-assisted thoracic surgery. W. Brown. ed. Saunders medical publishing, St-Louis, MO;301-304 :1994.

5. Bardini R, Segalin A, Ruol A, Pavanello M, Peracchia A. Videothoracoscopic enucleation of esophageal leiomyoma. Ann Thorac Surg 1992;54:576-7.

6. Collard JM, Lengele B, Malaise J, Otte JB, Kestens PJ. Management of thoracic duct injury by right thoracoscopy. In:Atlas of video-assisted thoracic

surgery. W. Brown. ed. Saunders Medical Publishing, St-Louis, MO;260-261,1994.

7.   Collard JM, Lengele B, Otte JB, Kestens PJ. En bloc and standard esophagectomies by thoracoscopy. Ann Thorac Surg 1993;56:675-9.

8.   Azagra JS, Ceuterick M, Goergen M. Thoracoscopy in oesophagectomy for esophageal cancer. Br J Surg 1993;80:320-1.

9.   Descottes B. Thoracoscopic esophagectomy. European Institute of Telesurgery, Strasbourg, France, October 1994, communication.

10.   Gossot D, Fourquier P, Cellerier M. Thoracoscopic esophagectomy:technique and initial results. Ann Thorac Surg 1993;56:667-70.

11.   Dexter SP, Martin IG, Mc Mahon M.J. Radical thoracoscopic esophagectomy for cancer. Surg. Endosc 1996;10:147-51.

12.   Akaishi T, Kaneda I, Higuchi N. et al. Thoracoscopic en bloc total esophagectomy with radical mediastinal lymphadenectomy. J Thorac Cardiovasc Surg 1996;112:1533-40.

13.   Law S, Fok M, Chu KM, Wong J. Thoracoscopic esophagectomy for esophageal cancer. Surgery 1997;22:8-14.

14.   Peracchia A, Rosati R, Fumagalli U, Bona S, Chella B. Thoracoscopic esophagectomy:are there benefits ? Semin Surg Oncol 1997;13:259-62.

15.   Buess GF, Becker HD, Naruhn MB. Endoscopic esophagectomy without thoracotomy. Problems in General Surgery 1991;8:478-86.

16.   Manncke K, Raestrup H, Buess G, Becker HD. Technique of endoscopic mediastinal dissection of the esophagus. In:Endosurgery, J Toouli, D Gossot, J.G Hunter, eds, Churchill Livingstone, New-York, USA;285-291,1996.

17.   Bumm R, Holscher AH, Siewert JR. Endoscopic esophagectomy:a better way to atraumatic surgery ? Dig Surg 1993;10:160-3.

18.   Depaula AL, Hashiba K, Ferreira EA, Depaula RA, Grecco E. Laparoscopic transhiatal esophagectomy with esophagogastroplasty. Surg Laparosc Endosc 1995;15:1-5.

19.   Luketich JD, Nguyen NT, Weigel T, Ferson P, Keenan R, Schauer P. Minimally invasive approach to esophagectomy. J Soc Laparoendosc Surg 1998;2:243-7.

20.   Swanstrom LL, Hansen P. Laparoscopic total esophagectomy. Arch Surg 1997;32:943-7.

21.   Yahata H, Sugino K, Takiguchi T, et al. Laparoscopic transhiatal esophagectomy for advanced thoracic esophageal cancer. Surg Laparosc Endosc 1997;7:13-6.

22.   Jagot P, Sauvanet A, Berthoux L, Belghiti J. Laparoscopic mobilization of the stomach for oesophageal replacement. Br J Surg 1996;83:540-2.

23.   Dallemagne B, Weerts JM, Jehaes C. et al. Subtotal oesophagectomy by thoracoscopy and laparoscopy. Min Invas Therap 1992;1:183-5.

24.   Liebermann-Meffert D, Lüscher U, Neff U, Rüedi TP, Allgöwer M. Esophagectomy without thoracotomy:is there a risk of intramediastinal bleeding ? Ann Surg 1987;206:186-92.

25.   Rice TW, Falk GW, Achkar E, Petras RE. Surgical management of high-grade dysplasia in Barrett's esophagus. Am J Gastroenterol 1993;88:1832-6.

26.   Kipfmuller K, Naruhn M, Melzer A, Kessler S, Buess G. Endoscopic microsurgical dissection of the esophagus. Results in an animal model. Surg Endosc 1989;3:63-9.

27.   Bumm R, Feussner H, Bartels H. et al. Radical transhiatal esophagectomy with two-field

lymphadenectomy and endodissection for distal esophageal adenocarcinoma. World J Surg 1997;21:822-31.

28.   Chui PT, Mainland P, Chung SC, Chung DC. Anaesthesia for three-stage thoracoscopic oesophagectomy:an initial experience. Anaesth Intensive Care 1994;2:593-6.

29.   Kawahara K, Maekawa T, Okabayashi K. et al. Video-assisted thoracoscopic esophagectomy for esophageal cancer. Surg Endosc 1999;13:218-23.

30.   Gossot D, Cattan P, Fritsch S, Halimi B, Sarfati E, Celerier M. Can the morbidity of oesophagectomy be reduced by the thoracoscopic approach ? Surg Endosc 1995;9:1113-5.

31.   Robertson GS, Lloyd DM, Wicks AC, Veith PS. No obvious advantages for thoracoscopic two-stage oesophagectomy. Br J Surg 1996;83:675-8.

32.   Müller JM, Erasmi H, Stelzner M, Zieren U, Pichlmayer H. Surgical therapy of oesophageal carcinoma. Br J Surg 1990;77:846-57.

33.   Matthews HR, Powell DJ, Mc Conkey CC. Effect of surgical experience on the results of resection for oesophageal carcinoma. Br J Surg 1986;73:621-3.

34.   Collard JM, Otte JB, Reynaert M, Michel L, Carlier MA, Kestens PJ. Esophageal resection and by-pass:a 6-year experience with a low postoperative mortality. World J Surg 1991;15:635-41.

35.   Shanian DM, Neptune WB, Ellis FH, Watkins E. Transthoracic versus extrathoracic esophagectomy: mortality, morbidity, and long-term survival. Ann Thorac Surg 1986;41:237-46.

36.   Houben JJ. Which approach to the oesophagus ? Third Eurosurgery Meeting, London, U.K, September 1993, Communication.

37.   De Kock M, Pichon G, Scholtes J.L. Intraoperative clonidin enhances postoperative morphine patient-controlled analgesia. Can J Surg 1992;39:537-544.

38.   Takemura M, Higashino M, Osugi H. et al. Changes of serum cytokine levels after thoracoscopic esophagectomy. JPN J Thorac Cardiovasc Surg 1998;46:1305-10.

39.   Collard JM, Tinton N, Malaise J, Romagnoli R, Otte JB, Kestens PJ. Esophageal replacement:gastric tube or whole stomach ? Ann Thorac Surg 1995;60:261-7.

40.   Collard JM, Romagnoli R, Hermans BP, Malaise J. Radical esophageal resection for adenocarcinoma arising in Barrett's esophagus. Am J Surg 1997;174:307-11.

41.   Collard JM, Giuli R. Surgical and multimodal approaches to cancer of the oesophagus:state of the art. Acta Gastroenterol Belg 1999;62:272-82.

41a   Collard JM, Otte JB, Finsse R, et al. Skeletonizing en bloc esophagectomy for cancer. Ann Surg 2000 : in press.

42.   Akiyama H, Tsurumaru M, Udagawa H, Kajiyama Y. Radical lymph node dissection for cancer of the esophagus. Ann Surg 1994;220:364-73.

43.   Dixit AS, Martin CJ, Flynn P. Port-site recurrence after thoracoscopic resection of oesophageal cancer. Aust N Z J Surg 1997;67:148-9.

44.   Segalin A, Bonavina L, Rosati R, Bettazza S. Parietal seeding of esophageal cancer after thoracoscopic resection. Dis Esoph 1994;7:64-5.

45.   Okumura M, Ohshima S, Kotabe Y, Morino H, Kikiu M, Yasumitsu T. Intraoperative pleural lavage cytology in lung cancer patients. Ann Thorac Surg 1991;51:599-604.

46.   Collard JM, Reymond MA. Video-assisted thoracic surgery (VATS) for cancer. Risk of parietal seeding and of early local recurrence. Int Surg 1996;81:343-6.

47.   Anderson JR. Laparoscopic staging of cancer of the esophagus. In:Minimally invasive surgery and new technology, FM Steichen and R Welter, eds. Quality Medical Publishing, St-Louis, USA; 532-7, 1994.

48.   UrscheL JD. Esophagogastric anastomotic leaks:the importance of gastric ischemia and therapeutic applications of gastric conditioning. J Invest Surg 1998;11:245-50.

49.   Nabeya K, Hanaoka T, Onozawa K, Nyumura T, Kimura O, Kaku C. Two-stage esophagogastrostomy for esophageal reconstruction. In:Diseases of the esophagus, malignant diseases, vol. 1, MK Ferguson, AG Little, and DB Skinner, eds. Futura, Mount Kisko, New-York, USA, 247-52, 1990.

50.   Inoue H, Mori M, Li J et al. Human oesophageal carcinomas frequently express the tumor-rejection antigens of MAGE genes. Int J Cancer 1995 ;63 :523-6.

6.5 MANAGEMENT OF POSTOPERATIVE COMPLICATIONS

Vera Rempe-Sorm, Ewout W. Steyerberg and Hugo W. Tilanus

1. INTRODUCTION

Surgery is the only possible curative therapy for esophageal carcinoma. Because 40-45% of the patients show advanced local or systemic disease at first presentation[33], only in about 50-65 % surgery with curative intention can be offered. Even in this selected patient group 5-year-survival rates vary from 10 – 80 %, depending mostly on pathological stage[1].

Esophagectomy with reconstruction once used to be the best palliative treatment to secure food passage, but nowadays non-surgical procedures, such as esophageal stenting[12,26] and brachytherapy[45] have become available and proven to be safe alternatives providing a comparable quality of life. Many authors argue that the goal of surgical treatment of esophageal carcinoma is locoregional control of 'at presentation' metastasized disease, and that this is only justified when morbidity and mortality are kept as low as possible. Regarding the relativity of the better prognosis of the resected patient group, it is important to realize, that the average reported mortality of this elective treatment nowadays varies from 4% in specialized centers to approximately 10% in most series[3,25].

The rate of postoperative morbidity after both curative and palliative surgical treatment for esophageal cancer is substantial[2]. Muller et al. reviewed the literature on surgical therapy of esophageal carcinoma between 1980 and 1988, and concluded that about 56 % of all patients presenting with esophageal carcinoma underwent resection and reconstruction. This treatment leads to an average of 12,5 % hospital mortality and in at least 36 % a complicated postoperative course. Particularly postoperative leakage of the anastomosis (12 %) and pulmonary complications (10 – 27 %) were analyzed, because these complications were related to the operative technique. They concluded from this review that impaired pulmonary function, defined as the existence of pneumonia, respiratory insufficiency or atelectasis, more often happened after transthoracic than after transhiatal resections[2]. A remark to this review is that they evaluated papers only if the majority of

the patients suffered from squamous cell carcinoma rather than adenocarcinoma, because the first type at that time was found to be by far the main malignant pathological entity in the esophagus.

Other authors suggest that transhiatal esophageal resection causes less morbidity and mortality especially for distal carcinomas than the transthoracic resection which should be reserved for more proximally localized, mostly squamous cell carcinomas[13]. Non-randomized studies showed a decrease of mortality[31] and morbidity in patients after transhiatal resection [3,8,10]. In contrast, in a review of Roth and Putnam there was no difference in mortality and morbidity rates between approaches with or without thoracotomy[15]. In a prospective randomized trial about transthoracic versus transhiatal esophagectomy from Goldminc et al.[28] and in a smaller prospective study from Chu et al[47] the results were equal.

Transthoracic esophagectomy (TTE) and transhiatal esophagectomy (THE) are regarded to be different approaches in terms of local radicality and the extent of the lymphadenectomy[44]. An intrathoracic lymph node dissection can only be performed by thoracotomy. A lymph node dissection in the transhiatal resection is only possible in the abdomen but a wide local excision of distal esophageal carcinoma is possible in both forms.

The principle aim of proponents of classical oncological values removal of the tumor as radical as possible to increase survival or the disease-free interval. Especially Japanese surgeons therefore advocate en-bloc resections in squamous cell carcinomas, which by Western surgeons is considered to be associated with high levels of postoperative morbidity[29,35]. Proponents of the transhiatal approach claim a lower incidence of postoperative mortality and morbidity (at least cardiopulmonary) with equal survival figures[8]. Reliable prospective data however are scarce.

The choice of surgical strategy is influenced by the tumor localization, as described by Siewert at al for adenocarcinoma of the esophagogastric junction[13]. They chose to treat distal esophageal carcinomas (usually arising from Barrett's epithelium) (type I)

357

H.W. Tilanus and S.E.A. Attwood (eds.), Barrett's Esophagus, 357–366.
© 2001 *Kluwer Academic Publishers. Printed in the Netherlands.*

TABLE 1. Morbidity and mortality of different surgical approaches for esophagectomy.

First author	Approach	No.pnts	In-hospital-mortality	Postoperative complications (%)				Survival after 5 years of follow up
				Anastomotic leakage	Pulmonary complications	Cardio-vascular complications	Recurrent nerve lesion	
Tilanus 1992[3]	THE vs TTE	152 vs 141	9 vs 5% °	26 vs 16%*	17 vs 34%*	n.m.	16 vs 6% *	25-45 vs 30-40%°
Orringer 1999[8]	THE	1085	4%	13%	2%	n.m.	7%	23%
Millikan 1995[24]	THE vs TTE	67 vs 71	4 vs 13%°	7 vs 4%°	15 vs 34%*	3 vs 4%°	n.m.	21%
Moon 1992[25]	THE vs TTE	63 vs 24	10 %	25 vs 12%*	13 vs 12%°	3 vs 4%°	10 vs12%°	15-86% (early vs advanced)
Fujita 1995[35]	TTE (two-vs three-field)	128 63 vs 65	2 vs 3%	11 vs 33%	57 vs 42%	2%	48 vs 70%	40 vs 36%
Gupta 1996[16]	THE	250	6 %	15%	3%	n.m.	14%	5%
Nishimaki 1998[25]	TTE	190	4,7 %	n.m.	22%	n.m	45%	41%
Kohl 1998[23]	TTE and THE	90	10%	6,7%	28,9%	1,1%	4,4%	n.m.
Karl 2000[17]	TTE	143	2,1 %	3,5%	19%	14%	n.m.	29,6%
Siewert 2000[13]	TTE vs THE	72 vs 315	7 vs 5%	n.m	n.m	n.m	n.m.	32,2% (overall)

THE = transhiatal esophagectomy
TTE = transthoracic esophagectomy   including respiratory distress syndrome, pneumonia, atelectasis, empyema
°= Not significant, * = significant
nm = not mentioned

TABLE 2. Distribution of surgical approaches 1978-2000 EUMCR

Surgical approach	1978-1984	1985-1989	1990-1994	1995-2000	Total
Exploratory laparotomy*	45 (13,7%)	72 (22,5%)	44 (13,4%)	37 (12,3%)	198 (15,5%)
Right dorsolateral thoraco-laparotomy, intrathoracic anastomosis⁺	138 (42,1%)	16 (5%)	7 (2,1)	42 (14,0%)	209 (14,2%)
Right anterolateral thoracotomy, cervical anastomosis	100 (30,5%)	64 (2%)	5 (1,5%)	12 (4,0%)	175 (13,3%)
Transhiatal resection, cervical anastomosis	-	151 (47,1%)	260 (79,3%)	205 (68,1%)	616 (48,2%)
Left thoraco-laparotomy	38 (11,6%)	2 (0,6%)	0	3 (1,0%)	43 (3,4%)
Gastrectomy, distal esophagectomy, esophagojejunostomy	0	10 (3%)	11 (3,4%)	2 (0,7%)	23 (1,8%)
Total	328 (100%)	320 (100%)	328 (100%)	301 (100%)	1277 (100%)

Percentages within period
*Peroperatively irresectable, no resection
⁺Ivor-Lewis
ᵃ No resection, palliative gastric tube bypass

with transthoracic en bloc esophagectomy with resection of the proximal stomach, carcinomas of the true esophagogastric junction (type II) and subcardial gastric carcinomas with proximal infiltration (type III) were preferably approached by extended total gastrectomy with transhiatal resection of the distal esophagus. They found a higher postoperative death rate after (transthoracic) esophagectomy than after total gastrectomy.

A summary of the literature restricted to series with more than 50 patients are shown in table 1.In our clinic, we changed our therapeutic approach of first choice for esophageal carcinoma in 1986 in an attempt to reduce postoperative mortality, which was considered mainly to be due to pulmonary insufficiency or failure of intrathoracic anastomosis. We altered our method from a laparotomy and a right-sided anterolateral thoracotomy with an intrathoracic anastomosis to transhiatal esophagectomy with blunt dissection and cervical anastomosis. The distribution of surgical approaches in our clinic through the years 1978-2000 is shown in table 2.

Nowadays, the incidence of squamous cell carcinoma seems to decrease, whereas the incidence of adenocarcinoma is increasing and has become the greater part of all esophageal cancers[5-7]. Another important issue is, whether careful preoperative selection of patients and assessment of risk factors for the development of postoperative

TABLE 3. Patient characteristics of 1277 esophagectomy procedures for malignancy, per diagnostic period. EMUCR 1978-2000.

Diagnostic period		1978-1984	1985-1989	1990-1994	1995-2000	Total
No. of patients		328	320	328	301	1277
Gender M:V		256:82	223:97	256:72	239:62	1277
Patients per age group	<50	43	34	34	33	144
	50-60	94	96	77	87	354
	60-70	114	108	133	100	455
	70-80	65	74	81	78	298
	>80	12	8	3	3	26
	total	328	320	328	301	1277
Co-morbidity	Cardial	28/325 (8,6%) (4 unknown)	42/320 (13,1%)	41/328 (12,5%)	50/300 (16,7%)	161/1273 (12,6%)
	Pulmonal	51/325 (15,7%) (4 unknown)	34/320 (10,6%)	53/328 (16,2%)	56/300 (18,7%)	195/1273 (15,3%)
	Vascular	16/325 (4,9%) (4 unknown)	11/320 (3,4%)	46/328 (14,0%)	58/300 (19,3%)	131/1273 (10,3%)
	Diabetes	13/325 (4%) (4 unknown)	9/320 (2,8%)	15/328 (4,6%)	21/300 (7%)	58/1273 (4,6%)
	Other malignancy	15/325 (4,6%) (4 unknown)	14/320 (4,4%)	14/328 (4,3%)	31/300 (10,3%)	74/1273 (5,8%)

complications, or even operative risk stratification could decrease the incidence rate of complications by more careful patient selection[4]. Improvements in preoperative selection, anaesthetic and critical care skills, and general supportive measures have reduced mortality and morbidity in esophageal surgery[2]. To define the current problems concerning postoperative complications of esophagectomy, we reviewed our prospectively established patient database as well as the current literature.

2. PATIENTS AND METHODS

Since 1978, 1880 patients with biopsy proven esophageal malignancies have been referred to our clinic. 1277 patients underwent surgery, 657 patients were offered other treatment or palliation. Patient characteristics of the surgery group are given in table 3. We divided the study period 1878-2000 into 4 consecutive periods, to analyze any historical changes in population characteristic or per- and postoperative results. In the consecutive periods comparable numbers of patients were offered surgery with curative intent. Sex ratio did not change significantly throughout the consecutive periods, on average 1 female to 3

male patients. Most patients were between their sixties and seventies, although 11% was younger than 50, and 25 % over 70. Comorbidity defined as preoperative pulmonary or cardiovascular disease, diabetes or a malignancy in the past, varied from 6-21% over the four periods. During the study period, changes regarding the malignant entities could be observed (table 4). As reported by other authors[5-7], in our series a significant shift in incidence of adenocarcinoma was noticed. The proportion of squamous cell carcinoma, that used to be the main malignant pathological entity of the esophagus, decreased with ca. 10 % during the past two decades. In contrast, a proportional raise of the amount of patients with adenocarcinoma of approximately 12 % was seen in the same period.

3. MORTALITY

Historically, esophagectomy has been associated with a high incidence of operative mortality. In the 1980 review from Earlam, concerning more than 80.000 esophagectomies for squamous cell carcinoma, a mortality rate of 29% was found, which made esophagectomy the procedure with the highest mortality risk in

TABLE 4: Shift in pathological entity. Erasmus University Medical Center Rotterdam 1978 - 2000

Period	1978 – 1984	1985 – 1989	1990 – 1994	1995 – 2000
Benign	2,3 %	0,4 %	2,0 %	0,7 %
Squamous cell carcinoma	48,8 %	39,7 %	38,8 %	38,1 %
Adenocarcinoma without Barrett's epithelium	33,6 %	39,7 %	42,0 %	41,8 %
Adenocarcinoma with Barrett's epithelium	7,9 %	11,9 %	11,8 %	12,7 %
Undifferentiated	3,9 %	5,4 %	3,2 %	2,3 %
Other	3,6 %	2,9 %	2,2 %	4,4 %
Total	100 %	100 %	100 %	100 %

TABLE 5. Mortality after esophagectomy for cancer

Authors	Year	Number	Squamous cell vs. Adenocarcinoma	Not-defined postoperative mortality	
				30 days mortality %	In-hospital mortality %
Earlam[10]	1980	Review >80000 patients	Mostly squamous	29 %	
Muller[1]	1990	Review >46000 patients	Squamous	13 %	
Bessel[11]	1996	53	Squamous	9 %	13 %
Tilanus[4]	1992	193	Both	Not given	9%(TTE) and 5%(THE)
Millikan[17]	1995	157	Both +cardia	7,6%	
Wijnhoven[9]	2000	252	Adenocarcinoma	Not given	4%
Gupta[16]	1996	250	Both	6 %	
Law[27]	1992	759	Both (625 vs 134)	4,8 vs 6,5%	16,5 vs 9,8%
Orringer[8]	1999	1085	Both + benign	Not given	4 %
Siewert[13]	2000	387	Esofagogastric junction	6,9 vs 4,8 %	Not given
Present study	2000	1277	Both	5,6 %	9,7%

general surgery at that time[10]. Ten years later, Muller at al. reviewed a similar number of resections of the esophagus and found a mortality rate of 13%[2]. Several authors from high-experienced clinics with large series of esophagectomies both for benign or malignant diseases of the esophagus, have published their mortality numbers in recent years, as summarized in table 5[1,4, 8-11,13,16,17,27]. Between 1987 and 1997, in-hospital mortality after surgery for esophageal cancer was 3,1-3,3 % in our clinic. Mortality numbers in literature are given as different variables; most authors publish them as 30-days-mortality, in-hospital-mortality (defined as the number of patients that died in the same hospital stay as the primary surgical procedure was performed in), or both. We defined mortality numbers as 30-days-mortality and 60-days-mortality and computed mortality rates in our clinic in the review period 1978-2000. 1277 esophagectomies for cancer were performed between 1978-2000; in this period, the total death was 1006 patients. 30-days-mortality was 5,6 % (71 patients), in-hospital-mortality was 9,7 % (124 patients). These numbers are comparable to reported mortality numbers in literature. Roth et al. reviewed several series of patients treated with three different types of resection (with or without thoracotomy) and did not find differences in mortality rates[15]. Bolton et al.[46] suggest that the decrease of operative mortality after esophagectomy in the last decade is correlated with the increased use of transhiatal instead of transthoracic approach. Few analyses concerned the matter of mortality risk factor [4,14]. Evident preoperative risk factors for higher postoperative mortality defined by most authors are age and preoperative pulmonary performance (FEV1/FVC) [4,14]. Other factors, like hypertension, previous cigarette smoking, are also thought to influence postoperative mortality rate[7.] In our series, there was a significant correlation for age and both 30-days- and 60-days-mortality (p=0,001), age and 30-days-mortality (p=0,008), but not for preoperative weight loss, cardiopulmonary diseases, diabetes mellitus or previous malignant diseases.

4. POSTOPERATIVE COMPLI-CATIONS-

The occurrence of postoperative complications was scored and prospectively recorded in a database. In 575 of 1277 patients, who underwent esophagectomy, there was no complication (45%). In 702 patients the postoperative course was in some way complicated (55%). Figure 1 shows the slight decrease in overall complications during the study period: 58,2% in 1978-1984, and 54,5% in 1995-2000, with the greatest decrease in the third period.

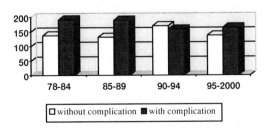

Figure 1. Esophagectomies with and without compli-cations 1978-2000

4.1 SURGERY RELATED COMPLI-CATIONS

We defined 8 postoperative complications as 'surgery related' because of the assumed direct relationship with surgical manipulation and technique. These complications were: hemorrhage requiring re-operation, chylothorax, anastomotic leakage, leakage of the jejunum feeding tube, recurrent nerve palsy, (abdominal or thoracic) wound infection, slow gastric tube passage and necrosis of the gastric tube requiring take-down. In table 6 the frequencies of these complications are summarized.

4.1.1. Hemorrhage
Postoperative bleeding that causes haemodynamic instability is rare and needs reoperation. Vascular tears during so-called 'blunt' dissection can cause mediastinal bleeding. These events are thought to diminish with increasing experience and with better direct vision through the enlarged hiatus[8,41]. In our series, in 48 patients (3%) a re-operation because of bleeding was required to stabilize haemodynamics. Twenty-five patients had a transhiatal resection (52,1%), 23 had a transthoracic procedure (47,9%); there was no significant difference. These numbers were comparable to or less than in the reviewed literature. The rate of this complication decreased significantly during the study period.

4.1.2 Chylothorax
Direct injury to the thoracic duct causes effusion of large amounts of chyle in the pleural cavity leading to respiratory failure and haemodynamic, nutritional and immunologic disturbances. It usually requires ligation via thoracotomy[42,55]. Thirty-eight patients in our series developed chyle leakage from the thorax (3,0%). Twenty of them had transhiatal, 18 transthoracic resection (52,2% vs 47,8%; p>0,05). This complication showed significantly increasing incidence possibly related to the introduction of the 2-field lymph node dissection in thorax and abdomen in a selected group.
Both conservative and intervention management can be considered depending on the overall status of the patient and the produced amount of chyle. In about 50% of the cases conservative measures such as drainage of pleural cavity and parenteral, short-chain fatty acid nutrition, will solve the chyle leakage eventually. Early re-operation in still 'fit' patients with elective ligation of the thoracic duct in the lower thorax imme-

TABLE 6. Surgery-related complications after esophagectomy. EUMCR 1978-2000

Period	Hemorrhage	Chylo-thorax	Anastomotic leakage	Leakage of jejunostomy	Recurrent nerve palsy		Wound infection	Delayed passage	Gastric tube necrosis
					unilateral	bilateral			
1978-1984	14/328 (4,3%)	3/328 (0,9%)	25/328 (7,6%)	6/328 (1,8%)	12/328 (3,7%)	7/328 (2,1%)	14/328 (4,3%)	12/328 (3,7%)	0
1985-1989	14/320 (4,4%)	9/320 (2,8%)	44/320 (13,8%)	0	27/320 (8,4%)	4/320 (1,3%)	7/320 (2,2%)	1/320 (0,3%)	0
1990-1994	13/328 (4,0%)	12/328 (3,7%)	20/328 (6,1%)	0	47/328 (14,3%)	6/328 (1,8%)	1/328 (0,3%)	0	11/328 (3,4%)
1995-2000	7/301 (2,3%)	14/301 (4,7%)	17/301 (5,6%)	2/301 (0,7%)	45/301 (15,0%)	11/301 (3,7%)	6/301 (2,0%)	0	8/301 (2,7%)
Total	48/1277 (3,0%)	38/1277 (3,0%)	106/1277 (8,3%)	8/1277 (0,6%)	131/1277 (10,3%)	28/1277 (2,2%)	28/1277 (2,2%)	13/1277 (1,0%)	19/1277 (1,5%)

diately solves the loss of chyle and is considered to be the most appropriate treatment[56].

4.1.3 Leakage of anastomosis

The clinical relevance of anastomotic leakage is largely dependent on the site of the anastomosis. Leakage of an intrathoracic anastomosis is associated with high morbidity and mortality rate due to mediastinitis and pleural empyema. Leakage of a cervical anastomosis however is, although more common, less fatal and requires in most cases no more than local drainage. The major predisposing factor for impaired healing of the esophagogastric anastomosis is considered to be the compromised blood supply of the proximal end of the gastric tube[21]. Etiologic factors are considered to be venous stasis in the upper part of the stomach, more than one attempt at anastomosis during operation, perioperative hypotension, portal hypertension, preoperative chemoradiotherapy and postoperative distension of the gastric tube. Some authors favor particular suturing techniques to diminish the risk of leakage[51-53]. In our series, overall anastomotic leakage rate was 8,3% (106 patients). 73% of these patients had a cervical anastomosis (n=78), out of a total number of cervical anastomoses of 754 (10,3%). From the 27 patients with leaking intrathoracic anastomosis (out of 523 intrathoracic anastomosis in total), 10 died (37%). Overall incidence of anastomotic leakage was increased in the first years after adopting the transhiatal procedure, but decreased then gradually to a lower level than before (23%-16%). The cervical anastomosis has become more common over the past decades. Avoiding the risk of complications of disruption of an intrathoracic anastomotic, it is thought to decrease the mortality of esophagectomy[8,20]. Detection is often by routine radiographic investigation without clinical symptoms. In clinically manifest cases there may be abscess formation with local inflammation and management usually involves bedside opening and local packing only[22,23]. Some authors report other treatment for cervical anastomotic leaks, such as endoscopic dilatation[30]. When the esophagogastric anastomosis is made within the thorax, leakage is rare, but the collection of leaked substances in the mediastinal compartment leads to a significant morbidity, i.e. mediastinitis or pleural empyema. Intrathoracic leakage therefore is the most serious surgical complication of esophagogastric reconstruction and is responsible for approximately 20 - 60 % of in-hospital mortality[17,18].

Managing intrathoracic leakage just by conservative measures, such as drainage of the empyema and parenteral nutrition or duodenal (tube) enteral feeding is rarely sufficient; only in early detected or mild cases a major mediastinal infection is prevented. Re-operation is clearly indicated for intrathoracic leaks from technical failure without gastric wall necrosis. A simple repair of the anastomosis is seldom possible; usually a takedown of the gastric tube, an esophageal fistula in the neck and closure of the distal end of the gastric tube is performed[17,18]. The chance of survival of the patient depends on the moment of detection, early re-operation, the septic status and response to proper antibiotic regimens.

4.1.4 Leakage of feeding jejunostomy

Routinely, a feeding jejunostomy is placed and feeding is generally started the first postoperative day. Problems with leakage or dislocation are rare: 8 patients (0,6%) in the whole study period.

In principle the jejunostomy is left in situ for at least 6 weeks after discharge, or longer if additional feeding is necessary.

4.1.5 Recurrent nerve paresis

Recurrent nerve paresis leading to vocal cord paralysis is seen especially in patients with cervical anastomosis and after extended lymphadenectomy[31,34,35]. The paresis is often unilateral and transient, but in bilateral and prolonged or persistent palsy it is a significant problem. It causes diminished coughing and hoarseness: pulmonary complications are often associated[34]. In our clinic, vocal cord movement is determined routinely by indirect laryngoscopy both preoperatively and postoperatively. Postoperatively, in 131 patients (10,3%) there was a unilateral recurrent nerve palsy, in 28 patients (2,2%) a bilateral palsy. This complication occurred more frequently later in the study period, conform the adoption of more transhiatal procedures with right cervicotomies (3,7% before, 8-15% in later periods). The incidence of this complication in our series is comparable to or lower than reported in the reviewed literature.

4.1.6 Wound infection

Wound infections after esophagectomy are rare. In 28 patients (2,2%) a superficial wound infection occurred, which could be solved with conservative measures, i.e. superficial opening and drainage. There was a significant decrease in incidence of this complication during the study period: 4,3 % in the first period, 2.0 % in the last.

4.1.7 Delayed passage of gastric tube>10 days

After either curative or palliative resection, recovery of normal oral food intake is an important goal. Delayed gastric emptying can be a significant postoperative problem. The necessity of a pyloric drainage procedure is controversial and possibly related to the diameter of the gastric substitute (i.e. total gastric interposition versus 'narrow' gastric tube[36,37]. In the beginning of the study period, a small percentage of patients (2%) had delayed passage (>10 days) through the gastric tube. This is probably related to the wider diameter of the gastric interposition at that time even after a pyloromyotomy in the

majority of patients. In the second half of the study period this complication did not occur anymore. During this period the gastric tube was reconstructed according to Akiyama with a 4-cm diameter. A pyloromyotomy was no longer performed. Sometimes medication is used to stimulate gastric emptying[32].

4.1.8 Necrosis of the gastric tube

Ischemia of the upper portion of the gastric tube is a risk of the scarce vascularization after mobilizing the stomach[21]. The worst possible result is necrosis of the gastric tip often requiring re-operation with take-down of the gastric tube, temporary cervical esophagostomy, prolonged feeding through the jejunostomy and eventually a reconstruction of the upper alimentary tract with bowel interposition[20].

In the last decade of the study period, 19 patients (1,5%) showed necrosis of the gastric tube. In our series 18 of the 19 patients with gastric tube necrosis had a cervical esophagogastric anastomosis. Seven of 19 patients died one because of non-surgical cause. Hospital stay was significantly prolonged in the survivors group (mean 59, range 17-173).

4.2 NON-SURGICAL COMPLICATIONS

Postoperative complications that typically could not be associated to the surgical technique included pulmonary impairment (pneumonia, atelectasis and ARDS), cardiovascular events (myocardial infarction, thrombo-embolism), sepsis and urinary tract infection.

In 462 patients (36,3%) one ore more of these complications occurred.

Table 7 gives an overview of these complications in our series.

4.2.1 Pulmonary complications

Postoperative pulmonary complications are frequently seen both after transthoracic and transhiatal esophagectomy[25,43,48]. Incidence numbers in literature vary up to 50% depending on the definition of minor and major pulmonary complications[25]. Pulmonary complications in our series are defined as postoperative impairment of pulmonary function requiring therapy such as antibiotics, prolonged mechanical ventilation or bronchoscopy. Pulmonary disease is often preoperatively present in patients requiring esophagectomy, and this has been described as a major predictive factor for postoperative outcome[38,39]. Although still controversial, avoiding thoracotomy in patients with poor

TABLE 7. Not-surgery related complications after esophagectomy. EUMCR 1978-2000

Period	Pneumonia/ atelectasis	ARDS	Myocardial infarction	Thrombosis or embolism	Sepsis	Urinary tract infection
% in 1277 patients	20,3%	5,3%	1,2%	1,6%	3,8%	2,5%

performance status by resecting the esophagus transhiatally, is said to diminish deterioration of (preexistent) pulmonary impairment[2,40].

In our series, where transhiatal esophagectomy was the procedure of first choice since 1986, irrespective of preoperative pulmonary status, pneumonia and atelectasis as revealed on a chest X-ray were more common after transhiatal (42%) than after transthoracic procedures (31%). ARDS requiring prolonged and aggressive mechanical ventilation on the contrary was seen more often after thoracotomy (12 % vs 8%).

Regardless of operative techniques, many authors underline the importance of preoperative assessment and, where possible, preoperative measurements (i.e. stop smoking, physiotherapeutic instructions) to prevent pulmonary complications[8,54].

4.2.2 Cardiovascular complications

Cardiovascular complications in our series defined as myocardial infarction or thromboembolism are rare after esophagectomy; these complications however do contribute to the in-hospital mortality. Several authors have reported among their complications other conditions such as arrhytmias and cardiac failure as well; these events are quite common after thoraco-abdominal surgery and usually respond very well to conservative or pharmacological measurements. In our series 15(1,2%) of the patients suffered from myocardial infarction, 8(0,6%) of them died in the postoperative phase. Thrombo-embolic complications (mostly pulmonary) occurred in 1,6%. In this group one patient died.

4.2.3 Infectious complications

The most serious infectious complication is sepsis, defined as bacteraemia with haemodynamic consequences requiring inotropic cardiovascular support. This is mostly secondary to an earlier complication like anastomotic leakage, pneumonia or abscess. In our series the rate of this complication was 3,8%. In this patient group in-hospital-mortality rate and hospital stay were significantly prolonged.

4.2.4 Benign anastomotic stricture

Dysphagia due to benign strictures of the esophagogastric anastomosis is the most common complication during follow-up, in our series in 23,5%. In the reviewed literature numbers varied from 10-35%. Poor vascularization of the tip of the gastric tube and anastomotic leakage, especially of the cervical anastomosis, are assumed to be the major causes[21,22,50]; the impact of different suturing techniques remain unclear[50,51]. Non-surgical treatment by endoscopic dilatation is thought to be the therapy of choice; even though repeated dilatational sessions are often required, this therapy is tolerated well and complications are scarce[49,50].

5. CONCLUSION

Resection of the esophagus for cancer with reconstruction in one session is a cervical, thoracic and abdominal procedure with significant of postoperative mortality and morbidity. Despite improvements in surgical techniques, anesthesiologic support and postoperative care during the last decades, postoperative course after esophagectomy is still complicated in approximately 50% of the cases.

Postoperative complications should be included in the decision making regarding surgical treatment versus non-surgical treatment and regarding the extent of surgery. Efforts to decrease levels of postoperative complications and deaths after this type of surgery based on pathofysiology, risk factors and management will contribute to the quality of life of the patients and to better survival.

REFERENCES

1. Mannel A, Becker PR. Evaluation of the results of oesophagectomy for oesophageal cancer. Br J Surg 1991;78:36-40.

2. Müller JM, Erasmi H, Stelzner M. Surgical therapy of oesophageal carcinoma. Br J Surg 1990;77:845-57.

3. Tilanus HW, Hop WCJ, Langenhorst BLAM et al. Esophagectomy with or without thoracotomy. Is there any difference? J Thor Cardiovasc Surg, 1993;105(5):898-903.

4. Ferguson MK, Martin TR, Reeder LB. Mortality after esophagectomy: risk factor analysis. World J Surg 1997;21:599-604.

5. Pera M, Cameron AJ, Trastek VF. Increasing incidence of adenocarcinoma of the esophagus and esophagogastric junction. Gastroenterology 1993;104:510-3.

6. Blot WJ,.Devesa SS, Kneller RW et al. Rising incidence of adenocarcinoma of the esophagus and gastric cardia. JAMA 1991;265:1287-9.

7. Reed PI. Changing pattern of oesophageal cancer. Lancet 1991;338:178.

8. Orringer MB, Marshall B, Iannettoni MD. Transhiatal esohagectomy: clinical experience and refinements. Ann Surg 1999; 230(3):392-403.

9. Wijnhoven BPI, Siersema PD, Hop WCJ et al. Adenocarcinoma of the distal oesophagus and gastric cardia are one clinical entity. Br J Surg 2000;86(4):529-35.

10. Earlam R, Cunha-Melo JP. Oesophageal squamous cell carcinoma: a critical review of surgery. Br J Surg 1080;67:382-90.

11. Bessel JR, Devitt PG, Gill PG, Goyal S, Jamieson GG. Prolonged survival follows resection of oesophageal squamous cell carcinoma downstaged by prior chemoradiotherapy. Aust NZ J Surg 1996;66:214-7.

12. Siersema PD, Hop WC, Dees J, Tilanus HW, van Blankenstein M. Coated self-expanding metal stents versus latex prostheses for esophagogastric cancer with special reference to prior radiation and chemotherapy: a controlled, prospective study. Gastroint Endosc 1998;47(2):113-20.

13. Siewert JR, Feith M, Werner M, Stein HJ.Adenocarcinoma of the esophagogastric junction. Results of surgical therapy based on anatomical/topographic classification in 1002 consecutive patients. Ann Surg 2000;232(3):353-361.

14. Liu JF, Watson DI, Devitt PG, Mathew G, Myburgh J, Jamieson GG. Risk factor analysis of post-operative mortality in oesophagectomy. Dis Esophagus 2000;13:130-5.

15. Roth JA, Putnam JB. Surgery for cancer of the oesofagus. Sem Oncology 1994;21(4):453-61.

16. Gupta NM. Oesophagectomy without thoracotomy:first 250 patients. Eur J Sur 1996;162(6):455-61.

17. Karl RC, Schreiber R, Boulware D. Factors affecting morbidity, mortality, and survival in patients undergoing Ivor Lewis esophagogastrectomy. Annals of Surgery 2000;231(5):635-43.

18. Agrawal S, Deshmukh SP, Patil PK. J Surgical Onc.1996;63(1):52-6.

19. Murakami M, Sugiyama A, Ikegami T. Revascularization using the short gastric vessels of the gastric tube after subtotal oesophagectomy for intrathoracic esophageal carcinoma. J Am Coll Surg 2000;190(1):71-7.

20. Iannetoni M, Whyte R, Orringer M. Catastrophic complications of the cervical esophagogastric anastomosis. J of Thor Cardiovasc Surg 1995;110(5):1493-1500.

21. Pierie JP, De Graaf PW, Poen H et al. Impaired healing of cervical oesophagogastrostomies can be predicted by estimation of gastric serosal blood perfusion by laser Doppler flowmetry. Eur J Surg 1994;160(11);599-630.

22. Lam TC, Fok M, Cheng SW et al. Anastomotic complications after esophagectomy for cancer: a comparison of neck and chest anastomoses. J Thor Cardiovasc Surg 1992;104:395-400.

23. Kohl P, Honore P, Gielen JL, Azzam C, Legrand M, Jacquet N. Surgery of esophageal cancer in Liege. Rev Med Liege 1998;53(4):187-92.

24. Millikan KW, Silverstein J, Hart V, Blair K, Bines S, Roberts J, Dolas A. A 15-year review of esophagectomy for carcinoma of the esophagus and cardia. Arch Surg 1995;130:617-24.

25. Katariya K, Harvey JC, Pina E, Beattie EJ. Complications of transhiatal esophagectomy. J Surg Onc 1994;17:157-63.

26. Lambert R. Treatment of esophagogastric tumors. Endoscopy 2000;32(4):322-30.

27. Law SY, Fok M, Cheng SW, Wong J. A comparison of outcome after resection for squamous cell carcinomas and adenocarcinomas of the esophagus and cardia. Surg Gyn Obst 1992;175(2): 107-12.

28. Goldminc M, Maddern G, Le Prise E, Meunier B, Campion JP, Launois B. Oesophagectomy by a transhiatal approach or thoracotomy, a prospective randomized trial. Br J Surg 1993;80(3): 367-70.

29. Akiyama H, Tsurumaru M, Kawamura T, Ono Y. Principles of Surgical treatment for carcinoma of the esophagus. Ann Surg 1981;194(4):438-45.

30. Basin DK, Sharma BC, Gupta, NM, Sinha SK, Singh K. Endoscopic dilatation for treatment of anastomotic leaks following transhiatal esophagectomy. Endoscopy 2000 Jun; 32(6): 469-71.

31. Rindani R, Martin CJ, Cox MR. Transhiatal versus Ivor-Lewis oesophagectomy; is there a difference? Austr N Z J Surg 1999;69(3):187-94.

32. Burt M, Scott A, Williard WC, Pommier R, Yeh S, Bains MS, Turnbull AD, Fortner JG, McCormack PM, Ginsberg RJ. Erythromycin stimulates gastric emptying after esophagectomy with gastric replacement: a randomized clinical trial. J Thor Cardiovasc Surg 1996;111(3):649-54.

33. Quint LE, Hepburn LM, Francis IR, Whyte RI, Orringer MB. Incidence and distribution of distant metastases from newly diagnosed esophageal carcinoma. Cancer 1995;576(7);1120-5.

34. Hulscher JBF, van Sandick JW, Devriese PP, van Lanschot JJB, Obertop H. Vocal cord paralysis after subtotal oesophagectomy. Br J Surg 1999; 86:1583-6.

35. Fujita H, Kakegawa T, Yamana H, Shima I, Toh Y, Tomita Y, Fujii T, Yamasaki K, Higaki K, Noake T, Ishibashi N, Mizutani K. Mortality and morbidity rates postoperative course, quality of life and proganosis after extended radical lymphadenectomy for esophageal cancer. Ann Surg 1995;222(5):654-62.

36. Gupta S, Chattopadhyay TK, Gopinath OG, Kapoor VK, Sharma LK. Emptying of the intrathoracic stomach with and without pyloroplasty. Am J Gastroenterology 1998;84(8): 921-3.

37. Fok M, Cheng SW, Wong J. Pyloroplasty vs no drainage in gastric replacement of the esophagus. Am J Surg 1991;162(5):447-52.

38. Marmuse JP, Maillochaud JH. Respiratory morbidity and mortality following transhiatal esophagectomy in patients with severe chronic obstructive pulmonary disease. Ann Chir 1999; 53(1):23-8.

39. Kuwano H, Sumiyoshi K, Sonoda D. Relationship between preoperative assessment of organ function and postoperative morbidity in patients with esophageal cancer. Eur J Surg 1998 Aug; 164(8): 581-586

40. Patti MG, Wiener JP, Way LW, Pellegrini CA. Impact of transhiatal esophagectomy on cardiac and respiratory function. Am J Surg. 1991 December, 162:563-566.

41. Matory YL, Burt M. Esophagogastrectomy: reoperation for complications. J Surg Onc. 1993 Sept; 54(1): 29-33.

42. Orringer MB, Bluett M, Deeb GM. Aggressive treatment of chylothorax complicating transhiatal esophagectomy without thoracotomy. Surgery 1988; 104:720-726.

43. Gandhi SK, Naunheim KS. Complications of transhiatal esophagectomy. Chest Surg Clin North Am 1997 Aug; 7(3): 601:610.

44. DeMeester TR. Esophageal Carcinoma: Current controversies. Sem Surg Onc 1997; 13:217-233.

45. Siersema PD, van Lanschot JJ, Fockens P, Tilanus HW. Gastrointestinal surgery and Gastroenterology. III. Diagnosis and treatment of esophageal carcinoma. Nederlands Tijdschrift voor Geneeskunde 1999 Sept 25; 143(39): 1947-1952.

46. Bolton JS, Ochsner JL, Abdoh AA. Surgical management of esophageal cancer. A decade of change. Ann Surg 1994 May; 219(5): 475-480.

47. Chu KM, Law SY, Fok M, Wong J. A preospective randomized comparison of transhiatal and transthoracic resection for lower-third esophageal carcinoma. Am J Surg 1997 Sept; 174(3): 320-4.

48. Jacobi CA, Zieren HU, Muller JM, Pichlmaier H. Surgical therapy of esophageal carcinoma: the influence of surgical approach and esophageal resection on cardiopulmonary function. Eur J Cardiothor Surg 1997 Jan; 11(1): 32-7.

49. Pierie JPEN, de Graaf PW, Poęn H, van der Tweel I, Obertop H. Incidence and management of benign anastomotic stricture after cervical oesophagogastrostomy. Br J Surg. 1993 Apr; 80; 471-4.

50. Honkoop P, Siersema PD, Tilanus HW, Stassen LP, Hop WC, van Blankenstein M. Benign anastomotic strictures after transhiatal esophagectomy and cervical esophagogastrostomy; risk factors and management. J Thor Cardiovasc Surg 1996 Jun; 111(6): 1141-6.

51. Bardini R, Bonavina L, Asolati M, Ruol A, Castoto C, Tiso E. Single-layered cervical esophageal anastomosis: a prospective study of two suturing techniques. Ann Thor Surg 1994; 58:1087-90.

52. Orringer MB, Marshall B, Iannettoni MD. Eliminating the cervical esophagogastric anastomotic leak with a side-to-side stapled anastomosis. J Thor Cardiovasc Surg 2000;119(2): 277-88.

53. Bisgaard T, Wojdemann M, Larsen H, Heindorff H, Gustafsen J, Svendsen LB. Double-stapled esophagogastric anastomosis for resection of esophagogastric or cardia cancer: a new application for an old technique. J Laparoendosc Adv Surg Techn 1999; 9(4): 335-9.

54. Gillinov AM, Heitmiller RF. Strategies to reduce pulmonary complications after transhiatal esophagectomy. Dis Es 1998;11:32-47.

55. Detry O, DeKoster G, Limet R. Le chylothorax et son traitement. Lyon Chir 1994;90(1):38-44.

56. Merrigan BA, Winter DC, O'Sullivan GG. Chylothorax. Br J Surg 1997;84:15-20.

6.6 MULTIMODALITY IN THE MANAGEMENT OF ADENOCARCINOMA OF THE ESOPHAGUS

Albert S. DeNittis, Richard Whittington and Lawrence Coia

1. BACKGROUND

Prior to 1980, due to the relatively low incidence of adenocarcinoma of the esophagus and the use of surgery as the primary modality of treatment, information regarding the efficacy of radiation in esophageal adenocarcinoma was limited. Reports in the literature as early as 1948, distinguish adenocarcinoma of the esophagus as a separate entity from the more commonly seen squamous cell carcinoma. A total of 18 cases of esophageal adenocarcinoma were reported in the literature pre-1980, which involved the use of radiation therapy (4 of which were treated preoperatively and 14 treated with radiotherapy alone). These earlier reports largely failed to report on the treatment schema or type of radiation used.

Many similarities as well as a few differences in the natural history of adenocarcinoma and squamous cell carcinoma have been demonstrated[1]. Both tumors are usually advanced at the time of presentation. Often the tumor penetrates the esophageal wall and invades regional lymph nodes. In addition, both tumors have a propensity for distant failure, including primarily lung, bone, pleura and liver. Adenocarcinoma has a slightly higher incidence of peritoneal seeding and brain metastases than squamous cell carcinoma[1]. Since the behavior of adenocarcinoma is relatively similar to that of esophageal squamous cell carcinoma, our management of adenocarcinoma has often been extrapolated from the treatment of squamous cell carcinoma. Unfortunately, the results of some studies are not reported by analyzing patients with squamous cell carcinoma separately from those with adenocarcinoma. Some prospective randomized studies have included patients with tumors of either histologic subtype but may have insufficient numbers of patients with adenocarcinoma to draw definitive conclusions regarding that entity. Thus optimal management and development of standards of care for adenocarcinoma of the esophagus is in evolution. This chapter will review the use of radiation as a component of either curative or palliative treatment of adenocarcinoma of the esophagus.

Moreover, ongoing trials and developing treatments will be addressed.

Initial case reports in the early 1950's published by Morson[2] and Allison[3] had found a variability in the location of esophageal adenocarcinoma, in that, patients presented with cancer in the cervical, thoracic, and distal esophagus. Interestingly, distal adenocarcinoma was often found in association with hiatal hernia. Several factors were determined to be potentially associated with the development of esophageal adenocarcinoma[4]. First, adenocarcinoma was shown to occur in areas where there are superficial and deep esophageal glands. Secondly, prominent foci of ectopic gastric mucosa erroneously left behind during embrylogic development were thought be a precursor of adenocarcinoma. And lastly, glandular metaplasia secondary to infection was also speculated as a causal factor.

Smithers in 1956, was the first to report both the incidence relative to squamous cell cancer and radiation response. Three hundred forty three patients seen at the Royal Marsden Hospital from 1936-1951 were diagnosed with carcinoma of the esophagus. Of the 343 patients, 26 or 8% had adenocarcinoma. Twenty-three of 26 patients did not have an association with a hiatal hernia. Two patients with adenocarcinoma were treated with radiotherapy preoperatively. The first patient had a 7-centimeter lesion of the lower third of the esophagus treated to unspecified dose in July of 1945. In December 1945 the patient underwent an esophagectomy because of stricture formation. Pathologic examination of the surgical specimen revealed no residual tumor. The second patient was treated in 1955 for an adenocarcinoma of the middle esophagus with 2 MeV x-rays to an unspecified dose. Esophagectomy in January 1956 showed no evidence of tumor.

In 1966, Raphael et al,[5] retrospectively reviewed 1,312 patients evaluated for surgical treatment with esophageal cancer at the Mayo Clinic from 1946-1963 and found 44 (3.3%) had primary adenocarcinoma. The reported incidence decreased from 3.3% to 0.76% when patients

H.W. Tilanus and S.E.A. Attwood (eds.), Barrett's Esophagus, 367–376.

with squamous cell carcinoma of the esophagus or primary gastric cancer were excluded.

Furthermore, a report by Turnbull and Goodner[6] from Memorial Sloan Kettering Cancer Center found 45 out of 1859 patients (2.4%) were diagnosed with adenocarcinoma. Of the 45 patients 33 were evaluable for outcome, 14 patients were treated with primary radiotherapy. Doses ranged from 2600-14,400 rad and toxicity was not reported. The radiotherapy patients were compared to a surgical group, and a group who received nothing but best supportive care (BSC). The average survival was 23.8 months, 12.5 months, and 5.2 months with surgery, radiotherapy and BSC respectively. The 5-year survival was 2.2%. Median survival for the patients with lower esophageal adenocarcinoma, was double that of patients with adenocarcinoma of the upper esophagus. The authors also reported a similar clinical course and outcome for epidermoid and adenocarcinoma in terms of patterns of failure and survival.

Jernstrom and Brewer[7] were the first to report on the use of preoperative radiotherapy (3000 rad) for the treatment of a patient with primary adenocarcinoma of the mid esophagus which had been related to hiatal hernia and reflux esophagitis. The patient expired in 4 months secondary to brain metastases.

Shafer[8] suggested that the columnar epithelium of the lower esophagus is a condition resulting from a protective response of the esophageal mucosa to repeated irritation from gastric acid. Furthermore, Bremner[9] seemed to make a convincing argument that chronic irritation of the distal esophagus with gastric acid was responsible for the formation of adenocarcinoma. A case report by Danoff[10] in 1978 demonstrated evidence for the radiosensitivity of adenocarcinoma of the esophagus. Repeat esophagrams showed tumor regression after treatment with radiation therapy.

2. CURATIVE TREATMENT

There are at present multiple potentially curative options for patients with esophageal adenocarcinoma. These include surgery alone, surgery plus pre or postoperative radiation therapy adjuvant therapy or chemoradiation alone. Surgery alone has been the mainstay of curative treatment however recent data has challenged this school of thought.

Comparisons of primary surgical versus chemoradiation approaches are difficult due to an absence of randomized studies and patient selection biases along with other factors. For instance patients with poor prognostic features (medically inoperable, locally unresectable disease or the presence of metastases) are often selected for nonsurgical therapies. Staging is not readily compared between patients treated surgically versus nonsurgically. Furthermore, there are several methods for esophagectomy and a variety of dose, fractionation and chemotherapy regimens used in chemoradiation approaches.

2.1 SURGERY AS PRIMARY TREATMENT

Surgery has been the standard treatment for esophageal carcinoma. Unfortunately most of the large series reporting on surgery alone have demonstrated poor overall survival. The two largest series quote a five year survival of 12-27%[11,12] and these studies have involved patients with squamous cell carcinoma with a median survival of 12 months. There are several randomized trials which report results of surgery alone arms[13-16]. The results of these trials can be seen in table 1. Three trials do include patients with adenocarcinoma [14-16]. The studies by Walsh et al, in which all patients had adenocarcinoma and Urba et al., in which 75% of patients had adenocarcinoma report 6% and 15% 3 year survival in the surgery alone arm respectively. In a recent study in which 55% of patients had adenocarcinoma, Kelsen et al report a 37% 2-year survival in the surgery alone arm but, there is high local failure. These results are quite similar to the results of the large surgical trials. However, poor patient outcome with surgery alone has led to the development of alternative primary treatment or adjuvant therapy in conjunction with surgery (Table 1).

2.2 PREOPERATIVE RADIATION THERAPY

The use of preoperative radiation therapy has theoretically potential biologic and physical advantages in the treatment of cancer. These include an increased tumor radioresponsiveness secondary to heightened tumor oxygenation and a decreased likelihood of dissemination at the time of surgery. The physical factors include an increased resectability and the ability to deliver higher doses of radiation preoperatively than postoperatively. There is only one reported randomized trial of preoperative radiation compared to surgery alone in the literature to date that includes patients with adenocarcinoma

TABLE 1. Comparison of Surgical Arms

Author	Year	Patients (total)	Patients (surgical)	Histology (% adenoca.)	Med.Surv. (months)	2 year Survival	3 year Survival
Walsh[14]	1996	110	55	100	11	26	6
Urba[15]	1997	100	50	74	18	N/A	15
Kelsen [16]	1998	221	103	55	16	37	N/A

and squamous cell carcinoma. Arnott et al[17] reported on 176 patients, 86 patients were treated with esophagectomy alone versus 90 patients who treated with preoperative radiation therapy. Adenocarcinoma comprised 65% of the overall patient population. Preoperative radiotherapy was administered by opposed fields using 4 MV photons. The superior margin included the suprasternal notch and the inferior margin included the cardia and fundus of the stomach. Total dose was only 2000 cGy at 200 cGy fraction. Resectability and local failure were not reported. This preoperative low dose radiation did not demonstrate a benefit in 5 year overall survival (17% vs 9% p=0.4) with surgery and preoperative radiation respectively. Analysis of survival by tumor histology did not demonstrate a difference between squamous cell or adenocarcinoma. Also in those patients with adenocarcinoma there was no benefit to preoperative radiation.

2.3. POSTOPERATIVE RADIATION

Accuracy in tumor staging and surgical accuracy in tumor location are potential advantages of surgery followed by postoperative radiation therapy rather than radiation preoperatively. This allows the radiation oncologist to treat areas at risk for recurrence while sparing otherwise normal radiosensitive structures and decreasing toxicity. In addition patients with pathologic stage T1-T2N0M0 or metastatic disease can be eliminated from treatment. As stated previously, the disadvantage of postoperative radiation is the limited tolerance of tissues after gastric pull up or intestinal interposition. Fok et al[18] reported on the results of 130 patients treated with postoperative radiation versus surgery alone for either adenocarcinoma (104 patients) or squamous cell carcinoma (26 patients). It should be noted that patients who underwent either curative and palliative resections were included in this trial. Radiation therapy was delivered to a total dose of 4900 cGy with 350 cGy fraction.

The dose fraction size is higher than generally used. The authors stated that this dose fraction was used due to heavy demand on treatment facilities. For patients who had undergone curative resection (all gross disease removed with negative margins) there was no difference in local control or median survival for postoperative radiation. In patients who had undergone a palliative resection, local failure was decreased from 46% to 20%, but there was no difference in median survival with postoperative radiation. In addition, there was a 7 fold increase in gastric toxicity with the use of postoperative radiation therapy. In subgroup analysis, patients with adenocarcinoma had showed no difference in survival with or without the use of radiotherapy (median survival 9.5 and 13.6 months, respectively; p=0.31). In summary, there is no evidence that postoperative radiation therapy improves survival, however, it is likely that it decreases local recurrence.

2.4. POSTOPERATIVE CHEMORADIATION

Whittington et al[19] performed a retrospective review of 165 patients with localized adenocarcinoma of the esophagus and gastroesophageal junction from 1972-1989. Optimum treatment regimens and their effect on local recurrence, median survival, and 2 year survival were analyzed. In table 2 the data shows that local recurrence had decreased from 71% for surgery alone and 100% for chemotherapy alone or radiation alone, to 48% for chemoradiation and to 15% for combined modality treatment consisting of surgery and postoperative chemoradiation. Median survival and 2 year survival were also improved with trimodality therapy. Aggressive use of combined modality therapy including surgery, chemotherapy and radiation therapy appears to produce an improved outcome. This study provides a basis for a change in philosophy toward a more aggressive approach for patients with adenocarcinoma of the esophagus.

TABLE 2. Different therapies and their outcome

Modality	N	Median survival	Local relapse (%)	2 year survival (%)
Surgery	50	15	71	31
XRT	25	5	100	5
CT	8		100	0
Chemo/XRT	26	10	48	15
Surgery + XRT	19	***	24	50
Surgery + CT	9	***	33	50
Surgery + CT/XRT	28	21	15	55

*** did not improve survival compared to surgery alone but superior to chemo/XRT

2.5. PREOPERATIVE CHEMORADIATION - NONRANDOMIZED TRIALS

There are several nonrandomized trials, which discuss the use of neoadjuvant or adjuvant chemoradiation (concurrent chemotherapy and radiation therapy). Early studies from Wayne State indicated promising results with preoperative chemoradiation for patients with squamous cell carcinoma. Forastiere et al from the University of Michigan[20] reported the use of preoperative chemoradiation in 43 patients with either histology. In that study 21 patients had adenocarcinoma and 22 had squamous cell carcinoma of the esophagus. Chemotherapy consisted of Cisplatin as a continuous 4 day IV infusion on days 1 and 17, with 5-FU added as a continuous infusion on days 1 to 21, and vinblastine given as IV bolus on days 1-4 and 17-20. Radiation therapy was delivered concurrently and consisted of 250 cGy for 5 days per week to 3750 cGy. Treatment was changed to 150 cGy twice a day to a total of 4500 cGy in an attempt to enhance the response rate. Transhiatal esophagectomy was performed 21 days after the completion of radiation and chemotherapy. Forty-one patients underwent resection. Median follow up was 29 months, 36 patients had a potentially curable resection. Patients who underwent a curable resection, 3 year survival rates were 36% and 43% for adenocarcinoma and squamous cell carcinoma respectively (p=0.589). Patients who had a complete pathologic response had a median survival duration of 70 months and 60% were alive at 5 years. Toxicity included severe leukopenia and was the chemotherapy dose limiting factor. The mean doses of chemotherapy achieved were 84% for all drugs. Kavanagh et al[20] reported the experience from Duke of 103 eligible patients receiving preoperative chemoradiation followed by surgery. A more conventional treatment regimen

was given consisting of 4500 cGy over 5 weeks given concurrently with 5-FU 1000 mg/m2/day x 4 days and Cisplatin 20 mg/m2/day x 5 days on weeks 1 and 5. The 26 patients with adenocarcinoma are reported together with 77 patients with squamous cell carcinoma treated with a different chemotherapy regimen so it is not possible to determine toxicity and patterns of failure of patients with adenocarcinoma. The median survival for patients with adenocarcinoma was 19 months and the 3-year survival was 27%. Forastiere et al[22], subsequently at Johns Hopkins Hospital, reported the use of a less intensive preoperative chemoradiation program than that used at the University of Michigan involving 45 patients. Adenocarcinoma was diagnosed in 31 patients and squamous cell in 12 patients. The study attempted to decrease toxicity and allow outpatient treatment. Chemotherapy consisted of a 4-week regimen of high dose infusional 5-FU 300 mg/m2/day days 1-30, infusional Cisplatin 26 mg/m2/day, days 1-5 and 26-30 and concurrent radiotherapy. Radiation consisted was delivered to a total dose of 4400 cGy at 200 cGy per day. Transhiatal esophagectomy was performed on week 8. There was a 42% complete response rate and an estimated 2-year survival of 56%. A study by Urba et.al[23] enrolled 24 patients diagnosed with localized esophageal adenocarcinoma were treated with 5-FU 300mg/m2/day continuous infusion for 96 hours and radiation therapy to 4900 cGy administered in 350 cGy per day, followed by transhiatal esophagectomy. Toxicity from this regimen was high and consisted of an extraordinarily large number of pericardial and pleural effusions (11/24 patients) with no survival benefit. The conclusion from this study was that this preoperative treatment regimen with large fraction size was too toxic and should be abandoned. The Trans Tasman Radiation Oncology Group (TROG)[24] published a study in

1996, to clarify the role of the management of esophageal carcinoma. Three hundred seventy three patients were analyzed treated on 3 prospective but nonrandomized protocols. The first protocol treated 92 patients preoperatively with 3500 cGy over 3 weeks and infusion 5 FU 500 mg/m2/day on days 1-5 and 28-33 and Cisplatin 80 mg/m2 on days 5 and 33. The chemotherapy was adjusted by deleting the second cycle of 5-FU and increasing the dose of 5-FU to 800mg/m2/day infused over days 1-4. The second protocol treated 57 patients definitively with chemoradiation. Six thousand cGy was delivered with two courses of the same chemotherapy as in protocol I. The third protocol treated 112 patients and consisted of the same regimen as in protocol II, but was delivered palliatively (patients with systemic metastases or poor performance status). In the preoperative study 45% had adenocarcinoma, 63% had squamous cell carcinoma. In the definitive study 20% had adenocarcinoma, 78% had squamous cell carcinoma, and in the palliative study 33% had adenocarcinoma, 60% had squamous cell carcinoma. The TROG had used a proportional hazard model to assess the importance of independent potential prognostic variables. The results of this study had demonstrated that for patients with adenocarcinoma, the type of treatment delivered determined patterns of local and systemic relapse. Of note, the cumulative incidence of local and systemic relapse were lower in patients with upper third tumors, regardless of modality, when compared to patients with lower third tumors. Patients in the definitive study had a lower systemic relapse at 3 years (30%) then those patients in the surgical study (50%). In palliatively treated patients, those with systemic metastases or poor performance status at presentation had a median survival of 4 months versus a median survival of slightly greater than a year in patients with good performance status or M0 disease. The authors concluded that concurrent chemoradiotherapy protocols might improve outcome in patients with good performance status.

Keller et al[25] report results of an eastern cooperative oncology group (ECOG) phase II study utilizing high dose chemoradiotherapy followed by esophagectomy for patients with stage I and II adenocarcinoma of the esophagus or gastroesophageal junction. Forty-six patients were accrued from 21 institutions with biopsy proven adenocarcinoma. Eight patients were stage I and 28 were stage II. External beam irradiation was delivered with megavoltage radiation and were treated 5 days/week at 200 cGy per day. Total dose was 6000 cGy. Within 24 hours after the start of radiation therapy chemotherapy was administered. 5-FU was infused continuously at 1000 mg/m2/day on days 2-5 and 28-31. On day 2 a 10 mg/m2 bolus of Mitomycin was injected intravenously. Esophagectomy was performed within 4-8 weeks after the completion of radiation therapy if the patient was medically fit or no evidence of metastatic disease was found. Eighteen patients achieved a complete response, 11 patients had a partial response, 8 patients had stable disease and 10 patients progressed. Esophagectomy was performed in 33 patients and 8 had a pathologic CR. Overall median survival was 16.6 months, 1-year survival was 57% and 2-year survival was 27%. Patients with a clinical complete response had a superior survival to those without a clinical complete response. Interestingly there was no difference in survival between patients with or without a pathologic complete response. Univariate analysis had demonstrated circumferential tumor growth as a prognostic variable (median 18.1 months versus 8.3 months; $p < 0.05$). In addition, there were 8 treatment related deaths related to therapy. The authors concluded that the treatment related morbidity and mortality was excessive in the cooperative group setting.

2.6. PREOPERATIVE CHEMORADIATION – RANDOMIZED TRIALS

Walsh et al[14] in the first randomized study compared surgery with preoperative Cisplatin, 5-FU, and concurrent radiation followed by surgery in 110 patients with adenocarcinoma of the esophagus. There were 55 patients assigned to multimodality therapy, and they received two courses of chemotherapy in weeks 1 and 6. Chemotherapy consisted of 5-FU 15 mg per kg of body weight daily for 5 days, and Cisplatin 75 mg per square meter of body area on day seven. Radiotherapy was given concurrently with the first course of chemotherapy. Patients were treated AP/PA (3 field in '94) to a total dose of 4000 cGy in 15 fractions. Surgery was performed using 5 separate approaches. Median survival was 16 months with preoperative chemoradiation compared to 11 months for the patients treated with surgery alone (p=01). The 1, 2, and 3 year survival rates were 52%, 37%, and 32% respectively for patients who received multimodality therapy and 44%, 26%, and 6%

for those patients assigned to surgery. The results were significant at 3 years (p=01).

A recent abstract by Urba et al[15] reported on 100 patients with resectable esophageal cancer randomized to receive preoperative chemoradiation followed by surgery versus surgery alone. Seventy five percent of the patients had adenocarcinoma and 25% of the patients had squamous cell carcinoma. Chemotherapy consisted of Cisplatin 20 mg/m2 on days 1-5 and 17-21, 5-FU 300 mg/m2 day 1-21, and vinblastine 1 mg/m2 day 1-4 and 17-20. Radiation was delivered 150 cGy BID for 3 weeks to a total dose of 4500 cGy. Surgery was performed on day 42. Tumors > 5 cm, age > 70, and squamous cell histology were associated with shorter survival. Three year survival was 15% in the surgery alone arm versus 32% in the combined modality arm (p=0.073). A review of the data at a median follow-up of 3.78 years shows a trend for survival advantage for the patients who received the chemoradiation and surgery.

2.7 CHEMORADIATION AS PRIMARY TREATMENT

The Fox Chase Cancer Center/University of Pennsylvania reported on a Phase II study in which 90 patients (57 stage I or II, 33 stage III or IV) with esophageal cancer had received primary chemotherapy and radiotherapy concurrently.[26,27] Treatment for patients with stage I and II disease received definitive radiation consisting of 60 Gy in 6 to 7 weeks with two 96 hour infusions of 5-FU (1 gm/m^2 on days 2 to 5, 29-32) and bolus Mitomycin C (10 mg/m2 on day 2). Patients with stage III and IV disease received palliative treatment of 50 Gy plus the same chemotherapy. Staging was based on clinical findings according to the 1978 AJC system. Ninety percent of all 90 patients had improvement in dysphasia with a median time of less than 2 weeks. The local relapse-free rate for patients with stage I and II disease was 73% at 12 months and 60% at three years. For stage I patients the local relapse-free rate was significantly better with a 3 year actuarial rate of 76% versus a rate of 55% for patients with stage II disease. The overall median survival was 18 months, and a 3 and 5 year survival of 29% and 18% respectively, for stage I and II patients. The actuarial cause specific survival for 3 and 5 years was 41% and 30% respectively. No difference was seen in overall and cause specific survival for patients with adenocarcinoma. More than two third of

the patients with a survival of greater than 1 year could tolerate at least a soft diet.

The use of radiotherapy alone demonstrates a predominant local failure pattern, however with the use of chemosensitized radiation, a predominant pattern of distant failure over local failure can be seen. This study found a local failure of 25% and a distant failure in 37% of patients. Patients with adenocarcinoma had a 35% local failure rate while patients with squamous cell carcinoma had a 22% local failure. Recurrent disease was seen in 29 patients. In these patients the median time to local failure was 7 months and the median time to distant failure was 10 months. Eighty percent of all failures occurred in 1 year. It is worthwhile to note that for patients who had recurrent disease 72% had distant failure as a component of failure.

Severe acute toxicity mainly in the form of esophagitis was seen in 11 (12%) of patients. Twenty patients needed a treatment break for 3 to 5 days. Three percent of patients required hospitalization secondary to treatment. They received fluids and parenteral nutrition for acute esophagitis.

Algan et al[28] in a Phase II study compared results of 35 patients with stage I or II potentially resectable adenocarcinoma of the esophagus treated with chemoradiation alone or chemoradiation followed by esophagectomy. Between 1981 and 1992, 11 patients were treated with radiation to 60 Gy with concurrent infusional 5-FU (1000 mg/m2/24 hours given over 96 hours starting day 2 and 29 and Mitomycin-C (10 mg/m^2) administered as a single bolus injection on day 2 alone) and 24 patients received the same chemoradiation plus planned esophagectomy. No difference was noted in median (19 months versus 15 months) or 3-year survival (36% versus 28%) for patients treated with chemoradiation versus chemoradiation and esophagectomy. Disease free survival (DFS) however was better for patients who received planned esophagectomy. At 3 years the DFS was 21% for chemoradiation and 42% for patients who had undergone the added esophagectomy. Forty-three percent of patients had acute toxicity while late toxicity was the same for both groups secondary to chemoradiation. There were added treatment related morbidity and death related to the surgery itself, including pneumonia, decreased wound healing and ARDS.

Interestingly 33% of patients undergoing surgery after chemoradiation had no evidence of

TABLE 3. Combined radiation therapy and chemotherapy

Author	Year	no. of patients	2 year survival	3 year survival	5 year survival	Median survival
Coia[27]	1991	90	NA	29%	18%	18 mo.
Algan[28]	1995	11	NA	28%	NA	15 mo.
Al-Sarraf [29,30]	1997	129	38%	NA	27%	12.5 mo.

malignancy in the surgical specimen and 50% of patients receiving the full planned dose of radiation had a pathologic complete response. The results of this retrospective study show that patients with adenocarcinoma of the esophagus have a similar survival and local control after chemoradiation plus or minus esophagectomy. In addition, higher morbidity with esophagectomy and the possibility of late surgical salvage without esophagectomy suggest that surgery should be limited to patients with residual disease or local failure. Herskovic et al[29] report results initiated by the Radiation Therapy Oncology Group (RTOG). This landmark phase III randomized intergroup study (RTOG 8501) compared concurrent Cisplatin, 5-FU and radiation to 50 Gy versus 60 Gy radiation alone. One hundred twenty-one patients with clinical stage I-III cancer of the esophagus were entered. Fifty-one (84%) patients had squamous cell carcinoma and 10 (16%) had adenocarcinoma. Chemotherapy was delivered over a planned 4 courses. It consisted of Cisplatin (75 mg/m2, week 1,5,8, and 11) and 5-FU (1000 mg/m2) as continuous 4 day infusion the same weeks as Cisplatin. Even though there was less radiation dose delivered in the concurrent arm, the results demonstrated a significant advantage of the combined arm over the radiation alone arm. The median survival in patients treated by radiation alone was 8.9 months compared to 12.5 months for those treated with chemoradiation. Two-year survival was improved from 10% to 38% with the addition of chemotherapy, and local recurrence was decreased from 24% to 16%. Distant metastases were decreased at 12 months were decreased from 38% to 22% with the addition of chemotherapy. The results were felt to be so superior that patient accrual was discontinued, and 60 additional patients were added to the combined arm. The study also had shown life threatening side effects involving, hematologic toxicity and fistula formation, were increased from 3% to 20 percent. In conclusion, this study had demonstrated a highly significant difference

in local recurrence, median and overall survival, and distant metastases with the addition of chemotherapy with the cost of increased side effects. An update of the Herskovic study by Al-Sarraf et al[30] included patients with minimum 5 year follow up and included data on the additional 69 nonrandomized patients accrued on the combined arm. Five-year survival in the radiation and chemotherapy arm was 27% compared to the radiation alone arm where no patient survived past three years. In the nonrandomized group of 69 patients, the survival results confirmed the outcome of the randomized arms. The median survival was 17 months with a 1 and 2 year survival of 63% and 35% respectively. Distant metastases were higher for the nonrandomized group (13% versus 8%), however there were a greater number of patients with stage T3 tumors in the nonrandomized group (26% versus 8%). This trial concluded that concurrent Cisplatin, 5-FU and radiation of 50 Gy followed by maintenance chemotherapy is superior to 64 Gy of radiation alone in patients with localized cancer of the esophagus. An intergroup study (RTOG 9405, INT 0123) of combined modality therapy for carcinoma of the esophagus, comparing 50.4 Gy to 64.8 Gy both with concurrent chemotherapy. The chemotherapy includes Cisplatin on weeks 1 and 5 repeated 4 weeks after the conclusion of radiotherapy along with 5-FU of 1 gm/m^2/day for 4 days the same weeks as Cisplatin. Preliminary analysis indicates little likelihood for superior outcome with higher radiation dose.

3. PALLIATIVE TREATMENT

3.1. DYSPHAGIA IMPROVEMENT

Radiation therapy has been used as an effective treatment modality for the palliation of esophageal carcinoma. Many studies in the literature demonstrate a 60-76 percent relief from dysphagia with the use of higher dose external beam radiation.[31-34] Doses of 50 Gy or more palliate symptoms better than doses less than 50 Gy, however, one must consider potential complications such as strictures or fistula formation as well as the need to deliver treatment in a relatively short time. Palliative chemoradiation is preferable to radiation alone for patients with advanced stage esophageal carcinoma who have a good performance status. Coia et al[35] performed a study to determine the impact of radiation and concurrent chemotherapy on swallowing function. Between 1980 and 1990 120 patients with carcinoma of the esophagus were treated at Fox Chase Cancer Center. Most patients had adenocarcinoma. They received treatment based on one of three prospective randomized protocols using concurrent chemotherapy and radiation therapy. Common to each protocol was the use of bolus Mitomycin C 10 mg/m2 on day 2 only and two 96 hour infusions of 5-FU 1 gm/m2/24 hon days 2-5 and 29-32. Protocol I included 58 patients with stage I or II carcinoma of the esophagus receiving the above chemotherapy with concurrent high dose radiation therapy (60 Gy on 30 fractions) as definitive treatment. Protocol II included 49 patients with stage III or IV disease. They also received the above chemotherapy and received concurrent conventional radiation therapy to a dose of 50 Gy in 25 fractions. Protocol III included 13 patients with adenocarcinoma of the esophagus who were treated with the above chemotherapy, high dose radiation therapy followed by surgery 4 weeks following radiation. In protocol three, only initial swallowing function and its change before surgery only were evaluated. The initial swallowing function of the majority of the 120 patients included some dysphagia to solid foods or could eat only soft food. Initially, 90 (88%) of the 102 patients had improvement in their dysphagia. For the 90 patients, median time to initial improvement was 2 weeks with 86% of these patients improving in 4 weeks. There was no improvement in overall percentage of dysphagia, in adenocarcinoma versus squamous cell carcinoma, in patients treated with curative or palliative intent. There was however a significant difference in relief of dysphagia for patients with distal thoracic tumors (95%) versus upper two-thirds tumors (79%). All but two patients were able to swallow at least soft or solid foods. Long term swallowing function was assessed in 25 patients who survived at least 1 year. At least 68% of these patients without recurrent disease were able to maintain or gain weight without parenteral support. More impressive is the low incidence of benign stricture of 12%. In the palliative protocol II improvement in swallowing function lasted until death in 67% of patients with a median duration of 7 months. In summary high dose radiation and concurrent chemotherapy provides rapid improvement in dysphagia and results in normal or near normal swallowing function in patients with adenocarcinoma of the esophagus. The role of brachytherapy in the management of adenocarcinoma of the esophagus is still being studied. Brachytherapy has long been advocated as a technique which allows a high dose of irradiation to a locoregional area of interest while sparing surrounding normal tissues. The other potential advantages when comparing brachytherapy to external beam radiation therapy include shortening of treatment time, patient convenience and quicker relief of dysphasia. These points are important due to the relative short time these patients have until death. Gaspar et al[36] reported a phase I/II study (RTOG 92-07) of external beam irradiation, brachytherapy and concurrent chemotherapy in localized cancer of the esophagus. This study included 48 patients with either squamous or adenocarcinoma. They were treated with external beam radiation therapy 50 Gy in 2 Gy fractions followed 2 weeks later by brachytherapy. The brachytherapy was either high dose rate (HDR) using 5 Gy x 3 at week 8,9 and 10 or low dose rate (LDR) 20 Gy at week 8. Chemotherapy was given concurrently and included Cisplatin 75 mg/m2 on day 1 and 5-FU 1 gm/m2/day on day 1-4. Only 70% of patients were able to complete the full course of therapy. Median survival and overall survival were comparable to chemoradiation alone. There was however, an increase in toxicity, with 29 patients developing severe or fatal events. Especially concerning was an increase in fistula formation with 12 percent of patients (3 deaths) experiencing this side effect of therapy. The overall conclusion was that the addition of brachytherapy used as a boost should be administered with extreme caution following concurrent external beam radiation therapy and chemotherapy. In 1997 the American Brachytherapy Society (ABS) consensus guidelines for brachytherapy of esophageal cancer were published.[37] The efficacy and toxicity of brachytherapy was determined by treatment related factors such as sequencing, timing, dose of chemotherapy or external beam radiotherapy. Brachytherapy parameters such as applicator diameter, dose rate, active length, interval, and fractionation were also determined. Their conclusions were for patients who have previously received external beam irradiation or have a short life expectancy; palliation of dysphagia can be achieved in the majority of patients with brachytherapy alone. HDR could be delivered in two to four fractions in doses of 15-20 Gy and LDR could be delivered at .4 Gy/hr to a total of 25-40 Gy. Brachytherapy could also be combined with external beam radiation (30 Gy in 10-12 fractions) to achieve similar or superior palliation in a less overall treatment time than for external beam alone. Total doses were 45-55 Gy. For patients with a life expectancy of greater than 6 months definitive treatment could provide prolonged dysphagia free survival. Treatment recommendations include external beam to 45-50 Gy with brachytherapy additional to 10 Gy with HDR or LDR 20 Gy 2-3 weeks from completion of external beam.

4. FUTURE DIRECTIONS

4.1. MULTIMODALITY THERAPY

Some key issues remain unresolved including:

(1) Is esophagectomy necessary following chemoradiation? If so can we identify which subsets of patients are likely to benefit? (2) Can introduction of newer chemotherapy agents such as Paclitaxel with radiation improve the results over standard chemoradiation with Cisplatin and 5-FU? (3) Will radiation dose escalation via brachytherapy or increase in fractionation decrease the local failure rate over standard treatment of 50 Gy and chemotherapy? (4) Can we prevent esophageal adenocarcinoma via dietary means or detect it at an earlier stage via screening of high risk populations? (5) Can we improve the applicability and prognostic values of the present staging system by incorporating tumor length and depth of circumference involvement to depth of wall penetration to nodal status.

SUMMARY

Advances in multimodality treatment have offered improved cure rates over surgery or radiation alone in patients with esophageal adenocarcinoma, a malignancy which has surpassed squamous cell carcinoma in incidence in many western industrialized nations.

REFERENCES

1. Law SY, Fok M, Cheng SW, et al A comparison of the outcome after resection for squamous cell carcinoma and adenocarcinoma of the esophagus and cardia. Surg Gynecol Obstet. 1992;175:107-12.
2. Morson BC, Belcher JR, Brit J Cancer 1952;6:127.
3. Allison PR, Johnstone AS, Thorax 1953;8:87.
4. Smithers DW, Adenocarcinoma of the oesophagus. Thorax 1956; 11:227.
5. Raphael HA, Ellis FH, Dockerty MB, Primary adenocarcinoma of the esophagus: 18 year review of the literature. Annuls of Surg 1966; 164(3):785-96.
6. Turnbull AD, Goodner JT, Primary adenocarcinoma of the esophagus. Cancer 1968;22(5):915-8.
7. Jernsrtrom P, Brewer LA, Primary adenocarcinoma of the mid-esophagus arising in ectopic gastric mucosa with associated hiatal hernia and reflux esophagitis (Dawson's syndrome). Cancer 1970;26(6):1343-8.
8. Shafer RB, Adenocarcinoma in Barrett's columnar-lined esophagus. Arch Surg 1971;103: 411-3.
9. Bremner CG, Lynch VP, Ellis FH, Barrett's esophagus: Congenital or Acquired? Surgery 1970;68:209-16.
10. Danoff B, Cooper J, Klein M, Primary adenocarcinoma of the upper oesophagus. Clin Radiol. 1978;29:519-22.
11. Earlam R, Cunha-melo JR. Oesophageal squamous cell carcinoma: I. A critical review of surgery. Br J Surg 1980;67: 381-90.
12. Whyte RI, Orringer MB, Surgery for carcinoma of the esophagus: The case for transhiatal esophagectomy. Sem Rad Oncol 1994;4(3):146-56.
13. Bosset JF, Gignoux M, Triboulet JP, Tiret E, Mantion G, Elias D, Lozach P, Ollier JC, Pavy JJ, Mercier M, Sahmoud T, Chemoradiotherapy followed by surgery compared with surgery alone in squamous cell cancer of the esophagus. NEJM 1997;337(3);161-7.
14. Walsh TN, Noonan N, Hollywood D, Kelly A, Kelling N, Hennessy TPJ A comparison of multimodality therapy and surgery for esophageal adenocarcinoma. NEJM 1996;335(7):462-7.
15. Urba S, Orringer M, Turrisi A, Whyte R, Iannettoni M, Forastiere A, A randomized trial comparing surgery to preoperative concomitant chemoradiation plus surgery in patients with resectable esophageal cancer: updated analysis. Proc Am Soc Clin Oncol 1997;16:277a.
16. Kelsen DP, Ginsberg R, Pajak TF, Sheahan DG, Gunderson L, Mortimer J, Estes N, Haller DG, Ajani J, Kocha W, Minsky BD, Roth JA, Chemotherapy followed by surgery compared with surgery alone for localized esophageal cancer. NEJM 1998;339(27):1979-84.
17. Arnott SJ, Duncan W, Kerr GR, et al Low dose preoperative radiotherapy for carcinoma of the oesophagus: results of a randomized trial. Radiotherapy and Oncol. 1992; 24:108-13.
18. Fok M, Sham JS, Choy D, Cheng S, Wong J, Postoperative radiotherapy for carcinoma of the esophagus: A prospective, randomised controlled study. Surgery 1993;113(2)138-147.
19. Whittington R, Coia LR, Haller DG, Rubenstein JH, Rosato EF, Adenocarcinoma of the esophagus and esophago-gastric junction: The effects of single and combined modalities on the survival and patterns of failure following treatment. IJROBP 1990;19:593-603.

20. Forastiere A, Orringer MB, Perez-Tamayo, C, Urba SG, Zahurak M, Preoperative chemoradiation followed by transhiatal esophagectomy for carcinoma of the esophagus:Final report. J Clin. Oncol. 1993;11:1118-23.

21. Kavanagh B, Anscher M, Leopold K, Deutsch M, Gaydica E, Dodge R, Allen K, Allen D, Staub W, Montana G, Crawford J, Wolfe W, Patterns of failure following combined modality therapy for esophageal cancer, 1984-1990 IJROBP 1992;24:633-42.

22. Forastiere A, Heitmiller DJ, Lee R, Abrams R, Zahuarak M, A 4 week intensive preoperative chemoradiation program for locoregional cancer of the esophagus. Proc Am Soc Clin Oncol. 1994;13:195a.

23. Urba SG, Orringer MB, Perez-Tamayo C, Bromberg J, Forastiere A, Concurrent preoperative chemotherapy and radiation therapy in localized esophageal carcinoma. Cancer 1991;69(2):285-91.

24. Denham JW, Burmeister BH, Lamb DS, Spry NA, Joseph Dj, Hamilton CS, Yeoh E, O'Brien P, Walker QJ, Factors influencing outcome following radio-chemotherapy for oesophageal cancer Radiotherapy and Oncology 1996;40:31-43.

25. Keller SM, Ryan L, Coia LR, Dang P, Vaught DJ, Diggs C, Weiner LM, Benson AB, High dose chemoradiotherapy followed by esophagectomy for adenocarcinoma of the esophagus and gastroesophageal junction. Cancer 1998;83(9):1908-16.

26. Coia LR, Engstrom PF, Paul A, Nonsurgical management of esophageal cancer: Report of a study of combined radiotherapy and chemotherapy. JCO 1987;5(11): 1783-90.

27. Coia LR, Engstrom PF, Paul AR, Stafford PM, Hanks GE, Long term results of infusional 5-FU, Mitomycin-C, and radiation as primary management of esophageal carcinoma. IJROBP 1991;20:29-36.

28. Algan O, Coia LR, Keller SM, Engstrom PF, Weiner LM, Schultheiss TE, Hanks GE, Management of adenocarcinoma of the esophagus with chemoradiation alone or chemoradiation followed by esophagectomy: results of sequential nonrandomized phase II studies. IJROBP 1994;32:753-61.

29. Herskovic A, Martz K, Al-Sarraf M, Leichman L, Brindle J, Vaitkevicius V, Cooper J, Byhardt R, Davis L, Emami B, Combined chemotherapy and radiotherapy compared with radiotherapy alone in patients with cancer of the esophagus. NEJM 1992;326(24):1593-8.

30. Al-Sarraf M, Martz K, Herskovic A, Leichman L, Brindle JS, Vaitkevicious V, Cooper J, Bryhardt R, Davis L, Emami B, Progress report of combined chemoradiotherapy versus radiothrapy alone in patients with esophageal cancer: an intergroup study. JCO 1997;15(1):277-84.

31. Langer M, Choi NC, Orlow E, Radiation therapy alone or in combination with surgery in the treatment of carcinoma of the esophagus. Cancer 1986;58:1208-13.

32. Wara WM, Mauch PM, Thomas AN, Palliation for adenocarcinoma of the esophagus. Radiology 1976; 121, 717-720.

33. Caspers RJL, Welvaart K, Verkes RJ, The effect of radiotherapy on dysphagia and survival in patients with esophageal cancer. Radiother Oncol 1988;12:15-23.

34. O'Rourke IC, Tiver K, Bull C, Swallowing performance after radiation therapy for carcinoma of the esophagus. Cancer 1988;61: 2022-6.

35. Coia LR, Soffen EM, Schultheiss TE, Martin EE, Hanks GE, Swallowing function in patients with esophageal cancer treated with concurrent radiation and chemotherapy. Cancer 1993;71(2): 281-5.

36. Gaspar LE, Qian C, Kocha WI, Coia LR, Herskovic A, Graham M, A phase I/Ii study of external beam irradiation, brachytherapy and concurrent chemotherapy in localized cancer of the esophagus (RTOG 92-07): Preliminary toxicity report. IJROBP 1997;37(3):593-9.

37. Gaspar LE, Nag S, Herskovic A, Mantravadi R, Speiser B, Clinical research committee ABS, American Brachyterapy Society (ABS) consensus guidelines for brachytherapy of esophageal cancer. IJROBP 1997;38(1):127-32.

6.7 ENDOSCOPIC MANAGEMENT OF DYSPHAGIA FROM ESOPHAGEAL CANCER

Peter D. Siersema

1. INTRODUCTION

More than 50% of patients with esophageal cancer present with locally advanced or metastatic disease, so that restoration of the ability to eat is the only possible therapy. Since most patients live no longer than 6 months, the aim of treatment is to relief the dysphagia rapidly, to maintain swallowing during life and to avoid serious complications. It is important to realize that treatment for incurable esophageal cancer should be individualized and based on tumor stage, medical condition and performance status and the patient's personal wishes. In addition, both the available expertise and equipment and results of prospective, randomized studies should be taken into consideration[1]. There is a wide variety of palliative techniques currently available (Table1).

TABLE 1. Palliative therapies in esophageal cancer

Modality	Method
Non-Endoscopic Techniques	
Surgery	
Radiation Therapy	External Beam
	Intraluminal (Brachytherapy)
Chemotherapy	
Endoscopic Techniques	
Dilatation	
Laser Therapy	Thermal
	Photodynamic
Electrocoagulation	BICAP Probe
Chemical Injection Therapy	
Intubation	Prosthetic Tube
	Self-Expanding Metal Stent
Nutritional support	Naso-Gastric Tube
	PEG Feeding

The main options can be divided into non-endoscopic modalities, of which radiation therapy is most commonly used, and endoscopic procedures, of which the most important are laser treatment and insertion of a self-expanding metal stent, that relieve obstruction. The use of surgery, radiation therapy and chemotherapy in the (palliative) treatment of esophageal cancer will be discussed in other chapters of this book. In brief, surgery can achieve an excellent quality of swallowing, but in patients with unresectable tumor such a major procedure is hard to justify in the light of the expected short survival of these patients. Radiation therapy may reduce the tumor bulk, however its effects are often delayed and unpredictable. Although different regimens of chemotherapy may offer some hope for the future, there are currently no publications having studied the effect of chemotherapy on the relief of malignant dysphagia. Each of the presently available, endoscopic palliative modalities will be discussed below. The main emphasis will be placed on (contra-)indications, (dis-)advantages and results of each palliative treatment, rather than on technical aspects of the method. The results achieved in different palliative regimens used in the combined modality programs will be summarized separately at the end of this chapter.

H.W. Tilanus and S.E.A. Attwood (eds.), Barrett's Esophagus, 377–386.
© 2001 *Kluwer Academic Publishers. Printed in the Netherlands.*

2. DILATATION

Dilatation can relieve dysphagia temporarily but it seldom provides palliation longer than a few days. It is frequently used to allow access through the tumor for different forms of endoscopic treatment. Dilatation is a simple, cheap and relatively safe procedure. The incidence of complications is 2.5-10% and these include perforation and haemorrhage[2,3]. The two most commonly used types of dilators are polyvinyl wire-guided bougies, of which the tapered Savary-Gilliard bougie is most frequently used, and through-the-scope hydrostatic balloons[4]. In theory, balloons are safer than bougies, since they exert a radial force instead of the longitudinal force exerted by bougies. Remarkably, the comparative efficacy of balloons and bougies in the dilatation of strictures in the esophagus has not been studied.

Since dilatation as a sole therapy needs to be repeated at frequent intervals, it should only be performed in extremely ill patients with a very short life-span.

3. LASER THERAPY - THERMAL

Treatment of obstructing esophageal cancer with the high-power neodymium yttrium-aluminium-garnet (Nd:YAG) laser was first described in 1982[5]. Since then, the procedure has become an accepted and effective method for the palliation of malignant dysphagia[6-16]. Laser therapy is carried out endoscopically with the patient sedated. Early investigators used a prograde technique, nowadays a retrograde approach with initial dilatation is preferred. A comparative study found that treatment with the retrograde technique was completed over a shorter period and there was a trend toward fewer treatment sessions[7]. Two to three treatment sessions are usually needed to establish an adequate lumen through the tumor. Recently, Mitty et al.[16] described effective palliation in one session using a retrograde approach under general anesthesia. Tumors that are relatively short (6 cm), non-angulated, exophytic, non-circumferential, and in the mid- or distal esophagus are most amenable to laser ablation. Laser treatment is unsafe for submucosal tumors, those causing extrinsic compression and angulated tumors, whereas circumferential tumors are vulnerable to stricture formation. In various studies, technical success ranges from 90-100%, whereas functional success ranges from 70-100%. Depending on the length of follow-up,

recurrent dysphagia occurs in 40-60% of patients between 4 to 10 weeks after initial treatment. Therefore, patients are usually reassessed at 4-6 weekly intervals. Complications include perforation, fistulas, hemorrhage and sepsis in 2-10% of patients. The median survival of patients treated with laser is 3-6 months. Barr al.[10] found an improvement in the overall quality of life in patients treated with laser for malignant dysphagia. If patients already had a poor pre-treatment performance, they were unlikely to attain complete functional relief of dysphagia, their rate of treatment-related complications was increased and survival time was limited[12]. In a prospective, randomized study comparing laser therapy with brachytherapy (intraluminal radiotherapy[17]), dysphagia and performance scores improved in approximately the same percentage of patients. Complication rates were not substantially different, however retreatments were more common with laser therapy.

4. LASER THERAPY - PHOTODYNAMIC

Photodynamic therapy (PDT) involves the local destruction of tumor tissue by light of a specific wavelength activating a previously administered photosensitiser which is retained in malignant tissue. Porphyrin compounds have been the most commonly used photosensitisers. As opposed to the thermal destruction induced by the Nd:YAG laser, the damage by PDT is initiated by a photochemical effect. One or two treatment sessions are usually required to establish an adequate tumor response. PDT may be useful for long tumors, for tumors that are narrow or angulated, and for flat infiltrating tumors[18-20]. Clinical experience with PDT for palliation of malignant dysphagia is limited. Nevertheless, encouraging results have been described in a few studies[21-23]. Relief of dysphagia has been reported in the majority of patients treated with PDT. The most frequent complication is prolonged skin photosensitivity with the most commonly used photosensitiser Photofrin®. Patients must avoid direct sunlight for at least 6 weeks after PDT, but normal levels of room lighting usually present no difficulty. Other side effects include fever, chest pain and pleural effusion, probably secondary to a transient, local inflammation, however these side effects are usually mild. Serious complications including perforation, fistulas and strictures have been reported in 10-20% of patients. At present, the high cost of a special laser unit in addition to a Nd:YAG source will confine the availability of PDT to a limited number of centers. The potential of PDT using the next generation of (less toxic) photosensitisers remains to be established. Two prospective, randomized studies have compared PDT with laser therapy[24,25]. Lightdale et al.[24] found equivalent improvements in dysphagia scores with a trend towards an improved response with PDT in tumors located in the upper and lower third of the esophagus, in long (> 10 cm) tumors and in patient who had prior therapy. More mild to moderate complications (including skin photosensitivity, nausea, fever and pleural effusion) followed PDT, whereas severe complications were equally divided between the two treatment groups. Heier et al.[25] found similar functional results and complication rates for PDT and laser therapy, however PDT resulted in an improved performance status and longer duration of response (84 vs. 57 days).

5. BICAP ELECTROCOAGULATION THERAPY

The BICAP tumor probe generates thermal energy in response to the passage of an electrical current through tissue. The probe consists of a metal olive with six electrodes arranged in a circumferential array. The depth of tumor destruction is highly predictable. An esophageal wall of at least 5 mm thickness should be documented by endoscopic ultrasound to avoid perforation. After inserting a guide wire, the obstruction is dilated so that the probe can pass under fluoroscopic control. As with laser therapy, two or three treatment sessions are required to achieve luminal patency. BICAP electrocoagulation is suitable for circumferential and submucosal tumors, and is particularly useful for tumors at the cardia[26,27].

In a few small series[28-30], more than 80% of patients demonstrate improved swallowing function after treatment. Complications vary between 10-20% and include perforation, fistulas and haemorrhage. Thermally-induced fibrous strictures may develop in 10% of patients. The mean duration of benefit before retreatment becomes necessary is 6-7 weeks.

BICAP electocoagulation therapy is cheap, however the BICAP probe never became very popular, as the procedure is rather cumbersome and technically demanding. In a prospective, non-randomized trial BICAP electrocoagulation therapy has been compared with laser therapy[31]. There were no clear differences in any of the outcome variables between the two treatment groups. however it was concluded that circumferential and submucosal tumors should be treated with BICAP electrocoagulation whereas exophytic tumors preferentially should be treated with laser therapy.

6. CHEMICAL INJECTION THERAPY

Chemically-induced tumor necrosis is also effective for palliation of malignant dysphagia. It is cheap and universally applicable since one does not require any special equipment. Treatment is usually performed by the injection of 100% ethanol in aliquots of 0.5-1 ml into the tumor. The mean number of treatment sessions varies between 2 and 3 sessions at intervals of 3-7 days. Exophytic tumors are most amenable to injection therapy, whereas firm and fibrotic tumors (after radiotherapy) prove difficult to inject[32-34]. Dysphagia may worsen over the first 1-3 days after the procedure owing to tissue swelling. Swallowing is restored 3-5 days after therapy when the tumor sloughs. An improvement in dysphagia score is obtained in 80-100% of patients. Minor complications include transitory retrosternal pain and low-grade fever. Major complications have only been described by Chung et al.[34] in 8% of their patients and included mediastinitis and fistula formation. Retreatment is necessary at 4-5 week intervals. A problem with endoscopic injection therapy is to judge the extent of tissue damage by the injection of a chemical. The injection of 3% polidocanol has been compared with laser therapy in a prospective, randomized trial[35]. Both methods were equally effective and safe with more than 80% of patients obtaining relief of dysphagia after the first treatment course. The need for further treatment was lower after endoscopic injection therapy.

7. INTUBATION – PROSTHETIC TUBES

Esophageal intubation with one of the inexpensive, commercially available prosthetic tubes is an inexpensive, rapid and durable method of restoring swallowing. The prostheses most frequently used have an internal diameter of 10-12 mm and an outer diameter of 20-25 mm at the midposition, a proximal funnel to prevent caudal migration and a distal flange to prevent cranial movement. Since the outer diameter of these devices is relatively large, prior dilatation to 18 mm is required (Figure 1).

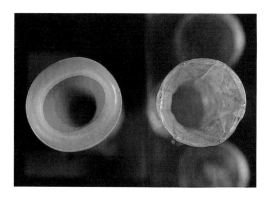

Figure 1: On the left is an example of a prosthetic tube (Celestin Pulsion Tube) which has an outer diameter of 22.5 mm at its proximal funnel and 20 mm at its distal funnel, while the inner diameter is 12 mm at its midposition. On the right is an example of a coated self-expanding metal stent (Gianturco-Z stent), which has an outer diameter of 18 mm at its midposition, while the proximal and distal ends are flared to a diameter of 25 mm.

Prosthetic tubes are particularly useful for long, asymmetric or tortuous tumors, tumors causing extrinsic compression, and as salvage therapy after other methods (radiotherapy, laser, etc.) have failed. High cervical tumors are often considered unsuitable for intubation because of foreign body sensation by the patient and proximal prosthesis migration[36-38]. In experienced hands, functional success after intubation ranges from 60-90%. Although with good counselling a soft nutritious diet is possible, swallowing after intubation never returns to normal. The complication rate associated with this procedure is variable, but has been reported to be as high as 35%. Complications include perforation (4-12%), hemorrhage (5-15%), aspiration (3-5%), erosion/ulcer at the end of the prosthesis (3-5%), fistula formation (3-5%) and severe pain (3-7%). The procedure-related mortality ranges from 3-15% and is often caused by perforation associated with preceding dilatation and/or placement of the prosthesis or life-threatening hemorrhage. Another problem is recurrent dysphagia which occurs in up to 35% of patients. Recurrent dysphagia is mainly due to migration of the prosthesis (10-25%), food bolus obstruction (5-15%) and tumor overgrowth (3-15%)[39-47].

8. INTUBATION – SELF EXPANDING METAL V STENTS

In an attempt to overcome the problems associated with prosthetic tubes, self-expanding metal stents have been introduced. Since 1990, 49 studies have reported on 1346 patients who received a metal stent for the palliation of obstructive esophageal cancer[48-96]. Metal stents have theoretical advantages over prosthetic tubes, since they can be inserted with a minimum of dilatation, the diameter of the delivery catheters being only 7-11 mm. After placement of the metal stent, the stent expands progressively, potentially decreasing subsequent stent-related complications. Moreover, the larger lumen achieved from 16 to 24 mm, and the flexibility of the stent should improve the quality of swallowing compared to prosthetic tubes (Figure 1). Two of the commercially available metal stents, the Ultraflex stent (Microvasive/Boston Scientific Corp., Watertown, USA)[48-58] and the Wall stent (Schneider AG, Bülach, Switserland)[59-74] are wire mesh stents constructed from stainless steel and nitinol, respectively. The third stent, the Gianturco-Z stent (Wilson-Cook Europe A/S, Bjaeverskov, Denmark)[75-89] with Korean (Song stent; Sooho Medi-tech, Seoul, Korea)[90,91] and Japanese (Soa-Tech, Showa, Himeji, Japan)[92] modifications, are assembled from interlocking stainless steel wires. The fourth stent, the Esophacoil, is a coiled spring made of nitinol[93-96]. The Gianturco-Z stent and later versions of the Ultraflex stent and the Wallstent are covered to prevent tumor ingrowth; the Esophacoil is not, but tumor ingrowth is avoided by the complete retraction of the broad spiral wire. Indications for placement of metal stents are not different from prosthetic tubes. Three randomized studies in patients with malignant dysphagia compared metal stents (the uncovered Ultraflex stent[55], the uncovered Wallstent[63] and the covered Gianturco-Z stent[88] with prosthetic tubes in 39, 42 and 75 patients, respectively. Technical success and improvement of dysphagia were similar in both treatment groups. Complications were more frequent with prosthetic tubes than with metal stents, but the incidence of recurrent dysphagia was the same for prosthetic tubes and metal stents. In the largest of these three studies it was found that prior radiation and/or chemotherapy increased the risk of device-related complications to the esophagus[88]. Recurrent dysphagia is observed with all types of stents and is usually caused by tumor ingrowth, tumor overgrowth and stent migration. A disadvantage of the first generation uncovered metal stents (uncovered Wallstents and Ultraflex stents) is tumor ingrowth through the wire mesh of the stent in 10-15% of patients.

Nowadays, this is avoided by the use of covered metal stents. However, migration rates are higher with covered metal stents than with uncovered metal stents (10-15% vs. 1%). A new design Wallstent, the covered Flamingo Wallstent, has been designed to reduce, if not eliminate, migration, and, in addition, to prevent tumor ingrowth through the wire mesh (Figure 2).

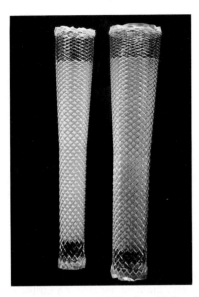

Figure 2: On the left is a small Flamingo Wallstent with a total length of 12 cm and proximal and distal diameters of 24 mm and 16 mm, respectively. On the right is a large Flamingo Wallstent with a total length of 14 cm and proximal and distal diameters of 30 mm and 20 mm, respectively. Note that there is a change in the braiding angle between the proximal and distal parts of the stent mesh and that they have a conical shape.

Migration with the Flamingo Wallstent is thought to be prevented by the proximal increase in diameter inherent to the conical shape. Moreover, the change in the braiding angle between the proximal and distal parts of the stent mesh might allow the distal part of the stent to stretch in response to peristaltic traction. Apart form one case of proximal migration in a patient with a distal carcinoma of 5 cm length after a prolonged period of vomiting, the Flamingo stent proved resistant to distal migration in all 40 patients stented by this new design metal stent[97]. At present, the major cause of recurrent dysphagia is overgrowth by the tumor at the proximal or distal end of the stent, despite the use of stents with an adequate length (Figure 3).

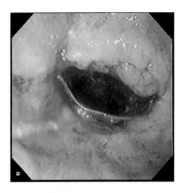

Figure 3. Tumor overgrowth at tha proximal end of a Gianturco Z-stent, which was placed for a stenotic esophageal carcinoma.

Prevention of tumor overgrowth should therefore be an important new issue in stent design. Possibly this could be achieved by the impregnation of metal stents with cytotoxic agents[98] or the incorporation of beta-emitting agents in stents. Esophagorespiratory fistulas, which are often difficult to manage and involve a significant reduction in the quality of life of patients, are a serious complication of malignant disease in the esophagus. The results in several small studies (including our own results in 16 patients) with different types of covered metal stents for palliation of malignant esophagorespiratory fistulas are promising (summarized in Table 2). Using covered metal stents, fistulas can effectively be occluded (Figure 4) and the high grade dysphagia in most patients suffering from malignant esophagorespiratory fistulas can be improved with an acceptable risk of complications[73,77,81,86,87,92,99-107]. It is not known which patients will benefit from which type of metal stent. In a retrospective study, Dorta et al.[108] found that the Wallstent was superior to the Ultraflex stent. In their series, 18 out of 49 Ultraflex stents failed to deploy completely despite balloon dilatation. In contrast, another retrospective, comparative study found that early complications and procedure-related mortality were significantly higher with the Wallstent than with the Ultraflex stent[109]. Our group performed a prospective, randomized study in 100 patients comparing the presently available covered metal stents, the Ultraflex stent, the Flamingo Wallstent and the Gianturco-Z stent (Figure 5).

TABLE 2. Coated metal stents for esophagorespiratory fistulas[73,77,81,86,87,92,99]

Stent type	N	Complete sealing (%)	Complications early (%)	late (%)	Survival (days)
Z-stent	89	86	3*	20*	36-121
Wallstent	61	87	13*	18*	59-157
Ultraflex stent	14	100	14	29	35-180
Esophacoil	4	100	0	0	78

*Complications not listed in all studies

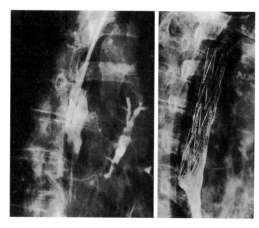

Figure 4: On the left an esophagobronchial fistula demonstrated by radiographic contrast examination. On the right a repeated radiographic contrast examination after placement of a Gianturco-Z stent, showing that the stent has occluded the fistula

There were no differences between the 3 stent types in the improvement of dysphagia and in the occurrence of complications and recurrent dysphagia (Table 3). It can be concluded from this study that all currently available covered metal stents offer the same degree of palliation of malignant dysphagia at the same risk. A major disadvantage of metal stents is their high costs. However, if these are weighed against superior palliation, their lower complication rates and short in-hospital stay[88], their use is probably economically well justified in this group of patients.

9. SUMMARY

Patients with nonresectable esophageal cancer have a life expectancy of 3-6 months only Effective palliation, i.e., restoration of the ability to swallow, has to ensure a good quality of life with minimal morbidity and mortality in these patients. The low complication rate, the ease of placement and the "long" lasting effect which are achieved with self-expanding metal stents, have made these an increasingly popular alternative compared to other methods in the treatment of esophageal tumors, tumors

causing extrinsic compression and esophagorespiratory fistulas. For patients with short (<6 cm) exophytic tumors, laser therapy is an alternative treatment to consider.

It remains to be established whether there is a role for so-called "new" monotherapies, i.e., chemical injection therapy, photodynamic therapy and electrocoagulation with the BICAP tumor probe in the palliative treatment of esophageal cancer. These treatment modalities should first be compared with the most commonly used techniques, i.e., laser therapy and placement of a self-expanding metal stent. They should only be applied if they provide better palliation, are associated with lower complication rates and if they proof to be a cheap alternative to the presently used palliative modalities.

It seems reasonable to consider a combination of palliative regimens, i.e., laser therapy or placement of a self-expanding metal stent plus chemotherapy or chemoradiation in patients with nonresectable esophageal cancer. However, before these combined modality regimens can be applied, it is important to compare local tumor control, complications, survival and patients' quality of life of these combinations in well-designed, prospective, randomized studies.

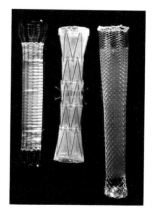

Figure 5: The presently available covered metal stents, the Ultraflex stent (left), the Gianturco-Z stent (middle) and the Flamingo Wallstent (right).

TABLE 3. Complications and recurrent dysphagia in 100 patients given an Ultraflex stent, a Flamingo Wallstent or a Gianturo-Z stent for palliation of esophagogastric cancer

	Ultraflex (n=34) (no. of patients) (%)	Flamingo Wallstent (n=33)	Gianturco-Z (n=33)
Complications*	8 (24)	6 (18)	12 (36)
≤ 7 days			
- Perforation	2	2	2
- Bleeding	0	0	2
- Fever	1	0	1
- Pressure necrosis	0	1	0
- Severe pain	0	0	1
≥ 7 days			
- Bleeding	5	3	6
Recurrent dysphagia*	11(32)	11(33)	8(24)
- Tumor overgrowth	4	5	4
- Migration of device	6	3	4
- Food-bolus impaction	1	3	0

*p=NS

REFERENCES

1. Lambert R. Palliation of carcinoma of the esophagus:is there a hope for cure? Am J Gastroenterol 1994;89:27-40.
2. Moses FM, Peura DA, Wong RKH, Johnson LF. Palliative dilation of esophageal carcinoma Gastrointest Endosc 1985;31:61-3.
3. Lundell L, Leth R, Lind T, Lönroth H, Sjövall M, Olbe L. Palliative dilation in carcinoma of the esophagus and esophagogastric junction. Acta Chir Scand 1989;155:179-84.
4. Tietjen TG, Pasricha PJ, Kalloo AN. Managemant of malignant esophageal stricture with esophageal dilation and esophageal stents. Gastrointest Endosc North Am 1994;4:851-62.
5. Fleischer D, Kessler F, Haye O. Endoscopic ND:YAG laser therapy for carcinoma of the esophagus:a new palliative approach. Am J Surg 1982;143:280-3.
6. Ell C, Demling L. Laser therapy of tumor stenoses in the upper gastrointestinal tract: an international inquiry. Lasers Surg Med 1987;491-4.
7. Pietrafitta JJ, Bowers GJ, Dwyer RM. Prograde versus retrograde endoscopic laser therapy for the treatment of malignant esophageal obstruction: a comparison of techniques. Lasers Surg Med 1988;8:288-93.
8. Radford CM, Ahlquist DA, Gosthout CJ, Viggiano TR, Balm RK, Zinsmeister AR. Prospective comparison of contact with concontact Nd:YAG laser therapy for palliation of esophageal carcinoma. Gastrointest Endosc 1989;394-7.
9. Mason RC, Bright N, McColl I. Palliation of malignant dysphagia with laser therapy: predictability of results. Br J Surg 1991;78:1346-7.
10. Barr H, Krasner N. Prospective quality-of-life analysis after palliative photoablation for the treatment of malignant dysphagia. Cancer 1991;68:1660-4.
11. Carter R, Smith JS, Anderson JR. Palliation of malignant dysphagia using the Nd:YAG laser. World J Surg 1993;17:608-14.
12. Alexander GL, Wang KK, Ahlquist DA, Viggiano TR, Gostout CJ, Balm R. Does performance staus influence the outcome of Nd:YAG laser therapy of proximal esophageal tumors? Gastrointest Endosc 1994;20:451-4.
13. Zittel TT, Allgaier D, Grund KE. Laser therapy for esophageal cancer. Results and additional endoscopic treatments. Surg Endosc 1994;8:1096-1100.
14. Spinelli P, Mancini A, Dal Fante M. Endoscopic treatment of gastrointestinal tumors: indications and results of laser photocoagulation and photodynamic therapy. Semin Surg Oncol 1995;11:307-18.
15. Maciel J, Barbosa J, Leal AS. Nd-YAG laser as palliative treatment for malignant dysphagia. Eur J Surg Oncol 1996;22:69-73.
16. Mitty RD, Cave DR, Birkett DH. One-stage retrograde approach to Nd:YAG laser palliation of esophageal carcinoma. Endoscopy 1996;28:350-5.
17. Low DE, Pagliero KM. Prospective randomized clinical trial comparing brachytherapy and laser photoablation for palliation of esophageal cancer. J Thorac Cardiovasc Surg 1992;104:173-9.
18. Overholt BF. Laser and photodynamic therapy of esophagal cancer. Semin Surg Oncol 1992;8:191-203.
19. Narayan S, Sivak Jr, MV. Palliation of esophageal carcinoma. Laser and photodynamic therapy. Chest Surg Clin North Am 1994;4:347-67.
20. Marcon NE. Photodynamic therapy and cancer of the esophagus. Semin Oncol 1994;6 Suppl 15:20-23.

21. Thomas RJ, Abbott M, Bhathal PS, St. John DJB, Morstyn G. High-dose photoirradiation of esophageal cancer. Ann Surg 1987;206:193-9.

22. McCaughan Jr, JS, Nims TA, Guy JT, Hicks WJ, Williams Jr, TE, Laufman LR. Photodynamic therapy for esophageal tumors. Arch Surg 1989;124:74-80.

23. Patrice T, Foultier MT, Yactayo S, Adam F, Galmiche JP, Douet MC, Le Bodic L. Endoscopic photodynamic therapy with hematoporphyrin derivative for primary treatment of gastrointestinal neoplasms in inoperable patients. Dig Dis Sci 1990;35:545-52.

24. Lightdale CJ, Heier SK, Marcon NE, McCaughan JS, Gerdes H, Overholt BF, Sivak, Jr, MV, Stiegmann GV, Nava HR. Photodynamic therapy with porfimer sodium versus thermal ablation therapy with Nd:YAG laser for palliation of esophageal cancer: a multicenter randomized trial. Gastrointest Endosc 1995;42:507-12.

25. Heier SK, Rothman KA, Heier LM, Rosenthal WS. Photodynamic therapy for obstructing esophageal cancer: light dosimetry and randomized comparison with Nd:YAG laser therapy. Gastroenterology 1995;109:63-72.

26. Reilly HF, Fleischer DE. Palliative treatment of esophageal carcinoma using laser and tumor probe therapy. Gastrointest Clin North Am 1991;20:731-42.

27. Laine L. Determination of the optimal technique for bipolar electrocoagulation treatment. Gastroenterology 1991;100:107-112.

28. Johnston JH, Fleischer D, Petrini J, Nord HJ. Palliative bipolar electrocoagulation therapy of obstructing esophageal cancer. Gastrointest Endosc 1987;33:349-53.

29. Conio M, Bonelli L, Martines H, Munizzi F, Aste H. Palliative bipolar electrocoagulation treatment of malignant gastresophageal strictures. Surg Endosc 1990;4:164-71.

30. Maunoury V, Brunetaud JM, Cochelard D, Boniface B, Cortot A, Paris JC. Endoscopic palliation for inoperable malignant dysphagia: long term follow up. Gut 1992;33:1602-7.

31. Jensen DM, Machicado G, Randall G, Tung LA, English-Zych S. Comparison of low-power YAG Laser and BICAP tumor probe for palliation of esophageal cancer strictures. Gastroenterology 1988;94;1263-70.

32. Moreira LS, Coelho RCL, Sadala RU, Dani R. The use of ethanol injection under endoscopic control to palliate dysphagia caused by esophagogastric cancer. Endoscopy 1994;26:311-4.

33. Nwokolo CU, Payne-James JJ, Silk DBA, Misiewisz JJ, Loft DE. Palliation of malignant dysphagia by ethanol induced tumor necrosis. Gut 1994;35:299-303.

34. Chung SCS, Leong HT, Choi CYC, Leung JWC, Li AKC. Palliation of malignant esophageal obstruction by endoscopic alcohol injection. Endoscopy 1994;26:275-7.

35. Angelini G, Fratta Pasini A, Aderle A, Castagnini A, Talamini G, Bulighin G. Nd:YAG laser versus polidocanol injection for palliation of esophageal malignancy: a prospective, randomized study. Gastrointest Endosc 1991;37:607-10.

36. Tytgat GNJ, den Hartog Jager FCA, Bartelsman JWFM. Endoscopic prostheses for advanced esophageal cancer. Endoscopy 1986;18 Suppl 3:32-9.

37. Parker CH, Peura DA. Palliative treatment of esophageal carcinoma using esophageal dilation and prosthesis. Gastroenterol Clin North Am 1991;20:717-29.

38. Reed CE. Atkinson tube placement. Chest Surg Clin North Am 1995;5:481-8.

39. Den Hartog Jager FCA, Bartelsman JFWM, Tytgat GNJ. Palliative treatment of obstructing esophageal malignancy by endoscopic positioning of a plastic endoprosthesis. Gastroenterology 1979;77:1008-14.

40. Ogilvie AL, Dronfield MW, Percuson R, Atkinson M. Palliative intubation of oesophago-gastric neoplasms at fiberoptic endoscopy. Gut 1982;23:1060-7.

41. Gasparri G, Casalegno PA, Camandona M, Dei Poli M, Salizzoni M, Ferrarotti G, Bertero D. Endoscopic insertion of 248 prostheses in inoperable carcinoma of the esophagus and cardia: short-term and long-term results. Gastrointest Endosc 1987;33:354-6.

42. Van den Brandt-Grädel V, den Hartog Jager FCA, Tytgat GNJ. Palliative intubation of malignant esophagogastric obstruction. J Clin Gastroenterol 1987;9:290-7.

43. Függer R, Niederle B, Jantsch H, Schiessel R, Schulz F. Endoscopic tube implantation for the palliation of malignant esophageal stenosis. Endoscopy 1990;22:101-4.

44. Liakakos TK, Ohri SK, Townsend ER, Fountain SW. Palliative intubation for dysphagia in patients with carcinoma of the esophagus. Ann Thorac Surg 1992;53:460-3.

45. Cusumano A, Ruol A, Segalin A, Norberto L, Baessato M, Tiso E, Perracchia A. Push-through intubation:effective palliation in 409 patients with cancer of the esophagus and cardia. Ann Thorac Surg 1992;53:1010-14.

46. Wilton A, Smith PM. Endoscopic intubation of oesophago-gastric malignancy. Eur J Gastroenterol Hepatol 1995;7:559-62.

47. Ho KY, Samarasinghe DA, Nicholson GI, Lane MR. Endoscopic palliation of esophageal carcinoma with Atkinson prosthesis. J Gastroenterol Hepatol 1995;10:56-9.

48. Raijman I, Walden D, Kortan P, Haber GB, Fuchs E, Siemens M, Kandel G, Marcon NE. Expandable esophageal stents: initial experience with a new nitinol stent. Gastrointest Endosc 1994;40:614-21.

49. Wagner HJ, Stinner B, Schwerk WB, Hoppe M, Klose KJ. Nitinol prostheses for the treatment of inoperable malignant esophageal obstruction. JVIR 1994;5:899-904.

50. Decker P, Jakschik J, Hirner A. Der selbstexpandierende Nitinol-Stent - Anwendung beim esophaguscarcinom. Chirurg 1995;66:1258-62.

51. Grund KE, Storek D, Becker HD. Highly flexible self-expanding meshed metal stents for palliation of malignant esophagogastric obstruction. Endoscopy 1995;27:486-94.

52. May A, Selmaier M, Hochberger J, Gossner L, Mühldorfer S, Hahn EG, Ell C. Memory metal stents for palliation of malignant obstruction of the esophagus and cardia. Gut 1995;37:309-13.

53. De Palma GD, Galloro G, Sivero L, Di Matteo E, Labianca O, Siciliano S, Abbruzzese P, Catanzano C. Self-expanding metal stents for palliation of inoperable carcinoma of the esophagus and gastresophageal junction. Am J Gastroenterol 1995;90:2140-2.

54. Winkelbauer FW, Schöfl R, Niederle B, Wildling R, Thurnher S, Lammer J. Palliative treatment of obstructing cancer with nitinol stents: value, safety, and long-term results. Am J Radiol 1996;166:79-84.

55. De Palma GD, Di Matteo E, Romano G, Fimmano A, Rondinone G, Catanzano C. Plastic prosthesis

versus expandable metal stents for palliation of inoperable esophageal thoracic carcinoma: a controlled prospective study. Gastrointest Endosc 1996;43:478-82.

56. Pocek M, Maspes F, Masala S, Squillaci E, Assegnati G, Moraldi A, Simonetti G. Palliative treatment of neoplastic strictures by self-expanding nitinol Strecker stent. Eur Radiol 1996;6:230-235.

57. Acuna B, Rozanes I, Akpinar S, Tunaci A, Tunaci M, Acuna G. Palliation of malignant esophageal strictures with self-expanding nitinol stents: drawbacks and complications. Radiology 1996;199:648-52.

58. Cwikiel W, Tranberg KG, Cwikiel M, Lillo-Gil R. Malignant dysphagia:palliation with esophageal stents: long-term results with 100 patients. Radiology 1998;207:513-8.

59. Domschke W, Foerster EC, Matek W, Rödl W. Self-expanding mesh stent for esophageal cancer stenosis. Endoscopy 1990;22:134-6.

60. Neuhaus H, Hoffman W, Dittler HJ, Niedermeyer HP, Classen M. Implantation of self-expanding stents for paliation of malignant dysphagia. Endoscopy 1992;24:405-10.

61. Bethge N, Knyrim K, Wagner HJ, Starck E, Pausch J, Kleist DV. Self-expanding stents for palliation of malignant esophageal obstruction - a pilot study of eight patients. Endoscopy 1992;24:411-5.

62. Fleischer DE, Bull-Henry K. A new coated self-expanding metal stent for malignant esophageal strictures. Gastrointest Endosc 1992;38:494-496.

63. Knyrim K, Wagner HJ, Bethge N, Keymling M, Vakil N. A controlled trial of an expansile metal stent for palliation of esophageal obstruction due to inoperable cancer. N Engl J Med 1993;329:1302-17.

64. Garcia M, D'Altorio RA, Glowacki D. Palliative treatment of malignant esophageal obstruction with metallic Wallstent. Dig Dis Sci 1994:39:2685-2688.

65. Ell C. Hochberger J, May A, Fleig WE, Hahn EG. Coated and uncoated self-expanding stents for malignant stenosis in the upper GI Tract: preliminary clinical experiences with wallstents. Am J Gastroenterol 1994;89:1496-1500.

66. Watkinson AF, Ellul J, Entwisle K, Mason RC, Adam A. Esophageal carcinoma: initial results of palliative treatment with covered self-expanding endoprostheses. Radiology 1995;195:821-7.

67. Ellul JPM, Watkinson JPM, Khan RJK, Adam A, Mason RC. Self-expanding metal stents for the palliation of dysphagia due to inoperable esophageal carcinoma. Br J Surg 1995;82:1678-81.

68. Vermeijden JR, Bartelsman JFWM, Fockens P, Meijer RCA, Tytgat GNJ. Self-expanding metal stents for palliation of esophagocardial malignancies. Gastrointest Endosc 1995;41:58-63.

69. Bethge N, Sommer A, von Kleist D, Vakil N. A prospective trial of self-expanding netal stents in the palliation of malignant esophageal obstruction after failure curative therapy. Gastrointest Endosc 1996;44:283-6.

70. Clements WDB, Johnston LR, McIlwrath E, Spence RAJ, McGuigan J. Self-expanding stents for malignant dysphagia. J R Soc Med 1996;89:454-6.

71. Feins RH, Johnstone DW, Baronos ES, O'Neil SM. Palliation of inoperable esophageal carcinoma with the Wallstent endoprosthesis. Ann Thorac Surg 1996;62:1603-7.

72. Moores DWO, Ilves R. Treatment of esophageal obstruction with covered, self-expanding esophageal Wallstents. Ann Thorac Surg 1996;62:963-7.

73. Nelson DB, Axelrad AM, Fleischer DE, Kozarek RA, Silvis SE, Freeman ML, Benjamin SB.

74. Raijman I, Siddique I, Lynch P. Does chemoradiation therapy increase the incidence of complications with self-expanding coated stents in the management of malignant esophageal strictures? Am J Gastroenterol 1997;92:2192-6.

Silicone-covered Wallstent prototypes for palliation of malignant esophageal obstruction and digestive-respiratory fistulas. Gastrointest Endosc 1997;45:31-7.

75. Kozarek RA, Ball TJ, Patterson DJ. Metallic self-expanding stent application in the upper gastrointestinal tract: caveats and concerns. Gastointest Endosc 1992;38:1-6.

76. Schaer J, Katon RM, Ivancev K, Uchida B, Rösch J, Binmoeller K. Treatment of malignant esophageal obstruction with silicone-coated metallic self-expanding stents. Gastointest Endosc 1992;38:7-11.

77. Wu WC, Katon RM, Saxon RR, Barton RE, Uchida BT, Keller FS, Rösch J. Silicone-covered self-expanding metallic stents for the palliation of malignant esophageal obstruction and esophagorespiratory fistulas: experience in 32 patients and a review of the literature. Gastrointest Endosc 1994;40:22-33.

78. Ell C, May A, Hahn EG. Gianturco-Z stents in the palliative treatment of malignant esophageal obstruction and esophagotracheal fistulas. Endoscopy 1995;27:495-500.

79. Saxon RR, Barton RE, Katon RM, Petersen BD, Lakin PC, Timmermans H, Uchida B, Keller FS, Rösch J. Treatment of malignant esophageal obstructions with covered metallic Z stents: long-term results in 52 patients. JVIR 1995;6:747-54.

80. Kozarek RA, Ball TJ, Brandabur JJ, Patterson DJ, Low D, Hill L, Raltz S. Expandable versus conventional esophageal prostheses: easier insertion may not preclude subsequent stent-related problems. Gastrointest Endosc 1996;43:204-8.

81. Kozarek RA, Raltz S, Brugge WR, Schapiro RH, Waxman I, Boyce W, Baillie J, Branch S, Stevens P, Lightdale CJ, Lehman GA, Benjamin S, Fleischer DE, Axelrad A, Kortan P, Marcon N. Prospective multicenter trial of esophageal Z-stent placement for malignant dysphagia and tracheesophageal fistula. Gastrointest Endosc 1996;44:562-7.

82. Kinsman KJ, DeGregorio BT, Katon RM, Morrison K, Saxon RR, Keller FS, Rösch J. Prior radiation and chemotherapy increase the risk of life-threatening complications after insertion of metallic stents for esophagogastric malignancy. Gastrointest Endosc 1996;43:196-203.

83. Demarquay JF, Conio M, Dumas R, Caroli-Bosc FX, Hastier P, Maes B, Delmont J. Fatal complication after placement of an esophageal self-expanding metal stent [letter]. Am J Gastroenterol 1996;91:178-9.

84. De Gregorio BT, Kinsman K, Katon RM, Morrison K, Saxon RR, Barton RE, Keller FS, Rösch J. Treatment of esophageal obstruction from mediastinal compressive tumors with covered, self-expanding metallic Z-stents. Gastrointest Endosc 1996;43:483-9.

85. Cook TA, Dehn TCB. Use of covered expandable metal stents in the treatment of esophageal carcinoma and tracheo-esophageal fistula. Br J Surg 1996;83:1417-1418.

86. Saxon RR, Morrison KE, Lakin PC, Petersen BD, Barton RE, Katon RM, Keller FS. Malignant esophageal obstructions and esophagoresoiratory fistula: palliation with a polyethylene-covered Z-stent. Radiology 1997;202:349-54.

87. Kozarek RA, Raltz S, Marcon N, Kortan P, Haber G, Lightdale C, Stevens P, Lehman G, Rex D, Benjamin S, Fleischer D, Bashir R, Fry S, Waxman I, Benson J, Polio J. Use of the 25 mm flanged esophageal Z stent for malignant dysphagia: a prospective multicenter trial. Gastrointest Endosc 1997;46:156-60.

88. Siersema PD, Hop WCJ, Dees J, Tilanus HW, Blankenstein M van. Coated self-expanding metal stents versus latex prostheses for esophagogastric cancer with special reference to prior radiation and chemotherapy: a controlled, prospective study. Gastrointest Endosc 1998;47:113-20.

89. Laasch H-U, Nicholson DA, Kay CL, Attwood S, Bancewicz J. The clinical effectiveness of the Gianturco esophageal stent in malignant esophageal obstruction. Clin Radiol 1998;53:666-72.

90. Song HY, Choi EK, Sohn KH, Cho BH, Ahn DS, Kim KS. Esophagogastric neoplasms: palliation with a modified Gianturco stent. Radiology 1991;180:349-54.

91. Song HY, Do YS, Han YM, Sung KB, Choi EK, Sohn KH, Kim HR, Kim SH, Min YI. Covered, expandable esophageal metallic stent tubes: experiences in 119 patients. Radiology 1994;193:689-95.

92. Miyayama S, Matsui O, Kadoya M, Yoshikawa J, Gabata T, Kitagawa K, Arai K, Takashima T. Malignant esophageal stricture and fistula: palliative treatment with polyurethane-covered Gianturco stent. JVIR 1995;6:243-48.

93. Goldin E, Beyar M, Safra T, Globerman O, Craciun I, Wengrower D, Fich A. A new self-expandable, nickel-titanium coil stent for esophageal obstruction: a preliminary report. Gastrointest Endosc 1994;40:64-8.

94. Axelrad AM, Fleischer DE, Gomes M. Nitinol coil esophageal prosthesis: advantages of removable self-expanding metallic stents. Gastrointest Endosc 1996;43:155-60.

95. Wengrower D, Fiorini A, Valero J, Waldbaum C, Chopita N, Landoni N. EsophaCoil: long-term results in 81 patients. Gastrointest Endosc 1998;48:376-82.

96. Olsen E, Thyregaard R, Kill J. Esophacoil expanding metal stent in the management of patients with nonresectable malignant esophageal or cardiac neoplasm: a prospective study. Endoscopy 1999;31:417-20.

97. Siersema PD, Hop WCJ, van Blankenstein M, Dees J. A new design metal stent (Flamingo stent) for palliation of malignant dysphagia: a prospective study. Gastrointest Endosc 2000;51:139-45.

98. Manifold DK, Maynard ND, Cowling M, Machan L, Mason RC, Adam A. Taxol coated stents in esophageal adenocarcinoma (abstract). Gastroenterology 1998;114:A27.

99. Fiorini AB, Goldin E, Valero JL, Bloom A, Beyar M, Pfeffer RP, Globerman O. Expandable metal coil stent for treatment of broncho-esophageal fistula. Gastrointest Endosc 1995;42:81-3.

100. Bethge N, Sommer A, Vakil N. Treatment of esophageal fistulas with a new polyurethane-covered, self-expanding mesh stent: a prospective study. Am J Gastroenterol 1995;90:2143-6.

101. Weigert N, Neuhaus H, Rösch T, Hoffmann W, Dittler HJ, Classen M. Treatment of esophagorespiratory fistulas with silicone-coated self-expanding metal stents. Gastrointest Endosc 1995;41:490-6.

102. Macken E, Gevers A, Hiele M, Rutgeerts P. Treatment of esophagorespiratory fistulas with a polyurethane-covered self-expanding metallic mesh stent. Gastrointest Endosc 1996;44:324-6.

103. Morgan RA, Ellul JPM, Denton ERE, Glynos M, Mason RC, Adam A. Malignant esophageal fistulas and perforations: management with plastic-covered metallic endoprostheses. Radiology 1997;204:527-32.

104. Raijman I, Lynch P. Coated expandable esophageal stents in the treatment of digestive-respiratory fistulas. Am J Gastroenterol 1997;92:2188-91.

105. Low DE, Kozarek RA. Comparison of conventional and wire mesh expandable prostheses and surgical bypass in patients with malignant esophagorespiratory fistulas. Ann Thorac Surg 1998;65:919-3.

106. May A, Ell C. Palliative treatment of malignant esophagorespiratory fistulas with Gianturco-Z stents. A prospective clinical trial and review of the literature on covered metal stents. Am J Gastroenterol 1998;93:532-5.

107. Dumonceau J-M, Cremer M, Lalmand B, Devière J. Esophageal fistula sealing: choice of stent, practical management, and cost. Gastrointest Endosc 1999;49:70-8.

108. Dorta G, Binek J, Blum AL, Bühler H, Felley CP, Koelz HR, Lammer F, Lang C, Meier R, Meyenberger C, Meyer-Wyss B, Michetti P, Protiva P, Scheurer U, Weber B, Wiesel P, Vogel S. Comparison bewteen the esophageal Wallstent and Ultraflex stents in the treatment of malignant stenoses of the esophagus and cardia. Endoscopy 1997;29(3):149-54.

109. Schmassmann A, Meyenberger C, Knuchel J, Binek J, Lammer F, Kleiner B, Hürlimann S, Inauen W, Hammer B, Scheurer U, Halter F. Self-expanding metal stents in malignant esophageal obstruction:a comparison between two stent types. Am J Gastroenterol 1997;92:400-6.

7.1 FUNCTION AND QUALITY OF LIFE AFTER ESOPHAGEAL RESECTION

Claude Deschamps, Francis C. Nichols, Daniel L. Miller, Mark S. Allen, Victor F.Trastek, James R. Headrick, Allison J McLarty, Peter C. Pairolero

1. FUNCTION AND QUALITY OF LIFE AFTER RESECTION FOR CARCINOMA

1.1 INTRODUCTION

Early detection and resection of esophageal carcinoma provide the best chance for cure[1]. Long-term survival is mostly stage dependent[2-4]. Five-year survival for resected stage I carcinoma varies between 50 and 85% and for resected stage II between 20% and 50%[1-5]. Because the incidence of adenocarcinoma of the esophagus and esophagogastric junction is increasing[6], endoscopic surveillance for Barrett's disease will very likely lead to earlier cancer detection and resection and possibly improved long-term survival[7-8]. However, little is known of the functional status and quality of life of long-term survivors after curative resection for esophageal carcinoma[9]. Success of curative treatment for esophageal cancer has been traditionally measured with survival. Few reports on quality of life after esophageal resection for cancer have been published. A review of the literature by Gelfand et al in 1992[9] revealed that of 7,569 publications written on the subject of esophageal carcinoma, only 44 dealt with quality of life (0.58 %). Clearly, a better understanding of the functional outcome and quality of life of long-term survivors is needed in this new era of health care. Appropriate tools to measure outcome, however, are limited and development of such instruments will become increasingly important in the future if surgeons are to better plan preoperative counseling, surgical approach and postoperative care.

We reviewed and analyzed both esophageal function and quality of life in patients who survived more than 5 years after resection of esophageal carcinoma[10]. Between January 1972 and December 1990, 359 patients underwent esophageal resection at the Mayo Clinic, Rochester, Minnesota for Stage I or II (A and B) carcinoma of the esophagus. One hundred and seven of these patients (30%) survived 5 or more years. The records of these patients were analyzed for functional outcome and quality of life. Follow-up data was obtained from patient's most recent clinic visit and a two part mail survey. Part one evaluated subjective digestive function as it relates to the esophagectomy patient. It specifically addressed the qualitative and quantitative estimate of dysphagia, the need for esophageal dilatation, the presence of heartburn and the need for medication. The size and number of daily meals, presence of dumping symptoms, bowel habits and weight change also were queried. Part two used the Medical Outcomes Study 36-Item Short-Form Health Survey (MOS SF-36)[11]. This national standardized questionnaire is a self-administered health assessment tool which permits group comparisons in eight conceptual areas covering general health (health perception), daily activities (physical functioning), work (role-physical), emotional problems (role-emotional), social activities (social functioning), nervousness/depression (mental health), pain (bodily pain), and vitality (energy/fatigue). A numerical score is arrived at for the answers in each of the conceptual areas. Means and standard deviation of the numerical score were determined and compared to national norms matched for age and sex. The MOS SF-36 survey was constructed to measure population differences in physical and mental health status, the health burden of chronic disease and the effect of treatments on general health status. It provides a common yardstick to compare those patients with chronic health problems to those sampled from the general population.

Relationship between variables was assessed using Chi-square tests for discrete factors and Wilcoxon Rank sum tests for continuous factors[12]. Evaluation of the patient's responses to the Health Status Questionnaire relative to a matched population (national norm) was done using the signed rank test[13]. A p value of less than 0.05 was considered significant.

H.W. Tilanus and S.E.A. Attwood (eds.), Barrett's Esophagus, 387–392.
© 2001 *Kluwer Academic Publishers. Printed in the Netherlands.*

The two-part written survey was sent to 80 patients believed to be alive at the beginning of this study. No response was obtained from 11 patients, seven of whom were later found to have died before the survey was sent. The remaining four patients were lost to follow-up. Sixty-nine patients returned the survey. Five patients were excluded because of incomplete data. Thus, complete data was available in 64 patients for a response rate of 80%. The results of part one written survey were combined with information obtained from our out-patient clinic to provide information on all patients.

There were 81 men and 26 women. At the time of esophagectomy, median age was 62 years (range, 30 to 81 years). The operation performed was an Ivor Lewis esophagogastrectomy in 77 patients (72%), transhiatal esophagectomy in 14 (13%), extended esophagectomy in 4 (4%), left thoracoabdominal esophagectomy in 4 (4%), partial esophagectomy and total gastrectomy in 3 (3%) and segmental esophageal resection in 5 (4%). Intestinal continuity was re-established with the stomach in 99 patients (93%), small bowel in 4 (4%) and isoperistaltic left colon in 3 (3%). One patient (1%) had a primary end-to-end esophageal anastomosis after a segmental resection of the cervical esophagus. Overall, 87 patients (81.3%) had an intrathoracic anastomosis and 20 patients (18.7%) had a cervical anastomosis. A pyloromyotomy was done in 52 (49%) and a pyloroplasty in 36 (34 %). The tumor was located at the gastroesophageal junction in 62 patients (58%), in the middle third of the esophagus in 43 (40%) and in the cervical region in 2 (2%). An adenocarcinoma was present in 72 patients (67%), squamous cell carcinoma in 28 (26%), leiomyosarcoma in 3 (3%), and hemangiopericytoma, small cell carcinoma, undifferentiated carcinoma and neuroendocrine carcinoma in one each. Thirty-two of the 72 patients with adenocarcinoma (44%) had histologically confirmed Barrett's mucosa. Thirty-four patients were postsurgically classified as stage I (32%), 65 as stage IIA (60%) and 8 as stage IIB (8%).

1.2 FUNCTIONAL OUTCOME

Information on functional esophageal outcome was available in all 107 patients. Seventeen patients (16%) were entirely asymptomatic.

Twenty-seven patients (25%) had dysphagia to solid food, 10 (9%) had pain on swallowing, 10 (9%) had dysphagia to a pureed diet and 3 (3%) had dysphagia to liquids. Forty-six patients (41%) underwent at least one postoperative dilatation. Sixty-four patients (60%) had heartburn which was intermittent in 58 and continuous in 6. Thirty-one patients (29%) required antacids for relief of heartburn. Forty patients (37%) ate smaller, more frequent meals. Fifty-two patients (49%) never regained lost weight following their operation, 27 (25%) maintained their initial preoperative weight and 6 (6%) gained weight above their preoperative weight. Fifty-three patients (50%) experienced symptoms of postprandial dumping, including 26 (24%) with diarrhea, 17 (16%) with abdominal cramps, 8 (8%) with nausea, 7 (7%) with dizziness, and 6 (6 %) with diaphoresis.

Factors affecting late functional outcome were analyzed. Patients with a cervical anastomosis had significantly less symptoms of reflux ($p<0.05$) than those with an intrathoracic anastomosis. Dumping symptoms occurred more frequently in younger patients ($p<0.05$) and in women ($p<0.01$). Neither the type of resection ($p = 0.82$) or the occurrence of a postoperative leak ($p = 0.56$) influenced the need for dilatation. The time interval since operation, tumor location, histology, adjuvant therapy, anastomotic leak and type or absence of gastric drainage did not significantly affect late functional outcome

1.3 QUALITY OF LIFE (Table 1)

Information on quality of life as assessed by the MOS SF-36 Health Survey Questionnaire was available in 64 patients (60%). A score was computed for each patient in each of the 8 conceptual areas. Data is expressed as mean (+/- standard deviation) for the group. Physical function scores were decreased significantly ($p<0.01$) compared to the national norm. Ability to work, social interaction, daily activities, emotional dysfunction scores, and perception of health were similar to the national norm. Level of energy was decreased compared to the national norm but the significance was borderline ($p = 0.05$). Our patients had higher scores in the area of mental health ($p<0.05$).

Factors affecting quality of life were also analyzed.

Table 1. Quality of Life Survey after esophagectomy for carcinoma (MOS SF-36)

Category	Patient Population	Normal Population
Health perception	65.3 (19.7)	69.9 (5.3)
Physical functioning	70.9 (25.8)*	80.5 (9.4)
Role-physical	76.2 (36.6)	75.8 (12.7)
Role-emotional	87.2 (25.8)	86.4 (6.2)
Social functioning	86.5 (23.6)	88.4 (4.4)
Mental health	80.5 (14.8)*	78.3 (1.6)
Bodily pain	79.3 (22.2)	76.2 (5.2)
Energy/Fatigue	56.5 (20.4)**	62.9 (3.5)

Scores are expressed as mean (standard deviation)
* $p<0.05$ when compared to normal population matched for age and sex
** $p = 0.05$

TABLE 2. Nine elements of a good quality of life after esophagectomy*

To be able to eat adequately and enjoy it
To be able to drink as desired, with moderate alcohol consumption
To be able to do both of the above socially
To have weight stability
To be able to sleep comfortably in a normal position
To be free of pain
To be able to earn one's living
To be able to participate in sports or hobbies
To have unimpaired libido

* J.D. Kirby

The occurrence of a postoperative anastomotic leak adversely affected the physical functioning and the health perception scores in our population (p < 0.05). Also, the need for postoperative dilatation adversely affected the social functioning score (p < 0.01). Age, sex, time interval since the surgery, location of lesion, histology, type of surgery, and adjuvant therapy did not significantly affect any of the 8 conceptual areas measured by the quality of life questionnaire.

1.4 DISCUSSION

Patient's perspective on quality of life is crucial. We are in an era during which health care outcome will increasingly be evaluated from the patient point-of-view.[11] J.D. Kirby, who founded the "Oesophageal Patients Association" suggested nine elements of a good quality of life after esophagectomy.[14] (Table 2)
Health outcome is better measured by using general health measures and traditional biomedical tools (i.e. disease-specific) synchronously.[11] We elected to combine a questionnaire aimed at upper and lower digestive functions with a quality of life survey. Our data demonstrate that when queried, the majority of patients were symptomatic years after esophagectomy. More than 50% complained of reflux symptoms, half had some degree of dumping and 46% had difficulty with swallowing. Moreover dumping was increased in younger patients and in women. These findings have been also reported by others[15-20]. In contrast to our functional outcome findings, however, esophagectomy for cancer did not appear to influence quality of life. Our patients were comparable to the national norm in all except physical functioning and actually scored significantly higher than the national norm in the area of mental health. One significant finding in our study revolves around the location of the anastomosis. The incidence of reflux is significantly reduced if the anastomosis is located in the neck. However, reduction in late reflux has to be balanced against an increased rate of fistula and recurrent nerve injury[3-4] associated with the cervical anastomosis in the early postoperative period. Moreover, the

occurrence of a postoperative leak had an adverse impact on quality of life scores that measure physical functioning and health perception. In addition, the need for dilatation postoperatively did adversely affect the social functioning score. Others have also shown that complications associated with cervical anastomosis can have long-lasting consequences[21]. No standardized tool exists for evaluating quality of life in esophageal carcinoma and the discrepancy in the results observed in the two parts of our study points to the difficulty in developing a valid questionnaire for a specific population of patients. Others have reported similar findings where symptoms specific to esophageal disease correlated poorly with quality of life scores[22-23] One possible explanation for the poor correlation is that despite symptoms secondary to their surgery, most patients can function at home or work and are happy to be alive and free of cancer[25].

2. FUNCTION AND QUALITY OF LIFE AFTER RESECTION FOR BARRETT'S WITH HIGH GRADE DYSPLASIA

We recently reviewed our experience with function and quality of life after esophagectomy for high-grade dysplasia in Barrett's esophagus.[25] From June 1991 through July 1997, 54 consecutive patients underwent esophageal resection for Barrett's esophagus with high-grade dysplasia (HGD) at the Mayo Clinic Rochester, Minnesota. Follow-up data was obtained from the patient's clinical record and a two-part mail survey which was mailed to all 46 patients thought to be alive in August 1999. We used the same two-part written survey described earlier. All 46 2-part written surveys were returned for a

response of 100%. Two patients were found to have died and their surveys were not completed. Complete data from the surveys was available for the remaining 44 patients. The follow-up was complete in all 54 patients. The median follow-up was 5.3 years (range, 6months to 9 years).

2.1 FUNCTIONAL OUTCOME

Long-term (greater than 2 years) functional outcome was available for 48 patients. Seven patients (13%) were entirely asymptomatic. Ten patients experienced no change in their weight. Thirty-one patients lost a median of 9 kg (range, 1-50 kg) and seven patients gained a median of 2kg (range, 1-5 kg). Thirty patients had no dysphagia. Mild, moderate, and severe dysphagia were seen in 15, 1, and 2 patients respectively. Reflux was present in 36 patients (68%). The majority had minimal symptoms with medical management. Dumping was present in 8 patients (15%).

Long-term functional outcome was significantly affected by the level of the anastomosis. Patients with a cervical anastomosis had significantly more dumping than those patients with an intrathoracic anastomosis (33.3% vs 6.7%), p=0.04. We were unable to detect any significant difference in dysphagia, reflux, or dumping with regards to age, gender, anastomotic location, and/or postoperative leaks.

2.2 QUALITY OF LIFE (Table 3)

Forty-four patients (82%) completed the MOS SF-36 Health Status Questionnaire. A score was competed for each patient for each of the eight conceptual areas.

TABLE 3. Quality of Life Survey after esophagectomy for HGD(MOS SF-36)

Category	HGD Patients	Normal Population
Physical functioning	76.0 (27.0)	80.74 (10.0)
Role-physical	76.7 (38.2)*	75.4 (13.9)
Role-emotional	86.5 (6.7)*	86.0 (25.5)
Social functioning	83.9 (26.4)	88.1 (4.9)
Mental health	76.9 (17.1)	78.5 (1.2)
Bodily pain	79.6 (20.3)	76.4 (5.5)
Energy/Fatigue	58.2 (19.6)	63.0 (4.4)
Health perception	62.8 (24.9)	69.6 (6.0)

Scores are expressed as mean (standard deviation)
* $p<0.05$ when compared to normal population matched for age and sex

If the patients with HGD only (i.e. no cancer) are compared to the national norm, significant differences in role-physical and role-emotional are identified (p<0.03). In both categories, our patients find themselves to be better than the norm. When factors affecting quality of life were analyzed, the occurrence of an anastomotic leak adversely affected the social functioning scores in our population (p=0.02).

Age is significantly correlated with physical functioning (p = 0.0007) and role-physical (p = 0.03). As our patients become older their physical function and physical performance at work are less than the norm. Time from surgery is significantly correlated with social functioning (p = 0.02). The further our patient population is out from surgery the better is their social function. We were unable to detect any difference in the categories of bodily pain, health perception, energy/fatigue, role-emotional, and mental health with the age, gender, time from surgery, anastomotic leak, reflux, or dumping.

Thirty-eight percent of patients had swallowing difficulties but in only six percent was this moderate to severe. Reflux was present in 68% of our patients. This, however, was well controlled with medication in the majority of patients. Dumping was present in 15% of patients. Interestingly in this patient group, neither dysphagia nor reflux was significantly related to the level of the anastomosis. In this group of patients, dumping was, much greater in patients with a cervical anastomosis in contrast to our patients with carcinoma where dumping was more common in younger patients and women. While the functional outcomes were acceptable but less than ideal, esophagectomy had no measurable negative impact on these patient's quality of life. While a postoperative leak adversely affected the social functioning score it improved significantly as the time interval from surgery increased.

In conclusion, long-term functional outcome following esophagectomy for carcinoma and Barrett's is affected by several factors. For those surviving five or more years, symptoms of reflux, dumping and dysphagia are not uncommon. However quality of life after resection as assessed by the patients themselves is similar to the national norm. The vast majority of patients will experience an acceptable functional outcome and a positive quality of life.

REFERENCES

1. O'Rourke I, Tait N, Bull C, Gebski V, Holland M, Johnson DC. Oesophageal cancer: outcome of modern surgical management. Aust.N.Z.J. Surg 1995; 65:11-16.
2. King RM, Pairolero PC, Trastek VF, Payne WS, Bernatz PE. Ivor Lewis esophagogastrectomy for carcinoma of the esophagus: early and late functional results. Ann Thorac Surg 1987;44:119-22.
3. Vigneswaran WT, Trastek VF, Pairolero PC, Deschamps C, Daly RC, Allen MS. Transhiatal esophagectomy for carcinoma of the esophagus. Ann Thorac Surg 1993;56:838-46.
4. Vigneswaran WT, Trastek VF, Pairolero PC, Deschamps C, Daly RC, Allen MS. Extended esophagectomy in the management of carcinoma of the upper thoracic esophagus. J Thorac Cardiovac Surg 1994;107:901-7.
5. Lizuka T, Isono K, Kakegawa T, Watanabe H. Parameters linked to ten-year survival in Japan of resected esophageal carcinoma. Chest 1989;96:1005-11.
6. Pera M, Cameron AJ, Trastek VF, Carpenter HA, Zinsmeister AR. Increasing incidence of adenocarcinoma of the esophagus and esophagogastric junction. Gastroenterology 1993;104:510-3.
7. Pera M, Trastek VF, Carpenter HA, Allen MS, Deschamps C, Pairolero PC. Barrett's esophagus with high-grade dysplasia: an indication for esophagectomy? Ann Thorac Surg 1992;54:199-204.
8. Edwards MJ, Gable DR, Lentsch AB Richardson JD. The rationale for esophagectomy as the optimal therapy for Barrett's esophagus with high-grade dysplasia. Ann Surg 1996;223:585-91.
9. Gelfand GAJ, Finley RJ. Quality of life with carcinoma of the esophagus. World J Surg 1994;18:399-405.
10. McLarty AJ, Deschamps C, Trastek VF, Allen MS, Pairolero PC, Harmsen WS. Esophageal resection for cancer of the esophagus: Long-term function and quality of life. Ann Thorac Surg 1997;63:1568-72.
11. Ware JE. SF-36 Health Survey. Manual and interpretation guide. Boston: Nimrod, 1993.
12. Dixon WJ, Massey Jr FJ. Introduction to statistical analysis. 3th ed. New-York: McGraw-Hill, 1969:77-80, 116-18, 156-63, 344-5, 509.
13. Siegel S. Nonparametric statistics for the behavioral sciences. 1st ed. New-York: Mc-Graw-Hill, 1956:63-83, 104-11, 161-72, 175-9, 184-93.
14. Kirby JD. Quality of life after oesophagectomy: the patient perspective. Dis Esophagus 1999;12:168-71.
15. Suzuki H, Shichisaburo A, Kitamura M, Hashimoto M, Izumi K, Sato H. An evaluation of symptoms and performance status in patients after esophagectomy for esophageal cancer from the viewpoint of the patient. Am Surg 1994;60:920-3.
16. Nishihira T, Watanabe T, Ohmori N et al. Long-term evaluation of patients treated by radical operation for carcinoma of the thoracic esophagus. World J Surg 1984;8:778-85.

17. Collard J-M, Otte J-B, Reynaert M, Kestens P-J. Quality of life three years or more after esophagectomy for cancer. J Thorac Cardiovasc Surg 1992;104:391-4.

18. De Leyn P, Coosemans W, Lerut T. Early and late functional results in patients with intrathoracic gastric replacement after oesophagectomy for carcinoma. Eur J of Cardiothorac Surg 1992;6:79-85.

19. Orringer MB, Marshall B, Stirling MC. Transhiatal esophagectomy for benign and malignant disease. J Thorac Cardiovasc Surg 1993;105:265-77.

20. Finley RJ, Lamy A, Clifton J, Evans KG, Fradet G, Nelems B. Gastrointestinal function following esophagectomy for malignancy. Am J Surg 1995;169:471-5.

21. Iannettoni MD, Whyte RI, Orringer MB. Catastrophic complications of the cervical esophagogastric anastomosis. J Thorac Cardiovasc Surg 1995;110:1493-1501.

22. Blazeby JM, Williams MH, Brookes ST, Alderson D, Farndon JR. Quality of life measurement in patients with oesophageal cancer. Gut 1995;37:505-8.

23. van Knippenberg FCE, Out JJ, Tilanus HW, Mud HJ, Hop WCJ, Verhage F. Quality of life in patients with resected oesophageal cancer. Soc Sci Med 1992;35:139-45.

24. Kuwano H, Ikebe M, Baba K, et al. Operative procedures of reconstruction after resection of esophageal cancer and the postoperative quality of life. World J Surg 17, 773-6, 1993.

25. Presented at the 37th Annual Meeting of the Society of Thoracic Surgeons, January 29-31, 2001; New Orleans, Louisiana. Manuscript submitted to Annals of Thorac Surg.

Index